T0141214

Nanotechnology and Drug Delivery

Volume 2: Nano-Engineering Strategies and Nanomedicines against Severe Diseases

Nanotechnology and Drug Delivery

Volume 2: Nano-Engineering Strategies and Nanomedicines against Severe Diseases

Editor

Professor Dr. José L. Arias

Department of Pharmacy and Pharmaceutical Technology
Faculty of Pharmacy
University of Granada
Granada
Spain

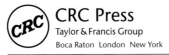

CRC Press
Taylor & Francis Group
Boca Raton London New York

CRC Press is an imprint of the
Taylor & Francis Group, an **informa** business

A SCIENCE PUBLISHERS BOOK

CRC Press
Taylor & Francis Group
6000 Broken Sound Parkway NW, Suite 300
Boca Raton, FL 33487-2742

First issued in paperback 2021

© 2016 by Taylor & Francis Group, LLC
CRC Press is an imprint of Taylor & Francis Group, an Informa business

No claim to original U.S. Government works

ISBN-13: 978-0-367-78314-3 (pbk)
ISBN-13: 978-1-4822-6271-1 (hbk)

Library of Congress Cataloging-in-Publication Data

Nanotechnology and drug delivery / [edited by] José L. Arias.
    p. ; cm.
    Includes bibliographical references and index.
    Summary: "Pharmacotherapy is often limited by the inefficient activity and severe toxicity of drug molecules. Nanotechnology offers a revolutionary and definitive approach for the efficient delivery of drug molecules to non-healthy tissues and cells. This first volume of a series of two volumes analyzes the basics in the development of drug-loaded nanoplatforms, the so-called nanomedicines. Special attention is given to physicochemical engineering, pharmacokinetics, biocompatibility and biodegradability, representative nanoplatforms (based on lipids, polymers, cyclodextrins, metals, carbon, silica, iron oxides, etc.), and advanced nano-engineering strategies for passive, ligand-mediated, and/or stimuli-sensitive drug delivery and release"--Provided by publisher.
    ISBN 978-1-4665-9947-5 (hardcover : alk. paper)
    I. Arias, José L., editor.
    [DNLM: 1. Drug Delivery Systems. 2. Nanoparticles. 3. Drug Design. 4. Nanotechnology--methods. QV 785]

RS420
615.1'9--dc23   2014013165

Visit the Taylor & Francis Web site at
http://www.taylorandfrancis.com

and the CRC Press Web site at
http://www.crcpress.com

Preface to The Book Series

Pharmacotherapy is frequently associated with inefficacy and toxicity problems limiting disease treatment and prognosis, and the quality of life of patients. Such incidents have been described even during the clinical use of new drug molecules, dosage forms, and more sophisticated treatment schedules. To beat the challenge, recent advances in drug therapy have involved the introduction of nanotechnology in the development of medicines. In fact, drug-loaded nanoplatforms (the so-called nanomedicines) are expected to become the definitive step toward a successful pharmacotherapy. These nanocarriers are wisely engineered to maximize drug accumulation into non-healthy tissues and cells, thus optimizing the pharmacokinetics and pharmacodynamics of active molecules, while minimizing their systemic side effects. In addition, new synthesis methodologies in nanomedicine formulation, the theranosis conceptualization, have made possible to combine disease diagnosis and therapy, thus opening the door to "personalized" medicines.

In line with all this revolutionary progress in the drug delivery field, "Nanotechnology and Drug Delivery" is a series of two volumes analyzing the fundamentals and more advanced aspects in the development of nanomedicines. The selected book chapter contributions have been written by well-known experts in the field, and comprise insights into the most promising moves toward superior drug-loaded nanoplatforms. Original concepts derived from advanced materials science, physical chemistry, and medicinal chemistry with critical applicability into the clinic are emphasized in the book series.

The first volume "Nanoplatforms in Drug Delivery" is focused on the physicochemical engineering of nanomedicines, their pharmacokinetics, biocompatibility and biodegradability aspects, representative nanoplatforms (based on lipids, polymers, cyclodextrins, metals, carbon, silica, iron oxides, etc.) for an efficient drug delivery, and advanced nano-engineering strategies for passive, ligand-mediated, and/or stimuli-sensitive drug targeting. As an ideal complement to this book, the second volume "Nano-Engineering Strategies and Nanomedicines against Severe Diseases" further discusses the possibilities of nanotechnology, in the context of nanomedicine, for oral, dental, topical and transdermal, pulmonary and nasal, ocular and otic, vaginal, and brain drug delivery and targeting. Furthermore, an updated point of view is given to nanomedicines against severe diseases, i.e., cancer, cardiovascular diseases, neurodegenerative disorders, infectious diseases, chronic inflammatory diseases, and metabolic diseases. Gene delivery and the recent concept of nanotheranosis are also analyzed in the book.

In my opinion, the book series will give a complete overview on the current state of the art, including more revolutionary conceptualizations, and future perspectives in nanotechnology and drug delivery. It will also be a vast source of knowledge not only for non-experts but also for senior researchers in the field of advanced drug delivery to severe diseases. Last but not least, I would like to thank all the contributors to the book series for the excellent work accomplished. It has been a privilege to work with them.

Professor Dr. José L. Arias

Preface to Volume 2

Nanomedicine development is revolutionizing the disease arena. Numerous preclinical and clinical investigations are demonstrating the possibilities coming from the vehiculization of therapeutic molecules into nanoparticulate platforms, not only in terms of improvement of the therapeutic effect but also by minimizing the associated toxicity. As a result, nanomedicines are being introduced into the clinic. Disease diagnosis has also taken advantage of the development of nanoplatforms capable of selectively accumulating diagnostic agents into non-healthy sites. The first volume "Nanoplatforms in Drug Delivery" of the book series "Nanotechnology and Drug Delivery" focused on the study of the representative physicochemical engineering approaches to the formulation of drug nanocarriers. In that book, special emphasis was given to those materials mainly used in nanoplatform formulation.

The second volume "Nano-Engineering Strategies and Nanomedicines against Severe Diseases" of the series of two volumes analyzes in depth the possibilities coming from the application of nanotechnology to the formulation of nanoplatforms to be administered through a route of drug administration, i.e., oral, dental, topical and transdermal, pulmonary and nasal, ocular and otic, vaginal, and even brain delivery and targeting. Special emphasis is given to the main aspects being considered when engineering a nanomedicine for a given route of administration, e.g., to the barriers that the drug nanocarrier will face before getting access to the bloodstream. The second part of the book will proportionate an updated vision of nanomedicines under clinical use or under development against severe diseases, i.e., cancer, cardiovascular diseases, neurodegenerative disorders, infectious diseases, chronic inflammatory diseases, and metabolic diseases. As a complementary image to the problem of the selective delivery of therapeutic agents, a chapter is focused on the use of nanoplatforms as carriers of genetic materials. Finally, attention is further given to the revolutionary concept of nanotheranosis, involving the design of nanoparticulate structures for a combined disease diagnosis and treatment. Such a promising approach was initially ascribed to the idea of image-guided drug delivery, but it is expected to be the definitive move toward the development of personalized medicines.

Chapter 1 (Emerging Technologies of Polymers for Nanomedicine Applications) focuses on a critical analysis of the use of polymeric nanomaterials in the development of drug delivery systems. Key properties of polymers to be considered and advances made in the field of drug delivery are brilliantly described by Prof. Souto and co-workers. The analysis of key aspects in the engineering of a nanomedicine to be administered orally is discussed in Chapter 2 (Nanotechnology for Oral Drug Delivery and Targeting, by the research group of Prof. Pinto Reis). Strategies are described to maximize drug delivery by the oral route and, therefore, drug bioavailability. Additionally, this contribution critically analyzes the challenges/opportunities found in the oral route, the breakthroughs in nanomedicine formulation, and the strategies being proposed to optimize drug delivery.

The rapidly emerging field of nanomedicine in dentistry is updated by Prof. Nguyen and co-authors (Chapter 3: Nanoparticulate Systems for Dental Drug Delivery). Special focus is given to liposomes, while the potential of other nanomaterials for use as dental drug delivery systems is also analyzed by the authors. In another interesting contribution, recent progress, benefits, practical limitations, and toxicity issues coming from the application of nanotechnology to transdermal and topical drug delivery are critically described by the research group of Prof. Roberts (Chapter 4: Nanotechnology for Topical and Transdermal Drug Delivery and Targeting). Special insight concerning the use of deformable liposomes and enhanced delivery devices to improve transdermal delivery of therapeutic molecules.

The pulmonary route of drug administration is also taking advantage on the engineering of nanoparticulate systems. Chapter 5 (Nanotechnology for Pulmonary and Nasal Drug Delivery) describes the engineering technologies involving not only traditional techniques but additionally more innovative processes to produce nanoparticles with a defined physical chemistry assuring an efficient nasal or pulmonary deposition. Prof. Williams III and his colleague further discuss the pulmonary and nasal physiologies correlated to particle deposition and absorption, and the clinical considerations of pulmonary and nasal delivery of nanoparticulate systems. A complementary contribution facilitating a detailed vision of the current state of the art in nanoparticulate-based pulmonary drug delivery has been written by Prof. Souto and co-authors (Chapter 6: Lipid Nanoplatforms for Pulmonary Drug Delivery). Their contribution is devoted to the in-depth study of novel therapeutic micro/nanostrategies generating satisfactory outcomes against some common diseases that affect the respiratory apparatus. Commonly used aerosol types and administration of micro/nanocarriers are analyzed, including their properties, applications, and toxicities.

Prof. Attama and co-workers (Chapter 7: Nanotechnology for Ocular and Otic Drug Delivery and Targeting) study the representative nanoparticulate structures for ocular/otic drug delivery and targeting that are overcoming the inherent limitations of conventional medicines. Current developments and applications to evade static and dynamic barriers associated with these organs are explored in depth. Nanoparticle-based approaches to the vaginal route of drug administration are updated in Chapter 8 (Nanotechnology for Vaginal

Drug Delivery and Targeting). Barriers to vaginal drug delivery and major aspects to be considered when engineering vaginal nanomedicines are studied in this contribution. Finally, Chapter 9 (Potential Nanocarriers for Brain Drug Delivery, by Prof. Holgado and co-workers) summarizes recent advances in drug delivery to the central nervous system. The contribution satisfactorily addresses the problem of circumventing/disrupting of the blood-brain barrier to deliver therapeutic agents into the brain.

At this point in the book (and in the book series) the reader would have gained a detailed overview of the basic and revolutionary conceptualizations in nanomedicine development, thus he/she will be ready to the study of those chapters devoted to the design and development of nanomedicines against severe diseases. Starting this section of the book, Prof. Prados and co-authors (Chapter 10: Nanomaterials and Cancer Therapy) explore in detail the nanomaterial-based medicines under development/clinical use against cancer. Special attention is given to advanced functionalization approaches being introduced in the nanocarrier structure that improve drug delivery to malignant cells. Then, Chapter 11 (Nanomedicine in Cardiovascular Disease, by Prof. Antoniades and co-workers) clearly analyzes the latest advances in nanotechnology reporting new possibilities against cardiovascular diseases, e.g., early detection and identification of atherosclerosis and treatment of acute vascular syndromes. Management of atherosclerosis by nanomedicinal approaches is brilliantly updated by the authors.

Chapter 12 [Nano(Neuro)Medicinal Interventions for Neurodegenerative Disorders: A Meta-Analysis of Concurrent Challenges and Strategic Solutions] summarizes recent nanomedicinal strategies against neurodegenerative diseases. The research group of Prof. Pillay provides a comprehensive analysis of representative investigations on the formulation and use of nanomaterials for imaging in the central nervous system, drug delivery to the brain and treatment of the neurological disorders, combined theranosis, and nano(neuro)toxicity. On the other hand, Chapter 13 (Nanomedicines against Infectious Diseases) studies in depth the development of nanomedicines against tuberculosis, malaria, leishmaniasis, and Chagas's disease. Prof. Romero and co-workers describe the relevant (micro/nano)approaches in the pharmaceutical and immunological fields involving the development of drug and vaccine delivery systems.

Chapter 14 (Nanomedicines against Chronic Inflammatory Diseases) highlights the possibilities coming from the design of nanoplatforms that can selectively deliver a therapeutic agent to the inflammation site. The authors present potential applications of nanomedicines toward the treatment of chronic inflammatory diseases, i.e., arthritis, inflammatory bowel diseases, chronic lung inflammatory diseases, and uveitis. Challenges, engineering innovations, and drug targeting opportunities in nanomedicine design are also discussed in detail. Finally, Prof. Sarmento and his colleague (Chapter 15: Nanomedicine Biopharmaceuticals for Metabolic Diseases) analyze the use of nanostructures in the formulation of safe and effective biopharmaceuticals for the treatment of metabolic diseases. The authors critically review recent advances on nanomedicine-based biopharmaceuticals for the treatment of diabetes, phenylketonuria, osteoporosis, growth hormone deficiency, Niemann-Pick disease, and Fabry disease.

Attention is finally given in the book to gene delivery and to the recent and revolutionizing concept of nanotheranosis. Prof. Aigner (Chapter 16: Nanotechnology in Gene Knockdown and *mi*RNA Replacement *In Vivo*) overviews the significant nanoparticle-based approaches for small interfering ribonucleic acid-mediated gene knockdown and micro ribonucleic acid replacement. Materials used in nanoplatform design, strategies for ligand-mediated targeted delivery, and *in vivo* applications of these nanomedicines are discussed. Regarding the promising development of theranostics, Prof. Lammers and co-authors (Chapter 17: Nanotheranostics) comprehensively review the current state of the art in the engineering of particulate systems as nanotools for combining disease diagnosis and therapy. The chapter compiles the advantages of nanotheranostics over conventional pharmacotherapeutic interventions, and the recent progress done in nanotheranostics and image-guided drug delivery.

In conclusion, it can be emphasized that the selected book chapter contributions to the second volume "Nano-Engineering Strategies and Nanomedicines against Severe Diseases" of the book series "Nanotechnology and Drug Delivery" are a rich source of updated background information and conceptualization to scientists involved in the formulation and clinical development of nanomedicines. At this point, I would like to thank all the authors for the outstanding contributions to this volume; I also thank them and the Editorial Office for their kindness and immense patience with my eye health problem that has delayed the edition of the book. In this line, and personally speaking, let me please take the opportunity to write one thought on my experience against the scariest adversary I ever faced, Acanthamoeba: *you never know how strong you are, until being strong is the only choice you have.* Finally, deep appreciation and love to my wife, María del Mar: *your continuous support helps me facing the adversity.*

Professor Dr. José L. Arias

Contents

CHAPTER 1

Emerging Technologies of Polymers for Nanomedicine Applications

Tatiana Andreani,[1,2,3,a] *Nagasamy Venkatesh,*[4]
Sandra F.V. Ferreira,[3,b] *Amélia M.L. Dias da Silva*[1,2,c] *and*
Eliana B. Souto[3,5,]*

ABSTRACT

Nanotechnology has attracted great attention in pharmacy regarding the development of drug-loaded nanoplatforms with a mean size smaller than 1,000 nm. Polymeric materials have been proposed as nanoparticulate drug carriers against diseases, improving the efficacy of pharmacotherapy. However, the efficiency of these nanosystems depends on their biological fate. New approaches have been developed on the basis of surface functionalization

---

[1] Department of Biology and Environment, University of Trás-os-Montes e Alto Douro (UTAD), Vila Real, Portugal.
[2] Centre for Research and Technology of Agro-Environmental and Biological Sciences, Vila Real, Portugal.
[3] Faculty of Health Sciences, Fernando Pessoa University, Rua Carlos da Maia, 296, P-4200-150 Porto, Portugal.
[a] Email: tatyandreani@hotmail.com
[b] Email: sandra_ferreira_89@hotmail.com
[c] Email: amsilva@utad.pt
[4] JSS College of Pharmacy, Department of Pharmaceutics, A Constituent College of JSS University, Mysore, Udhagamandalam - 643 001. Tamil Nadu, India.
Email: nagasamyvenkatesh@rediffmail.com
[5] Institute of Biotechnology and Bioengineering, Centre of Genomics and Biotechnology University of Trás-os-Montes and Alto Douro (CGB-UTAD/IBB), P.O. Box 1013, P-5001-801 Vila Real, Portugal.
* Corresponding author: emb.souto@gmail.com, souto.eliana@gmail.com

of the nanoparticulate system and on the precise control of the particle structure. In this regard, smart polymeric nanoparticles and nanoscale hydrogels have been engineered as stimuli-sensitive nanoplatforms to assure the controlled drug release at the specific site of action. This chapter highlights the most significant properties of polymers for the production of conventional nanoparticles and nanogels, as well as details the significant advances made in drug delivery.

Introduction

Nanoscale materials have been extensively used in diverse applications, such as electronics, textiles (Perelshtein et al. 2008), agriculture (Rai and Ingle 2012), and biomedicine (Parveen et al. 2012). Nanotechnology has attracted great attention in the pharmaceutical area with the development of drug-loaded particles with a diameter < 1,000 nm (Brigger et al. 2002). Nanoparticles (NPs) are solid systems classified into nanospheres and nanocapsules depending on the type of polymer, the localization of the active agent, and the production method (Fig. 1.1). Nanospheres are characterized by a matrix where the drug can be bound at the surface or dissolved into it. In contrast, nanocapsules are reservoir systems composed of a membrane, and the drug is confined into the

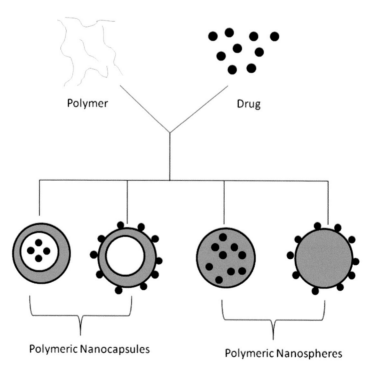

Polymer   Drug

Polymeric Nanocapsules   Polymeric Nanospheres

Figure 1.1. Polymeric nanostructures for drug delivery purposes. The drug can be entrapped inside or adsorbed on the surface of the nanocapsule/nanosphere.

inner liquid core or adsorbed at the surface (Reis et al. 2006). In this regard, many of the methodologies proposed for drug encapsulation in polymeric NPs require the presence of the drug in the reaction medium, which can lead to the inactivation of the drug, since several of these procedures use aggressive conditions, such as solvents or aggressive stirring (Reis et al. 2006). To overcome these limitations it has been proposed producing hydrogels in the absence of the drug, and then drug loading and NP formation due to the collapse of the gel.

In particular, polymeric NPs have been frequently used as particulate carriers for the diagnosis, prevention, and treatment of several diseases, improving the efficacy of insoluble drugs and thus, increasing their bioavailability (Kim et al. 2008). They can be obtained by using biomacromolecules derived from polysaccharides or proteins, or synthetic materials, such as poly(D,L-lactide) (PLA), poly(D,L-lactide-*co*-glycolide) (PLGA), and poly(ε-caprolactone) (PCL) (Mitra et al. 2001, Vrignaud et al. 2001, Musumeci et al. 2006, Cafaggi et al. 2008). However, some of these systems have demonstrated lack of specificity for drug delivery to the desired site of action (Sahoo et al. 2002). In fact, the therapeutic effect relies on the capability of these systems to overcome the resistance offered by physiological barriers, including external barriers (skin and mucosa), extracellular matrices, cellular and subcellular barriers, and blood clearance (Elsabahy and Wooley 2012). New approaches based on polymeric NPs have been developed for drug targeting thanks to the easy modification of their surface and the precise control of the polymer structure, permitting the synthesis of systems with different shapes, sizes, and surface charges to deliver the drug to the specific site of action. Size, surface charge, and hydrophobic character define the targeting ability of these nanosystems, since these factors can modulate the interaction with biological membranes and thus, can influence the intracellular uptake (Win and Feng 2005, Lorenz et al. 2010). Generally speaking, the gastrointestinal (GI) uptake seems to be more affected by NPs prepared from hydrophobic polymers in comparison to NPs based on hydrophilic polymers (Jung et al. 2000).

According to the biological environment conditions (pH, enzymatic activity, and oxidative and reductive conditions) (Colson and Grinstaff 2012), or external stimuli (temperature, light, ultrasounds) (Fomina et al. 2010, Rejinold et al. 2011, Fleige et al. 2012), polymer-based delivery systems can modulate drug release, being physiologically-responsive nanomaterials. These strategies have been developed for encapsulation of numerous anticancer drugs (Kalaria et al. 2009), especially for the oral route of administration (Dong and Feng 2005, Win and Feng 2005).

Due to their good mechanical integrity, biocompatibility, high water content, and three-dimensional structure, the development of hydrogels has attracted particular interest in tissue repair, and drug delivery (Hoare and Kohane 2008, Khaing and Schmidt 2012). Hydrogels can be confined to smaller dimensions (nanogels) that offer a tunable nanoscale size and a large surface area for the interaction with biological surfaces (Raemdonck et al. 2009), and thus could be a promising carrier in drug delivery.

Characteristics of Polymeric Nanoparticles for Drug Delivery

Regarding the target and control drug release, polymers based-nanomedicines are superior to conventional drug molecules. Drug targeting and delivery can be affected by several parameters, such as particle size and size distribution, surface properties, surface functionalization, and polymer nature (molecular weight, crystallinity, glass transition temperature (T_g), and polymer degradation) (Lenaerts et al. 1984, Arbós et al. 2003, Jeong et al. 2003, Mittal et al. 2007). Table 1.1 summarizes the main characteristics of polymers for the design and development of NPs in drug delivery.

Table 1.1. Effects of the most significant properties of polymeric NPs on drug delivery.

Characteristics	Effects on drug delivery	References
Size	Severe impact on toxicity and cellular uptake	Win and Feng 2005
Surface charge	Determine the opsonization, blood clearance, and biodistribution	Reis et al. 2006
Morphology (shape)	Critical factor that can influence particle function. Non-spherical particles can provide zero-order drug release, whereas particles with irregular shapes (and regions of different thicknesses) determine unique drug release behaviors due to shape changes over time	Hsieh et al. 1983, Champion et al. 2007
Surface modification/ long-circulating properties/targeting ligands	Hydrophilic polymer chains, such as poly(ethylene glycol) (PEG) can prevent opsonization processes, retarding particle recognition by the mononuclear phagocyte system (MPS). As a result, extended blood circulation times will be possible to the NPs. Smart ligands, such as monoclonal antibodies will facilitate a selective drug delivery and accumulation	Wood et al. 2005, Sheng et al. 2009, Shi et al. 2011
Drug release (mechanism)	Drug release profile can be modulated by using different stimuli-sensitive polymeric matrices	Leobandung et al. 2003, Sarmento et al. 2007

Effect of particle size and surface charge

Several methods have been employed for producing polymeric NPs with different geometries. These methods are based on two general processes: polymerization reactions or directly from a preformed polymer (Couvreur et al. 1995). The most relevant methods for polymeric NP preparation, as well the type of polymer and entrapped drugs are shown in Table 1.2.

The size and size distribution of NPs are the most important factors determining the interaction of these systems with cell membranes, as well as, their intracellular fate. Cell internalization is dependent on the type of biological barrier, targeted site, and circulation (Brannon-Peppas and Blanchette 2004). Cell uptake is mediated by the interaction between the particle and the components of cell surface leading to an invagination of the membrane followed by particle internalization into endocytic vesicles (Mukherjee et al. 1997). However, NP entrapment into these vesicles can result in drug release and drug degradation due to the low pH and to the presence of endosomal enzymes. The size of internalized vesicles can range from nanometers to micrometers, depending on the type of endocytosis, as well as the physiological conditions and the physicochemical characteristics of the particles.

Opsonization is the major obstacle to nanoparticulate carriers administered intravenously. Opsonin proteins can bind to the particle surface, being identifying by Kupffer cells (Frank and Fries 1991). These opsonins can be immunoglubulins, albumin, apolipoprotein, and fibrinogen (Dobrovolskaia and McNeil 2007a). Protein adsorption can destabilize the NP structure leading to premature drug release and, thus, can induce several side effects (Chen et al. 2008). Larger polymeric particles (≈ 500 nm in diameter) tend to agglomerate in high levels in the liver (Nagayama et al. 2007). Polymeric NPs with size ranging from 100 to 200 nm can circulate in the blood during a longer period of time, avoiding opsonization. Beyond removal by the reticuloendothelial system (RES), polymeric NPs must also avoid renal filtration. NPs with small diameters (mean size ≈ 10 nm) can escape from the renal system (Davis et al. 2008).

The NP surface charge is also an important parameter in drug delivery. Generally speaking, charged particles are rapidly opsonized by RES, resulting in particle aggregation, plasma clearance, and vessel occlusion (Xiao et al. 2011). Positive charge particles can promote immunological reactions and strong toxicity (Dobrovolskaia and McNeil 2007b). To overcome these processes, surface modification of polymeric NPs using hydrophilic polymers, such as PEG, and poly(ethylene oxide) (PEO) has been widely employed to modulate the hydrophilic character of the particle (Vittaz et al. 1996, Sheng et al. 2009).

Regarding the GI uptake, uncharged and positively charged NPs have high affinity for enterocytes, whereas polymeric NPs based on hydrophilic polymers and with negative charge can be absorbed by both M cells and enterocytes (Jani et al. 1989).

Active targeting

Active targeting of NPs is based on the attachment of smart ligands to the NP surface to enhance selective delivery to tumor tissues. Conjugation of

Table 1.2. Formulation methodologies to obtain polymeric NPs.

Method of preparation	Polymer	Loaded drug	Route of administration	Properties/Therapeutic effect	References
Emulsification/ internal gelation	Sodium alginate	Insulin	Oral	Decrease of blood glucose levels	Reis et al. 2007
Interfacial polymerization	Poly(alkylcyanoacrylate) (PACA)	Albumin	Oral	High entrapment efficacy, influenced by the amount of monomer used	Krauel et al. 2005
Emulsion polymerization	PACA	Doxorubicin (DOX)	Intravenous	DOX controlled release due to drug retention in the polymeric matrix	Alhareth et al. 2011
Solvent displacement	PLGA, poly(vinyl sulfonate-*co*-vinyl alcohol)-*graft*-poly(D,L-lactide-*co*-glycolide) [P(VS-VA)-g-PLGA]	Salbutamol	–	Smaller sizes lead to a greater drug encapsulation thanks to electrostatic interactions	Beck-Broichsitter et al. 2010
Interfacial deposition	PLA	Retinyl palmitate	Transdermal	Nanocapsules with high flexibility. Deep permeation of retinyl palmitate in the skin	Teixeira et al. 2010
Emulsification solvent evaporation	PLGA	Rifampicin	–	Initial burst drug release followed by a sustained drug release phase	Malathi and Balasubramanian 2011
Emulsification solvent diffusion	PLGA	Alendronate	–	Inhibition of raw macrophage. Inhibition of restenosis	Cohen-Sela et al. 2009
Polyelectrolyte complex	Chitosan and its derivatives	Insulin	Oral	Burst insulin release. Antibacterial effect against *Staphylococcus aureus*	Sadeghi et al. 2008
Ionotropic gelation	Chitosan and arabic gum	Insulin	Oral	Lower insulin release at pH 6.5 than at pH 7.2 and 1.2. Release mechanism can be controlled by non-Fickian diffusion	Avadi et al. 2010

antibodies fragments have been widely explored to promote the accumulation of NPs at the targeted site. However, the manufacturing processes involving antibodies molecules can be very complex and expensive, and can determine an increase in NP size (Alexis et al. 2008). Therefore, other strategies have been proposed on transport receptors overexpressed in malignant cells, such as transferrin and folate. PLGA NPs containing transferrin targeting ligand promoted the uptake by F-98 cells mediated caveolae and clathrin pathways. *In vivo* tests showed high levels of transferrin-NPs in an healthy brain (Chang et al. 2012). Currently, cyclodextrin-based NPs with transferrin molecules as the targeting moieties are in Phase I clinical trials for intravenous delivery of small interfering ribonucleic acid (*si*RNA) (Davis et al. 2010). In another study, 17-allylamino-17-demethoxygeldanamycin (17-AAG)-loaded PEGylated PLGA NPs surface functionalized with folate moieties (particle size ≈ 240 nm) demonstrated both higher uptake by MCF-7 human breast cancer cells and cytotoxicity effects in comparison to non-functionalized NPs (Saxena et al. 2012).

In summary, targeted NPs have the ability to accumulate in specific tissues or organs, playing an important role in the selective delivery of therapeutic agents with reduced side effects.

Bioadhesion

Bioadhesion is a general term which involves the adhesion between natural or synthetic materials to tissue surfaces. Mucoadhesive drug delivery systems utilize the ability of bioadhesion of the material to adhere to mucus membranes (Nagai and Machida 1985), targeting a drug to a particular mucus tissue for an extended period of time (Kamath and Park 1994) (Table 1.3).

Mucoadhesion is a complex phenomenon and the mechanisms responsible in the formation of bioadhesive bonds are not fully known. However, these mechanisms can be described by the combination of several theories (Huang et al. 2000, Smart 2005), such as electronic (Derjaguin et al. 1977), adsorption (Tabor 1977), diffusion (Mikos and Peppas 1986), wetting (Helfand and Tagami 1972) and fracture (Ponchel et al. 1987). Diverse factors can affect mucoadhesion, including the polymer properties and the physiological features, such as mucus turnover, mucus thickness, intestinal fluid volumes, pathological conditions, and pH (Mikos and Peppas 1986, Mortazavi and Smart 1993, Rubinstein and Tirosh 1994, Siccardi et al. 2005, Varum et al. 2008).

For the first generation of bioadhesive polymers, such as chitosan, alginate, and Carbopol® polymers, the mechanism of mucoadhesion is based on physicochemical interactions. Due to the presence of negative charges in the mucin, opposite electric charges are required to increase the residence time of particles and consequently to achieve a better drug absorption (George and Abraham 2006). It has been reported that chitosan binds to mucin due to the affinity of their positively charged amino groups for the negatively

Table 1.3. Mucoadhesion studies of various polymer-based nanosystems.

Assay	Polymer	Drug	Route of administration	References
In vivo	PGA, chitosan	Insulin	Oral	Sonaje et al. 2009
	Thiolated Eudragit®	Insulin	Oral	Zhang et al. 2012
	Eudragit®, PLGA	Salmon calcitonin	Oral	Cetin et al. 2012
	Albumin, cyclodextrin	Tacrine	Nasal	Luppi et al. 2011
	PLA, chitosan	5-fluorouracil (5-FU)	Ocular	Ramesh et al. 2010
	PLGA	Flurbiprofen	Ocular	Vega et al. 2006
	PEGylated chitosan	Insulin	Nasal	Zhang et al. 2008
In vitro	Thiolated chitosan	Docetaxel	Oral	Saremi et al. 2011
	Chitosan	Tenofovir	Intravaginal	Meng et al. 2011
	Thiolated chitosan	Leuprolide	Nasal	Shahnaz et al. 2012
	Chitosan	Natamycin	Ocular	Bhatta et al. 2012

charged sialic acid residues of glycoprotein, or by forming hydrogen bonds with mucin (Qaqish and Amiji 1999, Deacon et al. 2000, Dedinaite et al. 2005). However, some studies have reported that the use of anionic polymers leads to better mucosal adhesion than cationic polymers or non-ionic polymers (Chickering and Mathiowitz 1995). This observation can be attributed to the presence of numerous surface carboxyl groups on anionic polymers, generating strong bioadhesive interactions by hydrogen bonds with oligosaccharide chains of mucin (Bernkop-Schnurch 2002).

Lectins (carbohydrate-binding proteins) are the second generation of bioadhesives found in plants and microorganisms (Liener et al. 1986). Lectins have the ability to bind to specific sugar moieties on cell surfaces, playing an important role in the transport of drug across biological barriers (Clark et al. 2000, Bies et al. 2004). The potential use of *Lycopersicon esculentum* (tomato lectin) and *Triticum vulgare* (Wheat Germ Agglutinin, WGA) in oral drug delivery has been widely investigated, since they possess specificity for a specific site in the GI tract, have non-immunogenic properties, and are resistant to enzymatic degradation in the GI tract (Kompella and Lee 2001).

Polymeric NPs coated with lectins have become very popular in oral administration. For instance, Yin et al. (2006) investigated thymopentin-loaded WGA-conjugated PLGA NPs for oral delivery. The NPs were synthesized applying the emulsion-solvent evaporation process. These NPs produced a significant improvement on the oral absorption of the drug in comparison to the free drug (in aqueous solution) and NPs non-functionalized with WGA. In another study with lectin-coated PLGA NPs, Mishra et al. (2011) demonstrated a great potential for oral immunization against hepatitis B. These NPs made possible a strong immune response, as well as demonstrated a severe mucoadhesiveness in the bovine submaxillary mucin. Finally, PEGylated PLA NPs have also been decorated with WGA for nasal administration to improve the incorporation of the particles in the brain (Gao et al. 2006). The NP surface was coated with WGA by incorporating maleimide to the PEGylated polymer, leading to the interaction between thiol groups and lectin. Increased drug internalization into the brain was described for the WGA-polymeric NPs with negligible toxicity.

Glass transition temperature

T_g is the temperature at which the amorphous phase of the polymer is converted from a glassy to rubbery state. Regarding applications of polymeric matrices in drug delivery field, T_g can affect the controlled drug release. Since the mobility of the polymer chains is reduced (glassy state) below the T_g, a small amount of the drug will diffuse. In contrast, higher drug release rates are expected above the T_g, due to the relaxation of polymer chains (Siepmann and Peppas 2001). T_g of a system can be reduced when in contact with water or biological fluids. These solvents can act as a plasticizer by increasing the mobility of the polymeric chains, and thus higher drug amounts are released (Bikiaris et al. 2009, Papadimitriou and Bikiaris 2009).

Aliphatic polyesters have different melting points, varying from 46.7 to 166.4°C. Karavelidis et al. (2010) investigated the effect of melting point and T_g of ropinirole HCl-loaded polyester NPs on drug release behavior. Polyesters with high T_g (58.7°C) released the drug slowly compared to polyesters with low T_g (–57.8 and –53.1°C). According to Wu et al. (2009), polymer matrix can be greatly affected when the T_g is lower than body temperature leading to an increase in drug diffusion.

Hydroxypropyl methylcellulose (HPMC) is the most important hydrophilic polymer used for controlled drug release applications, due to its high swellability (Colombo 1993). In fact, the diffusion of encapsulated drug through the polymer results from the contact between the water or biological fluids and the polymeric matrix that leads to the relaxation of the polymer chains (Brannon-Peppas and Peppas 1990). Several studies have reported different T_g for HPMC using various thermal techniques, such as Differential Scanning Calorimetry (DSC), Differential Thermal Analysis (DTA), or thermomechanical analysis (TMA) (Doelker 1993).

Responsive behavior

As described above, polymeric NPs can possess stimuli-responsive properties. Responsive behavior of polymeric NPs can be characterized by a sequence of events, such as, reception of stimuli, changes in the material properties (dimension, structure, and interaction), and transduction of the changes in its aggregation state leading to drug release at the desired place.

Changes in pH are the biological stimuli more investigated. The pH of the polymeric matrix can be modulated by choosing of a polymer with a certain pKa. The incorporation of functional groups within the polymeric structure which can ionize at distinct pHs has been extensively used for pH-responsive polymeric NPs. Polymers based on cationic monomers and pKa > 7, at the physiological pH 7.4 will be protonated resulting in electrostatic repulsion between the polymer chains and drug expulsion. At pH above the pKa of the polymer, amino groups will deprotonate leading to high hydrophobic interactions and gel collapse. In contrast, polymers with acidic groups and pKa < 7, such as carboxylic groups, will exist in deprotonated state at above pH 7 resulting in water-soluble polymer chains, and consequently, drug release (Colson and Grinstaff 2012). Copolymers based on poly(methacrylic acid-*co*-ethylacrylate) have been used for drug delivery applications because they are insoluble at low pHs, whereas at high pHs their chains dissolve and release the incorporated drug (Foss et al. 2004). This strategy has been employed for the oral treatment of several pathological conditions, such as inflammatory bowel disease (Wang and Zhang 2012), as well as human immunodeficiency virus infection (De Jaeghere et al. 2000). Finally, poly(α,β-aspartic acid) derivatives have also been used for improving DOX release (Wang et al. 2012). PEG was conjugated to the copolymer structure to extend the plasma half-live. The cumulative DOX release was faster at pH 5.0 than at pH 7.4, thus optimizing the antitumor activity compared with a DOX solution.

In temperature-responsive polymers, the temperature can modulate the interactions between the polymeric chains and solvent, and the interactions between the monomers. These events are commonly represented by Lower Critical Solution Temperature (LCST) or Upper Critical Solution Temperature (UCST). Below LCST, the polymer is completely miscible, whereas above LCST hydrophobic interactions are the dominant effect. Regarding the UCST, above this temperature the polymer chains will be dissolved as the polymer-solvent interactions increases (Schmaljohann 2006). In another study, Rejinold et al. (2011) demonstrated that thermoresponsive chitosan-*graft*-poly(*N*-vinylcaprolactam) NPs (220 in size) can be a promising candidate for curcumin delivery. NPs were produced and a cumulative release test demonstrated a slow drug release profile and a specific anticancer activity above the LCST.

Oxidative stress is another biological change that can be advantageously used in drug delivery to non-healthy tissues. This is a process involving high levels of Reactive Oxygen Species (ROS), such as hydrogen peroxide, superoxide, and hydroxide. To control the concentration of these species, several enzymes can serve as antioxidants, including catalase, glutathione peroxidase, and superoxide dismutase. However, increasing ROS levels under some pathological conditions can result in lipid, protein, and deoxyribonucleic acid (DNA) damage. In a recent investigation, dextran NPs containing arylboronic esters were used for albumin delivery (Broaders et al. 2011). The ester groups were oxidized in the presence of ROS to phenols, resulting in the transformation of the hydrophobic particle into hydrophilic due to the exposure of the hydroxyl groups of dextran. Finally, Mahmoud et al. (2011) demonstrated that polythioether ketal-based NPs can undergo two chemical modifications. Firstly, the reaction between ether groups and ROS can lead to the formation of sulfones, and thus the particle becomes more hydrophilic. Secondly, the produced ketal groups are more susceptible to acidic-catalyzed degradation with intense protein release.

Nanogels as Drug Delivery Carriers

Hydrogels have been widely used in several biomedical applications, such as tissue engineering, drug delivery, and cell encapsulation (Hoffman 2002, Nguyen and Lee 2010). Hydrogels are generally synthesized from hydrophilic polymer networks with a three-dimension configuration enabling the incorporation of high amounts of water (Peppas and Mikos 1986, Gehrke and Lee 1990). The water absorption capability is attributed to the presence of hydrophilic compounds ($-NH_2$, $-OH$, $-SO_3H$) on the polymer surface (Peppas and Khare 1993). Hydrogels may also show a swelling behavior dependent on the external conditions, thus being physiologically-responsive systems (Peppas and Merrill 1976, Peppas 1991, Peppas and Mongia 1997). However, hydrogels present some limitations regarding drug delivery, since the presence of high content water and large pore size can define a burst drug release. The development of nanoscale hydrogel particles (nanogels) allows the immobilization of different drugs, acting as a drug reservoir for drug delivery purposes. Due to the combination of the gel properties and the colloidal characteristics, such as a structure with high heterogeneity, small size, and large surface area, nanogel particles are potential candidates for the clinical development of nanoformulations.

Diverse procedures have been developed to prepare nanogels (Table 1.4). These methods can be divided into two major syntheses routes: (i) nanogel formation using polymer precursors; and, (ii) nanogel preparation from monomer polymerization.

Nanogels have been extensively studied as pH sensitive platforms for the controlled delivery of chemotherapeutic agents. Nanogels based on methacrylic acid and ethylene glycol have been extensively investigated as bleomycin carriers (Blanchette and Peppas 2005). It was described that these nanogels can protect the drug against low pHs, and the release studies indicated a fast drug release at pH 7.4 after 1 hour.

Herceptin-conjugated cholesterol-modified pullulan nanogels are under investigation for vaccination against cancer, having finished a phase I clinical trial. Results indicated that this system can induce herceptin-specific humoral responses in patients with herceptin-expressing tumors after a subcutaneous injection (Kageyama et al. 2008). More recently, 5-FU-loaded chitin nanogels (120–140 nm in diameter) have shown a promising cytotoxicity against melanoma in a concentration ranging from 0.4 to 2.0 mg/mL. Skin permeation

Table 1.4. Major methodologies to prepare nanogels from polymeric precursor crosslinking.

Formulation procedure	Description	Size (nm)	References
Disulfide crosslinking	Crosslink between PEG and pyridyl disulfide	40–60	Ying-Quiao et al. 2011
Physical crosslinking	Host-guest interactions, electrostatics, aggregation, sol-gel transition	≈ 100	Teijeiro-Osorio et al. 2009, Shimoda et al. 2012
Amine crosslinking	Reaction between amino and carboxylic groups, and esters and iodides	50	Huang et al. 1998
Click chemistry crosslinking	Alkyl units with amino groups are immobilized to the corona via amidation of hydrophilic copolymer micelles	≈ 40	Joralemon et al. 2005
Photo-induced crosslinking	Technique used to stabilize polymers with functional groups that can polymerize	80–250	Lee et al. 2009
Nanogels from monomer polymerization crosslinking	Inverse water-in-oil (w/o) emulsion	≈ 200	Lee et al. 2007

assays demonstrated that these 5-FU-loaded nanogels can penetrate into deep layers of the skin (Sabitha et al. 2013).

Conclusions

Polymeric NPs have been extensively studied as drug carriers due to their biocompatibility, controlled drug release, and large versatility for surface modification. Several methods have been developed to prepare NPs. According to the physicochemical features of a drug, it is possible to choose the best preparation process, as well as the best polymer matrix to assure the best therapeutic effect. However, some limitations still have to be overcome. In fact, the presence of solvent residues and high energy input and the premature drug release in acidic pHs can affect the integrity of biomolecules loaded to the NPs.

Conjugation of certain smart moieties (e.g., PEG, antibodies, transferrin, and folate) and/or engineering smart NPs/nanogels, e.g., pH-responsive, can determine a preferential NP accumulation in tumor cells, thus optimizing the selectivity of drug delivery. Nevertheless, high costs of synthesis, inefficient translocation *in vivo*, as well lacks of toxicological concerns have limited the definitive introduction into the clinic of polymeric NPs against cancer. Therefore, it is necessary to address *in vitro* and *in vivo* the benefit-risk balance of these nanosystems not only with short-term exposure investigations, but also with long-term exposure studies.

Acknowledgements

Financial support from *Fundação para a Ciência e Tecnologia* is gratefully acknowledged (projects: PTDC/SAU-FAR/113100/2009 and PEst-C/AGR/UI4033/2011, and SFRH/BD/60640/2009 to Tatiana Andreani) and from European Union Funds (FEDER/COMPETE, project FCOMP-01-0124-FEDER-022696).

Abbreviations

17-AAG	:	17-allylamino-17-demethoxygeldanamycin
DNA	:	deoxyribonucleic acid
DOX	:	doxorubicin
DSC	:	differential scanning calorimetry
DTA	:	differential thermal analysis
5-FU	:	5-fluorouracil
GI	:	gastrointestinal
HPMC	:	hydroxypropyl methylcellulose
LCST	:	lower critical solution temperature
MPS	:	mononuclear phagocyte system
NP	:	nanoparticle
PACA	:	poly(alkylcyanoacrylate)
PCL	:	poly(ε-caprolactone)
PEG	:	poly(ethylene glycol)
PEO	:	poly(ethylene oxide)
PLA	:	poly(D,L-lactide)
PLGA	:	poly(D,L-lactide-*co*-glycolide)
P(VS-VA)-*g*-	:	poly(vinyl sulfonate-*co*-vinyl alcohol)-gra
PLGA		ft-poly(D,L-lactide-*co*-glycolide)
RES	:	reticuloendothelial system
ROS	:	reactive oxygen species
*si*RNA	:	small interfering ribonucleic acid
T_g	:	glass transition temperature
TMA	:	thermomechanical analysis
UCST	:	upper critical solution temperature
WGA	:	wheat germ agglutinin
w/o	:	water-in-oil

References

Alexis, F. and E. Pridgen, L.K. Molnar and O.C. Farokhzad. 2008. Factors affecting the clearance and biodistribution of polymeric nanoparticles. Mol. Pharm. 5: 505–515.

Alhareth, K. and C. Vauthier, C. Gueutin, G. Ponchel and F. Moussa. 2011. Doxorubicin loading and *in vitro* release from poly(alkylcyanoacrylate) nanoparticles produced by redox radical emulsion polymerization. J. App. Polym. Sci. 119: 816–822.

Arbós, P. and M.A. Campanero, M.A. Arangoa, M.J. Renedo and J.M. Irache. 2003. Influence of the surface characteristics of PVM/MA nanoparticles on their bioadhesive properties. J. Control. Release 89: 19–30.

Avadi, M.R. and A.M.M. Sadeghi, N. Mohammadpour, S. Abedin, F. Atyabi, R. Dinarvand and M. Rafiee-Tehrani. 2010. Preparation and characterization of insulin nanoparticles using chitosan and Arabic gum with ionic gelation method. Nanomedicine. 6: 58–63.

Beck-Broichsitter, M. and E. Rytting, T. Lebhardt, X. Wang and T. Kissel. 2010. Preparation of nanoparticles by solvent displacement for drug delivery: a shift in the "ouzo region" upon drug loading. Eur. J. Pharm. Sci. 41: 244–253.

Bernkop-Schnurch, A. Mucoadhesive polymers. pp. 147–165. *In*: S. Dumitriu [ed.]. 2002. Polymer Biomaterial. Marcel Decker, New York, USA.

Bhatta, R.S. and H. Chandasana, Y.S. Chhonker, C. Rathi, D. Kumar, K. Mitra and P.K. Shukla. 2012. Mucoadhesive nanoparticles for prolonged ocular delivery of natamycin: *in vitro* and pharmacokinetics studies. Int. J. Pharm. 432: 105–112.

Bies, C. and C.M. Lehr and J.F. Woodley. 2004. Lectin-mediated drug targeting: history and applications. Adv. Drug Deliv. Rev. 56: 425–435.

Bikiaris, D. and V. Karavelidis and E. Karavas. 2009. Novel biodegradable polyesters. Synthesis and application as drug carriers for the preparation of raloxifene HCl loaded nanoparticles. Molecules. 14: 2410–2430.

Blanchette, J. and N.A. Peppas. 2005. Oral chemotherapeutic delivery: design and cellular response. Ann. Biomed. Eng. 33: 142–149.

Brannon-Peppas, L. and N.A. Peppas. The equilibrium swelling behavior of porous and non-porous hydrogels. pp. 67–102. *In*: L. Brannon-Peppas and R.S. Harland [eds.]. 1990. Absorbent Polymer Technology. Elsevier, Amsterdam, The Netherlands.

Brannon-Peppas, L. and J.O. Blanchette. 2004. Nanoparticle and targeted systems for cancer therapy. Adv. Drug Deliv. Rev. 56: 1649–1659.

Brigger, I. and C. Dubernet and P. Couvreur. 2002. Nanoparticles in cancer therapy and diagnosis. Adv. Drug Deliv. Rev. 54: 631–651.

Broaders, K.E. and S. Grandhe and J.M. Fréchet. 2011. A biocompatible oxidation-triggered carrier polymer with potential in therapeutics. J. Am. Chem. Soc. 133: 756–758.

Cafaggi, S. and E. Russo, R. Stefani, R. Leardi, G. Caviglioli, B. Parodi, G. Bignardi, D. De Toreto, C. Ajello and M. Viale. 2008. Preparation and evaluation of nanoparticles made of chitosan or N-trimethyl chitosan and cisplatin-alginate complex. J. Control. Release. 121: 110–123.

Cetin, M. and M.S. Aktas, I. Vural and M. Ozturk. 2012. Salmon-calcitonin-loaded Eudragit and Eudragit-PLGA nanoparticles: *in vitro* and *in vivo* evaluation. J. Microencapsul. 29: 156–166.

Champion, J.A. and Y.K. Katare and S. Mitragotri. 2007. Making polymeric micro- and nanoparticles of complex shapes. PNAS. 104: 11901–11904.

Chang, J. and A. Paillard, C. Passirani, M. Morille, J.P. Benoit, D. Betbeder and E. Garcion. 2012. Transferrin adsorption onto PLGA nanoparticles governs their interaction with biological systems from blood circulation to brain cancer cells. Pharm. Res. 29: 1495–1505.

Chen, H. and S. Kim, W. He, H. Wang, P.S. Low, K. Park and J.X. Cheng. 2008. Fast release of lipophilic agents from circulating PEG-PDLLA micelles revealed by *in vivo* forster resonance energy transfer imaging. Langmuir. 24: 5213–5217.

Chickering, D.E. and E. Mathiowitz. 1995. Bioadhesive microspheres: I. A novel electrobalance-based method to study adhesive interactions between individual microspheres and intestinal mucosa. J. Control. Release. 34: 251–262.

Clark, M.A. and B.H. Hirst and M.A. Jepson. 2000. Lectin-mediated mucosal delivery of drugs and microparticles. Adv. Drug Deliv. Rev. 43: 207–223.

Cohen-Sela, E. and M. Chorny, N. Koroukhov, H.D. Danenberg and G. Golomb. 2009. A new double emulsion solvent diffusion technique for encapsulating hydrophilic molecules in PLGA nanoparticles. J. Control. Release. 133: 90–95.

Colombo, P. 1993. Swelling-controlled release in hydrogel matrices for oral route. Adv. Drug Deliv. Rev. 11: 37–57.

Colson, Y. and M.W. Grinstaff. 2012. Biologically responsive polymeric nanoparticles for drug delivery. Adv. Mater. 24: 3878–3886.

Couvreur, P. and C. Dubernet and F. Puisieux. 1995. Controlled drug delivery with nanoparticles: current possibilities and future trends. Eur. J. Pharm. Biopharm. 41: 2–13.

Davis, M.E. and Z. Chen and D.M. Shin. 2008. Nanoparticle therapeutics: an emerging treatment modality for cancer. Nat. Rev. Drug Discov. 7: 129–138.

Davis, M.E. and J.E. Zuckerman, C.H. Choi, D. Seligson, A. Tolcher, C.A. Alabi, Y. Yen, J.D. Heidel and A. Ribas. 2010. Evidence of RNAi in humans from systemically administered siRNA via targeted nanoparticles. Nature. 464: 1067–1070.

De Jaeghere, F. and E. Allémann, F. Kubel, B. Galli, R. Cozens, E. Doelker and R. Gurny. 2000. Oral bioavailability of a poorly water soluble HIV-1 protease inhibitor incorporated into pH-sensitive particles: effect of the particle size and nutritional state. J. Control. Release. 68: 291–298.

Deacon, M.P. and S. McGurk, C.J. Roberts, P.M. Williams, S.J.B. Tendler, M.C. Davies, S.S. Davis and S.E. Harding. 2000. Atomic force microscopy of gastric mucin and chitosan mucoadhesive systems. Biochem. J. 348: 557–563.

Dedinaite, A. and M. Lundin, L. Macakova and T. Auletta. 2005. Mucin-chitosan complexes at the solid-liquid interface: multilayer formation and stability in surfactant solutions. Langmuir. 21: 9502–9509.

Derjaguin, B.V. and Y.P. Toporov, V.M. Muller and I.N. Aleinikova. 1977. On the relationship between the molecular component of the adhesion of elastic particles to a solid surface. J. Colloid Interface Sci. 58: 528–533.

Dobrovolskaia, M.A. and S.E. McNeil. 2007a. Immunological properties of engineered nanomaterials. Nat. Nanotechnol. 2: 469–478.

Dobrovolskaia, M.A. and S.E. McNeil. 2007b. Immunological properties of engineered nanomaterials. Nat. Nanotechnol. 2: 469–478.

Doelker, E. 1993. Cellulose derivatives. Adv. Polym. Sci. 107: 199–265.

Dong, Y. and S.S. Feng. 2005. Poly(d,l-lactide-co-glycolide)/montmorillonite nanoparticles for oral delivery of anticancer drugs. Biomaterials. 26: 6068–6076.

Elsabahy, M. and K.L. Wooley. 2012. Design of polymeric nanoparticles for biomedical delivery applications Chem. Soc. Rev. 41: 2545–2561.

Fleige, E. and M.A. Quadir and R. Haag. 2012. Stimuli-responsive polymeric nanocarriers for the controlled transport of active compounds: concepts and applications. Adv. Drug Deliv. Rev. 64: 866–884.

Fomina, N. and C. McFearin, M. Sermsakdi, O. Edigin and A. Almutairi. 2010. UV and near-IR triggered release from polymeric nanoparticles. J. Am. Chem. Soc. 132: 9540–9542.

Foss, A. and T. Goto, M. Morishita and N.A. Peppas. 2004. Development of acrylic-based copolymers for oral insulin delivery. Eur. J. Pharm. Biopharm. 57: 163–169.

Frank, M. and L. Fries. 1991. The role of complement in inflammation and phagocytosis. Immunol. Today. 12: 322–326.

Gao, X. and W. Tao, W. Lu, Q. Zhang, Y. Zhang, X. Jianga and S. Fu. 2006. Lectin-conjugated PEG-PLA nanoparticles: preparation and brain delivery after intranasal administration. Biomaterials. 27: 3482–3490.

Gehrke, S.H. and P.I. Lee. Hydrogels for drug delivery systems. pp. 333–392. *In:* P. Tyle [ed.]. 1990. Specialized Drug Delivery Systems. Marcel Dekker, New York, USA.

George, M. and T.E. Abraham. 2006. Polyionic hydrocolloids for the intestinal delivery of protein drugs: alginate and chitosan—a review. J. Control. Release. 114: 1–14.

Helfand, E. and Y. Tagami. 1972. Theory of interface between immiscible polymers. J. Chem. Phys. 57: 1812–1813.

Hoare, T.R. and D.S. Kohane. 2008. Hydrogels in drug delivery: progress and challenges. Polymer. 49: 1993–2007.

Hoffman, A.S. 2002. Hydrogels for biomedical applications. Adv. Drug Deliv. Rev. 54: 3–12.

Hsieh, D.S.T. and W.D. Rhine and R. Langer. 1983. Zero-order controlled-release polymer matrices for micro- and macromolecules. J. Pharm. Sci. 72: 17–22.

Huang, H. and K.L. Remsen and K.L. Wooley. 1998. Amphiphilic core-shell nanospheres obtained by intramicellar shell crosslinking of polymer micelles with poly(ethylene oxide) linkers. Chem. Commun. 13: 1415–1416.

Huang, Y. and W. Leobandung, A. Foss and N.A. Peppas. 2000. Molecular aspects of muco- and bioadhesion: tethered structures and site-specific surfaces. J. Control. Release. 65: 63–71.

Jani, P. and C.W. Halbert, J. Langridge and A.T. Florence. 1989. The uptake and translocation of latex nanospheres and microspheres after oral administration to rats. J. Pharm. Pharmacol. 41: 809–812.

Jeong, J.C. and J. Lee and K. Cho. 2003. Effects of crystalline microstructure on drug release behavior of poly(ε-caprolactone) microspheres. J. Control. Release. 92: 249–258.

Joralemon, M.J. and R.K. O'Reilly, C.J. Hawker and K.L. Wooley. 2005. Shell click-crosslinked (SCC) nanoparticles: a new methodology for synthesis and orthogonal functionalization. J. Am. Chem. Soc. 127: 16892–16899.

Jung, T. and W. Kamm, A. Breitenbach, E. Kaiserling, J.X. Xiao and T. Kissel. 2000. Biodegradable nanoparticles for oral delivery of peptides: is there a role for polymers to affect mucosal uptake? Eur. J. Pharm. Biopharm. 50: 147–160.

Kageyama, S. and S. Kitano, M. Hirayama, Y. Nagata, H. Imai, T. Shiraishi, K. Akiyoshi, A.M. Scott, R. Murphy, E.W. Hoffman, L.J. Old, N. Katayama and H. Shiku. 2008. Humoral immune responses in patients vaccinated with 1-146 HER2 protein complexed with cholesteryl pullulan nanogel. Cancer Sci. 99: 601–607.

Kalaria, D.R. and G. Sharma, V. Beniwal and M.N.V. Ravi Kumar. 2009. Design of biodegradable nanoparticles for oral delivery of doxorubicin: *in vivo* pharmacokinetics and toxicity studies in rats. Pharm. Res. 26: 492–501.

Kamath, K.R. and K. Park. Mucosal adhesive preparations. pp. 133–163. *In:* J. Swarbrick and J.C. Boylan [eds.]. 1994. Encyclopedia of Pharmaceutical Technology. Marcel Dekker, New York, USA.

Karavelidis, V. and D. Giliopoulos, E. Karavas and D. Bikiaris. 2010. Nanoencapsulation of a water soluble drug in biocompatible polyesters. Effect of polyesters melting point and glass transition temperature on drug release behavior. Eur. J. Pharm. Sci. 41: 636–643.

Khaing, Z.Z. and C.E. Schmidt. 2012. Advances in natural biomaterials for nerve tissue repair. Neurosci. Lett. 519: 103–114.

Kim, J.H. and Y.S. Kim, K. Park, S. Lee, H.Y. Nam, K.H. Min, H.G. Jo, J.H. Park, K. Choi, S.Y. Jeong, R.W. Park, I.S. Kim, K. Kim and I.C. Kwon. 2008. Antitumor efficacy of cisplatin-loaded glycol chitosan nanoparticles in tumor-bearing mice. J. Control. Release. 127: 41–49.

Kompella, U.B. and H.L. Lee. 2001. Delivery systems for penetration enhancement of peptide and protein drugs: design considerations. Adv. Drug Deliv. Rev. 46: 211–245.

Krauel, K. and N.M. Davies, S. Hook and T. Rades. 2005. Using different structure types of microemulsions for the preparation of poly(alkylcyanoacrylate) nanoparticles by interfacial polymerization. J. Control. Release 106: 76–87.

Lee, H. and S. Mok, S. Lee, Y.K. Oh and T.G. Park. 2007. Target-specific intracellular delivery of siRNA using degradable hyaluronic acid nanogels. J. Control. Release. 119: 246–252.

Lee, J.I. and H.S. Kim and H.S. Yoo. 2009. DNA nanogels composed of chitosan and Pluronic with thermo-sensitive and photo-crosslinking properties. Int. J. Pharm. 373: 93–99.

Lenaerts, V. and P. Couvreur, D. Christiaens-Leyh, E. Joiris, M. Roland, S. Rollman and P. Speiser. 1984. Degradation of poly(isobutyl cyanoacrylate) nanoparticles. Biomaterials. 5: 65–68.

Leobandung, W. and H. Ichikawa, Y. Fukumori and N.A. Peppas. 2003. Monodisperse nanoparticles of poly(ethylene glycol) macromers and N-isopropyl acrylamide for biomedical applications. J. Appl. Polym. Sci. 87: 1678–1684.

Liener, I.E. and N. Sharon and I.J. Goldstein. 1986. The Lectins: Properties, Functions and Applications in Biology and Medicine. Academic Press, Orlando, USA.

Lorenz, S. and C.P. Hauser, B. Autenrieth, C.K. Weiss, K. Landfester and V. Mailänder. 2010. The softer and more hydrophobic the better: influence of the side chain of polymethacrylate nanoparticles for cellular uptake. Macromol. Biosci. 10: 1034–1042.

Luppi, B. and F. Bigucci, G. Corace, A. Delucca, T. Cerchiara, M. Sorrenti, L. Catenacci, A.M. Di Pietra and V. Zecchi. 2011. Albumin nanoparticles carrying cyclodextrins for nasal delivery of the anti-Alzheimer drug tacrine. Eur. J. Pharm. Sci. 44: 559–565.

Mahmoud, E.A. and J. Sankaranarayanan, J.M. Morachis, G. Kim and A. Almutairi. 2011. Inflammation responsive logic gate nanoparticles for the delivery of proteins. Bioconjug. Chem. 22: 1416–1421.

Malathi, S. and S. Balasubramanian. 2011. Synthesis of biodegradable polymeric nanoparticles and their controlled drug delivery for tuberculosis. J. Biomed. Nanotechnol. 7: 150–151.

Meng, J. and T.F. Sturgis and B.C. Youan. 2011. Engineering tenofovir loaded chitosan nanoparticles to maximize microbicide mucoadhesion. Eur. J. Pharm. Sci. 44: 57–67.

Mikos, A. and N.A. Peppas. 1986. Systems for controlled release of drugs. V. Bioadhesive systems. S.T.P. Pharma. Sci. 2: 705–716.

Mishra, N. and S. Tiwari, B. Vaidya, G.P. Agrawal and S.P. Vyas. 2011. Lectin anchored PLGA nanoparticles for oral mucosal immunization against hepatitis B. J. Drug Target. 19: 67–78.

Mitra, S. and U. Gaur, P.C. Ghosh and A.N. Maitra. 2001. Tumour targeted delivery of encapsulated dextran-doxorubicin conjugate using chitosan nanoparticles as carriers. J. Control. Release. 74: 317–323.

Mittal, G. and D.K. Sahana, V. Bhardwaj and M.N.V. Ravi Kumar. 2007. Estradiol loaded PLGA nanoparticles for oral administration: effect of polymer molecular weight and copolymer composition on release behavior *in vitro* and *in vivo*. J. Control. Release. 119: 77–85.

Mortazavi, S.A. and J.D. Smart. 1993. An investigation into the role of water movement and mucus gel dehydration im mucoadhesion. J. Control. Release 25: 197–203.

Mukherjee, S. and R.N. Ghosh and F.R. Maxfield. 1997. Endocytosis. Physiol. Rev. 77: 759–803.

Musumeci, T. and C.A. Ventura, I. Giannone, B. Ruozi, L. Montenegro, R. Pignatello and G. Puglisi. 2006. PLA/PLGA nanoparticles for sustained release of docetaxel. Int. J. Pharm. 325: 172–179.

Nagai, T. and Y. Machida. 1985. Mucosal adhesive dosage forms. Pharm. Int. 6: 196–200.

Nagayama, S. and K. Ogawara, Y. Fukuoka, K. Higaki and T. Kimura. 2007. Time-dependent changes in opsonin amount associated on nanoparticles alter their hepatic uptake characteristics. Int. J. Pharm. 342: 215–221.

Nguyen, M.K. and D.S. Lee. 2010. Injectable biodegradable hydrogels. Macromol. Biosci. 10: 563–579.

Papadimitriou, S. and D. Bikiaris. 2009. Novel self-assembled core-shell nanoparticles based on crystalline amorphous moieties of aliphatic copolyesters for efficient controlled drug release. J. Control. Release 138: 177–184.

Parveen, S. and R. Misra and S.K. Sahoo. 2012. Nanoparticles: a boon to drug delivery, therapeutics, diagnostics and imaging. Nanomedicine. 8: 147–166.

Peppas, N.A. and E.W. Merrill. 1976. PVA hydrogels: reinforcement of radiation-crosslinked networks by crystallization. J. Polym. Sci. Polym. Chem. Ed. 14: 441–457.

Peppas, N.A. and A.G. Mikos. Preparation methods and structure of hydrogels. pp. 1–27. In: N.A. Peppas [ed.]. 1986. Hydrogels in Medicine and Pharmacy. CRC Press, Boca Raton, USA.

Peppas, N.A. 1991. Physiologically responsive gels. J. Bioact. Compat. Polym. 6: 241–246.

Peppas, N.A. and A.R. Khare. 1993. Preparation, structure and diffusional behavior of hydrogels in controlled release. Adv. Drug Deliv. Rev. 11: 1–35.

Peppas, N.A. and N.K. Mongia. 1997. Ultrapure poly (vinylalcohol) hydrogels with mucoadhesive drug delivery characteristics. Eur. J. Pharm. Biopharm. 43: 51–58.

Perelshtein, I. and G. Applerot, N. Perkas, G. Guibert, S. Mikhailov and A. Gedanken. 2008. Sonochemical coating of silver nanoparticles on textile fabrics (nylon, polyester and cotton) and their antibacterial activity. Nanotechnology. 19: 245705.

Ponchel, G. and F. Touchard, D. Duchêne and A. Peppas. 1987. Bioadhesive analysis of controlled-release systems. I. Fracture and interpenetration analysis in poly(acrylic acid)-containing systems. J. Control. Release. 5: 129–141.

Qaqish, R. and M. Amiji. 1999. Synthesis of a fluorescent chitosan derivative and its application for the study of chitosan-mucin interactions. Carbohydr. Polym. 38: 99–107.

Raemdonck, K. and J. Demeester and S. De Smedt. 2009. Advanced nanogel engineering for drug delivery. Soft Matter. 5: 707–715.

Rai, M. and A. Ingle. 2012. Role of nanotechnology in agriculture with special reference to management of insect pests. Appl. Microbiol. Biotechnol. 94: 287–293.

Ramesh, N. and P.M. Singh, S. Kant, P. Maiti and J.K. Pandit. 2010. Chitosan coated PLA nanoparticles for ophthalmic delivery: characterization, *in-vitro* and *in-vivo* study in rabbit eye. J. Biomed. Nanotechnol. 6: 648–657.

Reis, C.P. and R.J. Neufeld, A.J. Ribeiro and F. Veiga. 2006. Nanoencapsulation I. Methods for preparation of drug-loaded polymeric nanoparticles. Nanomedicine. 2: 8–21.

Reis, C.P. and A.J. Ribeiro, S. Houng, F. Veiga and R.J. Neufeld. 2007. Nanoparticulate delivery system for insulin: design, characterization and *in vitro/in vivo* bioactivity. Eur. J. Pharm. Sci. 30: 392–397.

Rejinold, N.S. and M. Muthunarayanan, V.V. Divyarani, P.R. Sreerekha, K.P. Chennazhi, S.V. Nair, H. Tamura and R. Jayakumar. 2011. Curcumin-loaded biocompatible thermoresponsive polymeric nanoparticles for cancer drug delivery. J. Colloid Interface Sci. 360: 39–51.

Rubinstein, A. and B. Tirosh. 1994. Mucus gel thickness and turnover in the gastrointestinal tract of the rat: response to cholinergic stimulus and implication for mucoadhesion. Pharm. Res. 11: 794–799.

Sabitha, M. and N. Sanoj Rejinold, A. Nair, V.K. Lakshmanan, S.V. Nair and R. Jayakumar. 2013. Development and evaluation of 5-fluorouracil loaded chitin nanogels for treatment of skin cancer. Carbohydr. Polym. 91: 48–57.

Sadeghi, A.M.M. and F.A. Dorkoosh, M.R. Avadi, P. Saadat, M. Rafiee-Tehrani and H.E. Junginger. 2008. Preparation, characterization and antibacterial activities of chitosan, N-trimethyl chitosan (TMC) and N-diethylmethyl chitosan (DEMC) nanoparticles loaded with insulin using both the ionotropic gelation and polyelectrolyte complexation methods. Int. J. Pharm. 355: 299–306.

Sahoo, S.K. and J. Panyam, S. Prabha and V. Labhasetwar. 2002. Residual polyvinyl alcohol associated with poly (D,L-lactide-co-glycolide) nanoparticles affects their physical properties and cellular uptake. J. Control. Release. 82: 105–114.

Saremi, S. and F. Atyabi, S.P. Akhlaghi, S.N. Ostad and R. Dinarvand. 2011. Thiolated chitosan nanoparticles for enhancing oral absorption of docetaxel: preparation, *in vitro* and *ex vivo* evaluation. Int. J. Nanomedicine. 6: 119–128.

Sarmento, B. and A. Ribeiro, F. Veiga, P. Sampaio, R. Neufeld and D. Ferreira. 2007. Alginate/chitosan nanoparticles are effective for oral insulin delivery. Pharm. Res. 24: 2198–2206.

Saxena, V. and Y. Naguib and M.D. Hussain. 2012. Folate receptor targeted 17-allylamino-17-demethoxygeldanamycin (17-AAG) loaded polymeric nanoparticles for breast cancer. Colloids Surf. B Biointerfaces. 94: 274–280.

Schmaljohann, D. 2006. Thermo- and pH-responsive polymers in drug delivery. Adv. Drug Deliv. Rev. 58: 1655–1670.

Shahnaz, G. and A. Vetter, J. Barthelmes, D. Rahmat, F. Laffleur, J. Iqbal, G. Perera, W. Schlocker, S. Dünnhaput and A.B. Schürch. 2012. Thiolated chitosan nanoparticles for the nasal administration of leuprolide: bioavailability and pharmacokinetic characterization. Int. J. Pharm. 428: 164–170.

Sheng, Y. and C. Liu, Y. Yuan, X. Tao, F. Yang, X. Shan, H. Zhou and F. Xu. 2009. Long-circulating polymeric nanoparticles bearing a combinatorial coating of PEG and water-soluble chitosan. Biomaterials. 30: 2340–2348.

Shi, J. and Z. Xiao, N. Kamaly and O.C. Farokhzad. 2011. Self-assembled targeted nanoparticles: evolution of technologies and bench to bedside translation. Acc. Chem. Res. 44: 1123–1134.

Shimoda, A. and S. Sawada, A. Kano, A. Maruyama, A. Moquin, F.M. Winnik and K. Akiyoshi. 2012. Dual crosslinked hydrogel nanoparticles by nanogel bottom-up method for sustained-release delivery. Colloids Surf. B Biointerfaces. 99: 38–44.

Siccardi, D. and J.R. Turner and R.J. Mysny. 2005. Regulation of intestinal epithelial function: a link between opportunities for macromolecular drug delivery and inflammatory bowel disease. Adv. Drug Deliv. Rev. 57: 219–235.

Siepmann, J. and N.A. Peppas. 2001. Modeling of drug release from delivery systems based on hydroxypropyl methylcellulose (HPMC). Adv. Drug Deliv. Rev. 48: 139–157.

Smart, J.D. 2005. The basics and underlying mechanisms of mucoadhesion. Adv. Drug Deliv. Rev. 57: 1556–1568.

Sonaje, K. and Y.H. Lin, J.H. Juang, S.P. Wey, C.T. Chen and H.W. Sung. 2009. *In vivo* evaluation of safety and efficacy of self-assembled nanoparticles for oral insulin delivery. Biomaterials. 30: 2329–2339.

Tabor, D. 1977. Surface forces and surface interactions. J. Colloid Interface Sci. 58: 2–13.

Teijeiro-Osorio, D. and C. Remunan-Lopez and M.J. Alonso. 2009. New generation of hybrid poly/oligosaccharide nanoparticles for the nasal delivery of macromolecules. Biomacromolecules. 10: 243–249.

Teixeira, Z. and B. Zanchetta, B.A.G. Melo, L.L. Oliveira, M.H.A. Santana, E.J. Paredes-Gamero, G.Z. Justo, H.B. Nader, S.S. Guterres and N. Durán. 2010. Retinyl palmitate flexible polymeric nanocapsules: characterization and permeation studies. Colloids Surf. B Biointerfaces. 81: 374–380.

Varum, F.J.O. and E.L. McConnell, J.J.S. Souza, F. Veiga and A.W. Basit. 2008. Mucoadhesion and gastrointestinal tract. Crit. Rev. Ther. Drug Carrier Syst. 25: 207–258.

Vega, E. and M.A. Egea, M. Valls, M. Espina and M.L. García. 2006. Flurbiprofen loaded biodegradable nanoparticles for ophtalmic administration. J. Pharm. Sci. 95: 2393–2405.

Vittaz, M. and D. Bazile, G. Spenlehauer, T. Verrecchia, M. Veillard, F. Puisieux and D. Labarre. 1996. Effect of PEO surface density on long-circulating PLA-PEO nanoparticles which are very low complement activators. Biomaterials. 17: 1575–1581.

Vrignaud, S. and J. Benoit and P. Saulnier. 2001. Strategies for the nanoencapsulation of hydrophilic molecules in polymer-based nanoparticles. Biomaterials. 32: 8593–8604.

Wang, X.Q. and Q. Zhang. 2012. pH-sensitive polymeric nanoparticles to improve oral bioavailability of peptide/protein drugs and poorly water-soluble drugs. Eur. J. Pharm. Biopharm. 82: 219–229.

Wang, X. and G. Wu, C. Lu, W. Zhao, Y. Wang, Y. Fan, H. Gao and J. Ma. 2012. A novel delivery system of doxorubicin with high load and pH-responsive release from the nanoparticles of poly(α,β-aspartic acid) derivative. Eur. J. Pharm. Sci. 47: 256–264.

Win, K.Y. and S.S. Feng. 2005. Effects of particle size and surface coating on cellular uptake of polymeric nanoparticles for oral delivery of anticancer drugs. Biomaterials. 26: 2713–2722.

Wood, K.C. and S.R. Little, R. Langer and P.T. Hammond. 2005. A family of hierarchically self-assembling linear-dendritic hybrid polymers for highly efficient targeted gene delivery. Angew. Chem. Int. Ed. 44: 6704–6708.

Wu, M. and L. Kleiner, F.W. Tang, S. Hossainy, M.C. Davies and C.J. Roberts. 2009. Nanoscale mechanical measurement determination of the glass transition temperature of poly(lactic acid)/everolimus coated stents in air and dissolution media. Eur. J. Pharm. Sci. 36: 493–501.

Xiao, K. and Y. Li, J. Luo, J.S. Lee, W. Xiao, A.M. Gonik, R.G. Agarwal and K.S. Lam. 2011. The effect of surface charge on *in vivo* biodistribution of PEG-oligocholic acid based micellar nanoparticles. Biomaterials. 32: 3435–3446.

Yin, Y. and D. Chen, M. Qiao, Z. Lu and H.Y. Hu. 2006. Preparation and evaluation of lectin-conjugated PLGA nanoparticles for oral delivery of thymopentin. J. Control. Release. 116: 337–345.

Ying-Quiao, Z. and R. Zhang, F.S. Du, D.H. Liang and Z.C. Li. 2011. Multi-responsive nanogels containing motifs of ortho ester, oligo(ethylene glycol) and disulfide linkage as carriers of hydrophobic anti-cancer drugs. J. Control. Release. 152: 57–66.

Zhang, X. and H. Zhang, Z. Wu, Z. Wang, H. Niu and C. Li. 2008. Nasal absorption enhancement of insulin using PEG-grafted chitosan nanoparticles. Eur. J. Pharm. Biopharm. 68: 526–534.

Zhang, Y. and X. Wu, L. Meng, Y. Zhang, R. Aj, N. Qi, H. He, H. Xu and X. Tang. 2012. Thiolated Eudragit nanoparticles for oral insulin delivery: preparation, characterization and *in vivo* evaluation. Int. J. Pharm. 436: 341–350.

CHAPTER 2

Nanotechnology for Oral Drug Delivery and Targeting

Catarina Pinto Reis,[1], Nuno Martinho[1],[a] and Christiane Damgé[2]*

ABSTRACT

The oral route is the most attractive pathway for drug delivery since it is easy for administration, and will clinically improve patient compliance while reducing the overall healthcare costs. Over the last decades there has been a relentless pursuit in improving clinical delivery of therapeutics by the oral route but low clinical translation has been observed. Therapeutics such as peptides, proteins, and nucleic acids face a great challenge in drug delivery and several technological endeavors have to be surpassed before reaching clinical products. Although only a small portion of nanoparticles has been shown to be absorbed, this technology has clearly demonstrated their ability to protect the drugs, reach the bloodstream, and improve the bioavailability of poorly permeable drugs. Moreover, these carriers have shown to be able to induce immunization compared to other administration routes, and reduce side effects commonly found by conventional drug delivery systems. This chapter will approach the general considerations underlying the oral route in terms of its physiology and main mechanisms of permeation. Furthermore, it is meant to enlighten main challenges and opportunities found in the oral route, the major breakthroughs in nanomedicine for oral administration, and the strategies used to improve drug delivery. This kind of technology shows countless possibilities to be further explored to improve oral drug delivery.

[1] CBIOS - Research Center for Biosciences and Health Technologies, Universidade Lusófona de Humanidades e Tecnologias, Lisboa, Portugal; and, IBEB - Biophysics and Biomedical Engineering, Faculty of Sciences, Universidade de Lisboa, Lisboa, Portugal.
[a] Email: nunomartinho@hotmail.com
[2] Faculty of Pharmacy, University Henry Poincaré, EA3452, Nancy, France.
  Email: christiane.damge@medecine.u-strasbg.fr; damge@unistra.fr
* Corresponding author: catarinapintoreis@ulusofona.pt; catarinapintoreis@gmail.com

Introduction

The design of a pharmaceutical dosage form has always taken into account the bioavailability of the therapeutic at the target site. Each dosage form is unique and reveals its intricacies related to the intended use. These variations in terms of formulations not only raise problems related to the limitations of the administration route but also to the specificities of each drug. The proper design of a formulation has to therefore take into account both considerations of the physicochemical and biological characteristics of the route of administration.

It is estimated that ≈ 40% of marked drugs and 40 to 60% of new drugs from high-throughput screening belong to the Biopharmaceutics Classification System (BCS) class II and IV (Panchagnula and Thomas 2000). The poor solubility leads to ineffective absorption and therefore the therapeutic value is rather defined by their physicochemical properties (instead of pharmacological activity), leading to early abandonment and having reduced their potential for clinical use. On the other hand, there are molecules that have good physicochemical properties but fail to resist the harsh environment of the gastrointestinal tract (GIT). Additionally, with the advents of biotechnological processes, therapeutic proteins and peptides have become widely available. However, these fail to provide acceptable oral bioavailability due to their extended degradation in the GIT milieu combined with their inherent low permeability. The parenteral administration of these therapeutics is therefore the common way to overcome these limitations but is usually tedious (especially in diseases that require long-term treatment), painful and discomforting for the patient, causing anxiety and difficulties in compliance. As a result, the possibility of administration by the oral route would constitute an exceptional advantage over these formulations.

The oral route has always been known to be the patients' preference route of drug administration, particularly when chronic usage is required. The oral route has obvious advantages and ultimately enhances patient compliance and treatment management especially for therapeutics where careful monitoring is required. The use of controlled release systems by means of an oral formulation would also bring benefits for drugs whose concentration should be maintained for prolonged periods of time including hormones, analgesic, and anti-inflammatory drugs. These systems would therefore restrict the interaction of the drug with the mucosal epithelium avoiding common problems such as GIT irritation. Also, the use of combinatory multidrug treatments in one system would bring benefit for treatments that require different release of therapeutics at different time scale. However, to accomplish these goals several biological and technical difficulties arise from this route.

To overcome the potential deficiencies of drug absorption several innovative formulations have been employed to improve solubility, rate and extent of absorption, and reduce local side effects. Among the technologies that have been envisioned, one of the most promising tools for oral delivery of therapeutics is their incorporation into nanoparticulate systems. The tools from nanotechnology offer many advantages over conventional dosage forms introducing a new concept of nanomedicine.

Gastrointestinal tract physiology: general background

To reach the blood in sufficient concentration, drugs must overcome the biological barriers that compose the GIT. To be absorbed they must rely on physicochemical properties that favor a Hydrophilic–Lipophilic Balance (HLB), low Molecular weight (M_w), resist to acid and slightly alkaline environment, avoid pre-degradation by enzymes, and diffuse through the mucus barrier.

The different organs that compose the GIT display differentiated structures and cells as well as physicochemical features. This composition forms a complex and efficient barrier to most of the molecules and macromolecules that are presented at their surface. The GIT is not only able to transform and absorb simple molecules from food into the bloodstream but also protect against potential hazardous molecules, particles, and microorganisms. In the stomach, the digestion is initiated with the breaking down by enzymes and the acidic environment. Although the stomach does not contribute as much as the small intestine, some molecules can diffuse through. Following the digestion, the intestine is the main site for absorption where small peptides, disaccharides, fatty acids, and monoglycerides are taken in. This structure presents an increased area which favors the absorption. The intestinal epithelium is composed of a cell monolayer of enterocytes (allow the absorption of nutrients) and goblet cells (responsible for the secretion of the mucus layer). These cells are tightly connected by tight junctions (composed of claudins, occludins, and junctional adhesion molecules) forming a strong barrier that hinder the passage of different molecules and pathogens. In the intestine there are also many enzymes and efflux transporters that excrete the substrates to the lumen, and therefore contribute for the poor absorption of drugs. In the apical brush border membrane of the enterocytes great amounts of peptidases are present (such as adsorbed pancreatic enzymes) that hydrolyze proteins into amino acids (Langguth et al. 1997). Moreover, glycoproteins (80% of which is composed of mucins) cover the mucosa forming the mucus layer. The thickness of this mucus layer varies along the GIT (higher in the stomach and lower in the colon) and forms a significant barrier to particulate forms and microorganism (Ensign et al. 2012).

Due to the exposure to the external environment and pathogenic entities, the mucosa is enriched beneath the epithelial layer by a primary lymphoid mucosa (primary immune system of the GIT) called the *organized associated lymphoid mucosa tissue* (O-MALT) or the *gut associated lymphoid tissue* (GALT) (Buda et al. 2005). These are composed by intraepithelial lymphocytes, dendritic cells, and the lymphoid nodules. The lymphoid tissue is organized either as individually (called isolated lymphoid follicles) or aggregated/ clusters so-called Peyer's patches in which membranous cells (microfold cells or *M* cells) are located. Even though *M* cells only compose 5% of the Peyer's patches (and less than 1% the total intestine), they have gained particular focus due to their transport ability of particles into the underlying lymphoid tissue (des Rieux et al. 2007a). In fact, M cells are a route for many dietary particles and antigen to access the gut lumen and immune cells as well as many pathogens (bacteria, protozoa, and virus) (des Rieux et al. 2006). As a result, many studies have developed strategies to efficiently target M cells.

Nanoparticles as Carriers

Since drug absorption is highly dependent on physicochemical properties of the therapeutics, the commercial value of potent drugs is hampered by defective means of promoting their absorption.

To overcome the previously described barriers of the GIT, various strategies have been proposed. Common approaches usually employ enhancement of drug solubility and permeation (through permeation enhancers, dissolution aid systems, or drug analogs), inhibition of reflux transporter or enzymes, or even delaying the release of the drug to protect from premature degradation. However, those strategies are not ideal since most of them can disturb mucosal cell surface or disturb the natural processes of GIT, and therefore increasing drug side effects or unexpected drug effects. Others may fail to protect the enzymatic degradation and may require unrealistic doses to improve the absorption of sensitive and low permeation therapeutics such as proteins. Even well established commercial products are not necessarily well formulated causing frequent and adverse side effects such as ulcers (e.g., non-steroidal anti-inflammatory drugs). As a result, an ideal drug delivery system would be able to effectively enhance the bioavailability of the therapeutic agent (whether systemic or local) with minimal interaction with the normal physiology of the GIT.

By virtue of their small size and surface area available for contact, nanoparticles (NPs) display many interesting features that make them suitable for a variety of application including the oral delivery of a wide variety of both hydrophilic and hydrophobic drugs. NPs have extended the concept of drug delivery due to their unique properties. Among the various nanomedicine technologies available for oral delivery, the term nanocarrier includes many technological tools such as cyclodextrin (CD)-drug complexes, liposomes, polymer-therapeutic conjugates, polymer micelles, quantum dots, fullerenes, carbon nanotubes, nanocrystals, gold NPs, dendrimers, and polymeric NPs.

NPs alter the dissolution, solubility, permeability, and distribution of the drugs. These are common features that will ultimately increase the bioavailability at the targeting site. These features allow the possibility of specific release (either locally in the GIT or to systemic circulation), altered half-life (which will ultimately determine the interval of administration and consequently alter the convenient time interval), and alter the residence time with the mucosa (offering the possibility of a protective effect). Moreover,

NPs can specially be designed to avoid specific side effects such as irritation/ damage of the gastric mucosa (Surnar and Jayakannan 2013), thus extending the therapeutic window of drugs.

The principle of enhancing the contact area and improving drug bioavailability was applied in the commercial technology of NanoCrystal Technology which uses a technique of wet milling to reduce the powder of the drug to the desired size of the nanoscale. In this product, the crystalline nano-sized drug is stabilized with stabilizer agents to prevent agglomeration and aggregation, and to enhance drug permeability. These technologies allow reducing the time to achieve maximum concentration as well as increase the bioavailability. Several commercial products for a variety of drugs have been approved based on this technology such as Megace ES® (Megestrol acetate), TriCor® (Fenofibrate), Emend® (Aprepitant), and Rapamune® (Sirolimus). Nanocrystals have also shown an interesting feature for oral delivery since they can eliminate the effect of food in the bioavailability of the drug (Junghanns and Muller 2008). This technique has also been applied to insulin, producing particles for which the size could be controlled by the milling time. Although, these nano-sized particles were able to induce a prolonged hypoglycemic effect with a rapid onset (Merisko-Liversidge et al. 2004), high quantities were required revealing that other tools are required to effectively deliver this kind of therapeutic.

Other common techniques to improve the release and permeation profile of drugs is the inclusion of CDs complex within the polymeric matrix of NPs. CDs are oligosaccharides that have the ability of forming non-covalent complexes with a variety of drugs including proteins and peptides (complex with the hydrophobic domains). These systems have shown to enhance the encapsulation efficiency, alter the hydration of the matrix, and modify the drug stability, solubility, release kinetics, bioavailability, and absorption across mucosal surfaces (Loftsson et al. 2004).

Polymeric NPs due to their higher stability in GIT environment and relatively low toxicity can be applied to a wide range of drugs with the possibility of functionalization (addition of active moieties to render specific targeting). This offers a major advantage over liposomes since these are generally destabilized in the GIT. Another advantage of polymeric carriers is their biodegradability and biocompatibility such as poly(D,L-lactide-*co*-glycolide) (PLGA) NPs which offer an interest approach in oral delivery due to their relatively safe use (Kumari et al. 2010). Also, due to their versatile application, they can be incorporated in many platforms of drug formulation development (some of their potential application are listed in Table 2.1).

Many polymers and copolymers are currently available for oral drug delivery and should be chosen to meet the needs and specificities of the drug to be associated. For the majority of intended drugs (peptides, nucleic acids, and BCS class III and IV), the selecting criteria should be bioavailability and

Table 2.1. Potential applications of NPs in pharmaceutical formulations.

Protection from external environment (moisture, light, heat, oxidation, enzymatic degradation)	Reduction or elimination of gastric irritation, increase of gastric tolerance
Controlled release (chemical or enzymatically triggered, prolonged constant release)	Co-administration of incompatible drugs
Site-specific target	Co-administration of incompatible drugs and excipients
Enhancement of drug dispersion and/or dissolution in the medium, and permeation	Enhancement of power flow
Reduce drug doses and frequency of administration, increase patient compliance	Mask bad flavors
Reduction of drug accumulation in non-intended organs (thus reducing side effects)	Enhance pharmacological activity (e.g., vaccination)
Enhancement of pharmacokinetic and biopharmaceutic parameters: half-life, bioavailability	Avoid fed/fasted variations
Multidrug encapsulated in one particulate system and with different hydrophilic–lipophilic profiles	Enhance therapeutic index
Reduction aids of dissolution including strong acids or bases	Avoids infection complications of parenteral delivery
Enhancement of drug stability (e.g., reduction of volatility) and increase shelf-life	Enhance drug stability in the controlled medium of the core
Reduce multidrug resistance effect on drugs	Use of "original drugs" (no need for prodrugs, salt forms)

biocompatibility as well as low variability in response with cellular (except for vaccines) and protein interaction (e.g., adsorption of constituents or inhibition of an enzyme that will affect the metabolism of nutrients). Also, the duration of drug treatment should be evaluated as some strategies are useful for temporary use (e.g., enzymatic inhibitors, opening of tight junctions, and use of permeation enhancers) but could fail in chronic use (chronic uptake of toxins with accumulation in long-term treatments). After meeting these criteria, other factors must be taken into account including controlled release (dependent on the drug type), target ligands to be used, known fate of clearance and degradation process as well as ease of production and scale up. Moreover, when choosing a targeting model, it is important to consider the differences between the *in vivo* model used and its correlation to humans. Furthermore, the physicochemical properties of the polymer will determine the manufacturing process as well as size, surface charge, and drug release profile, among others. Nevertheless, each case has to be evaluated depending on their need, because for some drugs a prolonged release of days or months will be suitable (e.g., hormones) while others need a rapid absorption with a controlled release of hours (e.g., insulin). This drug release can be modulated by means of the polymer choice [e.g., chitosan (CS) vs. PLGA vs. poly(ε-caprolactone) (PCL)] and manufacturing processes (e.g., formation of pores in the drying process). In the first case, the physicochemical properties of the polymer will determine the solubility at different pH values (e.g., Eudragit® polymers), the interactions between drug-polymer (e.g., different charges), and degradation profile by means of intrinsic degradation (e.g., PCL vs. PLGA), enzymatic induced-degradation (e.g., CS), or the response to internal (e.g., temperature) or external (e.g., magnetic, electric, or ultrasound) physical stimuli. On the other hand, the manufacturing process will determine the stability of the carrier (e.g., freeze-drying, amount of surfactant) or change the intrinsic characteristics of the polymer (conjugations, copolymers) to meet the above mentioned criteria. Finally, although no signals of inflammation should arrive due to the use of NPs, the inducing of an immunogenic response will depend on its application (e.g., vaccines). Besides carrying high drug payloads, NPs can also display biological activity for their own. As an example, CS and derivates have been shown to have anti-microbial action, regenerative properties, absorption of toxic metals, enzymatic inhibition as well immunostimulation for its adjuvant properties (Agnihotri et al. 2004).

There are several mechanisms that have been explored for oral delivery by NPs. Due to their smaller size, they display a large surface area that favors their absorption compared to higher particles such as microparticles. Polymeric NPs can also be further tailored to change their properties such as hydrophobic character, bioadhesive properties, surface charge, dissolution, release and degradation profile as well as grafting with specific targets [e.g., arginine-glycine-aspartic acid (RGD) peptide]. All these strategies can be used to improve cellular uptake, enhance absorption in the specific target organ, or be altered to give a favorable pharmacokinetic profile with controlled release profile, simply enhance the residence time by adherence to cell apical surface, and/or reduce their side effects. These features combined with the protection of their loaded cargo from the harsh environment of GIT make them ideal for oral delivery of sensitive drugs.

After absorption through intestinal mucosa it is important to evaluate the biodistribution of the drug but also the carrier, their intracellular trafficking (the particles can be completely digested releasing their content in the cell), and the metabolic fate of both over time. Also, careful attention has to be taken in the effect of NPs in the gut flora since this is an important part of the normally functionality of the GIT. Bacteria present in colon produce enzymes that are capable of digestion of polysaccharides polymers such as pectin, guar gum, and CS (Ren et al. 2005). Nevertheless, this property can be explored to trigger targeting to the colon to exploit the digestion of undigested particles.

Finally, the specificities of the disease have to be taken into account when formulating the NPs. As an example, in the infection caused by *Helicobacter pylori*, urease is released in the gastric medium. This enzyme was found to enhance the degradation process of poly(alkylcyanoacrylate) (PACA) NPs and therefore this nanoparticulate system can be designed for specific targeting, releasing higher amounts of the drug by chemical triggering (Fontana et al. 2001).

Although, low clinical translation of nanomedicine tools for oral delivery have been achieved, a lot of progress is being performed for improvement of particle uptake, and in the future new promise tools will revolutionize the market.

Consideration on techniques of production

The techniques of production have a fundamental role in the nanoparticulate systems since they can influence the morphological and internal structure, stability, degradation rate, and therefore several parameters have to be assessed. The properties of the polymeric NPs produced will ultimately influence their uptake, and therefore the techniques of production play a major role in obtaining functional NPs that can resist the harsh environment of GIT milieu and promote absorption.

The method of production can be either top-down or down-top (Fig. 2.1). The miniaturization from bigger powder is an example of the top-down technology which starts from a large-size drug powder to be reduced in size. However, the majority of NP production employs down-top procedures by using natural or synthetic monomers or pre-formed polymers to form

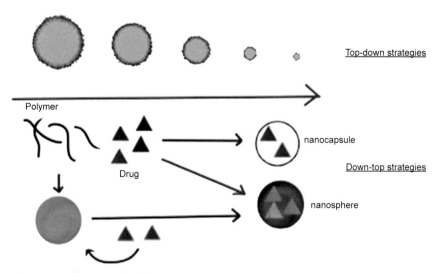

Figure 2.1. Different methods for NP preparation based on top-down and down-top strategies.

complex NPs. These can be further combined with surfactants to increase the stability, reduce aggregation (which is very important for their uptake), or with targeting ligands to improve specific uptake (Pinto Reis et al. 2006).

Polymeric NPs can be prepared by a variety of methods depending on the intended application and physical characteristics. Such examples include emulsion, polymerization, interfacial polymerization and polycondensation, solvent displacement and interfacial deposition, emulsification/solvent diffusion, salting out, multiple emulsions, nanoprecipitation, ionic gelation, and reverse micellar methods (Pinto Reis et al. 2006). Choosing the right method assumes the right protocol for elimination of residues (e.g., monomers or solvents) and other contaminants, since their presence can raise health issues and also they can affect the stabilization of the encapsulated drug or hinder the therapeutic effect.

For polymeric NPs, the drug can be dispersed, entrapped in the inner core, adsorbed, or attached to the matrix. This creates two major categories named nanospheres (matrix particles) and nanocapsules (covering a core of water or oil). Depending on the intended use, major adjustments have to be performed to choose from composition to the intended release profile. The methods should be initially selected according to the drug either to be hydrophilic [e.g., water-in-oil-in-water (w/o/w), nanoprecipitation] or lipophilic [e.g., oil-in-water (o/w)], but also should take into account the intrinsic properties of the polymer including its relative solubility for the drug. This is particularly important for drugs with a similar charge since it is difficult to achieve high encapsulation efficiencies.

The drugs can be added during the manufacturing process (incorporation) or after particle formation (incubation). The choice of the step in which the drug will be added depends on the possible interaction or if they are sensitive within the manufacturing process (e.g., solvents, temperature, pH, cross-linking agent) (Agnihotri et al. 2004), or on the specificities of the drug such as using it as a targeting moiety. However, adsorbed drugs (as well as drugs near the surface) will rapidly be released when in contact with the GIT medium, thus originating burst releases. The manufacturing process will also depend on the stability and interaction of the drug with the polymer matrix. The choice of the method should provide high encapsulation efficiencies, but ultimately lead to high payloads as high concentrations of polymer must balance with the required dose without inducing toxicity. The chosen method should be simple, easy to scale up, provide low polydispersity index (which represents the homogeneity of a population of particles), use minimal organic solvents, not alter or destabilize the drug, and be highly reproducible without being time consuming. Most importantly, the resultant system should maintain the biological activity of the drug as it is essential to maintain the pharmacological activity (the so-called pharmacological efficiency) which is particularly difficult to achieve by sensitive macromolecules such as proteins and nucleic acids (Damgé et al. 1997, Reis et al. 2007). Another important parameter should be the assessment of residual organic solvents and surfactants, since they can alter the drug uptake and also induce potential hazardous reactions. It must be evaluated since even non-toxic polymers such as PLGA can carry contaminated substances that can induce cell damage or elicit an immune response, e.g., variable levels of lipopolysaccharide contaminants in NPs induced macrophage activation (Oostingh et al. 2011).

Technologically, many factors may contribute to the success of the method chosen. As a result, in the design of a new formulation it is important to evaluate different parameters such as aqueous/oil ratios, concentration of different process intervenient (monomers, surfactants, drug, polymer, molecular aids of solubilization, additives, etc.), viscosity, M_W of the polymers as well as degree of substitution (e.g., deacetylation in CS), influence of the temperature on manufacturing and solvent removal, shear conditions (homogenization cycles and stirring rate), the pH influence, and the recovery process. All factors will ultimately determine the physicochemical and morphological features including NP size, surface charge, stability, release and degradation profile as well as toxicity. As an example, the variation of the drug: polymer ratio showed differences in the duration of the biological effect (Damgé et al. 1997).

In terms of encapsulation material, natural polymers such as CS, alginate (ALG), guar gum, and cellulose derivates have gained focus due to their biodegradable and biocompatible properties. These polymers find a wide range of applications in the pharmaceutical field and can be easily self-assembled by complexation between opposite charges [e.g., CS, ALG, or sodium tripolyphosphate (STPP)] forming polyelectrolyte complexes. The conjugation of diverse properties of different polymers can provide specific release within the GIT. As an example, CS can be used with a variety of other polymers such as Eudragit® and poly(γ-glutamic acid) to combine different properties including solubility, charge, affinity to cells, and mucus adhesiveness. Built on this assumption these polymer combinations can efficiently tailor the stability of the polymer within the GIT milieu allowing the modification of the release kinetics and biological response. The combination of CS and ALG is an example of combinatory properties since CS is soluble at low pHs and insoluble at higher pHs, while ALG has the opposite effect. Therefore, the structure shrinks forming impermeable networks and allowing the controlled drug release (Chaudhury and Das 2010). Another approach that can be optimized is the chemical alteration of the polymer to enhance some characteristics while maintaining others. In such cases, trimethyl CS cystein conjugate was produced to have high solubility at neutral/higher pH values while keeping the high bioadhesion properties of CS (Yin et al. 2009).

Limitations and difficulties in nanoparticle oral uptake

The oral administration of macromolecules or low soluble/permeable drugs is desirable but faces considerable challenges regarding the normal function of the GIT. To this matter, the drug delivery system should be able to protect the drug and avoid interactions with luminal content, while enhancing drugs permeability throughout the mucosa. Even though NPs have shown promising drug oral delivery as well as oral immunization, they have many challenges that need to be overcome to prevent erratic absorption. A long standing issue regarding oral delivery is to deliver the correct dosage with a safe therapeutic window, and not at the expense of increasing the toxicity (e.g., concentration of polymer or surfactant) or disruption of normal physiology. This is particularly important for particulate designs that have a low payload of the drug, and therefore high doses have to be used.

The first element to effectively deliver these therapeutic agents is to resist the highly acidic environment of the stomach and the hydrolytic enzymes (particularly pepsin) that can induce the degradation (Damgé et al. 1997). In fact, different nanocarriers such as PACA NPs were able to effectively protect insulin from proteolytic enzymes (Damgé et al. 1997). Also, the progression of pH which NPs contact during their passage through GIT can induce NP aggregation, compromising the size-dependent absorption and toxicity (Nafee et al. 2009).

On the other hand, for strategies that pursue enzymatic inhibition or opening of tight junctions, long-term use should be evaluated as it can increase the absorption of potential toxic substances. Polymers such as CS are able to transiently open the tight junctions and increase the paracellular transportation of drugs. The reversibility of tight junction opening should be evaluated as well as the time it takes to recover (e.g., by measuring the transepithelial resistance).

The mucus layer is another important barrier that can limit the absorption of both drugs and NPs (Hillery and Florence 1996). The extent of particle absorption depends on the ability of the carrier to diffuse through the mucus becoming accessible for contact with the cells (enterocytes and M cells). This poses a primary limitation for carriers that show strong interaction with the mucus layer (either by electrostatic repulsion, hydrophobic interactions, or mucus entrapment), as these are cleared by the continuous natural turnover of mucus. Moreover, the administration protocol of NPs should be carefully taken into account as it has been reported that the amount of buffer in which NPs are suspended can significantly dilute the mucus and therefore change the outcomes (O'Hagan 1996, Ensign et al. 2012).

However, even after diffusion through the mucus, the negatively charged cell membrane will prevent the diffusion of molecules with anionic surface. On the other hand, in the apical side of M cells, esterases are present and they are responsible for NP degradation, such as in the case of PACA NPs (Pinto-Alphandary et al. 2003). Also the potential toxicity of NPs can rise by interaction with the components expressed at the cell surface.

After interaction with the cell, NPs are trapped and taken up by internalizing structures (early and late endosomes) that will be directed to lysosomal degradation. The low pH found in this compartment together with several enzymes including proteases and nucleases will induce the degradation of both the drug and the polymeric NP. For an effective drug delivery, the NPs must be able to prevent the degradation of the drug by lysosomes and must be able to perform and endosomal/lysosomal evasion (Richardson et al. 2008). Here, the physicochemical characteristics of the polymer play an important role as polyelectrolite complexes of CS can be unstable and disintegrate, while polyethyleneimine (PEI) can sustain its properties.

Since modifying the characteristics of production (size, surface, charge, attachment of ligands, and coating the surface with surfactants) can alter the NP absorption, the properties of particulate systems should therefore be evaluated in their full behavior in order to draw effective conclusions related to their influence on GIT absorption (i.e., specificity for *M* cells and avoidance of defense mechanisms, as well as toxicity).

The structure of NPs can be easily modified during the production and the stability can influence their efficacy *in vivo*. As the surface of NPs can be easily modified by adsorption of molecules, in the GIT it is probable that these molecules will desegregate and "new" molecules/enzymes will be adsorbed at the surface (Fig. 2.2). Consequently, it is important to understand this interaction within the biological milieu to further correlate to intestinal absorption, interaction with blood components (e.g., induction of hemolysis), and understand their cellular interaction (as well as localization within

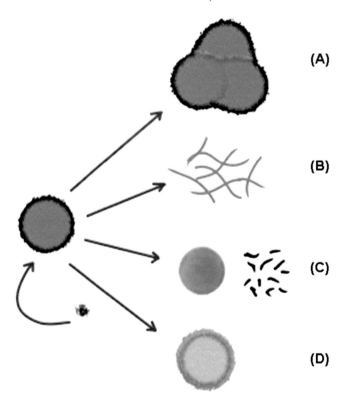

(A)

(B)

(C)

(D)

Figure 2.2. Possible fates of NPs within the GIT: (A) aggregation, (B) disintegration, (C) desorption of coating materials, and (D) adsorption of GIT compounds.

cellular compartments). On the other hand, the chronic use of NPs should be evaluated since it can cause disruption of natural processes, such as observed for carboxylated NPs which have shown to disrupt the iron transport (Mahler et al. 2012).

To bring the full benefits of NPs as an alternative to parenteral formulations, there are still some parameters that should be well characterized. A good *in vitro/in vivo* correlation is a fundamental requirement for evaluation of the carrier systems. There are several *in vitro* models that can evaluate the potential of NP uptake. Using monocultures of Caco-2 cells to mimic the enterocytes is the most common assay to evaluate the transport of NPs across cells. However, this system lacks the complexity of GIT and different permeation profiles are observed depending on the characteristics of the particles and the different cell model used (Woitiski et al. 2011). As a result, co-cultures of Caco-2 have been studied as models of NP uptake. Since the mucus plays an important role in trapping NPs as well as in the release of their content, MTX-E12 or HT29 cells have been co-cultured to simulate the goblet cells (the second most representative in the GIT) (Woitiski et al. 2011). Another method for evaluating NP transport across the membrane is by using Raji-B or lymphocytes from Peyer's patches to stimulate Caco-2 cells to form *M* cells (des Rieux et al. 2007a, Garinot et al. 2007). The comparison between monoculture and co-culture with *M* cells allows the understanding between the non-specific and specific transportation (Garinot et al. 2007). Recently, tri-cultures have been used to evaluate the combined intervenient of the GIT (Mahler et al. 2012). From these results, it is clearly observed (when employing co-cultures with *M* cells) that NP uptake is performed in a much greater extent.

There are important conditions that should be evaluated to correctly evaluate NP uptake. Before using NPs, these systems should be well characterized in terms of their stability, size and surface charge in different media (pH and viscosity), as well as to evaluate their sedimentation profiles. Moreover, it is important when studying the influence of size on NP uptake to obtain a homogenous population with low polydispersity index, because otherwise there will be a heterogeneous population with different surface area properties. It is also important to study the aggregation of NPs in different media and pH values since it will inevitably influence the NP uptake (Loh et al. 2010, Powell et al. 2010). Details of protein adsorption (forming the so-called "corona") is another area that should be checked as it can hinder the targeting moieties, surface charge, induce aggregation, and inhibit particle uptake. For all reasons stated, this implies an evaluation of the NP design for their specific applications. On the other hand, the relative difficulty in obtaining high loadings, the cost of polymers and targeting molecules, and the *in vivo* inter-subject variation have hampered the clinical translation. Even though only a small percentage of the administered dose of NPs have been reported to be absorbed, given the broader application of fields and promising results that have been obtained, the use of NPs to effectively deliver molecules of high therapeutic value (including insulin) will open a new era of drug delivery by the oral route and revolutionize the marketplace.

Strategies and uptake mechanism of nanoparticles by GIT

It has been observed for a long time that particulate matter can be absorbed across the intestinal mucosa. The first step of particle uptake requires the interaction with the cells surface/membrane, and it depends on charged interactions with negatively cell membranes or receptors (Yin et al. 2009). Over the last decades, various strategies have been explored to enhance the absorption of therapeutic valuable drugs. Several parameters affecting the extent of NP uptake *in vitro* and *in vivo* have been identified (Table 2.2), and considering their size and unique surface properties, polymeric NPs have demonstrated their ability to: (i) alter the release profile of therapeutics (e.g., prolong drug explosion); (ii) control the targeting of therapeutics through active and passive targeting (e.g., targeting *M* cells); (iii) avoid degradation in GIT mileu; (iv) enhance drug absorption and deliver therapeutics to the blood circulation; (v) induce immune responses; and, (vi) protect the GIT mucosa and avoid side effects.

Table 2.2. Factors determining the extent of NP uptake *in vitro* and *in vivo*.

Particle size and polydispersity
Loading capacity
Dose of particles administered
Particle surface (hydrophobic character, surface charge, targeting ligands)
Carrier (polymer vs. lipid-based vs. surface characteristics)
Stability of the carrier
Bioadhesive properties and mucus entrapment
Food intake and volume of administration
Species under investigation (rabbits vs. rats vs. humans)
Degradation profile
Release profile
Residence time, contact time
Enterocytes vs. *M* cells

The epithelial cells of the GIT constitute an efficient barrier against the external environment. Cells are very well interconnected with only small intercellular spaces. There are three possible mechanisms by which NPs can be absorbed/transported or increase the absorption of drugs across the intestinal mucosa (Fig. 2.3): (i) via paracellular pathway (transport through the spaces between cells); (ii) unspecific transcytosis or receptor-mediated

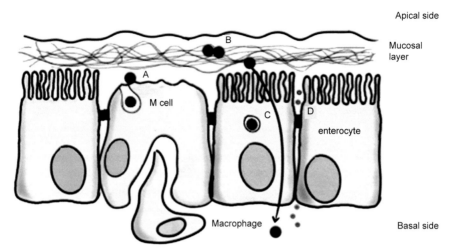

Figure 2.3. Schematic model of the GIT epithelium and the possible mechanisms by which NPs can be uptaken. (A) NP uptake by *M* cells. (B) NPs trapped within the mucus. (C) transcytosis through enterocytes. (D) paracellular transport through intercellular spaces.

(transport through cells); and, (iii) specific transcytosis through *M* cells. Paracellular transport through the tight junctions plays an important role in drug absorption, but in a lesser extent for the carrier since the size of commonly used particles exceeds the size of the gaps. Also for macromolecules that have high M_w this uptake pathway is limited. Nevertheless, NPs can be prepared to release the drug in a pH sensitive trigger release and explore the intrinsic properties of a transiently open of the tight junctions (e.g., CS). The common pathway for NP uptake is transcellularly which can be performed by normal intestinal enterocytes (although in a lesser extent) and through active capture by *M* cells. Various transports are available and can be explored utilizing natural uptake mechanism such as the one for vitamin B_{12}.

The protection of drugs from degradation to improve the transmucosal transport is particularly important for proteins since they are easily unstable within the GIT environment. Size and surface chemistry (including HLB) are the major determinants for NP uptake, distribution, and clearance (des Rieux et al. 2006). It has been found that NPs are uptaken in a size-dependent manner with smaller particles having a higher rate of absorption until they reach an ideal size of 50 to 200 nm (des Rieux et al. 2007b). It has also been observed that NPs are absorbed systemically while microparticles remain in the Peyer's patches (Desai et al. 1996). On the other hand, the lipophilic character of the particles as well as the surface charge will determine the availability at the cell surface and their uptake extent and localization within the cell compartment. These two parameters are greatly influenced by the polymer composition, but can also be modulated by grafting ligands. Particles with diverse surface characteristics show different uptake and association with cells (e.g., polystyrene vs. CS or PLGA in Caco-2 cells) (Behrens et al. 2002, Gaumet et al. 2009). These properties have to balance between reducing the uptake of particles and being trapped in the mucus which represents a major obstacle for NP diffusion (Behrens et al. 2002). The mucoadhesive properties can be explored and although they delay the absorption of NPs, they can increase the residence and contact time positively (Sandri et al. 2007).

The transcelullar transport occurs by an active process of endocytic uptake in the apical side of both enterocytes and *M* cells. Several mechanisms of endocytosis have been described for NPs (des Rieux et al. 2006, Mahler et al. 2012): (i) pinocytosis; (ii) macropinocytosis; (iii) caveolae-mediated endocytosis; and, (iv) clathrin-mediated endocytosis. These are energy-dependent, specific, saturable, and highly regulated processes, and will be determined by both the size and the physiochemical properties of the carrier (Behrens et al. 2002). For instance, when PACA particles linked to poloxamer 188 were given intragastrically, clusters of them were observed in the glycocalyx matrix of the brush border of enterocytes. On the other hand, NPs with poloxamer 188 absorbed at the surface were also seen in the intercellular spaces formed by phagocytic cells (Pinto-Alphandary et al. 2003).

Uptake mechanism of nanoparticles by M cells

M cells posses a high translocation capacity of particles, including NPs, to the underlying lymphoid tissue being able to induce an immune response. *M* cells are an important defense mechanism against toxic substances and inducing mucosal immunity (Mahler et al. 2012). They exhibit irregular microvilli at the apical surface and a pocket in the basolateral side that contains both B and T lymphocytes and a small number of macrophages (Buda et al. 2005, Garinot et al. 2007). Several *M* cell surface targeting moieties have been proposed (e.g., sialyl Lewis A antigen, and cathepsin E) and these can therefore be valuable for specific targeting of NPs. *M* cells also lack closely packed microvilli and have a reduced brush border glycocalyx and associated proteins. In contrast to other parts of the GIT, *M* cells are covered less by mucus and have a reduced expression of hydrolases as well as the number of lysosomes (des Rieux et al. 2007b). For all these reasons, it has been proposed that these conditions could facilitate the interaction with NPs by improving contact with cells and the uptake of intact therapeutics (des Rieux et al. 2007b). Therefore, *M* cells are the main absorption pathway for oral delivery of low permeating drugs such as macromolecules as well as to induce immunization responses with oral antigens. However, the extrapolation of results from *in vitro* (15 to 30% *M* cells) and *in vivo* models (30 to 50% for pigs and rabbits, 10% for rodents) has to be carefully evaluated, since *M* cells in human account for *ca.* 5% of the Follicle-Associated Epithelium (FAE) (O'Hagan 1996, Buda et al. 2005, des Rieux et al. 2007a). Nevertheless, the importance of *M* cells for NP uptake is without a doubt the most effective way to deliver NPs orally. This has been shown *in vivo* since after their administration, NPs are commonly found in Peyer's patches where *M* cells are located. Also, they are able to transport antigens from NPs to the underlying mucosa, thus inducing a successful immunization. Due to their significance in NP absorption, these factors will be further explored.

Size effect on nanoparticle uptake

Particle size has shown to be one of the most important parameters to effectively deliver drugs to the systemic circulation or to induce immune responses. Despite some disparities in defining the upper limit for NP absorption, a size-dependent absorption has been observed. *In vitro* and *in vivo* experiments have shown that smaller particles are absorbed in a greater extent than bigger particles (Win and Feng 2005). Also, the usual size found for an efficient delivery has been defined in the range between 50 and 200 nm. A series of very monodispersed population of both PLGA and polystyrene NPs with similar hydrophilic character ranging from 100 to 2000 nm were evaluated for their uptake in Caco-2 cells. From the results size- and concentration-dependent responses were observed with only 100 nm-sized particles (and 300 nm-sized for polystyrene NPs) being internalized while others only interacted with cell membranes (Gaumet et al. 2009). *In vivo* experiments corroborate these results, since they have also shown that 50 nm- and 100 nm-sized particles are more likely to be internalized than microparticles (Desai et al. 1996). Also, in co-cultures up to 500 nm-sized NPs were uptaken, even though in a smaller extent compared to 200 nm-sized (des Rieux et al. 2005). Moreover, greater particle uptake was found in Peyer's patches compared to other parts of the tissue, and a greater uptake was found in the ileum region compared to duodenum (Desai et al. 1996). On the other hand, particles up to 3–5 μm are taken up by *M* cells and can reach the lymphatic pathway (Desai et al. 1996). These results confirm the high ability of *M* cells for transcytosis of particulate matter. Also, it was found that 200 nm-sized particles were uptaken through non-specific endocytosis even when tight junctions are open (des Rieux et al. 2007a), while 50 nm-sized particles are predominantly transported by paracellular pathway (Mahler et al. 2012). Higher uptake and deeper in the tissue were found for 100 nm- and 300 nm-sized particles, while 3 μm-sized particles had a lower and more superficial uptake (Desai et al. 1996, Shakweh et al. 2005). On the other hand, particles greater than 5 μm were retained in the Peyer's patches and they were not absorbed (O'Hagan 1996).

Physicochemical properties, hydrophobic character, and surface charge

Together with size, the surface characteristics will determine NPs fate within the GIT medium, and therefore they are critical for the uptake. NPs can display different charges and HLB depending on the characteristics of the polymer used as well as the surfactant and molecules adsorbed to their surface. Early studies have demonstrated that the hydrophobic character plays a direct role in the particle uptake. Hydrophobic particles when given orally were more prone to be absorbed by *M* cells (in Peyer's patches) than hydrophilic counterparts (Eldridge et al. 1990). This fact was further evidenced by coating hydrophobic particles with more hydrophilic coatings since a reduction in the uptake was observed (Hillery and Florence 1996). However, straight observation that the hydrophobic particles will guarantee an efficient uptake cannot be drawn since the surface charge and NP stability and intrinsic properties also influence particle absorption (Gaumet et al. 2009). Grafting copolymers to the NP surface can result in alteration of the uptake. For example, positively charged PLGA-PEI NPs were uptaken in a smaller extent compared to PLGA-polyvinyl alcohol (PVA) and PLGA-hydrophobically modified hydroxyethylcellulose which both display a negative surface (Shakweh et al. 2005). Surface charge is not only important to increase the interactions with the negatively charged membranes but also because this can result in entrapment within the negative moieties of mucin as well as interactions and adsorption of molecules of the GIT milieu (des Rieux et al. 2005). In the case of mucoadhesive polymers such as CS, particle adhesion to the outer mucus surface can limit drug absorption (Ensign et al. 2012). On the other hand, negatively charged NPs have shown the ability to bind to molecules of the gut lumen, being absorbed into Peyer's patches through *M* cells (Mahler et al. 2012). Also, since the stabilization of the particle depends on the surface, it is related to its uptake as it can form aggregates, agglomerates, or disintegration (e.g., polyelectrolyte complexes) (Sonaje et al. 2009). Furthermore, it is implied that the nanocarrier should be stable in various conditions. The steric stabilization of the NPs is a fundamental tool for clinical practice because it can increase the stability in the biological environment such as the use of poly(ethylene glycol) (PEG).

Strategies to increase residence time

The duration of NP exposure to cell has shown to positively influence drug and NP uptake both on *M* cells and enterocytes (Win and Feng 2005). *In vivo*, this can be achieved by increasing the retention within the mucus. Several polymers display mucoadhesive properties, including CS and poly(acrylates). These usually display protonated groups that confer a global positive charge and increase the interaction with mucin, thus these NPs have been observed in intimate contact with the GIT membrane (Damgé et al. 2007, Lopedota et al. 2009). PACA NPs have been shown to increase the bioavailability of drugs not by enhancing the permeation of NPs but by increasing the residence time (Allemann et al. 1998).

CS is the major polymer used to increase the NP residence time due to its mucoadhesive properties. However, difficulties have been observed in peptide and protein delivery in the intestine due to its high solubility in acidic medium (Chaudhury and Das 2010), especially for CS polyelectrolyte complexes that easily destabilize and low solubility at higher pH values (Yin et al. 2009). As a result, derivates from the CS have been employed. One of the most known derivates is the thiolated version of CS that exhibited a 6–100-fold enhancement of the mucoadhesive properties and enhanced paracellular permeation compared to CS, resisting both the effect of acidic and neutral pH environments (Chaudhury and Das 2010). One of the common techniques for thiol conjugation is the use of cysteine or reduced glutathione (GSH). The thiomers are rich in thiol groups that can interact with the cysteine-rich glycoproteins mucus layer through disulfide bonds. Trimethyl CS NPs loaded with insulin showed higher penetration into the duodenum and jejunum tissues due to their strong mucoadhesive properties (Chaudhury and Das 2010). CS and its thiol version have a strong interaction with mucus (negatively charged mucin containing sulfate and sialic acid groups) (Behrens et al. 2002). Even though a large amount of NPs are associated with the mucus due to its strong interaction, they are able to be absorbed by cells (Behrens et al. 2002). Also, it is essential for the protein to be correctly delivered so that the particle uptake is not too delayed. These prolonged effects are generally due to an increased residence time and continuous arrival of particles from the stomach.

Triggered drug release

The use of a triggered release is based on the intrinsic dissolution/degradation properties of the polymer or copolymers that enable specific release at a determined site. As an example, Eudragit® polymers display dissolution profiles that are pH-dependent and therefore can resist the harsh environment of the stomach releasing their content only in the intestine. This mechanism can benefit both drugs that are sensible to low pH values or that cause irritation to gastric mucosa. On the other hand, CS can release their content in the colon triggered by biodegradation of the colonic bacterial flora (Ren et al. 2005). Thus, the instability of the polymer at determined pH values can be designed to selectively deliver their contents. As an example, CS complexed with heparin was used to selectively deliver their contents in *H. pylori* infection in the stomach (Lin et al. 2009). This last complex was unstable at pH 7.0. Furthermore, as previously mentioned a specific enzyme produced by *H. pylori* was able to increase the degradation of PACA NPs, thus enhancing the effectiveness of the drug delivery (Fontana et al. 2001).

Functionalization and targeting of nanoparticles

Although NPs display many intrinsic properties that enable a better permeation of drugs, some still show deficiencies related to non-specific targeting (non-absorptive tissues or mucus entrapment) or low permeation. Grafting molecules to alter the properties of the NPs is a common strategy employed to enhance various applications from drug carriers to adjuvant of vaccines. Surface modification can be performed to enhance the stability, biodegradation profile, enhance targeting selection and transport, enhance residence time, or even enhance the biological effect of the therapeutic agent.

Certain molecules can be either adsorbed (e.g., polyelectrolyte complex) or chemically grafted (by covalent bonds or hydrophobic insertion) to the surface of NPs to change their characteristics. Grafting or adsorption of molecules can be done prior to the formation of the particles or after the NPs are formed. Several surface coatings have been described from PEG, surfactants (such as poloxamers, polysorbates, and poloxamines), phosphatidylinositol, dextran, thiol groups, and cholate to specific ligands such as molecules that can inhibit the enzymatic degradation. Also, various polymers can be conjugated to obtain and conjugate certain features that lack on the original polymer per se. These processes allow the modification of the HLB as well as steric hindrance and targeting properties, therefore enhancing their abilities to successfully deliver drugs. The coating process is important since it can be easily removed, degraded, or chemically (oxidized) modified in the GIT thus preventing the proper alteration of the particle.

Surfactants

Although initial concerns in their usage, surfactants have proven an important role both technologically and biologically in oral delivery formulations. Technologically, surfactants exert an important role as they can give stabilization of the carrier (preventing aggregation), enhance drug loading, and modify the particle size, charge surface, and HLB. Biologically, they can avoid or specifically adsorb molecular constituents, increase circulation half-life, avoid non-specific targeting, and interact with cells. Surfactants can also enhance the transcellular transport by enhancing the membrane permeability. Permeation enhancers if adsorbed to the NP surface can readily be desorbed in the GIT milieu and be absorbed more rapidly than the NPs (Bernkop-Schnurch et al. 2003). However, for some stabilizers, their removal is difficult mainly due to a strong interaction between the polymer and the surfactant (Galindo-Rodriguez et al. 2004).

Poloxamers are non-ionic block copolymeric surfactants that are relatively safe and do not cause gastric mucosal damage as observed after five days of feeding poloxamer-coated polystyrene NPs to rats (Hillery and Florence 1996). Poloxamer 188 is a common stabilizer used for NP production since it can prevent NP aggregation, and it is regarded as being safe to use. Due to their versatility, poloxamers can be tailored to perform different functions and display different properties. Depending of the hydrophobic properties of the polymer used, poloxamer can reduce the absorption. Coating polystyrene NPs with poloxamer lead to a more hydrophilic profile causing a reduction in intestinal uptake compared to free-poloxamer particles (Hillery and Florence 1996). On the other hand, poloxamers with longer polyoxyethylene chains can display greater mucoadhesive properties which can enhance the NP interaction. In fact, the coating of PACA NPs with poloxamer 188 greatly improved the bioadhesive properties by 14- to 44-folds (Bravo-Osuna et al. 2007). Furthermore, poloxamer 188 can also induce the phaghocytic activity of macrophages which can be used in the design of vaccines. It has been observed that the length of polyoxyethylene chain can define the immunostimulatory pathway, since low HLB values can induce the destabilization of lysosomes' membranes while high HLB disrupt lipid bilayers channeling their efficacy through the major histocompatibility complex (MHC) class II (Moghimi and Hunter 2000).

Another interesting surfactant that has been employed in nanoparticulate systems for oral drug delivery is vitamin E D-α-tocopheryl PEG succinate (Italia et al. 2009). It has shown greater stability and bioadhesion properties resulting in improved uptake.

PEGylation

PEG functionalization is one of the most used and useful strategies applied for surface modification. In fact, PEG, a linear or branched hydrophilic polymer, can be employed in several technological tools for drug improvement (e.g., drug-PEG conjugates in clinical use), and specifically in NPs it has been used to improve their stability, avoid cellular interactions, enhance absorption, as well as enhance the half-life. PEGylation can be either achieved by PEG adsorption or grafting to the surface. Several copolymers have been synthesized with PEG chains, and the latter have been preferentially observed at the NP surface. PEGylation of NPs produces a shielding effect that is able to reduce the interaction and adsorption of blood proteins, increasing the residence time. This is especially important in avoiding enzymes and other molecules to be absorbed, therefore reducing the degradation, aggregation, while enhancing the availability of the targeting ligand. As an example, grafting PEG to PLA (PEG-block-PLA) NPs showed *in vitro* stability in simulated GIT medium as well as human serum medium (des Rieux et al. 2007b). On the other hand, PEGylation of NPs has shown reduced interaction with cellular membranes in Caco-2 cells, when compared with non-PEGylated NPs (Behrens et al. 2002). However, GIT is a complex system and other cells participate in the NP incorporation such as M cells. This can be observed by the five-fold increase of helodermin absorption in co-culture of Caco-2 cells with Raji-B cells (with an 18-fold increase in transport of intact helodermin) compared to monoculture (des Rieux et al. 2007b). It is proposed that PEG stabilizes these NPs thereby avoiding the protein/enzyme adsorption and protecting against degradation and aggregation (des Rieux et al. 2007b). The mechanism by which PEG prevents absorption of proteins is due to the formation of a steric barrier which has been observed to increase the plasma half-life when given systemically (des Rieux et al. 2006). The steric hindrance of PEG depends on the M_w as it will modify the PEG conformation and therefore prevent the interaction and adsorption of mucin.

Targeting moieties

Grafting molecules to target specific uptake mechanisms is a reasonable strategy since there will be an enhanced interaction at the site of absorption and an enhanced NP uptake by cells (Fig. 2.4). One of the strategies that have been employed is the grafting of the particle surface with molecules to target M cells. *Ulex europaeus* 1 lectin and sialyl Lewis A antigen have shown the ability to target M cells (Buda et al. 2005), and therefore this strategy has been used for vaccination strategies. Other lectins such as *Sambucus nigra* and *Viscum album* have a wider range being able to target both enterocytes and M cells from human FAE (Buda et al. 2005). A number of other lectins have been used to bind to a range of receptors [concanavalin A, peanut agglutinin, *Lens culinaris* agglutinin, Wheat Germ Agglutinin (WGA)]. Lectin WGA strongly interacts with N-acetylglucosamine which is expressed in the apical side of epithelial cells (Behrens et al. 2002). The β_1-integrin is also expressed in the human FAE with increased expression in human ileal FAE, and it is a potential target. Indeed, the RGD peptide sequence that bind to the integrin receptors (Garinot et al. 2007), and thus NPs can be highly bound to cells expressing these integrins. As an example, PEGylated PCL NPs linked to RGD sequence were found to be taken up 3.5-times compared to non-functionalized PEGylated PCL NPs by M cells (co-culture), while no differences were observed in monocultures (Garinot et al. 2007). Cell-penetrating peptides show enhanced intestinal absorption and their conjugation to NPs potentially increases their interaction with cells. Although these strategies can find useful peptide sequences with enhancing properties of NPs in the case of peptide sequence, these can fail to provide effective strategies since they can be degraded in the harsh environment of GIT (Fievez et al. 2009).

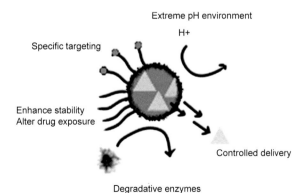

Figure 2.4. Modulating factors for the protection and controlled delivery of therapeutics by nanoparticulate systems.

Drugs of interest

Nanoparticulate strategies can be adapted to a wide range of therapeutics. While most of the drugs are intended for systemic absorption others can be used for topical delivery in the GIT. However, it is in treatments in which only parenteral route is available that there are the major blockbusters that would revolutionize the drug delivery and a great investment has been made in order to improve the bioavailability.

Peptides

The recent development of new biotechnological techniques allowed the production of a variety of peptides and proteins, which in turn allowed a wide range of therapeutics have become available. Peptides and proteins are especially useful for treatment as they are highly specific and potent at low concentrations. Also, they can be used in a wide range of therapies. The proteolytic degradation is mainly responsible for protein low bioavailability since 94 to 98% of the total proteins are completely degraded through GIT (Langguth et al. 1997), where several enzymes are associated such as pepsin, trypsin, α-trypsin, α-chymotrypsin, elastase, carboxipeptidases A and B, and endopeptidases and exopeptidases (Langguth et al. 1997, Allemann et al. 1998). Various technologies and strategies have been envisioned in the last decades to increase peptide absorption and reduce their degradability. The use of chemical peptide modifications (such as lipophilic derivates), PEGylation, peptidomimetics (replace of amide functions to non-hydrolyzable bonds), inhibitors of proteolytic enzymes, absorption enhancers, bile salts, emulsions, CDs, complexation with polymers, bioadhesive systems, site-specific delivery systems (e.g., colon targeting), hydrogel, bioadhesive carriers, and encapsulation in particulate systems have been some of the strategies that have been proposed.

One of the most desirable peptides for oral delivery is insulin. The daily subcutaneous administrations are uncomfortable and stressful and may cause infections. Oral administration of free insulin results in only less than 0.5% being absorbed (Damgé et al. 1997). After absorption, insulin undergoes the first passage by the liver, triggering a first response in inhibiting glucose production (Damgé et al. 2007, Reis et al. 2008), an effect similar to the physiological route therefore avoiding the complications associated with peripheral hyperinsulinemia. Many efforts have been made to enhance insulin absorption. Due to the controlled release of NPs, these systems have the potential to mimic the normal basal secretion of insulin, and they have proven to reduce the glucose levels. In the early studies, PACA NPs loaded with insulin had a reduction in glycemia by 50 to 60%, but this effect only appeared two days after administration and was prolonged for 20 days (Damgé et al. 1988). However, these results showed that particles were able to protect insulin from degradation. Another strategy employed for insulin delivery was the use of a "suicidal" targeting such as albumin to be preferentially digested, and therefore protect insulin from degradation by proteolysis (Reis et al. 2008). Also, this coating has been demonstrated to be important for the permeation of NPs through different cell models (Woitiski et al. 2011), and the use of dextran sulfate prevented insulin degradation at low pH values (Reis et al. 2008).

Administration of particles can suffer from a rapid delivery to the blood while the majority of the particles are still in the GIT. As an example, 2 hours after the intragastric administration of PACA NPs containing insulin, the majority of insulin was found in the GIT while merely 15% of this biomolecule reached the blood (Damgé et al. 1997). The site of administration also influences the effect obtained, since PACA NPs showed higher hypoglycemic effects and were observed in higher amounts in the ileum (Michel et al. 1991) which may be related to a higher absorption at this place. Trimethyl CS conjugated with cysteine induced a hypoglycemic effect for 12 hours (with an insulin dose of 50 IU/Kg), and a more pronounced effect was observed when given directly into the ileum (Yin et al. 2009). However, in the case of PACA NPs it was observed that the hypoglycemic effect was due to greater residence of insulin rather than NP uptake (Lowe and Temple 1994). CS NPs were also extensively used for protein delivery (Chaudhury and Das 2010). CS polyelectrolyte NPs with STPP containing insulin and coated with poloxamer 188 were found to deliver insulin and reduce the glycemia of rats (Pan et al. 2002). However, this effect could only be observed after 6 to 10 hours, and a dose effect was observed with prolonged effects for $\approx$ 20 hours. However, the dose effect observed was attributed to the size of the particles since bigger particles (*ca.* 300 nm) had difficulties in dissolving in the acidic medium and therefore a higher protection was feasible (Pan et al. 2002). Similarly, ionic cross-linking with hydroxipropyl methylcellulose phthalate have shown better stability than STPP and enhanced the hypoglycemic effect (Makhlof et al. 2011). Nevertheless, a dose-dependent hypoglycemic effect (15 IU/Kg vs. 30 IU/Kg) was observed for insulin-loaded CS-PGA NPs with a prolonged effect of 10 hours (Lin et al. 2007), and similar effects were observed for ALG/CS NPs (25 IU/Kg vs. 50 and 100 IU/Kg) (Sarmento et al. 2007), and PCL/Eudragit® RS (the 25 IU/Kg was ineffective) (Damgé et al. 2007), and a multilayer particulate system consisting of ALG/dextran sulfate/CS-PEG coated with albumin (Reis et al. 2008). On the other hand, for PACA NPs (mean diameter: 250–300 nm) of 12.5, 25, and 50 UI/Kg, a similar reduction in glycemia was observed after two days of intragastric administration, but a dose-dependent effect was observed for the duration of the effect (Damgé et al. 1990). The dose of NPs is important since it was suggested that the inefficacy at 25 IU/Kg could be due to degradation or that it was not released from NPs (Damgé et al. 2007). Therefore, these results suggest that the delivery of insulin through NPs is dependent on the polymer characteristics and conjugation. More than just reducing the glucose levels, NPs have also demonstrated their ability to reduce polydipsia and proteinuria

(Reis et al. 2008), and also prevented glycemia increase after glucose challenge (Damgé et al. 2007, Reis et al. 2008).

Salmon calcitonin is another interesting peptide for oral delivery. It is marketed in injectable and nasal spray forms to treat osteoporosis and hypercalcemia. Salmon calcitonin has a low stability at physiological pH values (Guggi et al. 2003), and a small amount of intact calcitonin is absorbed in the GIT (Sakuma et al. 2001). The same principles applied to insulin are applied to calcitonin, and include the protection of calcitonin from enzymatic degradation and enhance its transport across the mucosa while avoiding side effects. Although NPs have not reached clinical trials, several systems have improved calcitonin delivery *in vivo*. Different CS coating liposomes NPs and microparticles can deliver calcitonin, lowering in *ca.* 10% calcium levels. The depression of calcium levels was maintained for a prolonged period of time, and the bioavailability of calcitonin was dependent upon the particle size and the CS surface (Takeuchi et al. 2005). PEG was grafted to CS, and the nanoparticulate system was given to deliver calcitonin. The PEG grafting reduced the toxicity of the system while enhancing the stability in gastrointestinal fluids (Prego et al. 2006). CS has also been used to coat PLGA NPs and thus it enhanced particle uptake (Kawashima et al. 2000).

Another peptide with great commercial interest is cyclosporine A. This is an immunosuppressive cyclic oligopeptide that is very lipophilic. Moreover, this peptide is a substrate for the *P*-glycoprotein and suffers from high presystemic metabolism (Faulds et al. 1993). Several nanoformulations have been developed to compensate the poor absorption characteristics of cyclosporin A and reduce its side effects (e.g., nephrotoxicity) (Italia et al. 2007). As an example, PLGA NPs (smaller than 200 nm) increased the bioavailability of cyclosporine A, with reduced nephrotoxicity compared to commercial formulations in rats (Italia et al. 2007).

Nucleic acids

Genes are very promising therapeutic agents to be delivered since they can profoundly alter the pathogenesis of the majority of diseases, and as a result a vast range of applications can be achieved with those systems. However, similar to peptides and proteins, nucleic acids are extensively degraded in the external environment (nucleases are present in the GIT). Moreover, they require internalization in the cell nucleus while escaping the lisosomal activity of the cell. Nanocarriers developed for gene delivery are generally classified as viral and non-viral platforms. The use of viruses raises concerns related to their safety of risk of insertional mistakes and activation of proto-oncogenes, self-viral replication, and strong immune and inflammatory responses. Thus, non-viral NPs are a suitable alternative to protect and deliver the nucleic acid to the cells. In this field, CS is again an attractive polymer due to its positive charge that facilitates the formation of stable complexes with nucleic acids (which are negatively charged) (Li et al. 2009). However, its use is hampered by low transfection efficiency. It has been demonstrated that CS NPs can protect deoxyribonucleic acid (DNA) from the action of DNase, from a wide range of pH values (3 to 9), and showed a moderate immunostimulatory effect (Li et al. 2009). On the other hand, another cationic polymer that it is frequently used for transfection studies is PEI. Despite its good transfection efficiency, its use is reduced due to its toxicity. To effectively transfect a cell, the nanocarrier has to interact with the cell, be transported to the interior of the cell, resist the hurdle environment of lysosomes, and effectively deliver the gene to the cytoplasm, or if necessary by trafficking to the nucleus compartment (Agnihotri et al. 2004). As the majority of the strategies employing NPs were used for vaccination therapies, this will be further explored later.

Nanoparticles as potential vaccination adjuvants

Vaccination remains the most successful prophylaxis approach against infectious diseases. The GIT is well covered by primary lymphoid tissue being a potential target for immunization. The importance of the presence of M cells in the Peyer's patches is thereby stressed by sometimes being called "specialized antigen-sampling epithelial cells" since they promote direct delivery to the GALT making it a potential site to approach the immunization strategies. The underlying tissue is specialized in antigen processing, thus promoting both mucosal and systemic immunization responses with the production of both mucosal immunoglobulin (Ig) A and circulating Ig G. For immunization, NPs can either carry the antigen to the GALT or act as adjuvants for low immunogenicity antigens (Kanchan and Panda 2007). As antigens are usually proteins, they suffer degradation in the luminal side and therefore they show reduced antigenicity. To elicit an immune response NPs have to be efficiently uptaken. Thus, NPs should efficiently deliver the antigen/DNA vaccine to the Peyer's patches through M cells protecting it from degradation in the GIT and inducing both T and B cell immunities.

Several studies have explored NPs to promote *in vivo* immune responses. In general, these systems were able to incite immune responses with both inductions of Ig A and Ig G. Moreover, an increasing Ig G2a secretion inducing a T helper type-1 cell response was observed (increase levels of interferon γ). The cytokine profile stimulation is also important as interleukin 4, interleukin 10, and transforming growth factor β are known to inhibit antigen presenting cells (Porporatto et al. 2005). CS polymer has shown to induce interleukin 10 and transforming growth factor β release, and therefore inducing the production of Ig A (Porporatto et al. 2005).

Size also compromises an important feature in immunization. In similarly composed liposomes, smaller sizes induced higher cellular and humoral immune responses, and it was proposed that differences in the size could alter endocytosis and consequently the presentation of the antigen (Milicic et al. 2012). However, general rules related to the size cannot be easily draw since 100 nm-sized NPs elicited a greater Ig G production against tetanus toxoid compared to bigger particles (Jung et al. 2001), while 1 µm-sized particles elicited higher Ig G against bovine serum albumin compared to 200 nm- and 500 nm-sized particles (Gutierro et al. 2002). The latter particles were tested in three models of administration (subcutaneous, oral, and intranasal) and although 1000 nm-sized particles were able to induce an Ig G production compared to the subcutaneous route of administration, a higher dose of antigen had to be provided (Gutierro et al. 2002). Other set of experiments with particles with sizes ranging from 20 to 2000 nm found that 40 nm was the optimal size to induce T cell production against ovalbumin (Fifis et al. 2004). Also, comparison between microparticles and NPs reveled higher Ig G for microparticles but with differences in the Ig G_1/Ig G_2a ratios (microparticles had a higher ratio with an increase in interleukin 4 secretion and therefore a preferential profile towards T helper type-2 cells) suggesting preferential elicitation of humoral response for microparticles (Kanchan and Panda 2007).

NPs have the advantage to deliver the antigen to both MHC class I and II pathways eliciting both humoral and cellular responses while micron-sized counterparts are only able to promote humoral responses (Kanchan and Panda 2007). The oral immunization elicits Ig A secretion which subcutaneous injections fail to provide. Only systems that induced mucosal Ig A and systemic Ig G responses are able to provide a full immune response. Moreover, they can also provide better responses for low immunogenic antigens (acting as adjuvants) and could replace multi-administration by providing constant levels of antigen to the GALT (Kanchan and Panda 2007). DNA vaccination has been explored to modify the immunitary response from T helper type-2 cells to T helper type-1 cells, and therefore being able to treat allergic diseases such as asthma and atopic dermatitis (Li et al. 2009). Finally, NPs are interesting since antigen and adjuvant can be co-encapsulated, being present at the same time in antigen presenting cells.

Conclusions

The oral route for drug administration has been a field that has been remarkably explored to enhance the bioavailability of poorly absorbed therapeutic agents, or to enhance the efficacy of well-established therapeutics. New recent tools allow the use of drugs that otherwise would not be delivered by conventional formulations. This has opened a new field of opportunities and although only a small portion of particles has been reported to be absorbed, new efforts will certainly enhance the bioavailability of therapeutics in a controlled fashion. Nevertheless, NPs have proven to be able to protect and bypass the hurdles of the GIT and deliver drugs to the intended site. Moreover, NPs have shown the ability to enhance immune responses, thus eliciting both humoral and cellular responses that cannot be achieved by the parenteral route. As a result, it will not take long until clinical trials of NPs will be favorable and revolutionize the clinical practice.

Abbreviations

ALG	:	alginate
BCS	:	Biopharmaceutics Classification System
CD	:	cyclodextrin
CS	:	chitosan
DNA	:	deoxyribonucleic acid
FAE	:	follicle-associated epithelium
GALT	:	gut associated lymphoid tissue
GIT	:	gastrointestinal tract
GSH	:	glutathione
HLB	:	hydrophilic–lipophilic balance
Ig	:	immunoglobulin
M cell	:	microfold cell
MHC	:	major histocompatibility complex
M_W	:	molecular weight
NP	:	nanoparticle
O-MALT	:	organized associated lymphoid mucosa tissue;
o/w	:	oil-in-water
PACA	:	poly(alkylcyanoacrylate)
PCL	:	poly(ε-caprolactone)
PEG	:	poly(ethylene glycol)
PEI	:	polyethyleneimine
PLGA	:	poly(D,L-lactide-*co*-glycolide)
PVA	:	polyvinyl alcohol
RGD	:	arginine-glycine-aspartic acid
STPP	:	sodium tripolyphosphate
WGA	:	wheat germ agglutinin
w/o/w	:	water-in-oil-in-water

References

Agnihotri, S.A. and N.N. Mallikarjuna and T.M. Aminabhavi. 2004. Recent advances on chitosan-based micro- and nanoparticles in drug delivery. J. Control. Release. 100: 5–28.

Allemann, E. and J. Leroux and R. Gurny. 1998. Polymeric nano- and microparticles for the oral delivery of peptides and peptidomimetics. Adv. Drug Deliv. Rev. 34: 171–189.

Behrens, I. and A.I. Pena, M.J. Alonso and T. Kissel. 2002. Comparative uptake studies of bioadhesive and non-bioadhesive nanoparticles in human intestinal cell lines and rats: the effect of mucus on particle adsorption and transport. Pharm. Res. 19: 1185–1193.

Bernkop-Schnurch, A. and C.E. Kast and D. Guggi. 2003. Permeation enhancing polymers in oral delivery of hydrophilic macromolecules: thiomer/GSH systems. J. Control. Release. 93: 95–103.

Bravo-Osuna, I. and C. Vauthier, A. Farabollini, G.F. Palmieri and G. Ponchel. 2007. Mucoadhesion mechanism of chitosan and thiolated chitosan-poly(isobutyl cyanoacrylate) core-shell nanoparticles. Biomaterials. 28: 2233–2243.

Buda, A. and C. Sands and M.A. Jepson. 2005. Use of fluorescence imaging to investigate the structure and function of intestinal M cells. Adv. Drug Deliv. Rev. 57: 123–134.

Chaudhury, A. and S. Das. 2010. Recent advancement of chitosan-based nanoparticles for oral controlled delivery of insulin and other therapeutic agents. AAPS Pharm. Sci. Tech. 12: 10–20.

Damgé, C. and C. Michel, M. Aprahamian and P. Couvreur. 1988. New approach for oral administration of insulin with poly(alkyl cyanoacrylate) nanocapsules as drug carrier. Diabetes. 37: 246–251.

Damgé, C. and C. Michel, M. Aprahamian, P. Couvreur and J.P. Devissaguet. 1990. Nanocapsules as carriers for oral peptide delivery. J. Control. Release. 13: 233–239.

Damgé, C. and H. Vranckx, P. Balschmidt and P. Couvreur. 1997. Poly(alkyl cyanoacrylate) nanospheres for oral administration of insulin. J. Pharm. Sci. 86: 1403–1409.

Damgé, C. and P. Maincent and N. Ubrich. 2007. Oral delivery of insulin associated to polymeric nanoparticles in diabetic rats. J. Control. Release. 117: 163–170.

des Rieux, A. and E.G.E. Ragnarsson, E. Gullberg, V.R. Préat, Y.J. Schneider and P. Artursson. 2005. Transport of nanoparticles across an *in vitro* model of the human intestinal follicle associated epithelium. Eur. J. Pharm. Sci. 25: 455–465.

des Rieux, A. and V. Fievez, M. Garinot, Y.J. Schneider and V. Preat. 2006. Nanoparticles as potential oral delivery systems of proteins and vaccines: a mechanistic approach. J. Control. Release. 116: 1–27.

des Rieux, A. and V. Fievez, I. Theate, J. Mast, V. Preat and Y.J. Schneider. 2007a. An improved *in vitro* model of human intestinal follicle-associated epithelium to study nanoparticle transport by M cells. Eur. J. Pharm. Sci. 30: 380–391.

des Rieux, A. and V. Fievez, M. Momtaz, C. Detrembleur, M. Alonso-Sande, J. Van Gelder, A. Cauvin, Y.J. Schneider and V. Preat. 2007b. Helodermin-loaded nanoparticles: characterization and transport across an *in vitro* model of the follicle-associated epithelium. J. Control. Release. 118: 294–302.

Desai, M.P. and V. Labhasetwar, G.L. Amidon and R.J. Levy. 1996. Gastrointestinal uptake of biodegradable microparticles: effect of particle size. Pharm. Res. 13: 1838–1845.

Eldridge, J.H. and C.J. Hammond, J.A. Meulbroek, J.K. Staas, R.M. Gilley and T.R. Tice. 1990. Controlled vaccine release in the gut-associated lymphoid tissues. I. Orally administered biodegradable microspheres target the peyer's patches. J. Control. Release. 11: 205–214.

Ensign, L.M. and R. Cone and J. Hanes. 2012. Oral drug delivery with polymeric nanoparticles: the gastrointestinal mucus barriers. Adv. Drug Deliv. Rev. 64: 557–570.

Faulds, D. and K.L. Goa and P. Benfield. 1993. Cyclosporin. A review of its pharmacodynamic and pharmacokinetic properties, and therapeutic use in immunoregulatory disorders. Drugs. 45: 953–1040.

Fievez, V. and L. Plapied, A.D. Rieux, V. Pourcelle, H. Freichels, V. Wascotte, M.L. Vanderhaeghen, C. Jerôme, A. Vanderplasschen, J. Marchand-Brynaert, Y.J. Schneider and V. Préat. 2009. Targeting nanoparticles to M cells with non-peptidic ligands for oral vaccination. Eur. J. Pharm. Biopharm. 73: 16–24.

Fifis, T. and A. Gamvrellis, B. Crimeen-Irwin, G.A. Pietersz, J. Li, P.L. Mottram, I.F. McKenzie and M. Plebanski. 2004. Size-dependent immunogenicity: therapeutic and protective properties of nano-vaccines against tumors. J. Immunol. 173: 3148–3154.

Fontana, G. and M. Licciardi, S. Mansueto, D. Schillaci and G. Giammona. 2001. Amoxicillin-loaded polyethylcyanoacrylate nanoparticles: influence of PEG coating on the particle size, drug release rate and phagocytic uptake. Biomaterials. 22: 2857–2865.

Galindo-Rodriguez, S. and E. Allemann, H. Fessi and E. Doelker. 2004. Physicochemical parameters associated with nanoparticle formation in the salting-out, emulsification-diffusion, and nanoprecipitation methods. Pharm. Res. 21: 1428–1439.

Garinot, M. and V. Fievez, V. Pourcelle, F. Stoffelbach, A. des Rieux, L. Plapied, I. Theate, H. Freichels, C. Jerome, J. Marchand-Brynaert, Y.J. Schneider and V. Preat. 2007. PEGylated PLGA-based nanoparticles targeting M cells for oral vaccination. J. Control. Release. 120: 195–204.

Gaumet, M. and R. Gurny and F. Delie. 2009. Localization and quantification of biodegradable particles in an intestinal cell model: the influence of particle size. Eur. J. Pharm. Sci. 36: 465–473.

Guggi, D. and C.E. Kast and A. Bernkop-Schnurch. 2003. *In vivo* evaluation of an oral salmon calcitonin-delivery system based on a thiolated chitosan carrier matrix. Pharm. Res. 20: 1989–1994.

Gutierro, I. and R.M. Hernandez, M. Igartua, A.R. Gascon and J.L. Pedraz. 2002. Size dependent immune response after subcutaneous, oral and intranasal administration of BSA loaded nanospheres. Vaccine. 21: 67–77.

Hillery, A.M. and A.T. Florence. 1996. The effect of adsorbed poloxamer 188 and 407 surfactants on the intestinal uptake of 60-nm polystyrene particles after oral administration in the rat. Int. J. Pharm. 132: 123–130.

Italia, J.L. and D.K. Bhatt, V. Bhardwaj, K. Tikoo and M.N. Kumar. 2007. PLGA nanoparticles for oral delivery of cyclosporine: nephrotoxicity and pharmacokinetic studies in comparison to Sandimmune Neoral. J. Control. Release. 119: 197–206.

Italia, J.L. and M.M. Yahya, D. Singh and M.N. Ravi Kumar. 2009. Biodegradable nanoparticles improve oral bioavailability of amphotericin B and show reduced nephrotoxicity compared to intravenous Fungizone. Pharm. Res. 26: 1324–1331.

Jung, T. and W. Kamm, A. Breitenbach, K.D. Hungerer, E. Hundt and T. Kissel. 2001. Tetanus toxoid loaded nanoparticles from sulfobutylated poly(vinyl alcohol)-graft-poly(lactide-co-glycolide): evaluation of antibody response after oral and nasal application in mice. Pharm. Res. 18: 352–360.

Junghanns, J.U. and R.H. Muller. 2008. Nanocrystal technology, drug delivery and clinical applications. Int. J. Nanomedicine. 3: 295–309.

Kanchan, V. and A.K. Panda. 2007. Interactions of antigen-loaded polylactide particles with macrophages and their correlation with the immune response. Biomaterials. 28: 5344–5357.

Kawashima, Y. and H. Yamamoto, H. Takeuchi and Y. Kuno. 2000. Mucoadhesive DL-lactide/glycolide copolymer nanospheres coated with chitosan to improve oral delivery of elcatonin. Pharm. Dev. Technol. 5: 77–85.

Kumari, A. and S.K. Yadav and S.C. Yadav. 2010. Biodegradable polymeric nanoparticles based drug delivery systems. Colloids Surf. B Biointerfaces. 75: 1–18.

Langguth, P. and V. Bohner, J. Heizmann, H.P. Merkle, S. Wolffram, G.L. Amidon and S. Yamashita. 1997. The challenge of proteolytic enzymes in intestinal peptide delivery. J. Control. Release. 46: 39–57.

Li, G.P. and Z.G. Liu, B. Liao and N.S. Zhong. 2009. Induction of Th1-type immune response by chitosan nanoparticles containing plasmid DNA encoding house dust mite allergen Der p 2 for oral vaccination in mice. Cell Mol. Immunol. 6: 45–50.

Lin, Y.H. and F.L. Mi, C.T. Chen, W.C. Chang, S.F. Peng, H.F. Liang and H.W. Sung. 2007. Preparation and characterization of nanoparticles shelled with chitosan for oral insulin delivery. Biomacromolecules. 8: 146–152.

Lin, Y.H. and C.H. Chang, Y.S. Wu, Y.M. Hsu, S.F. Chiou and Y.J. Chen. 2009. Development of pH-responsive chitosan/heparin nanoparticles for stomach-specific anti-Helicobacter pylori therapy. Biomaterials. 30: 3332–3342.

Loftsson, T. and M.E. Brewster and M. Másson. 2004. Role of cyclodextrins in improving oral drug delivery. Am. J. Drug Deliv. 2: 261–275.

Loh, J.W. and G. Yeoh, M. Saunders and L.Y. Lim. 2010. Uptake and cytotoxicity of chitosan nanoparticles in human liver cells. Toxicol. Appl. Pharmacol. 249: 148–157.

Lopedota, A. and A. Trapani, A. Cutrignelli, L. Chiarantini, E. Pantucci, R. Curci, E. Manuali and G. Trapani. 2009. The use of Eudragit® RS 100/cyclodextrin nanoparticles for the transmucosal administration of glutathione. Eur. J. Pharm. Biopharm. 72: 509–520.

Lowe, P.J. and C.S. Temple. 1994. Calcitonin and insulin in isobutylcyanoacrylate nanocapsules: protection against proteases and effect on intestinal absorption in rats. J. Pharm. Pharmacol. 46: 547–552.

Mahler, G.J. and M.B. Esch, E. Tako, T.L. Southard, S.D. Archer, R.P. Glahn and M.L. Shuler. 2012. Oral exposure to polystyrene nanoparticles affects iron absorption. Nat. Nanotechnol. 7: 264–271.

Makhlof, A. and Y. Tozuka and H. Takeuchi. 2011. Design and evaluation of novel pH-sensitive chitosan nanoparticles for oral insulin delivery. Eur. J. Pharm. Sci. 42: 445–451.

Merisko-Liversidge, E. and S.L. McGurk and G.G. Liversidge. 2004. Insulin nanoparticles: a novel formulation approach for poorly water soluble Zn-insulin. Pharm. Res. 21: 1545–1553.

Michel, C. and M. Aprahamian, L. Defontaine, P. Couvreur and C. Damgé. 1991. The effect of site of administration in the gastrointestinal tract on the absorption of insulin from nanocapsules in diabetic rats. J. Pharm. Pharmacol. 43: 1–5.

Milicic, A. and R. Kaur, A. Reyes-Sandoval, C.K. Tang, J. Honeycutt, Y. Perrie and A.V.S. Hill. 2012. Small cationic DDA: TDB liposomes as protein vaccine adjuvants obviate the need for TLR agonists in inducing cellular and humoral responses. PLoS One. 7: e34255.

Moghimi, S.M. and A.C. Hunter. 2000. Poloxamers and poloxamines in nanoparticle engineering and experimental medicine. Trends Biotechnol. 18: 412–420.

Nafee, N. and M. Schneider, U.F. Schaefer and C.M. Lehr. 2009. Relevance of the colloidal stability of chitosan/PLGA nanoparticles on their cytotoxicity profile. Int. J. Pharm. 381: 130–139.

O'Hagan, D.T. 1996. The intestinal uptake of particles and the implications for drug and antigen delivery. J. Anat. 189: 477–482.

Oostingh, G.J. and E. Casals, P. Italiani, R. Colognato, R. Stritzinger, J. Ponti, T. Pfaller, Y. Kohl, D. Ooms, F. Favilli, H. Leppens, D. Lucchesi, F. Rossi, I. Nelissen, H. Thielecke, V.F. Puntes, A. Duschl and D. Boraschi. 2011. Problems and challenges in the development and validation of human cell-based assays to determine nanoparticle-induced immunomodulatory effects. Part. Fibre Toxicol. 8: 8.

Pan, Y. and Y.J. Li, H.Y. Zhao, J.M. Zheng, H. Xu, G. Wei, J.S. Hao and F.D. Cui. 2002. Bioadhesive polysaccharide in protein delivery system: chitosan nanoparticles improve the intestinal absorption of insulin *in vivo*. Int. J. Pharm. 249: 139–147.

Panchagnula, R. and N.S. Thomas. 2000. Biopharmaceutics and pharmacokinetics in drug research. Int. J. Pharm. 201: 131–150.

Pinto-Alphandary, H. and M. Aboubakar, D. Jaillard, P. Couvreur and C. Vauthier. 2003. Visualization of insulin-loaded nanocapsules: *in vitro* and *in vivo* studies after oral administration to rats. Pharm. Res. 20: 1071–1084.

Pinto Reis, C. and R.J. Neufeld, A.J. Ribeiro and F. Veiga. 2006. Nanoencapsulation I. Methods for preparation of drug-loaded polymeric nanoparticles. Nanomedicine. 2: 8–21.

Porporatto, C. and I.D. Bianco and S.G. Correa. 2005. Local and systemic activity of the polysaccharide chitosan at lymphoid tissues after oral administration. J. Leukoc. Biol. 78: 62–69.

Powell, J.J. and N. Faria, E. Thomas-McKay and L.C. Pele. 2010. Origin and fate of dietary nanoparticles and microparticles in the gastrointestinal tract. J. Autoimmun. 34: J226–J233.

Prego, C. and D. Torres, E. Fernandez-Megia, R. Novoa-Carballal, E. Quiñoá and M.J. Alonso. 2006. Chitosan-PEG nanocapsules as new carriers for oral peptide delivery. Effect of chitosan pegylation degree. J. Control. Release. 111: 299–308.

Reis, C.P. and A.J. Ribeiro, S. Houng, F. Veiga and R.J. Neufeld. 2007. Nanoparticulate delivery system for insulin: design, characterization and *in vitro/in vivo* bioactivity. Eur. J. Pharm. Sci. 30: 392–397.

Reis, C.P. and F.J. Veiga, A.J. Ribeiro, R.J. Neufeld and C. Damge. 2008. Nanoparticulate biopolymers deliver insulin orally eliciting pharmacological response. J. Pharm. Sci. 97: 5290–5305.

Ren, D. and H. Yi, W. Wang and X. Ma. 2005. The enzymatic degradation and swelling properties of chitosan matrices with different degrees of N-acetylation. Carbohydr. Res. 340: 2403–2410.

Richardson, S.C. and K.L. Wallom, E.L. Ferguson, S.P. Deacon, M.W. Davies, A.J. Powell, R.C. Piper and R. Duncan. 2008. The use of fluorescence microscopy to define polymer localisation to the late endocytic compartments in cells that are targets for drug delivery. J. Control. Release. 127: 1–11.

Sakuma, S. and M. Hayashi and M. Akashi. 2001. Design of nanoparticles composed of graft copolymers for oral peptide delivery. Adv. Drug Deliv. Rev. 47: 21–37.

Sandri, G. and M.C. Bonferoni, S. Rossi, F. Ferrari, S. Gibin, Y. Zambito, G. Di Colo and C. Caramella. 2007. Nanoparticles based on N-trimethylchitosan: evaluation of absorption properties using *in vitro* (Caco-2 cells) and *ex vivo* (excised rat jejunum) models. Eur. J. Pharm. Biopharm. 65: 68–77.

Sarmento, B. and A. Ribeiro, F. Veiga, P. Sampaio, R. Neufeld and D. Ferreira. 2007. Alginate/ chitosan nanoparticles are effective for oral insulin delivery. Pharm. Res. 24: 2198–2206.

Shakweh, M. and M. Besnard, V. Nicolas and E. Fattal. 2005. Poly(lactide-co-glycolide) particles of different physicochemical properties and their uptake by peyer's patches in mice. Eur. J. Pharm. Biopharm. 61: 1–13.

Sonaje, K. and Y.H. Lin, J.H. Juang, S.P. Wey, C.T. Chen and H.W. Sung. 2009. *In vivo* evaluation of safety and efficacy of self-assembled nanoparticles for oral insulin delivery. Biomaterials. 30: 2329–2339.

Surnar, B. and M. Jayakannan. 2013. Stimuli-responsive poly(caprolactone) vesicles for dual drug delivery under the gastrointestinal tract. Biomacromolecules. 14: 4377–4387.

Takeuchi, H. and Y. Matsui, H. Sugihara, H. Yamamoto and Y. Kawashima. 2005. Effectiveness of submicron-sized, chitosan-coated liposomes in oral administration of peptide drugs. Int. J. Pharm. 303: 160–170.

Win, K.Y. and S.S. Feng. 2005. Effects of particle size and surface coating on cellular uptake of polymeric nanoparticles for oral delivery of anticancer drugs. Biomaterials. 26: 2713–2722.

Woitiski, C.B. and B. Sarmento, R.A. Carvalho, R.J. Neufeld and F. Veiga. 2011. Facilitated nanoscale delivery of insulin across intestinal membrane models. Int. J. Pharm. 412: 123–131.

Yin, L. and J. Ding, C. He, L. Cui, C. Tang and C. Yin. 2009. Drug permeability and mucoadhesion properties of thiolated trimethyl chitosan nanoparticles in oral insulin delivery. Biomaterials. 30: 5691–5700.

CHAPTER 3

Nanoparticulate Systems for Dental Drug Delivery

Sanko Nguyen,[1,] Gro Smistad,[1,a] Morten Rykke[2] and Marianne Hiorth[1,b]*

ABSTRACT

The most common oral ailments we face today are dental caries and periodontal diseases. In our modern society, tooth wear and xerostomia-induced caries have recently gained increased attention as these problems seem to prevail and have been associated with changes in our behavior and lifestyle. Conventional methods that are used in the prevention and therapy of these problems are numerous, focusing mainly on eliminating the source of infection (antimicrobial therapy) and remineralization and strengthening of teeth (topical application of fluoride). However, the efficacy of commercial oral care products is limited due to physiological challenges with the delivery of therapeutics into the oral cavity. With the continuous secretion of saliva, the functional processes of mastication and swallowing, and the rich microbial flora, the oral cavity presents a complex and dynamic environment for any foreign agent introduced. To optimize the effect of prevailing methods, nanoparticulate drug delivery have been explored. Nanoparticulate systems have also the potential to carry novel drug substances to introduce alternative and/or new treatment in the area of dental pharmacotherapy.

[1] P.O. Box 1068 Blindern, 0316 Oslo, Norway.
[a] Email: gro.smistad@farmasi.uio.no
[b] Email: marianne.hiorth@farmasi.uio.no
[2] P.O. Box 1109 Blindern, 0317 Oslo, Norway.
  Email: morten.rykke@odont.uio.no
* Corresponding author: s.h.nguyen@farmasi.uio.no

Liposomes, often consisting of phospholipids, are spherical vesicles that have received the most attention as nano-sized drug delivery system. Extensive research in liposomes as drug carriers has resulted in commercial liposomal products. Based on the success in medicine, research and development of liposomes for use as nanocarriers in dentistry is therefore highly anticipated. The potential of other nanoparticulate structures, such as polymer-based micelles and nanoparticles, are also considered for use as dental drug delivery systems. The present chapter aims to provide an early glimpse on the future implications of the rapidly emerging field of nanomedicine in dentistry.

Introduction

The majority of diseases in the oral cavity are related to the teeth and gum. Dental disorders are considered a public health burden worldwide, although tremendous improvement has been made in the last two decades in both levels of personal oral hygiene and professional dental care (Petersen et al. 2005, Baghramian et al. 2009). The most prevalent oral diseases today are dental caries (tooth decay) and periodontal diseases (tooth loss). Historically, these dental ailments have always been the main threat to human oral health. In recent years, concern of tooth wear has gained increased attention due to the changes in behavior and life style with our modern society. Aberrant activity of oral functions may also inflict damage to the teeth. One important example is the reduced production of saliva leading to xerostomia (dry mouth) and serious complications of xerostomia-induced caries and increased tooth wear.

The international trend in clinical dental practice today, especially in caries management, is to move away from the operative intervention and towards a preventive approach or a minimal invasive dental treatment. The aim is to get better control with the initiation and progression of the disease over a person's lifetime. Dental caries is a chronic disease that progresses slowly in most people. Prolonged therapy is therefore required to repair the enamel. Since restorative treatment tend to have short durability due to recurrent caries, and being far more expensive, more emphasis has been laid on the prevention of caries management. In order to find and develop pharmaceutical strategies to prevent and treat tooth-related conditions, a better understanding into the pathophysiologic basis of the dental problems is essential. A brief description of the four most common causes to dental problems is hereby presented.

Common causes to dental problems

Dental caries

Dental caries is defined as localized destruction of susceptible dental hard tissues by acidic by-products from bacterial fermentation of dietary carbohydrates (Marsh and Martin 2009). The cariogenic bacteria metabolize especially small molecular carbohydrates, such as glucose, sucrose, and fructose. The disease is a result from an imbalance in the physiological equilibrium between tooth minerals and fluids in the oral microbial biofilms (Fig. 3.1). The production of organic acids by the cariogenic bacteria causes local pH values to fall below a critical value resulting in demineralization of the enamel and dentin. However, initial demineralization can be reversed in its early stages through the uptake of calcium, phosphate, and fluoride. In this case, saliva acts as a buffer and quickly restore pH by the supply of the inorganic ions. Whether dental caries progresses, stops, or reverses, is thus, dependent on the demineralization (destruction) and remineralization (repair) processes (Selwitz et al. 2007). These two processes take place frequently during the day, however, over time it will lead to either cavitation within the tooth, repair of the initial enamel lesion, or maintenance of the status quo. Dental caries is a complex disease with the interplay of many factors. The main factors involved are tooth, bacteria in biofilm, diet, and time. Oral environmental factors, including salivary flow, the exposure to fluoride and the consumption of dietary sugars, also play important roles.

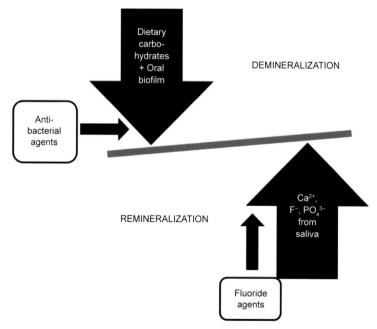

Figure 3.1. The balance of the caries process. Therapeutic target areas of dental caries are inhibition of demineralization by antibacterial agents and/or facilitation of remineralization by application of fluoride agents.

Periodontal diseases

Periodontal diseases are a collective term to denote diseases in the surrounding and supportive structures of the teeth, including the gum, periodontal ligament, and bone, caused by oral bacteria. The diseases are often divided into two categories: gingivitis and periodontitis. In gingivitis, pathogenic bacteria cause inflammation of the gingiva (the gum tissues) with symptoms such as bleeding, redness, and swollen gums. Periodontitis is characterized by chronic inflammation and infection of the periodontium. Thus, it is a more advanced stage (into the deeper structures) and aggressive form of the disease. One characteristic feature is the formation of periodontal pockets where the condition is ideal for anaerobic bacteria to harbor and proliferate. The condition can be severe and lead to periodontal destruction and tooth loss.

Tooth wear

Unlike dental caries and periodontal diseases, tooth wear is the loss of tooth substance not associated with oral microorganisms. Wear can occur by two distinct mechanisms: those of physical origin (abrasion and attrition) and those of chemical origin (erosion). The mechanical removal of dental hard tissues by abrasion is defined by a foreign material in repeated contact with the teeth. This could be abrasive food or dentifrices with abrasives. Attrition is caused by the direct contact between teeth without any third substance intervening. Tooth erosion is the loss of dental hard tissue following chemical dissolution by acid where the acid source is not derived from oral bacteria. Acid can stem directly from the intake of acidic foods and beverages or from gastric acid due to medical conditions, such as gastroesophageal reflux disease and eating disorders. Erosive demineralization softens the enamel so that the tooth surface is more vulnerable to mechanical impacts thereby able to enhance physical wear. The clinical outcome of tooth wear is, thus, often a combined result of attrition, abrasion, and erosion. Recent focus on tooth wear, particularly erosion, is due to life style changes in our modern society as erosion has been associated with changes in people's eating and drinking habits. There is also a tendency to develop more wear with age. As tooth wear is a cumulative process and there is a tendency of an aging population, the importance of a lifetime protection of the teeth is becoming more evident.

Xerostomia

Xerostomia is defined as a subjective complaint of dry mouth that most often is a result from salivary gland dysfunction with a decrease in the production of saliva (hyposalivation) (Cotrim et al. 2013). Most patients do not complain about dry mouth symptoms until the salivary secretion has dropped to 50% of the normal when damages, such as recurrent caries and tooth wear, are already severe. Hyposalivation may be due to radiotherapy for cancer treatment of the head and neck region and certain systemic autoimmune diseases, e.g., Sjögren's syndrome. Xerostomia is also a common side effect of a large array of medications, including antidepressants, antihistamines, antihypertensives, tranquilizers, diuretics, and analgesics. Elderly people typically use more of these types of medications. The issue with polypharmacy is another reason why the geriatric population often suffer from medication-induced xerostomia. Xerostomia is associated with difficulties in chewing, swallowing, tasting, and speaking. The condition may lead to loss or reduced activity of the protective functions of saliva in the oral cavity, including lubrication of the oral surfaces, clearance of unfavorable substances, buffer capacity, and remineralization of the teeth. Continuous salivary secretion therefore plays an important inhibitive role in the early phase of caries lesion development. Thus, the lack of saliva can rapidly lead to adverse oral complications such as dental caries, tooth wear, and fungal infections.

Challenges with Drug Delivery to the Oral Cavity

Dental problems can greatly impair an individual's well being and thereby have a negative impact on the individual's health and quality of life. There are two main strategies for the current prevention and treatment of dental caries and periodontal diseases: by inhibiting the acid production in dental plaque and reducing periodontal infections by the use of antibacterial agents, or by promoting remineralization by the use of fluoride agents (Fig. 3.1). The prevention of tooth wear and xerostomia-induced caries is also closely related to these strategies as they also imply demineralization and the softening of tooth substance. In both the prevention and treatment of dental problems, many pharmaceutical products for local delivery of active substances are on the market for self-administered care. They exist mostly in the form of toothpaste, mouth rinse, gel, and varnish. The most familiar products are fluoride toothpastes and chlorhexidine mouth rinses. The main disadvantage of the conventional formulations is the short residence time in the oral cavity leading to inadequate pharmacotherapeutic effect. Evidently, there is a great demand for optimization and the development of more efficient products. From a pharmaceutical point of view, the delivery of active substances to the oral cavity is challenging due to the complex and dynamic intraoral environment. There are three main factors contributing to this condition: the oral microbial flora, salivary secretions, and oral functions.

Microbial flora

The oral cavity shelters a rich and diverse microbial flora. The healthy oral cavity is normally colonized by microorganisms like fungi, viruses, and a great number of bacteria in a natural balance. It has been estimated that 700 bacterial species reside in the mouth (Aas et al. 2005); some are beneficial but some other are or may become pathogenic to the human host. *Streptococcus mutans* and lactobacilli are the most common causes for the development of dental caries. The co-existence of complex populations found on the tooth surface is often embedded in an extracellular matrix of polymers of host and microbial origin, resulting in the formation of an oral biofilm. This type of biofilm is also known as dental plaque (Fig. 3.2). Dental plaque is the key factor in the development of dental caries and periodontal diseases, because cariogenic bacteria are associated in dental plaques rendering them increased protection and resistance to antimicrobial agents. Besides adhering to oral surfaces, oral bacteria may attach to other substrates, including drug substances, interfering with their therapeutic action in the oral environment.

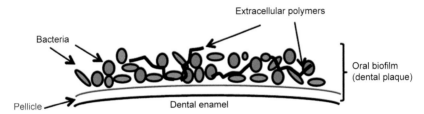

Figure 3.2. A schematic illustration of the dental plaque. The biofilm ecosystem protects the cariogenic bacteria and makes them resistant against antimicrobial agents.

Salivary secretion

Saliva is a watery secretion from the three major paired glands (parotid, submandibular, and sublingual glands) in addition to a numerous minor mucous glands. A very small fraction of saliva ($\approx 1\%$), constituting of organic (proteins, carbohydrates, and lipids) and inorganic constituents (sodium, potassium, calcium, hydrogen carbonate, phosphate, chloride, and fluoride), is responsible for many of saliva's physiological functions (Ferguson et al. 1999). The inorganic ions calcium, phosphate, and fluoride are important in the remineralization of teeth, while hydrogen carbonate enables saliva's buffering properties. The large array of proteins is the most important organic portion, contributing to lubrication of oral surfaces by mucins, initiation of digestion by the enzymes lipase, amylase, and protease, and antibacterial activity by immunoglobulins (Igs), lactoferrin, and lactoperoxidase. Determination of the exact amount and composition of saliva is difficult, because the secretion of saliva is highly variable and dependent on a number of factors, including the type of secreting gland, the time of the day, the flow rate, and the nature and duration of the stimulation. Both inter-and intraindividual variations also occur. These salivary variables often make it difficult to correlate *in vitro* studies to *in vivo* performance of potential drug candidates.

The oral surfaces are thus continuously bathed in a fluid consisting of an intricate mixture of oral bacteria, leukocytes, desquamated epithelial cells, food remnants, salivary secretions, and crevicular fluid. This oral fluid, often referred to as whole saliva or mixed saliva, is the transporting vehicle within the oral environment. This is a pivotal aspect of drug delivery into the oral cavity as interaction with whole saliva is inevitable. Any foreign substances, including drug and drug components, introduced to the oral cavity can be inactivated or diluted and subsequently cleared from the oral cavity by saliva. This so-called salivary clearance is beneficial for oral health since it can rapidly remove exogenous harmful substances. However, rapid clearance is unfavorable for drug therapy in the oral cavity since it often clears away the drug agents before an adequate therapeutic effect is obtained. This remains the main limitation and a formulation challenge with drug delivery to the oral cavity.

Oral functions

The oral cavity consists of various structures (buccal mucosa, tongue, teeth, gingival, and palate) representing both soft and hard tissues. Common for all is that they are continuously covered by saliva and have evolved to perform the important biological functions of eating, drinking, and breathing, in addition to speaking, tasting, and infection control. Related to these activities, the environment in the oral cavity undergoes substantial changes due to the consumption of exogenous food and drink materials, the masticatory process, and fluctuations in the salivary secretion. Food and drink substances may directly interact with drugs, and interfere with their intended therapeutic action. Oral enzymes, which are important in the initiation of digestion, may potentially cleave and degrade drug compounds. Together with the individual's eating and drinking behavior, personal factors such as the overall general health and physical activity also influence the oral state. The oral cavity, thus, presents a physically harsh and chemically hostile environment for drug compounds to sustain.

Nanoparticulate Systems for the Prevention and Treatment of Dental Problems

Nano-sized structures possess unique physical properties and thereby behave significantly different than their larger counterparts. Many biological functions are carried out at this length scale and the application of nanostructures has therefore gained much interest in medical science. Nanoparticles (NPs), preferentially from 10 to 100 nm in size, have high surface area per unit of mass and have the ability to pass cell membranes. In the last two decades, extensive research has been focused on the use of nanomaterials for a specific diagnostic or therapeutic purpose (Boulaiz et al. 2011, Doane and Burda 2012). NPs have been developed to function as drug delivery systems with the main objective to optimize the therapeutic effect of the drug while reducing the negative side effects. The characteristics of NPs can be manipulated to promote targeted and/or controlled drug delivery for an enhanced effect. Nano-sized systems have therefore been greatly investigated as the platform for the delivery of anticancer agents (Chauhan and Jain 2013, Wang et al.

2013). Research in modern dentistry has also discovered the potential use of nanomaterials (Allaker 2010, Hannig and Hannig 2010 and 2012). For instance, to mimic the natural biomineralization process, hydroxyapatite (HA) nanorods have been synthesized to artificially create the dental enamel (Chen et al. 2005). NPs have been successfully employed in dental resin-based composites and as fillers in impression materials for improved appearance and mechanical properties (Xia et al. 2008, Chen 2010). The use of nanostructures in the domain of dental therapy has recently been explored as well (Renugalakshmi et al. 2011). Nanoparticulate systems can be used to encapsulate and specifically deliver active agents to the dental tissues, and/or to overcome the challenges associated with dental delivery.

The natural development of improved oral care products is often based on the reformulation of conventional agents by implementing advances in pharmaceutical technology. Nanoparticulate systems can be utilized to load classical active compounds, known to be effective, to specifically direct them to teeth, gum tissues, or dental plaque (targeting function). They can be developed to retain the drug in the place of action to achieve sufficient therapeutic level (bioadhesive function), thus, overcoming the saliva clearance. For example, the application of fluoride toothpaste has proven to be the most effective self-care preventive measure of dental caries. It has been shown that the continuous presence of fluoride, even in low concentrations, is favorable in the inhibition of caries (Duckworth 1993). With infrequent administration of fluoride, it is therefore a great advantage to maintain constant level of fluorides in the oral cavity (sustained delivery), necessitating the optimization of fluoride delivery. Long-term activity or oral substantivity is also a desirable property for other therapeutic agents, such as antimicrobials, due to the aforementioned challenges with drug delivery to the oral cavity.

A new and alternative therapy to conventional antibiotics in the treatment of dental caries is the use of antibacterial peptides. These small molecules, such as histatins and defensins, are able to disrupt the bacterial cell membrane. They can be used in the specific targeting to organisms in the oral cavity as well as for a broad spectrum of antibacterial activity. With these new emerging drug substances, there are also many pharmaceutical challenges to be met, such as short half-life, low *in vivo* stability and bioavailability, the susceptibility to proteases, low safety margin, and high levels of oral clearance (Pepperney and Chikindas 2011). Nanocarriers can be applied to overcome these shortcomings since they can operate as stability-enhancing systems for the drug substance (protective function). Advantages associated to the use of nanoparticulate drug delivery systems to the teeth are summarized in Fig. 3.3.

Various types of nano-sized structures have been developed, the morphology stretching from hollow nanotubes and nanorods to spherical NPs and branched dendrimers. In the context of dental drug delivery, this chapter will focus on spherical vehicles, i.e., polymeric NPs, micelles, and liposomes with emphasis on the latter (Fig. 3.4). Broad knowledge and experience have been acquired with liposomes due to extensive research in liposomal

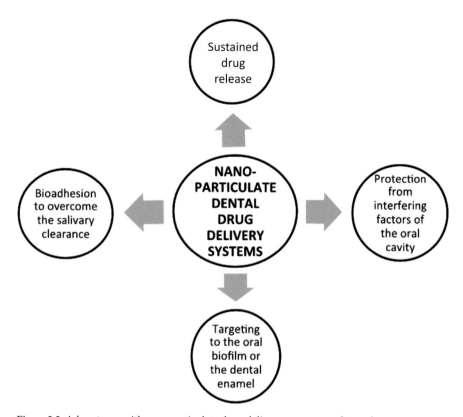

Figure 3.3. Advantages with nanoparticulate drug delivery systems to the teeth.

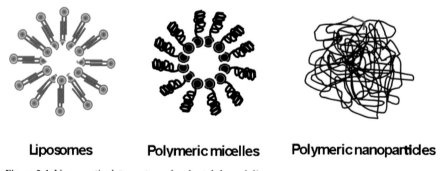

Liposomes   **Polymeric micelles**   **Polymeric nanoparticles**

Figure 3.4. Nanoparticulate systems for dental drug delivery.

technology in the past four decades. Today, liposomes stand as the most successful nanoparticulate drug delivery system having obtained a clinical established role. Since late 1990s, approved liposomal products have been on the pharmaceutical market for the treatment of cancer and infectious diseases (e.g., Doxil®, Ambisome®). Therefore, liposomes often present a classic model for nanoparticulate drug delivery. The basic principles behind the application of liposomes can often be transferred to other nanostructures. Principal ideas in the development of nanoparticulate systems, with emphasis on liposomes, in dental delivery are presented followed by studies reported in the literature to support the concepts.

Liposomes

Liposomes are vesicles comprising of lipids, most often phospholipids, of natural or synthetic origin, concentrated in one or more bilayers. The lipid molecules, each of which typically consists of a hydrophilic headgroup and two hydrophobic hydrocarbon tails, spontaneously self-assemble in the presence of an aqueous environment. Hydrophilic molecules can be entrapped in the aqueous core, while lipophilic molecules can be incorporated in the lipid bilayer. Hence, liposomes are able to function as drug carriers, carrying both water-soluble and water-insoluble compounds. Liposomes are biocompatible and biodegradable, and are versatile systems as they are easy to design and target for a specific purpose. They are mainly used as drug carriers in the delivery of anticancer agents due to their potential to reduce serious systemic side effects, while maintaining or enhancing the efficacy of the drug (Kaasgaard and Andresen 2010, Slingerland et al. 2012). Other areas that also use liposomal nanocarriers are in dermal, ophthalmic and gene therapy, diagnostic imaging, and in the cosmetic industry (Goins 2008, Patravale and Mandawgade 2008, Balazs and Godbey 2011, Mishra et al. 2011, Pierre and Costa 2011).

The potential application of liposomes in dental therapy can be based on two main principles: chemical or physical protection of the teeth, or both. The main focus of conventional dental pharmacotherapy has been the chemical protection of teeth with the aim to modify the demineralization and remineralization processes by the use of antibacterial and/or fluoride agents. To improve targeting and enhancing drug delivery to the teeth, liposomes may function as carriers for both conventional and new active substances. Three chemical approaches are possible: (i) to inhibit demineralization process by interfering with bacterial activity (acid production in the dental plaque) by using the combination of liposomes and antibacterials for targeting to oral bacteria or biofilm; (ii) to facilitate the remineralization process by the use of liposomes and inorganic ions such as fluoride, calcium, and phosphate; and, (iii) to immunize against dental caries by the use of liposome-based vaccines.

Inhibiting demineralization with liposomes

Better understanding in oral microbiology has lead to the targeting of antibacterials to oral biofilms instead of planktonic bacteria in the combat of infectious dental diseases. Already in the late 1990s, investigations on the use of liposomes to deliver the bactericides triclosan and chlorhexidine against the oral biofilm was initiated (Jones et al. 1997, Kaszuba et al. 1997). It was shown that liposomes adsorbed to a bacterial surface. Because most bacteria have a net negative surface charge, cationic liposomes attract to bacteria by electrostatic interactions. Anionic liposomes are also able to interact with bacteria, however, by a different mechanism (hydrogen bonding). Follow-up studies demonstrated a rapid release of bactericides from the liposomes allowing drug penetration into the biofilm (Jones et al. 1997). Compared to free bactericides, superior delivery was observed with liposomal bactericides. Direct targeting to dental plaque by using liposomes as vehicles to deliver antibacterials may therefore be a more efficient method to utilize the drug, possibly reducing the concentration needed to obtain a therapeutic effect.

The liposome surface can be easily modified by conjugating monoclonal antibodies or ligands for more specific binding, e.g., to antigens expressed on the cell surface of bacteria. These so-called immunoliposomes, functioning as highly specific targeting vehicles, can be used to carry antibacterials for selective inhibition of the oral bacteria. Specific targeting is necessary to limit killing to the disease-causing bacteria and not the commensal species existing in parallel in the oral cavity. Based on the fact that certain oral bacteria are known to be initial colonizers of the tooth surface, targeting antimicrobial agents to these species may provide a better way to control the development of plaque bacteria implicated in dental caries and periodontal diseases. By the use of monoclonal antibodies, it was demonstrated that immunoliposomes had a better affinity to the oral bacterium *Streptococcus oralis*, which is a predominant early tooth colonizer, than liposomes bearing no antibodies (Robinson et al. 1998). The immunoliposomes prepared were physically stable with regard to size distribution. Since the antibody is an essential factor in this regard, ensuring antibody specificity and affinity in the formulation is important in the development of immunoliposomes.

Facilitating remineralization with liposomes

Nanoparticulate systems, such as liposomes, offer new avenues to remineralize the teeth. The outmost layer of the teeth, the dental enamel, is the hardest substance in the human body. The dental enamel is highly mineralized: the inorganic content ($\approx 96\%$ by weight) consists of crystalline calcium phosphate, also termed HA. Liposomes can be coated with calcium phosphate to increase the chemical recognition of the dental hard tissues. It has been investigated whether it is possible to deposit such nanocoatings on the liposomes (Fig. 3.5) (Schmidt et al. 2004). The researchers showed that it was feasible to prepare stable, discretely coated liposomes, and they suggested that these particles could be used in the delivery of bone and dental therapeutics due to the high content of calcium and phosphate. With increased targetability to the dental hard tissues, the calcium phosphate-coated liposomes could potentially entrap anticaries agents in their interior and deliver them directly on the tooth surface for a remineralizing action. More research is necessary to investigate the release mechanisms from the coated liposomes and the appropriate coating thickness of these particles to evaluate their potential as dental drug delivery systems.

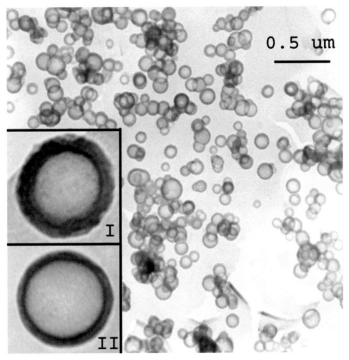

Figure 3.5. Transmission electron microscopy (TEM) images of calcium phosphate-coated liposomes. *I* and *II*: differences in the thickness of the coating layer. Bar length: 0.5 μm. Reprinted with permission from Schmidt et al. (2004). Copyright American Chemical Society (2004).

A modern trend in preventive dentistry is the use of biomimetic nanomaterials. Liposomes have been exploited as mediators for the mineral precipitation onto enamel surfaces based on a bioinspired strategy (Murphy and Messersmith 2000). Calcium and phosphate ions were separately entrapped in temperature-sensitive liposomes before they were mixed together. The liposome mixture was applied to warm human dentin and to the enamel surfaces. By an increase in the environmental temperature (to body temperature), the membrane of the liposomes became more permeable, thus leading to leakage of the entrapped ions. Outside the liposomes, the calcium and phosphate ions reacted to form calcium phosphate mineral, which deposited onto the surface of the tissue substrates. The idea with these so-called thermo-sensitive liposomes was to induce rapid inorganic mineral formation on tooth surfaces to facilitate remineralization, particularly in patients with incipient caries. Based on this concept, it was managed to deposit enamel-like HA on the enamel surface by mixing these thermo-sensitive calcium- and phosphate-loaded liposomes with a synthesized amelogenin-inspired peptide (Luo et al. 2012). Amelogenin has shown to be an important protein in the growth and nucleation of HA during enamel formation and enable HA to form well-organized prism patterns. The purpose of adding an amelogenin-like peptide was therefore to control the enamel remineralization and better mimicking the process that occurs during natural mineralized tissue formation.

Immunization with liposomes

S. mutans is one of the primary causative agents of dental caries in humans, using sucrose as a substrate to form a cariogenic biofilm. Once a biofilm is formed, susceptibility to antibiotics is significantly reduced, making it difficult to kill the bacteria. This has lead to other strategies to eliminate the source of contagion, such as immunological prevention methods. *S. mutans* possesses various cell-surface substances that play important roles in the interactions between the organism and its host, e.g., serotype-specific polysaccharide antigens, lipoteichoic acids, glucosyltransferases (GTFs), and glucan-binding proteins (Koga et al. 2002). By binding and blocking these substances, the initial adhesion and subsequent accumulation (plaque formation) by *S. mutans* on the dental enamel can be inhibited. Thus, cell-surface substances on cariogenic bacteria function as antigens and appear to be possible targets for a vaccine against dental caries. Immunological intervention enables another approach for the specific killing of cariogenic bacteria rather than the commensal bacteria. There are two methods of immunization: active immunity that induces salivary Ig A by providing antigens to the host through mucosal immunization, and passive immunity where a specific antibody against *S. mutans* is produced externally and applied to the oral cavity.

Many of the substances that are possible candidates for a dental vaccine are sensitive to degradation when delivered naked to the oral cavity. To optimize the immunization potential, nanocarrier systems have been utilized in the formulation of a mucosal vaccine. A liposome-based vaccine against dental caries with GTF was investigated (Childers et al. 1994). GTF is a key enzyme in the conversion of sucrose to glucans. Glucans are necessary for the accumulation of *S. mutans* on the tooth surface and the induction of caries. Thus, GTF presents as an important virulence factor of *S. mutans*. Salivary glands produce antigen-specific secretory Ig A antibodies that are secreted into saliva. By delivering GTF incorporated into liposomes, the aim was to intensify the induction of salivary Ig A immune response in humans that can protect against dental caries (active immunity). In this investigation, it was reported that the oral immunization of seven individuals by a liposomal GTF vaccine was effective in eliciting a secretory Ig A antibody response. This was one of the first studies presenting liposomes as adjuvants in the design of a caries vaccine. Although immunization provide a means to significantly reduce caries incidence, the development of a dental vaccine has been slow facing other issues than formulation challenges. The most likely target group for a caries vaccine is young children. Since no vaccine is absolutely safe, there is a great concern whether it is ethical to put healthy children at this risk since the disease does not affect survival rate. Moreover, the cost of large clinical trials are high and often requires financial support. Because dental infections are considered non-life-threatening diseases, low priority has been given to this type of clinical research (Taubman and Nash 2006, Smith 2010). Nonetheless, prospects of a dental caries vaccine remains promising as new technologies are emerging and government regulations are moving towards requiring and providing incentives for the conduct of pediatric clinical trials.

Physical protection by liposomes

Due to their small size, liposomes may also offer physical protection of the teeth. This strategy is based on another bioinspired concept. A thin proteinaceous layer termed the acquired pellicle is formed on all oral hard tissues from the oral fluid after tooth eruption or thorough tooth cleaning. The pellicle layer has many important functions to protect the dental surfaces; it serves as a physical barrier against demineralizing acids, modifies the attachment of cariogenic bacteria to the teeth, and lubricates the dental surfaces against normal wear (Hannig and Joiner 2006). It has been reported that phosphoproteins from saliva associate into micelle-like structures, from 100 to 500 nm in size, adsorbing to tooth surfaces forming the dental pellicle (Rykke et al. 1995). Thus, structures that morphologically resemble the salivary micelle-like globules can potentially mimic the properties of the natural protective mechanisms in the oral cavity. Casein micelles from bovine milk have long been known to have caries protective effects (Guggenheim et al. 1999). Globular casein micelles exhibited as single units with a size of ≈ 80 to 120 nm, appearing to be similar to human salivary micelle-like structures. Casein phosphopeptides derived from milk has been used to stabilize calcium and phosphate, forming complexes termed casein phosphopeptide-amorphous calcium phosphate. These nano-sized bioinspired particles have the ability to remineralize carious lesions in the dental enamel (Cross et al. 2007). By a similar bioinspired mechanism, liposomes can easily be designed to approximate the protective actions of the salivary micelle-like globules. In recent studies, phospholipid liposomes were formulated to adsorb to synthetic HA and later to the human dental enamel in order to investigate their potential as dental drug delivery systems (Nguyen et al. 2010, 2011, 2013). The prepared liposomes were ≈ 200 nm in size, since this is the same size range as the micelle-like globules of the pellicle (Fig. 3.6). The surface of HA is amphoteric, exhibiting both calcium and phosphate ions at the surface, allowing for electrostatic interactions at the HA interface. Nguyen et al. (2010) observed that cationic liposomes adsorbed better to HA than their charged opposites. This was due to the predominance of negatively charged phosphate ions on the HA surface at neutral pH, enabling a strong attraction of the cationic liposomes. This study indicates the importance of the surface properties of the nanosystems in the physical protection of the dental enamel.

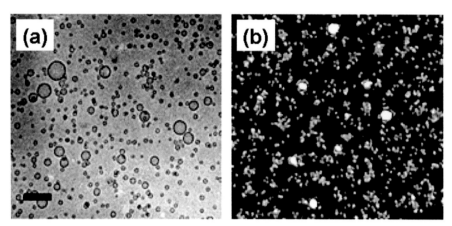

Figure 3.6. The resemblance of (a) liposomes to (b) the micelle-like structures of saliva. (a) Cryo-electron microscopy image of liposomes: the liposome dispersion was vitrified in a thin film and observed at –170°C in a transmission electron microscope. (b) Atomic force microscopy image of parotid saliva. Diluted parotid saliva was applied to freshly cleaved mica, air-dried, and observed in intermittent contact mode. Bar length: 100 nm.

Clearly, combining several mechanism for tooth protection would provide a better means to prevent and treat dental problems, in particular preventing tooth wear and reducing sypmtoms associated with a dry mouth. Adsorption of liposomes on tooth surfaces provide a physical layer that can minimize abrasion/attrition and acts as a tangible barrier against acids and mineral loss in tooth wear. This liposomal coat may also help to moisturize oral surfaces to reduce oral discomfort in xerostomic patients. A dual effect can be obtained when these liposomes encapsulate a chemical agent, e.g., a remineralization compound, to reduce erosion and/or prevent the development of caries. This synergism provide a more optimized therapy in patients vulnerable to tooth wear and xerostomia, or especially applied to patients at high risk of erosion.

Liposomes have been surface modified with mucoadhesive polymers, such as Carbopol® and chitosan (CS), to increase the bioadhesivity of the liposomes (Karn et al. 2011). Bioadhesive drug delivery systems help to maintain the drug in place of action to improve drug bioavailability. Bioadhesion in the oral cavity is useful to avoid the rapid elimination of pharmaceutics due to the constant flushing of saliva. Nguyen et al. (2011, 2013) prepared liposomes coated with the polymer pectin intended for dental drug delivery. They found that pectin-coated liposomes adsorbed and retained on the dental enamel despite being exposed to a flow rate similar to that of normal stimulated saliva. Bioadhesive liposomes may also be utilized in conditions such as xerostomia where prolonged lubrication is desirable. Saliva substitutes are often used to relieve xerostomic symptoms. The main disadvantage with available products is that they have to be used in a frequent manner to obtain a continuous effect. To overcome this problem, bioadhesive liposomes may be formulated to adhere to oral surfaces, increasing the retention time in the oral cavity and provide prolonged lubrication. However, this remains to be investigated.

Other nanostructured materials

Polymeric micelles

Micelles are vesicles composed of amphiphilic copolymers. They self-assemble under aqueous conditions and form a spherical core-shell structure. In order to form micelles the concentration of the polymer must be above the critical micelle concentration (CMC). The CMC is dependent upon the chemical structure of the polymer as well as the molecular weight of each block of the polymer (Tyrell et al. 2010, Ebrahim Attia et al. 2011). The micelles have a hydrophilic corona and a hydrophobic core where drugs with low water solubility can be dissolved. The size of the micelles ranges from 10 to 100 nm (Tyrrell et al. 2010). Micellar systems have been extensively studied in the field of drug delivery, particularly in cancer therapy, but yet no polymeric micelle product is registered on the market despite several botential formulations are under clinical trials (Talelli and Hennink 2011, Gong et al. 2012). One of the most studied polymeric micelles is commercialized under the name Pluronic®. These micelles are formed from the block copolymers of hydrophilic poly(ethylene oxide) and hydrophobic poly(propylene oxide) (Ebrahim Attia et al. 2011).

The potential of using micelles in dental therapy seems in many ways to be the same as for the liposomes, but the research is mainly concentrated around chemical protection of the teeth. Special focus has been on inhibiting the demineralization process by using the combination of micelles and antibacterials for targeting the biofilm. A biomineral-binding moiety (alendronate) was covalently attached to Pluronic® P85 and Pluronic® P123 and micelles of ≈ 100 nm in size were produced (Chen et al. 2009). Alendronate was used to obtain high affinity to HA and thereby increase targetability and binding to the tooth surfaces. Farnesol, an anti-caries agent with low water solubility, was successfully encapsulated in these micelles. The study showed that the affinity for HA was higher for the micelles with alendronate compared to the micelles without this moiety and ethanol solutions of farnesol. The drug showed a sustained release over a period of 48 hours. A follow-up study incorporated triclosan, also a drug with low water solubility, into these mineral binding micelles (Chen et al. 2010). The *in vitro* ability of this formulation to inhibit biofilm formation by S. mutans was then tested. The micelles released triclosan in a sustained manner over 48 hr and were superior to the blank control in inhibiting the biofilm formation at both an early and mature stage of the biofilm development. Thus, polymeric micelles seem promising for dental delivery of drugs with low water solubility.

Polymeric nanoparticles

Polymeric NPs can be produced both from synthetically derived polymers, such as Pluronics® and poly(D,L-lactide-*co*-glycolide) (PLGA), as well as from biopolymers, such as CS and alginate. Different methods exist for producing

NPs from polymers, but all NPs for pharmaceutical purposes should be in the range from 40 to 400 nm (Dinarvand et al. 2011).

PLGA is a synthetic biodegradable polymer commonly used in drug delivery. Different drug products containing this polymer have been approved by the Food and Drug Administration (FDA), and the research on this compound is tremendous (Fredenberg et al. 2011). Formulations such as microparticles, pellets, and implants have been investigated. NPs from this polymer can be produced by several methods, but all methods include starting with an emulsified system (Dinarvand et al. 2011). Then, several routes can be followed to obtain NPs. The potential of using PLGA NPs in dental therapy seems to be the same as for the micelles. PLGA NPs loaded with triclosan have been proposed as a potential drug delivery system for the treatment of periodontal diseases (Pinon-Segundo et al. 2005). However, the research conducted on PLGA NPs is mainly concentrated on antimicrobial photodynamic therapy (aPDT) and killing of the bacteria embedded in the biofilm. aPDT is a relatively new treatment modality in dentistry using a photosensitizer in combination with light to obtain a bactericidal effect (Konopka and Goslinski 2007). This treatment modality can be useful in the treatment of dental caries and periodontal diseases due to several advantages: the treatment has direct effect on the oral biofilm by disrupting the plaque structures, it has an effect against antibiotic resistant and antibiotic-susceptible bacteria, and there is a low risk of drug resistance development. NPs have been used as carrier systems to target and deliver the photosensitizers to microorganisms. NPs may also protect the photosensitizers from being ineffective and enhance their solubility because many photosensitizers are very hydrophobic. Nanoparticulate systems that have been suggested in the aPDT literature besides from polymeric NPs are liposomes, micelles, and cyclodextrins (Tsai et al. 2009, Pagonis et al. 2010, Hegge et al. 2012, Longo et al. 2012).

In a recent study, methylene blue, a well-established photosensitizer for targeting oral bacteria, was encapsulated in poly(ethylene oxide)-PLGA NPs (Pagonis et al. 2010). The toxicity against *Enterococcus faecalis*, a microorganism associated with endodontic infections, and the ability to deliver the photosensitizer to the root canal system were investigated. The study showed that the NPs adhered to the bacteria (Fig. 3.7) and that the viability both in the planktonic phase and in the root canal was reduced. In a follow-up study, methylene blue was encapsulated in both anionic and cationic PLGA NPs and tested on dental plaque samples (Klepac-Ceraj et al. 2011). The study showed that the cationic methylene blue-loaded NPs developed the highest toxicity against both planktonic and biofilm bacteria. However, the toxicity was not significantly higher than the anionic methylene blue-loaded NPs and free methylene blue. The explanation could be that methylene blue was not released in sufficient concentrations to allow a significant difference in the bacteria killing. Nonetheless, cationic PLGA NPs are still promising nanocarriers for biofilm uptake and more research is needed to optimize the delivery for use in aPDT.

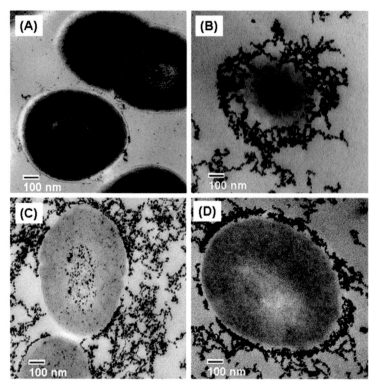

Figure 3.7. TEM images of: (A) *E. faecalis*, and PLGA NPs adhering to the cell walls of the bacteria after 2.5 minutes (B), 5 minutes (C), and 10 minutes (D) of incubation. Bar lengths: 100 nm. Reprinted with permission from Pagonis et al. (2010). Copyright American Association of Endodontists (2010).

CS is a biopolymer mainly composed of β-1,4-linked glucosamine and N-acetyl-D-glucosamine, and is derived from the exoskeleton of crustaceans. CS is a cationic biopolymer and is considered as non-toxic (Roberts 1992). In addition to its mucoadhesive properties, CS has both antibacterial and antifungal activity (Rabea et al. 2003). CS has been studied in many different formulations for drug delivery such as microparticles, coatings, and pellets. CS NPs can be prepared from different methods; one of the most common is ionotropic gelation with divalent ions such as sodium tripolyphosphate (Dash et al. 2011). The potential of NPs derived from CS seems to be the same as for the other polymeric nanostructures, namely inhibiting the formation of the biofilm. NPs derived from CS have been evaluated as a delivery system for root canal disinfection (Kishen et al. 2008). In this study, the antibacterial and antibiofilm effect of CS NPs, zinc oxide NPs, a combination of zinc oxide and CS NPs, and zinc oxide NPs coated with CS were investigated. All types of NPs showed antibacterial effect against *E. faecalis*. When the NPs were mixed with a sealer, the antibacterial effect of the sealer improved together with its flow characteristics. To examine the ability of the NPs to prevent bacterial adherence on root canal dentin, dentin was first treated with different irrigants and then the nanoformulations were added. Root canal dentin irrigated with chlorhexidine, which was found to render maximum reduction in bacterial adherence, and later treated with NPs showed a consistent reduction (approx. 97%) in bacterial adherence. This confirmed the positive antibiofilm effect of the NPs.

Potential limitations with nanoparticulate drug delivery systems

Despite the numerous advantages with nanoparticulate structures, there are some challenges that might occur and limit their development as dental drug delivery systems.

Formulation instabilities

Stability problems are one of the main hurdles in pharmaceutical manufacturing, requiring the product to tolerate handling and transportation and still remain stable during shelf life. There are three different processes for instability: chemical, physical, and biological. With nanopharmaceutics such as liposomes, chemical degradation can occur by hydrolysis of the ester bond or oxidation of unsaturated phospholipids. Both reactions can lead to increased permeability of the lipid bilayers and premature leakage of the drug. Methods such as freeze-drying can be applied in the manufacturing process in order to improve liposomal *in vitro* stability. Physical processes that affect shelf life include loss of the entrapped drug within the nanosystem as well as changes in particle size due to aggregation and fusion. Aggregation is the reversible formation of larger units of nanoparticulate material, while fusion is an irreversible process where the nano-units are coming together and form new colloidal structures. Biological stability refers to the stability of the nanosystems in biological fluids. For drug delivery to the teeth, the systems are influenced by the intraoral environment, such as salivary macromolecules, enzymes, pH variation, food substances, and salivary flow rates. Hence, there is a minute balance between overcoming oral obstacles to obtain a therapeutic effect without negatively interfering the biological system and its physiological functions (safety concern). For liposomes, stability can be controlled by manipulating formulation factors such as phospholipid composition, size distribution, and surface properties to improve the *in vivo* stability.

Safety concern

The small dimension of nanosystems renders them novel properties, making it difficult to predict the toxicity of nanosystems from the toxicity known for the chemical entity itself. The type of nanomaterials used need also to be addressed, such as their biocompatibility and biodegradability. The associated risks of using nanoparticulate carriers, especially long-term use, are not yet clear. There is still a major need to fully understand how nanoparticulate carriers interact with the body's system, and how they are distributed and transported across compartmental barriers in the body.

Other considerations

Other challenges faced by the general use of nanoparticulate carriers are feasibility of mass production, regulation, and social issues such as ethics and public acceptance. These issues should be addressed early in the development of a nanoparticulate product.

Conclusions

The use of nanoparticulate systems is an emerging field in medicine as well as in dentistry. Nanopharmaceutics are promising in providing more efficient prophylactic measures and in improving dental pharmacotherapeutic outcomes. It therefore has the potential to bring significant benefits to health. The application of nanomedicine in dentistry is still in its infancy and further research is necessary to elucidate the issues of translating stable nanoformulations from the laboratory into the clinics. As with all pharmaceutics, nanomedicinal products need also to demonstrate efficacy, quality, and safety before they can be used to provide better dental care to the public. The implication of nanoparticulate systems in modern dental practice will become clearer as research efforts are put through, involving interdisciplinary collaboration and expertise of scientists in dentistry, pharmacy, chemistry, and biology.

Abbreviations

aPDT	:	antimicrobial photodynamic therapy
CMC	:	critical micelle concentration
CS	:	chitosan
FDA	:	food and drug administration
GTF	:	glucosyltransferase
HA	:	hydroxyapatite
Ig	:	immunoglobulin
NP	:	nanoparticle
PLGA	:	poly(D,L-lactide-*co*-glycolide)
TEM	:	transmission electron microscopy

References

Aas, J.A. and B.J. Paster, L.N. Stokes, I. Olsen and F.E. Dewhirst. 2005. Defining the normal bacterial flora of the oral cavity. J. Clin. Microbiol. 43: 5721–5732.

Allaker, R.P. 2010. The use of nanoparticles to control oral biofilm formation. J. Dent. Res. 89(11): 1175–1186.

Baghramian, R.A. and F. Garcia-Godoy and A.R. Volpe. 2009. The global increase in dental caries. A pending public health crisis. Am. J. Dent. 23: 3–8.

Balazs, D.A. and W.T. Godbey. 2011. Liposomes for use in gene delivery. J. Drug Deliv. 2011: 326497.

Boulaiz, H. and P.J. Alvarez, A. Ramirez, J.A. Marchal, J. Prados, F. Rodriguez-Serrano, M. Peran, C. Melguizo and A. Aranega. 2011. Nanomedicine: application areas and development prospects. Int. J. Mol. Sci. 12: 3303–3321.

Chauhan, V.P. and R.K. Jain. 2013. Strategies for advancing cancer nanomedicine. Nat. Mater. 12: 958–962.

Chen, H. and B.H. Clarkson, K. Sun and J.F. Mansfield. 2005. Self-assembly of synthetic hydroxyapatite nanorods into an enamel prism-like structure. J. Colloid Interface Sci. 288: 97–103.

Chen, F. and X.-M. Liu, K.C. Rice, X. Li, F. Yu, R.A. Reinhardt, K.W. Bayles and D. Wang. 2009. Tooth-binding micelles for dental caries prevention. Antimicrob. Agents Chemother. 53: 4898–4902.

Chen, F. and K.C. Rice, X.M. Liu, R.A. Reinhardt, K.W. Bayles and D. Wang. 2010. Triclosan-loaded tooth-binding micelles for prevention and treatment of dental biofilm. Pharm. Res. 27: 2356–2364.

Chen, M.H. 2010. Update on dental nanocomposites. J. Dent. Res. 89: 549–560.

Childers, N.K. and S.S. Zhang and S.M. Michalek. 1994. Oral immunization of humans with dehydrated liposomes containing *Streptococcus mutans* glucosyltransferase induces salivary immunoglobulin A2 antibody responses. Oral Microbiol. Immunol. 9: 146–153.

Cotrim, A.P. and C. Zheng and B.J. Baum. 2013. Xerostomia. pp. 233–248. *In*: S.T. Sonis and D.M. Keefe [eds.]. Pathology of Cancer Regimen-Related Toxicities Springer, New York, USA.

Cross, K.J. and N.J. Huq and E.C. Reynolds. 2007. Casein phosphopeptides in oral health—chemistry and clinical applications. Curr. Pharm. Des. 13: 793–800.

Dash, M. and F. Chiellini, R.M. Ottenbrite and E. Chiellini. 2011. Chitosan—A versatile semi-synthetic polymer in biomedical applications. Prog. Polym. Sci. 36: 981–1014.

Dinarvand, R. and N. Sepehri, S. Manoochehri, H. Rouhani and F. Atyabi. 2011. Polylactide-co-glycolide nanoparticles for controlled delivery of anticancer agents. Int. J. Nanomedicine. 6: 877–895.

Doane, T.L. and C. Burda. 2012. The unique role of nanoparticles in nanomedicine: imaging, drug delivery and therapy. Chem. Soc. Rev. 41: 2885–2911.

Duckwroth, R.M. 1993. The science behind caries prevention. Int. Dent. J. 43: 529–539.

Ebrahim Attia, A.B. and Z.Y. Ong, J.L. Hedrick, P.P. Lee, P.L.R. Ee, P.T. Hammond and Y.Y. Yang. 2011. Mixed micelles self-assembled from block copolymers for drug delivery. Curr. Opin. Colloid Interface Sci. 16: 182–194.

Ferguson, D.B. and A. Shuttleworth and D.K. Whittaker. 1999. Oral Bioscience. Churchill Livingstone, New York, USA.

Fredenberg, S. and M. Wahlgren, M. Reslow and A. Axelsson. 2011. The mechanisms of drug release in poly(lactic-co-glycolic acid)-based drug delivery systems—a review. Int. J. Pharm. 415: 34–52.

Goins, B.A. 2008. Radiolabeled lipid nanoparticles for diagnostic imaging. Expert Opin. Med. Diagn. 2: 853–873.

Gong, J. and M. Chen, Y. Zheng, S. Wang and Y. Wang. 2012. Polymeric micelles drug delivery system in oncology. J. Control. Release. 159: 312–323.

Guggenheim, B. and R. Schmid, J.M. Aeschlimann, R. Berrocal and J.R. Neeser. 1999. Powered milk micellar case in prevents oral colonization by *Streptococcus sobrinus* and dental caries in rats: a basis for the caries-protective effects of dairy products. Caries Res. 33: 446–454.

Hannig, M. and A. Joiner. The structure, function and properties of acquired pellicle. pp. 29–64. *In*: R.M. Duckworth [ed.]. 2006. The Teeth and Their Environment. Monogr. Oral Sci. Karger, Basel, Switzerland.

Hannig, M. and C. Hannig. 2010. Nanomaterials in preventive dentistry. Nat. Nanotechnol. 5: 565–569.

Hannig, M. and C. Hannig. 2012. Nanotechnology and its role in caries therapy. Adv. Dent. Res. 24: 53–57.

Hegge, A.B. and T.T. Nielsen, K.L. Larsen, E. Bruzell and H.H. Tønnesen. 2012. Impact of curcumin supersaturation in antibacterial photodynamic therapy—effect of cyclodextrin type and amount: studies on curcumin and curcuminoides XLV. J. Pharm. Sci. 101: 1524–1537.

Jones, M.N. and Y.H. Song, M. Kaszuba and M.D. Reboiras. 1997. The interaction of phospholipid liposomes with bacteria and their use in the delivery of bactericides. J. Drug Target. 5: 23–34.

Kaasgaard, T. and T.L. Andresen. 2010. Liposomal cancer therapy: exploiting tumor characteristics. Expert Opin. Drug Deliv. 7: 225–243.

Karn, P.R. and Z. Vanić, I. Pepić and N. Škalko-Basnet. 2011. Mucoadhesive liposomal delivery systems: the choice of coating material. Drug Dev. Ind. Pharm. 37: 482–488.

Kaszuba, M. and A.M. Robinson, Y.H. Song, J.E. Creeth and M.N. Jones. 1997. The visualization of the targeting of phospholipid liposomes to bacteria. Colloids Surf. B Biointerfaces. 8: 321–332.

Kishen, A. and Z. Shi, A. Shrestha and K.G. Neoh. 2008. An investigation on the antibacterial and antibiofilm efficacy of cationic nanoparticulates for root canal disinfection. J. Endod. 34: 1515–1520.

Klepac-Ceraj, V. and N. Patel, X. Song, C. Holewa, C. Patel, R. Kent, M.M. Amiji and N.S. Soukos. 2011. Photodynamic effects of methylene blue-loaded polymeric nanoparticles on dental plaque bacteria. Lasers Surg. Med. 43: 600–606.

Koga, T. and T. Oho, Y. Shimazaki and Y. Nakano. 2002. Immunization against dental caries. Vaccine. 20: 2027–2044.

Konopka, K. and T. Goslinski. 2007. Photodynamic therapy in dentistry. J. Dent. Res. 86: 694–707.

Longo, J.P.F. and S.C. Leal, A.R. Simioni, M.F.M. Almeida-Santos, A.C. Tedesco and R.B. Azevedo. 2012. Photodynamic therapy disinfection of carious tissue mediated by aluminum-chloride-phtalocyanine entrapped in cationic liposomes: an *in vitro* and clinical study. Lasers Med. Sci. 27: 575–584.

Luo, J.J. and T.Y. Ning, Y. Cao, X.P. Zhu, X.H. Xu, X.Y. Tang, C.H. Chu and Q.L. Li. 2012. Biomimic enamel remineralization by hybridization calcium- and phosphate-loaded liposomes with amelogenin-inspired peptide. Key Eng. Mater. 512: 1727–1730.

Marsh, P. and M.V. Martin. 2009. Oral Microbiology. 5th Edition. Churchill Livingstone Elsevier, Oxford, UK.

Mishra, G.P. and M. Bagui, V. Tamboli and A.K. Mitra. 2011. Recent applications of liposomes in ophthalmic drug delivery. J. Drug Deliv. 2011: 863734.

Murphy, W. and P.B. Messersmith. 2000. Compartmental control of mineral formation: adaptation of a biomineralization strategy for biomedical use. Polyhedron. 19: 357–363.

Nguyen, S. and L. Solheim, R. Bye, M. Rykke, M. Hiorth and G. Smistad. 2010. The influence of liposomal formulation factors on the interactions between liposomes and hydroxyapatite. Colloids Surf. B Biointerfaces. 76: 354–361.

Nguyen, S. and M. Hiorth, M. Rykke and G. Smistad. 2011. The potential of liposomes as dental drug delivery systems. Eur. J. Pharm. Biopharm. 77: 75–83.

Nguyen, S. and M. Hiorth, M. Rykke and G. Smistad. 2013. Polymer coated liposomes for dental drug delivery - Interactions with parotid saliva and dental enamel. Eur. J. Pharm. Sci. 50: 78–85.

Pagonis, T.C. and J. Chen, C.R. Fontana, H. Devalapally, K. Ruggiero, X. Song, F. Foschi, J. Dunham, Z. Skobe, H. Yamazaki, R. Kent, A.C. Tanner, M.M. Amiji and N.S. Soukos. 2010. Nanoparticle-based endodontic antimicrobial photodynamic therapy. J. Endod. 36: 322–328.

Patravale, V.B. and S.D. Mandawgade. 2008. Novel cosmetic delivery systems: an application update. Int. J. Cosmet. Sci. 30: 19–33.

Pepperney, A. and M.L. Chikindas. 2011. Antibacterial peptides: opportunities for the prevention and treatment of dental caries. Probiotics & Antimicro. Prot. 3: 68–96.

Petersen, P.E. and D. Bourgeois, H. Ogawa, S. Estupinan-Day and C. Ndiaye. 2005. The global burden of oral diseases and risks to oral health. Bull. World Health Organ. 83: 661–669.

Pierre, M.B. and I. Dos Santos Miranda Costa. 2011. Liposomal systems as drug delivery vehicles for dermal and transdermal applications. Arch. Dermatol. Res. 303: 607–621.

Pinon-Segundo, E. and A. Ganem-Quintanar, V. Alonso-Perez and D. Quintanar-Guerrero. 2005. Preparation and characterization of triclosan nanoparticles for periodontal treatment. Int. J. Pharm. 294: 217–232.

Rabea, E.I. and M.E.T. Badawy, C.V. Stevens, G. Smagghe and W. Steurbaut. 2003. Chitosan as antimicrobial agent: applications and mode of action. Biomacromolecules. 4: 1457–1465.

Renugalakshmi, A. and T.S. Vinothkumar and D. Kandaswamy. 2011. Nanodrug delivery systems in dentistry: a review on current status and future perspectives. Curr. Drug Deliv. 8: 586–594.

Roberts, G.A.F. Preparation of chitin and chitosan. pp. 54–84. *In*: G.A.F. Roberts [ed.]. 1992. Chitin Chemistry. The Macmillian Press Ltd., London, UK.

Robinson, A.M. and J.E. Creeth and M.N. Jones. 1998. The specificity and affinity of immunoliposomes targeting to oral bacteria. Biochim. Biophys. Acta. 1369: 278–286.

Rykke, M. and G. Smistad, G. Roella and J. Karlsen. 1995. Micelle-like structures in human saliva. Colloids Surf. B Biointerfaces. 4: 33–44.

Schmidt, H.T. and B.L. Gray, P.A. Wingert and A.E. Ostafin. 2004. Assembly of aqueous-cored calcium phosphate nanoparticles for drug delivery. Chem. Mater. 16: 4942–4947.

Selwitz, R.H. and A.I. Ismail and N.B. Pitts. 2007. Dental caries. Lancet. 369: 51–59.

Slingerland, M. and H.J. Guchelaar and H. Gelderblom. 2012. Liposomal drug formulations in cancer therapy: 15 years along the road. Drug Discov. Today 17: 160–166.

Smith, D.J. 2010. Dental caries vaccines: prospects and concerns. Expert Rev. Vaccines 9: 1–3.

Talelli, M. and W.E. Hennink. 2011. Thermosensitive polymeric micelles for targeted drug delivery. Nanomedicine (Lond.). 6: 1245–1255.

Taubman, M.A. and D.A. Nash. 2006. The scientific and public-health imperative for a vaccine against dental caries. Nat. Rev. Immunol. 6: 555–563.

Tsai, T. and Y.T. Yang, T.H. Wang, H.F. Chien and C.T. Chen. 2009. Improved photodynamic inactivation of gram-positive bacteria using hematoporphyrin encapsulated in liposomes and micelles. Lasers Surg. Med. 41: 316–322.

Tyrrell, Z.L. and Y. Shen and M. Radosz. 2010. Fabrication of micellar nanoparticles for drug delivery through the self-assembly of block copolymers. Prog. Polym. Sci. 35: 1128–1143.

Wang, R. and P.S. Billone and W.M. Mullett. 2013. Nanomedicine in action: an overview of cancer nanomedicine on the market and in clinical trials. J. Nanomater. 2013: 1–12.

Xia, Y. and F. Zhang, H. Xie and N. Gu. 2008. Nanoparticle-reinforced resin-based dental composites. J. Dent. 36: 450–455.

CHAPTER 4

Nanotechnology for Topical and Transdermal Drug Delivery and Targeting

Elizabeth Ryan,[1,a] *Jeffrey E. Grice*[1,b] and
Michael S. Roberts[1,2,3,]*

ABSTRACT

The application of nanotechnology to transdermal and topical delivery and targeting has heralded a new era in the delivery of therapeutics through the skin and in cosmetic applications. Progress in the field of topical and transdermal drug delivery in the last number of decades has been remarkable, with the development of an array of therapeutic nanoparticles. The skin's inherent barrier function limits the delivery routes available to many nanoparticles; however some concern has been raised regarding the ability of some nanoparticles to penetrate the *stratum corneum* and reach the viable epidermis. The intercellular route is proposed as being the main path for nanoparticle delivery across intact skin, along with the hair follicles. Transdermal nanoparticle delivery is also being enhanced using delivery devices called microneedles and other technologies such as electroporation. One of the most recent developments of note in the field of nanotechnology is the formulation of deformable liposomes which enhance penetration efficacy

[1] Therapeutics Research Centre, School of Medicine, University of Queensland, Translational Research Institute, Princess Alexandra Hospital, Woolloongabba QLD 4102, Australia.
[a] Email: e.ryan@uq.edu.au
[b] Email: jeff.grice@uq.edu.au
[2] Therapeutics Research Centre, School of Pharmacy and Medical Sciences, and Sansom Institute for Health Research, University of South Australia, Adelaide SA 5001, Australia.
[3] The Basil Hetzel Institute for Translational Health Research, The Queen Elizabeth Hospital, Woodville South SA 5011, Australia.
* Corresponding author: m.roberts@uq.edu.au

through the skin, and also allow targeted delivery to cells. Although the interest in nanotechnology for transdermal and topical delivery has grown significantly, there are still a number of practical limitations and toxicity issues which must be addressed.

Introduction

The application of nanotechnology to medicine has already had a significant impact in many areas. Within the last two decades, a number of nanoparticle (NP)-based therapeutic and diagnostic agents have been developed for the treatment of cancer, diabetes, pain, asthma, allergy, and infections. Currently, more than 20 NP-based therapeutics are in clinical use, validating the ability of NPs to improve the therapeutic index of drugs (Zhang et al. 2007). Nanotechnology is the engineering and manufacturing of materials at the atomic and molecular scale, i.e., a structure in the 1 to 100 nm size range in at least one dimension, although nanotechnology is commonly used to describe structures that are up to several micrometers in size (Farokhzad and Langer 2009). Various types of NPs have been applied to a range of medicinal purposes, including liposomes, polymeric micelles, quantum dots (QDs), gold (Au) and silicon polymer shells, dendrimers, carbon nanotubes, and fullerenes (DeLouise et al. 2012, Liu et al. 2012).

The application of nanotechnology to drug delivery is already changing the landscape of the pharmaceutical and biotechnological industries, due to its broad ranging advantages over conventional therapeutics. These advantages include the possible improved delivery of poorly water soluble drugs, the cell or tissue specific targeted delivery of drugs, the transcytosis of drugs across endothelial and epithelial barriers, the delivery of macromolecules to intracellular sites of action, the co-delivery of two or more drugs for combination therapies, the visualization of sites of drug delivery by combining therapeutic agents with imaging modalities, and the real time analysis of *in vivo* therapeutic efficacy. A major limitation includes the complexity of manufacture of these systems, which may cause difficulty for generic companies (Farokhzad and Langer 2009, Liu et al. 2012).

In terms of transdermal delivery, the skin provides a natural barrier against particle penetration; however certain opportunities exist to deliver NPs to and through the skin, specifically in diseased skin and the openings of hair follicles (Prow et al. 2011). For topical products, such as sunscreens, it has been accepted that NPs such as zinc oxide (ZnO) and titanium dioxide (TiO_2) can be detected in the *stratum corneum* (*SC*) layer of the skin. However, the penetration of NPs into the viable layers of the skin may cause adverse toxicological effects (Nohynek et al. 2007). A substantial amount of research is now being focused on proving the safety of these topical sunscreen formulations.

Recent advances in NP-based therapeutics have been in three main areas: skin cancer imaging and targeted therapeutics, immunomodulation and vaccine delivery, and antimicrobials and wound healing. Nanotechnology has been applied to skin cancer therapy for imaging and therapeutic purposes, with a major focus on diagnosing and treating metastatic melanoma. One of the main advantages of nanotechnology in this area is that NPs allow selective delivery of the therapeutic entity to the melanoma cells, thereby removing the problem of wide scale chemotherapeutic drug cytotoxicity to healthy cells. NPs also allow for insoluble drugs to be loaded within them. A large range of drugs and high loading efficiencies can be obtained with NP formulations (DeLouise 2012). The skin provides both innate and adaptive immune responses. The use of NPs in transcutaneous immune modulation has been receiving much interest with recent publications showing the ability of NPs to carry antigens and to accumulate in hair follicles following mechanical agitation (Toll et al. 2004, Lademann et al. 2007). The third main advancing area in NP technology is the application of NPs for antimicrobial and wound healing purposes. Much work has been focused on the use of silver (Ag) and Au NPs due to the inherent antimicrobial properties of Ag ions and the antimicrobial and odor reducing properties of nano-Au (DeLouise 2012). The amount and depth of NP penetration into hair follicles is dependent on many factors, but the particle size has received much attention (Vogt et al. 2006, Lademann et al. 2007).

Design considerations of NPs, including their geometry and surface functionalization are the parameters which influence their transport and adhesion to each other and to biological milieu. An emerging area in NP technology is the fabrication of NPs that can actively change their shape and properties based on their local environment. This would improve the biological specificity in diagnosis and therapies through a precise control of agent delivery. Stimuli responsive nanoplatforms are being developed which will release their payload following an external stimulus such as pH, temperature, light or magnetic field, depending on the characteristics of each specific nanoplatform (Liu et al. 2012). Recent advances in this area include the use of pH- and heat-sensitive NPs to target tumor sites (Soppimath et al. 2007).

The Application of Nanotechnology to Transdermal and Topical Drug Delivery

The benefits of nanotechnology are many. The physicochemical properties of nanomaterials are often distinctly different from their bulk form. These physicochemical traits can then be harnessed to provide the required therapeutic effect. Nanomaterials and devices are expected to become faster, smaller, more efficient, and more powerful. Consequently, treatments are expected to become more efficacious, more flexible and specific, and devices and drugs are expected to be more customized, versatile and cost effective (Nasir 2010). NPs can be fabricated from a wide range of organic and inorganic materials such as emulsions, solid lipid nanoparticles (SLNs), nanocapsules, nanospheres, micelles, liposomes, dendrimers, QDs, fullerenes and carbon nanotubes. These materials are being used to encapsulate and solubilize therapeutic agents for improved drug delivery *in vivo*, or provide unique optical, magnetic, and electrical properties for imaging and therapy. Liposomes and SLNs have both been applied to transcutaneous drug delivery, with some being commercialized and many more in clinical trials (DeLouise 2012).

The application of any molecule (pharmaceutical system, cosmetic preparation, or sunscreen) to the skin is basically divided into three distinct delivery areas: topical, the skin itself (epidermis or dermis) or the systemic circulation. The surface of the skin may be a target when considering delivery of antiseptics, insect repellents, sunscreens, or cosmetics. This is called topical delivery. Targeting the various layers of the skin is relevant when the disease state is present within the organ itself; this is called regional delivery. Examples of regional delivery include treating neoplasias, inflammatory disorders, and microbial infections of the skin (Brown et al. 2006). Transdermal or percutaneous delivery, whereby the systemic circulation is the principal target, is being considered as an alternative to conventional systemic and oral routes of administration.

The skin is an attractive site for the systemic delivery of pharmaceuticals (Gupta and Sharma 2009), as well as for more localized delivery. There are many advantages offered by the transdermal route when compared to other non-invasive delivery routes. These advantages include the avoidance of the first pass hepatic metabolism, the potential for continuous drug administration, the reduction in side effects associated with systemic toxicity, improved patient acceptance and compliance, direct access to target diseased site for treatment of skin disorders such as eczema and psoriasis, easy dose termination in the event of any adverse reaction, convenient and painless administration, and the availability of an alternative treatment type for when other dosing is not possible (Brown et al. 2006). Although the skin provides a formidable barrier to drug delivery, due almost completely to the SC, over 35 transdermal products (16 approved molecules) were approved in 2008 (Tanner and Marks 2008). The active pharmaceutical ingredients which have the ability to permeate the SC share a number of characteristics including being highly potent, small (< 500 Da), reasonably water-soluble, and relatively highly lipophilic (Magnusson et al. 2004, Coulman et al. 2009).

The skin is the largest and one of the most complex organs in the human body and is designed to carry out a wide range of functions (Fig. 4.1) (Chuong et al. 2002). The barrier properties of the skin ensure that the underlying organs are protected from external stresses, whether they are physical, chemical, or microbial. The skin contains specialized cells to defend against ultraviolet (UV) radiation and mop up free radicals. The deeper layers of the skin contain nerve endings for sense, and a highly developed vasculature, which plays an important role in nourishing the skin and in thermoregulation. Vitamin D synthesis is another key function performed by this organ (Menon 2002).

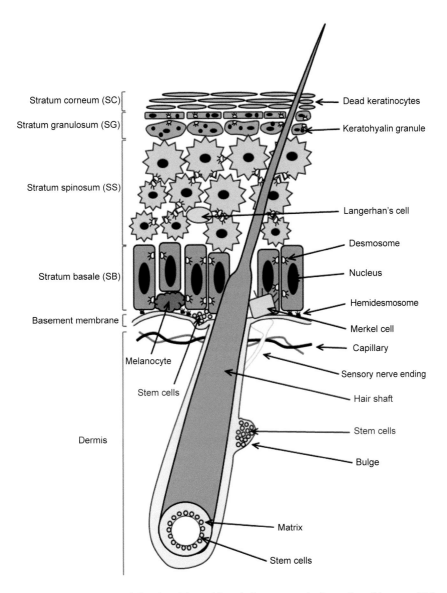

Figure 4.1. The structure of the skin. The epidermis is composed of a series of layers which are characterized by differences in cellular structure. The dermis sits beneath the epidermis. *SC: stratum corneum; SG: stratum granulosum; SS: stratum spinosum; SB: stratum basale.*

The *SC* is the outermost layer of the skin and is considered the main barrier to the percutaneous absorption of exogeneous material (Roberts and Cross 2008). The thickness of this layer in humans is typically 10 μm when dry, although factors such as the degree of hydration and skin location influence its thickness. The *SC* on the palms and soles can be, on average,

400 to 600 μm thick, whilst hydration can result in a four-fold increase in thickness (Roberts and Walters 2008). The *SC* consists of 10 to 25 layers of dead keratinocytes, now called corneocytes, embedded in the secreted lipids from lamellar bodies (Roberts and Walters 2008). Following a two week migration through the *SC*, corneocytes are sloughed off in a process known as desquamation (Egelrud 2000). The corneocytes are flattened, elongated, dead cells, lacking nuclei and other organelles (Benson 2005). The cells are joined together by desmosomes which maintain the cohesiveness of this layer (Menon 2002). The heterogeneous structure of the *SC* is composed of ≈ 75–80% proteins, 5–15% lipids, and 5–10% unidentified on a dry weight basis (Roberts and Walters 2008).

The cutaneous appendages include the pilosebaceous follicles, apocrine glands, and eccrine sweat glands. The pilosebaceous unit consists of the hair follicle, hair shaft, associated *arrector pili* muscle, and associated sebaceous gland. Hairs can be pigmented or non-pigmented and can extend more than 3 mm into the hypodermis (Meidan et al. 2005). The density of these units varies with body region. Follicular openings can account for up to 10% of the surface area on the face, whilst on other parts of the body, these orifices make up only 0.1% of the surface area (Meidan et al. 2005). The sebaceous gland secretes sebum which lubricates the skin surface and maintains skin surface pH at ≈ 5 (Singh and Singh 1993). The eccrine glands play an important part in thermoregulation and respond to increased temperature and stress by releasing sweat. The eccrine glands are located in the dermal tissue and are distributed throughout the body surface, with particular concentrations on the hands and feet. They are connected to a duct which ascends towards the surface (Bronaugh and Maibach 1989, Singh and Singh 1993). Humans have ≈ 3 to 4 million eccrine glands on their skin, which produce as much as 3 L/hour of sweat (Tobin 2006). The apocrine glands reside closer to the epidermal-dermal boundary and are associated with the axillae, and ano-genital regions. Their ducts are connected to the skin surface via hair follicles (Singh and Singh 1993, Tobin 2006).

The Langerhans cells are targeted in skin applied vaccine delivery as they are antigen presenting cells with immune function. They are generated in the bone marrow and migrate to and localize in the *SB*. They migrate from the epidermis to the dermis when activated by the binding of an antigen to the cell surface. From the dermis, they migrate to the regional lymph nodes and sensitize to the *T* cells where an immune response is generated. Melanocytes produce melanin which provides pigmentation of the skin, hair, and eyes. Melanin also absorbs UV radiation and therefore minimizes the liberation of free radicals. Merkel cells are associated with nerve endings, being concentrated in the fingertips and lips. It has been suggested that their primary function is cutaneous sensation (Benson 2012).

The Application of Nanotechnology to Cosmetic Formulations

NPs in cosmetic formulations have received much attention in recent years (Table 4.1), with the addition of TiO_2 and ZnO NPs to sunscreen formulations being a main area of interest. Active sunscreen ingredients can attenuate the damaging effect of overexposure to UV radiation, but can also elicit a range of side effects that have not yet been fully considered (Otberg et al. 2004). The original reason for metal oxide NP addition to sunscreens was to allow for transparent sunscreen formulations to be produced. ZnO particles which are normally opaque and greasy, become transparent and feel smooth when broken down into NPs. Emulsions are also commonly used in cosmetics. Those which are fragmented into nanometer-sized are less oily, have a smoother texture, and penetrate the hair and skin more deeply when incorporated into emollients and hair conditioners (Nasir 2010). The debate as to whether such formulations may allow penetration of NPs into the viable epidermis is ongoing.

Table 4.1. NPs found in topical consumer products. Adapted with permission from Robertson et al. (2010). Copyright American Scientific Publishers (2010).

NP	Dermal application	Total of consumer products	Other applications
TiO_2	Sunscreen, cosmetics	50	Cleaning products, sporting goods
ZnO	Sunscreen, cosmetics	30	Mineral supplement
Au	Cosmetics	27	Mineral supplement
Ag	Antibacterial, burn dressing, cosmetics	259	Clothing, cooking, toys, hair straightener, curler
Copper	Cosmetics	10	Mineral supplement
Manganese dioxide	Sunscreen (impurity)	1	–
Magnesium oxide, magnesium ascorbate	Cosmetics (magnesium ascorbate)	6	Mineral supplements, sporting goods
Aluminum oxide	Cosmetics	4	Antibacterial bathroom spray
Cerium oxide (CeO_2)	Proposed in sunscreens	1	Diesel catalyst
Platinum, platinum dioxide	Cosmetic	4	Colloidal supplement, fuel catalyst

A recent review paper by Pardeike et al. (2009) illustrated how recent developments in nanotechnology have impacted on cosmetic science, in particular SLNs and nanostructured lipid carriers (NLCs). Such lipid nanocarriers can form monolayer films on the skin. These films are hydrophobic and have an occlusive effect on the skin to prevent water loss by evaporation.

The size of the particles is proportional to the degree of occlusion. This is defined by the occlusion factor; at identical lipid content, reducing the particle size results in an increase in the number of particles. Also, at a set particle size, increasing the lipid concentration will also increase the number of particles. An increase in the number of particles consequently results in a more dense film, therefore enhancing the degree of occlusion. Smaller particle size results in a more effective evaporation barrier. The lipidic NP suspensions form dense films via particle fusion when pressure is applied to them on application to the skin. The capillary forces involved in evaporation promote this fusion. The hydration properties of NPs may also improve skin elasticity. The occlusive properties of lipidic particles have also been shown to influence the skin penetration of active ingredients. Muller and Dingler (1998) showed that the penetration of coenzyme Q_{10} and α-tocopherol applied in lipid microparticles or NPs varied significantly, with 40% more penetration occurring when NPs were used. Lipid NPs also provide excellent lubrication. Formulation aspects such as whitening and chemical stabilization can also be improved by using lipidic NPs. SLNs and NLCs are composed of a solid matrix capable of stabilizing active ingredients which are chemically labile. Lipid NPs have also been shown to have a synergistic effect on UV scattering when used in combination with molecular sunscreens, which may allow the reduction in the required concentration of molecular sunscreen. Super-loaded NLCs were developed which had a sunscreen loading of 70%. Other cosmetic applications of these lipidic carriers include encapsulants for perfumes, fragrances, and repellents.

Combinatorial Delivery Strategies

NPs must readily penetrate the *SC* to be therapeutically effective. For this reason, many enhancement strategies and technologies have been employed to assist in the disruption of this barrier. These technologies include methods which result in ablation or poration of the *SC* (Cevc and Vierl 2010). Examples of such technologies include tape stripping, microneedles (MNs), sonophoresis, electroporation, and gene gun technologies (Lindemann et al. 2003, Polat et al. 2011). Mechanoporation is the most common of all these techniques due to the advances in micron scale delivery devices (i.e., MNs) since the late 1990s.

MNs allow for the microporation of biological membranes for enhanced transdermal delivery. The application of such systems to the skin results in the creation of transport pathways of micron dimensions (Kaushik et al. 2001). MNs consist of an array of micro-projections, generally ranging from 25 to 2000 µm in height, of different shapes, which are attached to a base support (Garland et al. 2011). The most common type of MNs available include: (i) polymeric dissolvable MNs which include their payload within the needles themselves; (ii) coated MNs, which are usually prepared from materials like stainless steel and the payload is coated onto the needles; or, (iii) hollow MNs, through which a liquid formulation is injected through a pressurized system.

These micron pathways should readily permit the transport of macromolecules, as well as possibly supramolecular complexes and microparticles and NPs (Prausnitz 2004). The enhancement of delivery of drugs and biomolecules with a wide variety of physicochemical properties has been demonstrated in *in vitro*, *ex vivo*, and *in vivo* experiments. MN devices are also being developed for the convenient and pain-free delivery of vaccines across the skin barrier layer (Pearton et al. 2010, Chen et al. 2011). MN delivery systems are advantageous compared to other disruption techniques due in part to their simplicity of use, which results in patient friendly administration, and their low fabrication costs. Altering the geometry and fabrication material of MNs enables the control of drug release into the skin. In this way, drug delivery can be optimized to obtain the best therapeutic effect. MNs have been shown to penetrate the skin, across the SC, and into the viable epidermis. This can be achieved without causing pain, as they are unable to contact the nerve fibers which reside in the dermal layer (Kaushik et al. 2001). Recent MN publications have examined the enhancement of transdermal NP delivery using this technology. A recent paper by Coulman et al. (2009) showed the successful enhancement of delivery of fluorescent polystyrene (PS) NPs through MN treated skin. This paper used the traditional method, whereby MNs were just used to produce porations in the skin and the NP formulation was then applied. Another study by Donnelly et al. (2010) showed the successful delivery of nile red-loaded poly(D,L-lactide-*co*-glycolide) NPs into the skin using polymeric MNs. This system utilized a dissolvable MN system into which the NPs were incorporated. Other recent advances in MN technology include Mark Kendall's nanopatch system, consisting of arrays of densely packed microprojections which are designed to target vaccines. The nanopatches are coated with antigens, adjuvants, and/or deoxyribonucleic acid (DNA) payloads and have been successfully applied to vaccine delivery (Prow et al. 2010).

Skin flexing and massage has been shown to influence topical delivery and the toxicology of NPs through the skin. For drug delivery, hair follicles are of special interest because they are surrounded by blood capillaries, dendritic cells, and host stem cells (Lademann et al. 2009). A study by Tinkle et al. (2003) examined how mechanical stress on the skin affected NP penetration. Human skin was 300 to 400 µm thick and stored under constant hydration. It was treated with 0.5 µm and 1 µm beads, and the skin was fixed to a flexing device with double sided tape and flexed at 45°C, 20 flexes per minute or left flat for 15, 30, or 60 minutes. Control samples were not flexed. Following experimental manipulation, the skin samples were rinsed in phosphate buffered saline, fixed overnight in 10% buffered formalin, and flash frozen in liquid nitrogen. 0.5 µm beads and 1 µm beads penetrated into the epidermis in two of 11 skin samples (18%) flexed for 15 minutes, in five of 12 samples (41%) flexed for 30 minutes, and in nine of 16 samples (56%) flexed for 60 minutes. Penetration into the dermis occurred in two samples after flexing 60 minutes. Rouse et al. (2007) showed that flexing in fresh porcine skin increased the rate of penetration of 3.5 nm modified fullerenes. Skin was dermatomed to a thickness of 400 µm and was fixed to a flexing apparatus designed to flex skin at ± 45°C at a frequency of 20 flexes per minute. Following the application of the NP formulation, skin was flexed for 60 or 90 minutes. A non-flexed sample was used as a control. The fullerenes were primarily localized in the epidermal layers of non-flexed skin. Greater dermal penetration was seen in the 60 minute-samples and dermal penetration was seen in the 90 minute-samples. In this study, Transmission Electron Microscopy (TEM) allowed the visualization of the fullerenes localized within the intercellular spaces of the epidermis, suggesting that migration through the skin occurred intercellularly.

Greater penetration of NPs may be enabled in a formulation, skin type, and massage mechanism dependent manner (Prow et al. 2011). These findings are important in terms of the enhancement of NP penetration but accordingly, they must be considered with respect to the possibility of NP penetration into the skin from cosmetic and sunscreen formulations. The manner in which the general public applies such formulations to the skin and the way in which the skin naturally flexes on certain parts of the body may actually be increasing the possibility of NP penetration and therefore increasing possible adverse toxicological effects.

Considerations of the Skin as a Delivery Route for Nanoparticles

Following 15 years of investigation, there is still a debate as to whether NPs can penetrate healthy or impaired skin barriers. The wide variability seen in results from *in vitro* and *in vivo* skin studies between research groups, the limitations of certain analytical instruments to detect isolated NPs and the diverse range in NP types all add to the uncertainty of this debate. However, a number of trends have begun to emerge and it is generally accepted that healthy skin provides an effective barrier to NP penetration, NPs may congregate at the hair follicles (especially after skin massage and flexing, as described above) and the surface charge of the NPs influences skin interactions (DeLouise 2012). The fact that most environmental NPs (viruses, bacteria, dust, or allergens) do not penetrate human skin, proves what a formidable barrier the skin is. When the skin barrier is compromised, as in aged or diseased skin, there may be potential for enhanced particle penetration (Prow et al. 2011).

The intercellular route is the most favorable for the majority of penetrating molecules (Fig. 4.2). Small lipophilic molecules have the ability to freely move within these intercellular spaces. The rate of diffusion of such molecules is controlled by both their lipophilic character and their physiochemical characteristics, such as the ability to hydrogen bond, molecular weight, and solubility in a given vehicle (Potts and Guy 1995).

It is widely accepted that one of the main determinants of dermatological and systemic penetration across the skin is the delivery or flux of solutes across the skin. The maximum dose of a solute that can be delivered through the skin

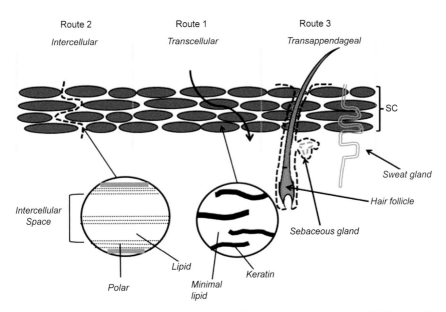

Figure 4.2. The possible routes of delivery for transdermal products across the SC. Route 1: the transcellular pathway. Route 2: the intercellular pathway. Route 3: the trans-appendageal pathway (across hair follicles, sweat glands, and sebaceous glands).

is defined by its maximum flux from a given vehicle. A paper by Magnusson et al. (2004) determined that the molecular size was the main determinant of maximum flux across the skin, with melting point, log octanol solubility, and molecular volume being less important parameters. As the skin barrier capacity is controlled by the lipids that fill the extracellular space, a number of studies have looked at lipid packing within the SC. Using conventional electron microscopy, Madison et al. (1987) reported that the SC lipid material or "lipid matrix" displays 13 nm-sized repeating units of broad:narrow:broad electron lucent bands. Garson et al. (1991) analyzed human SC using X-ray diffraction to show one 4.5 nm and one 6.5 nm diffraction peak related to lipids. White et al. (1988) and Bouwstra et al. (1991) reported the presence of 13 nm-sized repeating units in mouse and human SC. More recently, McIntosh (2003) showed the asymmetric distribution of cholesterol within model systems composed of reconstituted SC lipids extracted from pig skin. Iwai et al. (2012) used high magnification cryo electron microscopy, molecular modeling, and electron microscopy simulation to determine the molecular organization of the skin lipid matrix. This work concluded that the lipid organization is a stacked bilayer structure of ceramides in the fully extended (splayed chain) conformation with cholesterol associated with the ceramide sphingoid moiety. It consists of a bilayer rather than an arrangement of stacked monolayers. An important consideration for NP transport is the limiting size of the lipid channels within the SC, which have been measured as being

19 nm and 73 nm in width from two different studies (van der Merwe et al. 2006, Baroli et al. 2007). Another important consideration is the cyclical removal of corneocytes by desquamation. The *SC* is turned over in an average of 14 days (Reddy et al. 2000). This continuous movement of corneocytes to the surface layer of the skin is regarded as an added protective mechanism which assists in the elimination of foreign bodies, including NPs, cancer cells, or pathogens from the *SC* (Marks 2004). The ability of different types of permeants to penetrate the *SC* and the routes through which they pass has been an area of differing opinion. Traditionally, it was thought that polar and non-polar solutes used different paths to pass through the *SC* (with polar solutes traveling via the transcellular route and non-polar through the intercellular lipids) (Scheuplein 1965). Following an array of histological and theoretical studies, it was deduced that transcellular partitioning through both lipophilic and hydrophilic components would be too difficult. Therefore, the intercellular lipid route is generally accepted to be the most likely route for all solutes (Elias and Friend 1975, Albery and Hadgraft 1979, Grice et al. 2010). Hair follicles (appendages) are sparsely distributed across the skin but are thought to be a realistic delivery route across the *SC* (Lademann et al. 2007). The follicles extend deep into the skin and the thickness of the *SC* is reduced at these points. There is also a capillary blood supply available to transport solutes diffusing out of the follicle (Roberts and Walters 2008). Recent studies have looked at the contribution of the follicular route to drug penetration and targeting, with successful follicular penetration observed for liposomes and PS NPs (Lieb et al. 1992, Shim et al. 2004, Alvarez-Roman 2004). Vogt et al. (2006) showed that 40 nm-sized particles penetrated the skin via the follicular route and possibly into the perifollicular dermis, and entered epidermal Langerhan's cells. In contrast, 750 nm-sized and 1500 nm-sized NPs aggregated in hair follicle openings. The skin used in this study was not hydrated, i.e., fresh skin samples were used and the samples were tape stripped twice prior to application of beads (Fig. 4.3).

The surface pH of the skin is 4.2–5.6 and is defined by the term "acid mantle" (Schmid-Wendtner and Korting 2006). A range of factors such as sex, anatomical site, sweat, sebum, and hydration can influence the pH of the skin (Krien and Kermici 2000, Hanson et al. 2002). There is a sharp pH gradient across the *SC*, with the pH approaching neutral in the upper layers of the viable epidermis, i.e., *SG*. A study by Hanson et al. (2002) used two photon fluorescence lifetime imaging of a pH-dependent fluorophore applied to the skin of hairless rats. Acidic microdomains were observed in the extracellular matrix which became less frequent away for the surface of the viable epidermis. The acid mantle's functions include antimicrobial defense (Janssens et al. 1996), the maintenance of the skin's permeability barrier (Genotelle et al. 2004), the preservation of optimal corneocyte integrity and cohesion regulated by pH sensitive proteolytic enzymes (Li et al. 2005), and the restriction of inflammation by restricting the release of pro-inflammatory cytokines (Terreno et al. 2008). There is a clear association between elevated skin pH values and diseases such as atopic dermatitis, with significant pH

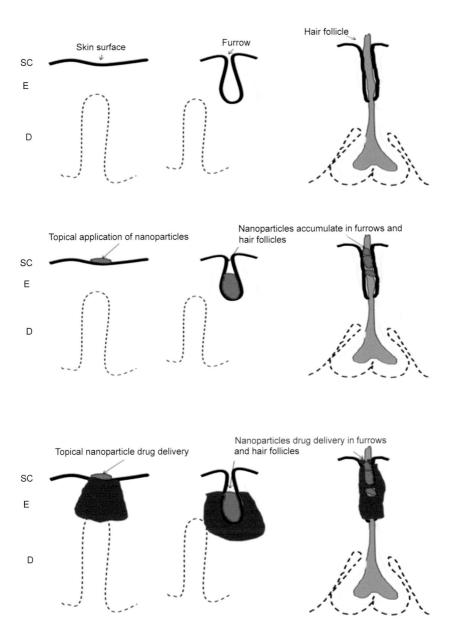

Figure 4.3. Sites in skin for NP delivery. Topical NP drug delivery takes place in three major sites: *stratum corneum* (*SC*) surface, furrows (dermatoglyphs), and openings of hair follicles (infundibulum). The NPs are shown in blue and the drug in red. Other sites for delivery are the viable epidermis (*E*) and dermis (*D*). Adapted with permission from Prow et al. (2011). Copyright Elsevier (2011).

differences between affected and unaffected skin (Seidenari and Giusti 1995). The acid mantle may also contribute to the skin's barrier to NP distribution. It has been shown that carboxylate PS NPs aggregate upon lowering of pH due to the reduction in electrostatic interactions (Murphy et al. 2010). The acid mantle may allow targeted skin delivery and the control of release properties of polymeric pH-sensitive NPs.

Fate of nanomaterials on the skin

The skin functions as a chemical and metabolic carrier, as well as a physical barrier. The skin enzymes are mainly located in the basal layer of the viable epidermis, the extracellular spaces of the *SC*, and the appendages in the dermis (Guy et al. 1987, Oesch et al. 2007). Whether NPs are affected by these processes, depends on their ability to pass the *SC* and enter these areas. Many NPs are biodegradable through hydrolysis, enzyme activity, and physical forces which may cause NPs to bind with the intercellular lipids (Bouwstra and Honeywell-Nguyen 2002). The skin metabolism following topical delivery has been referred to as first pass, analogous to that in the liver (Roberts and Walters 2008). Depending on the physiochemical composition of the NPs, the skin metabolism may contribute to their destruction, and therefore release the active compound. All these factors may be tailored for targeted and controlled delivery of active agents from their nanoparticulate carrier. If NPs can access these areas, as they have been shown to access the hair follicles, there is a potential for skin metabolism to be exploited for NP delivery purposes, as soft-drugs and pro-drugs have been (Gysler et al. 1999).

Cellular targets of nanoparticles for skin cancer therapy

The application of nanotechnology to skin cancer has prompted the design of new therapeutic approaches. Most chemotherapeutics are administered systemically and are cytotoxic to healthy cells. The severe side effects caused by this non-selective therapy have prompted the development of NPs which selectively deliver drugs or small interfering ribonucleic acid (*si*RNA) specifically to melanoma cells (Chen et al. 2010a,b, Yao et al. 2011).

Metastatic melanoma tumors have been shown to be selectively targeted by homing ligands attached to NPs on a number of occasions. Kim et al. (2010) demonstrated the use of gold nanocages (AuNCs) which were bioconjugated with [Nle[4], D-Phe[7]]-α-melanocyte-stimulating hormone for imaging of tumors. Conventional imaging methods are generally not sensitive or specific enough and have low spatial resolution and shallow penetration depths. In this paper, high-resolution photoacoustic tomography was used in combination with these conjugated AuNCs. The bioconjugated AuNCs enhanced contrast $\approx 300\%$ more than the control, AuNCs surface coated with poly(ethylene glycol) (PEG, PEGylated). Lu et al. (2009) developed hollow gold nanospheres (HAuNSs) to specifically target melanoma cells. HAuNSs were stabilized with a PEG coating and attached to an [Nle^4, D-Phe^7]-α-melanocyte-stimulating hormone, which is a potent agonist of the melanocortin type-1 receptor overexpressed in melanoma. The intracellular uptake of the PEGylated HAuNSs and the distribution of β-arrestin were examined in murine B16/F10 melanoma cells. It was found that the NPs were specifically taken up by melanoma cells, which initiated the recruitment of β-arrestins, the adapters to link the activated G-protein-coupled receptors to clathrin, indicating the involvement of receptor-mediated endocytosis. This resulted in enhanced extravasation of these conjugated nanospheres from tumor blood vessels and their dispersion into tumor matrix, compared to non-specific PEGylated HAuNSs.

QDs have also been used as an immunofluorescent label for biomedical imaging in cancer cells. Highly fluorescent CdSe/ZnS QDs were capped with PEG-COOH and conjugated with streptavidin. These nanoconjugates were used to target the cell adhesion molecule CD146 and the labeling of these cells with them resulted in high brightness, photostability, and selectivity, making them excellent candidates for the detection of melanoma cells in biomedical applications (Zheng et al. 2010).

Analytical methods for the detection of nanoparticles in the skin

Tape stripping is a well-defined and widely used method for studying the penetration of topically applied formulations (including NPs) to the SC. The amount of topically applied substance removed by each tape strip can be determined by analytical methods such as Inductively Coupled Plasma Mass Spectrometry (ICP-MS). These amounts can then be correlated with their location within the skin, and in this way, accurate penetration profiles can be determined (Lindemann et al. 2003). An alternative and perhaps more accurate method of looking NP penetration is by taking a biopsy and analyzing by freezing in liquid nitrogen and sectioning using a cryostat. Skin slices can then be analyzed using a laser scanning microscope. By superposition of the resulting images, the penetration depths can be analyzed (Patzelt et al. 2011).

Confocal imaging has been used widely to evaluate NP penetration, delivery, toxicity, and localization (Prow et al. 2011). Multiphoton imaging offers a non-invasive method for the direct visualization of skin structures and dermal penetration of NPs (Fig. 4.4). In multiphoton imaging, excitation of the fluorophores relies on the simultaneous absorption of two or more photons of lower energy in longer wavelengths, usually in the near-infrared spectrum. It is a promising method for studying penetration of the skin barrier. Geusens et al. (2012) used the skin's autofluorescence to facilitate identification of morphological features in the skin sample into and through which the penetration of ultradeformable liposomes (SECosomes) was evaluated. These NPs were found to efficiently deliver *si*RNAs in cultured primary melanocytes and keratinocytes.

Inductively Coupled Plasma Atomic Emission Spectroscopy (ICP-AES) and ICP-MS are commonly used techniques for the quantification of

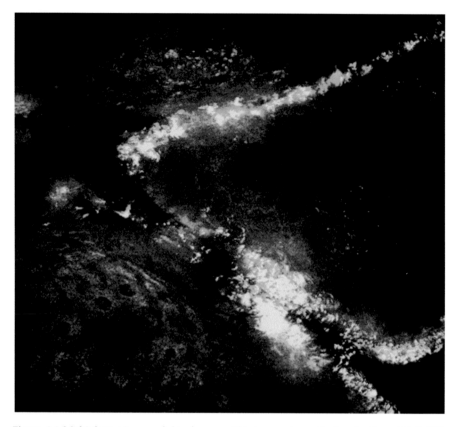

Figure 4.4. Multiphoton image of skin furrows. This image shows the localization of ZnO NPs which have accumulated at the skin furrows. Thanks to Dr. W. Sanchez for permitting the publication of the image.

internalized NP's composition. ICP-AES is used to detect trace metals and ICP-MS is capable of detecting metals and several non-metals at concentrations as low as one part in 10^{12}. Many *in vitro* nanotoxicity studies have used ICP-AES to assess uptake of NPs composed of Au, CeO_2, and iron oxide. This is done by the isolation of cells from the culture media followed by acidic digestion, dilution, and ICP-AES analysis (Marquis et al. 2009).

A widely used *in vivo* assay for toxicity is the examination of histological changes for given cells/tissues/organs following NP exposure. Histological examinations are carried out on tissues that have been fixed after sacrifice of the animal, and changes in the tissue and cell morphology are examined with light microscopy. Following fixation, the tissue is cut into sections and stained with hematoxylin and eosin strain. Problems with this method include the addition of artifacts during the processes of fixation, embedding, sectioning, or staining (Marquis et al. 2009).

In studies which look at NPs targeting melanoma cells, standardized cell culture experiments are used. For example, Benezra et al. (2011) used cell culture techniques to assess the particle binding of silica NPs to human melanoma cells M1 and M2, by radiolabeling them and accessing cell binding using an automatic gamma counter. This paper also used flow cytometry and anti-adhesion studies for further quantification.

TEM can provide very detailed information with regard to *in vitro* NP uptake and localization. It allows both visualization of the NPs' location within a cell or tissue, and in combination with certain spectroscopic methods, the composition of the NPs can be characterized. Electron-dense nanomaterials such as metal NPs are most easily imaged using TEM. High resolution TEM can be used to describe crystalline structures and has been used to identify superparamagnetic structures (Marquis et al. 2009). TEM has been used to show the cellular uptake of carbon nanotubes into intracytoplasmic vacuoles of human epidermal keratinocytes (Montiero-Rivere et al. 2005).

TEM or Scanning Electron Microscopy (SEM) in combination with a microanalysis system such as Electron Dispersive X-ray (EDX) analysis can be used to identify the chemical composition of NPs in a biological sample. One reason why elemental analysis is so important is because the staining procedures used to visualize biological samples may introduce electron dense nano-sized aggregates as artifacts (Marquis et al. 2009). Zvyagin et al. (2008) demonstrated the use of SEM-EDX to image and quantify ZnO NPs in the skin.

Proliferation assays allow the determination of the number of cells that are growing in the absence or presence of certain proliferation effecting agents. The 3-(4,5-dimethylthiazol-2-yl)-2,5-diphenyltetrazolium bromide (MTT) assay is a very commonly used technique which has been used to assess the *in vitro* toxicity of a range of nanostructures. It works by assessing the cellular reduction in MTT to produce formazan-based dyes. The formazan dyes are monitored by optical absorbance as a measurement of cellular metabolism. This in turn is used to calculate the percentage of metabolically active cells. Although MTT assays have many advantages over other assays, including minimal manipulation of model cells and fast reproducible results, there are also limitations with this technique. These include an NPs' unclear cellular mechanism for the reduction of tetrazolium salts and changes in the media pH or the culture media additives, which can alter measurements. Other commonly used assays include, necrosis assays, apoptosis assays, DNA damage assay, and oxidative stress assays (Marquis et al. 2009).

Toxicological aspects of nanoparticle delivery to the skin

As with any new type of technology, there are disadvantages. The application of nanotechnology to dermatology has resulted in the development of entirely new classes of irritants, allergens, haptens, cross-reactants, and unanticipated particle-particle interactions (Nasir 2010). There are many factors which must be taken into account when considering NP toxicity. The ability of specific types of NPs to pass the *SC* and reach the viable tissue is the most obvious factor. If the NP manages to bypass this barrier, then factors such as particle size, size distribution, agglomeration state, shape, crystal structure, chemical composition, surface area, surface chemistry, surface charge, and porosity must be considered (Oberdorster et al. 2005). As NPs decrease in size, they occupy less volume but their surface area per unit mass increases. This dramatically increases the availability of surface groups for biological interaction (Nasir 2010). This enhances potential toxic mechanisms (and can also provide useful properties), including hydrophobic interactions, redox handling, and free radical formation. It has been estimated that a 20 nm-sized particle has roughly 100 times the inherent toxicity of a 2 μm-sized particle in an equivalent dose based on mass and assuming a direct relationship with surface area. The surface properties can affect the pharmacokinetics of NPs, by influencing particle aggregation. Small particles with large surface areas are more prone to aggregation than larger particles (Emerich and Thanos 2007). Limited information is available about the biological effects induced by exposure to NPs; however Montiero-Riviere et al. (2005) reported that exposure of human epidermal keratinocytes to walled carbon nanotubes initiated a pro-inflammatory response, indicated by the release of interleukin 8. This group later published a work which examined the limitations associated with current cell culture toxicity assays (Montiero-Riviere et al. 2009). They reported that classical dye-based assays such as MTT and neutral red that determine cell viability produce invalid results with some nanomaterials due to interactions between the NP and dye and/or nanomaterial adsorption of the dye/dye products.

Recent advances in deformable and charged liposome skin delivery

Liposomes are sub-microscopic vesicular structures of amphipathic lipids arranged in one or more concentric bilayers with an entrapped aqueous core (Venuganti and Perumal 2009). They generally consist of a natural or synthetic phospholipid, and a stabilizer such as cholesterol. The physiochemical properties of the entity to be encapsulated generally dictate where in the liposome it will be loaded. Hydrophilic drugs are incorporated into the aqueous core whereas amphiphilic, lipophilic, and charged hydrophilic drugs can be entrapped or associated within the vesicle lipid bilayer by hydrophobic and/or electrostatic interactions (Venuganti and Perumal 2009, González-Rodríguez and Rabasco 2011). Liposomes are often favored as drug carriers for topical applications due to the compatibility of phospholipids with biological constituents (Tamilvanan et al. 2008).

In terms of transdermal and topical delivery, conventional liposomes are mainly confined to the *SC* (Lasch et al. 1992), while flexible liposomes and deformable liposomes have been shown to possess the characteristics required for skin penetration (Song and Kim 2006). These types of liposomes can overcome the skin barrier due to their increased capacity for deformability and flexibility. This allows them to squeeze through intercellular hydrophilic pathways in the skin (Cevc and Blume 1992, Cevc and Blume 2004). Geusens et al. (2010) recently published a study in which SECosomes successfully transport *si*RNA through intact human skin.

Charged liposomes have received much attention as drug carriers. The external charge on a liposome, along with other physiochemical and structural characteristics, will dictate its route of passage through the skin, the type of payload it can carry, and how it interacts with its target site. A recent review paper examined the potential of charged liposomes as skin permeation enhancers (González-Rodríguez and Rabasco 2011). It focused on the development of new and more advanced liposome formulations, as well as the development of more advanced preparation methods. Liposomal formulations have been extended to include a range of deformable liposomes. The flexible structure of these NPs improves their ability and their payload's ability to penetrate through the *SC* lipid lamellar regions. This phenomenon is generally thought to be a result of the hydration or osmotic force in the skin. The osmotic gradient in the skin is caused by the difference in water content between the skin surface and skin interior. The hydrophilic character of the phospholipid head groups in the bilayer results in the liposomes avoiding dry surroundings. The swollen vesicles on the surface of the skin will attempt to follow the local moisture gradient. This facilitates movement towards the deeper layers of the skin. It has also been suggested that the lipid composition of these liposomes is similar to the composition of the epidermis, therefore enabling them to penetrate the epidermal barrier (Cevc and Vierl 2010, González-Rodríguez and Rabasco 2011).

In general, deformable liposome literature has classified them in terms of their constituents. Cevc (2012) stated that the deformable bilayer vesicle class is more diverse than previously thought. Deformable liposomes can now be classified into three generations, according to the bilayer constituents. First generation deformable liposomes are the phospholipid or phospholipid surfactant blends. Second generation liposomes are a refined version of the first and contain synergistic phospholipid-amphiphat or drug mixtures. They exhibit improved drug payload and adaptability compared to first generation liposomes. Finally, third generation deformable liposomes are the most recent development in deformable liposomes, that include amphipathic combinations with appropriate effective tail cross sections. They utilize a novel mechanism of controlling bilayer properties by distributing hydrophilic modulators near the bilayer. It is suggested that these hydrophilic entities replicate the function of surfactant molecules in first and second generation deformable liposomes. Hydrophilic modulators can increase vesicle adaptability, stability, and drug payload.

Lipid molecules are arranged in a bilayer formation with the hydrophilic head groups in contact with the external aqueous medium, the double lipophilic tail ends form the bilayer and an internal aqueous compartment exists inside this lipid bilayer. Depending on the permeability of the bilayer, when molecules are added to the liposomes externally, they will either adsorb to the liposome structure or migrate across the lipid bilayer and absorb onto the inner surface (González-Rodríguez and Rabasco 2011). A study by Liu et al. (2001) looked at the effect of varying the ratios of cationic palmitoyloleoyl-phosphatidylglycerol and zwitterionic palmitoyloleoyl-phosphatidylcholine (POPC) and found that the absorption of the cationic dye malachite green increased linearly with the fraction of negatively charged lipids in the bilayer. Another paper by Colletier et al. (2002) described the encapsulation efficiency of proteins to liposomes prepared from the lipids POPC and 1-palmitoyl-2-oleoyl-*sn*-glycero-3-phosphoserine. It concluded that the interactions of the protein acetylcholinesterase with the lipid bilayer, and hence the encapsulation efficiency, increased with higher lipid concentrations. Both studies illustrated how the surface charge density of a liposome will influence the success of complexation and encapsulation efficiency. The lipid composition and consequently the surface charge of the liposomes will also influence the route of liposome permeation and the site of liposome delivery.

The theories by which liposomes penetrate into the skin include penetration enhancement, as illustrated by ultrastructure changes in the SC following application of a liposome preparation to the SC. Hofland et al. (1995) observed adsorption of the liposomes onto the outer surface of the SC. The authors concluded that the complexity of the phospholipid headgroup controlled the headgroup interactions with the SC. The success of drug complexation, encapsulation, and eventually drug penetration is influenced by modifying the surface electrical charge of liposomes. Strategies employed to modify the surface charge of liposomes include: (i) using charged phospholipids such as 1,2-dioleoyl-3-trimethylammonium-propane (chloride salt) within the liposome preparation method; (ii) coating the liposomes with polymers; and, (iii) the addition of charge inducer agents (González-Rodríguez and Rabasco 2011).

Limitations of nanoparticles and nanocarriers as delivery vehicles

As discussed by Prow et al. (2011), there are a number of limitations associated with the production, design, and characterization of nanoparticulate systems. At present, we are unable to fabricate highly reproducible NP geometries. We have difficulty in achieving optimal drug loading or controlling the rate of drug release from the vesicles. Lastly, the design of stable materials which do not cause any toxicity concerns has yet to be optimized. The toxicity concerns regarding the possible penetration of NPs into the skin and systemic circulation from cosmetic or other topical formulations are also a potential concern. The potential toxicity of NPs on and within the skin depends on a number of factors, including the ability of the particles to penetrate the skin, where these particles are going (i.e., cellular level or systemic circulation), how the NPs are breaking down, what types of toxic byproducts are being formed, if any, and at what levels and how the body is eliminating these toxic byproducts. Until each of these concerns are answered for all nanoparticulate systems, any questions regarding the safety profiles of NPs on and in the skin cannot be settled.

Conclusions

Despite the enormous commercial interest, topical and transdermal delivery applications of nanotechnology are still in their infancy. Consequently, there are a number of limitations yet to be overcome in order to reach their full potential. For instance, current technology does not give sufficient control to allow fabrication of highly reproducible particle shapes or sizes, while further improvements in achieving optimal drug loading and better control of the rate and site of payload release are needed. The potential toxicity of these technologies is of major importance to consumers, researchers, commercial interests, and regulators. Hence, it is essential that very careful studies on penetration of particles into the viable epidermis and their eventual fate, including targets, routes of elimination, and breakdown products, are undertaken.

One of the most exciting prospects for this technology is in the field of skin cancer, where targeted delivery is expected to be used for tumor recognition and treatment. Other future directions include the use of novel skin delivery routes, such as furrows, sweat ducts, and hair follicles, as well as nanoplatforms which can be primed to release their payload in response to specific stimuli.

Abbreviations

Au	:	gold
AuNC	:	gold nanocage
CeO_2	:	cerium oxide
DNA	:	deoxyribonucleic acid
EDX	:	electron dispersive X-ray
HAuNS	:	hollow gold nanosphere
ICP-AES	:	inductively coupled plasma atomic emission spectroscopy
ICP-MS	:	inductively coupled plasma mass spectrometry
MN	:	microneedle
MTT	:	3-(4,5-dimethylthiazol-2-yl)-2,5-diphenyltetrazolium bromide
NLC	:	nanostructured lipid carrier
PEG	:	poly(ethylene glycol)
POPC	:	palmitoyloleoyl-phosphatidylcholine
PS	:	polystyrene
QD	:	quantum dot
SB	:	*stratum basale*
SC	:	*stratum corneum*

SEM	:	scanning electron microscopy
*si*RNA	:	small interfering ribonucleic acid
SG	:	*stratum granulosum*
SLN	:	solid lipid nanoparticle
SS	:	*stratum spinosum*
TEM	:	transmission electron microscopy
TiO_2	:	titanium dioxide
UV	:	ultraviolet
ZnO	:	zinc oxide

References

Albery, W.J. and J. Hadgraft. 1979. Percutaneous absorption: theoretical description. J. Pharm. Pharmacol. 31: 129–139.

Alvarez-Roman, R. and A. Naik, Y.N. Kalia, R.H. Guy and H. Fessi. 2004. Skin penetration and distribution of polymeric nanoparticles. J. Control. Release. 99: 53–62.

Baroli, B. and M.G. Ennas, F. Loffredo, M. Isola, R. Pinna and M.A. Lopez-Quintela. 2007. Penetration of metallic nanoparticles in human full-thickness skin. J. Invest. Dermatol. 127: 1701–1712.

Benezra, M. and O. Penate-Medina, P.B. Zanzonico, D. Schaer, H. Ow, A. Burns, E. DeStanchina, V. Longo, E. Herz, S. Iyer, J. Wolchok, S.M. Larson, U. Wiesner and M.S. Bradbury. 2011. Multimodal silica nanoparticles are effective cancer-targeted probes in a model of human melanoma. *J. Clin. Invest.* 121: 2768–2780.

Benson, H.A.E. 2005. Transdermal drug delivery: penetration enhancement techniques. Curr. Drug Deliv. 2: 23–33.

Benson, H.A.E. Skin structure, function, and penetration. pp. 3–22. *In*: H.A.E. Benson and A.C. Watkinson [eds.]. 2012. Topical and Transdermal Drug Delivery. Wiley, New Jersey, USA.

Bouwstra, J.A. and G.S. Gooris, A. Weerheim, J. Kempenaar and M. Ponec. 1991. Structural investigations of human *stratum corneum* by small-angle X-ray scattering. J. Invest. Dermatol. 97: 1005–1012.

Bouwstra, J.A. and P.L. Honeywell-Nguyen. 2002. Skin structure and mode of action of vesicles. Adv. Drug Deliv. Rev. 54: 41–55.

Bronaugh, R.L. and H.I. Maibach. 1989. Percutaneous Absorption. 2nd Ed. Marcel Dekker. New York, USA.

Brown, M.B. and G.P. Martin, S.A. Jones and F.K. Akomeah. 2006. Dermal and transdermal drug delivery systems: current and future prospects. Drug Deliv. 13: 175–187.

Cevc, G. and G. Blume. 1992. Lipid vesicles penetrate into intact skin owing to the transdermal osmotic gradients and hydration force. Biochim. Biophys. Acta. 1104: 226–232.

Cevc, G. and G. Blume. 2004. Hydrocortisone and dexamethasone in very deformable drug carriers have increased biological potency, prolonged effect, and reduced therapeutic dosage. Biochim. Biophys. Acta. 1663: 61–73.

Cevc, G. and U. Vierl. 2010. Nanotechnology and the transdermal route: a state of the art review and critical appraisal. J. Control. Release. 141: 277–299.

Cevc, G. 2012. Rational design of new product candidates: the next generation of highly deformable bilayer vesicles for noninvasive, targeted therapy. J. Control. Release. 160: 135–146.

Chen, Y. and X. Zhu, X. Zhang, B. Liu and L. Huang. 2010a. Nanoparticles modified with tumor-targeting scFv deliver siRNA and miRNA for cancer therapy. Mol. Ther. 18: 1650–1656.

Chen, Y. and S.R. Bathula, Q. Yang and L. Huang. 2010b. Targeted nanoparticles deliver siRNA to melanoma. J. Invest. Dermatol. 130: 2790–2798.

Chen, X. and G.J.P. Fernando, M.L. Crichton, C. Flaim, S.R. Yukiko, E.J. Fairmaid, H.J. Corbett, C.A. Primiero, A.B. Ansaldo, I.H. Frazer, L.E. Brown and M.A.F. Kendall. 2011. Improving the reach of vaccines to low-resource regions, with a needle-free vaccine delivery device and long-term thermostabilization. J. Control. Release. 152: 349–355.

Chuong, C.M. and B.J. Nickoloff, P.M. Elias, L.A. Goldsmith, E. Macher, P.A. Maderson, J.P. Sundberg, H. Tagami, P.M. Plonka, K. Thestrup-Pedersen, B.A. Bernard, J.M. Schröder, P. Dotto, C.H. Chang, M.L. Williams, P.A. Maderson, K.R. Feingold, L.E. King, A.M. Kligman, J.L. Rees and E. Christophers. 2002. What is the "true" function of skin? Exper. Dermatol. 11: 159–187.

Colletier, J.P. and B. Chaize, M. Winterhalter and D. Fournier. 2002. Protein encapsulation in liposomes: efficiency depends on interactions between protein and phospholipid bilayer. BMC Biotechnol. 2: 1–8.

Coulman, S.A. and A. Anstey, C. Gateley, A. Morrissey, P. McLoughlin, C. Allender and J.C. Birchall. 2009. Microneedle mediated delivery of nanoparticles into human skin. Int. J. Pharm. 366: 190–200.

Cross, S.E. and B. Innes, M.S. Roberts, T. Tsuzuki, T.A. Robertson and P. McCormick. 2007. Human skin penetration of sunscreen nanoparticles: *in vitro* assessment of a novel micronized zinc oxide formulation, Skin Pharmacol. Physiol. 20: 148–154.

DeLouise, L.A. 2012. Applications of nanotechnology in dermatology. J. Invest. Dermatol. 132: 964–975.

Donnelly, R.F. and D.I.J. Morrow, F. Fay, C.J. Scott, S. Abdelghany, R.R. Singh, M.J. Garland and A.D. Woolfson. 2010. Microneedle-mediated intradermal nanoparticle delivery: potential for enhanced local administration of hydrophobic pre-formed photosensitisers. Photodiagnosis Photodyn. Ther. 7: 222–231.

Egelrud, T. 2000. Desquamation in the *stratum corneum*. Acta Derm Venereol. Suppl. (Stockh). 208: 44–45.

Elias, P.M. and D.S. Friend. 1975. The permeability barrier in mammalian epidermis. J. Cell Biol. 65: 180–191.

Emerich, D.F. and C.G. Thanos. 2007. Targeted nanoparticle-based drug delivery and diagnosis. J. Drug Target. 15: 163–183.

Farokhzad, O.C. and R. Langer. 2009. Impact of nanotechnology on drug delivery. ACS Nano. 3: 16–20.

Garland, M.J. and K. Migalska, T.T. Mahmood, T.R. Singh, A.D. Woolfson and R.F. Donnelly. 2011. Microneedle arrays as medical devices for enhanced transdermal drug delivery. Expert Rev. Med. Devices. 8: 459–482.

Garson, J.C. and J. Doucet, J.T. Leveque and G. Tsoucaris. 1991. Oriented structure in human *stratum corneum* revealed by X-ray diffraction. J. Invest. Dermatol. 96: 43–49.

Genotelle, N. and T. Lherm, O. Gontier, C. Le Gall and D. Caen. 2004. Right uncontrollable haemothorax revealing a liver injury with diaphragmatic rupture. Ann. Fr. Anesth. Rèanim. 23: 831–834.

Geusens, B. and M. Van Gele, S. Braat, S.C. De Smedt, M.C.A. Stuart, T.W. Prow, W. Sanchez, M.S. Roberts, N.N. Sanders and J. Lambert. 2010. Flexible nanosomes (SECosomes) enable efficient siRNA delivery in cultured primary skin cells and in the viable epidermis of *ex vivo* human skin. Adv. Funct. Mat. 20: 4077–4090.

González-Rodríguez, M. and A. Rabasco. 2011. Charged liposomes as carriers to enhance the permeation through the skin. Expert Opin. Drug Deliv. 8: 857–871.

Grice, J.E. and S. Ciotti, N. Weiner, P. Lockwood, S.E. Cross and M.S. Roberts. 2010. Relative uptake of minoxidil into appendages and *stratum corneum* and permeation through human skin *in vitro*. J. Pharm. Sci. 99: 712–718.

Gupta, H. and A. Sharma. 2009. Recent trends in protein and peptide drug delivery systems. Asian J. Pharm. 3: 69–75.

Guy, R.H. and J. Hadgraft and D.A. Bucks. 1987. Transdermal drug delivery and cutaneous metabolism. Xenobiotica. 17: 325–343.

Gysler, A. and B. Kleuser, W. Sippl, K. Lange, H.C. Korting and H.D. Holtje. 1999. Skin penetration and metabolism of topical glucocorticoids in reconstructed epidermis and in excised human skin. Pharm. Res. 16: 1386–1391.

Hanson, K.M. and M.J. Behne, N.P. Barry, T.M. Mauro, E. Gratton and R.M. Clegg. 2002. Two photon fluorescence lifetime imaging of the skin *stratum corneum* pH gradient. Biophys. J. 83: 1682–1690.

Hofland, H.E.J. and J.A. Bouwstra, H.E. Bodde, F. Spies and H.E. Junginger. 1995. Interactions between liposomes and human *stratum corneum in vitro*: freeze fracture electron microscopical visualization and small angle X-ray scattering studies. Br. J. Dermatol. 132: 853–866.

Iwai, I. and H. Han, L. den Hollander, S. Svensson, L.G. Öfverstedt, J. Anwar, J. Brewer, M. Bloksgaard, A. Laloeuf, D. Nosek, S. Masich, L.A. Bagatolli, U. Skoglund and L. Norlén. 2012. The human skin barrier is organized as stacked bilayers of fully extended ceramides with cholesterol molecules associated with the ceramide sphingoid moiety. J. Invest. Dermatol. 132: 2215–2225.

Janssens, J. and D. Communi, S. Pirotton, M. Samson, M. Parmentier and J.M. Boeynaems. 1996. Cloning and tissue distribution of the human P2Y1 receptor. Biochem. Biophys. Res. Commun. 221: 588–593.

Jung, S. and A. Patzelt, N. Otberg, G. Thiede, W. Sterry and J. Lademann. 2009. Strategy of topical vaccination with nanoparticles. J. Biomed. Opt. 14: 021001.

Kaushik, S. and A.H. Hord, D.D. Denson, D.V. McAllister, S. Smitra, M.G. Allen and M.R. Prausnitz. 2001. Lack of pain associated with microfabricated microneedles. Anesth. Analg. 92: 502–504.

Kim, C. and E.C. Cho, J. Chen, K.H. Song, L. Au, C. Favazza, Q. Zhang, C.M. Cobley, F. Gao, Y. Xia and L.V. Wang. 2010. *In vivo* molecular photoacoustic tomography of melanomas targeted by bioconjugated gold nanocages. ACS Nano. 4: 4559–4564.

Kim, Y.C. and J.H. Park and M.R. Prausnitz. 2012. Microneedles for drug and vaccine delivery. Adv. Drug Deliv. Rev. 64: 1547–1568.

Krien, P.M. and M. Kermici. 2000. Evidence for the existence of a self-regulated enzymatic process within the human *stratum corneum*—an unexpected role for urocanic acid. J. Invest. Dermatol. 115: 414–420.

Lademann, J. and H. Richter, A. Teichmann, N. Otberg, U. Blume-Peytavi, J. Luengo, B. Weiss, U.F. Schaefer, C.M. Lehr, R. Wepf and W. Sterry. 2007. Nanoparticles—an efficient carrier for drug delivery into the hair follicles. Eur. J. Pharm. Biopharm. 66: 159–164.

Lademann, J. and A. Patzelt, H. Richter, C. Antoniou, W. Sterry and F. Knorr. 2009. Determination of the cuticula thickness of human and porcine hairs and their potential influence on the penetration of nanoparticles into the hair follicles. J. Biomed. Opt. 14: 021014.

Lasch, J. and R. Laub and W. Wohlrab. 1992. How deep do intact liposomes penetrate into human skin. J. Control. Release. 18: 55–58.

Lee, J.W. and J.H. Park and M.R. Prausnitz. 2008. Dissolving microneedles for transdermal drug delivery. Biomaterials. 29: 2113–2124.

Lieb, L.M. and C. Ramachandran, K. Egbaria and N. Weiner. 1992. Topical delivery enhancement with multilamellar liposomes into pilosebaceous units: I. *In vitro* evaluation using fluorescent techniques with the hamster ear model. J. Invest. Dermatol. 99: 108–113.

Lindemann, U. and K. Wilken, H.J. Weigmann, H. Schaefer, W. Sterry and J. Lademann. 2003. Quantification of the horny layer using tape stripping and microscopic techniques. J. Biomed. Opt. 8: 601–607.

Liu, Y. and E.C.Y. Yan and B. Eisenthal. 2001. Effects of bilayer surface charge density on molecular adsorption and transport across liposome bilayers. Biophys. J. 80: 1004–1012.

Liu, Y. and J. Tan, A. Thomas, D. Ou-Yang and V.R. Muzykantov. 2012. The shape of things to come: importance of design in nanotechnology for drug delivery. Ther. Deliv. 3: 181–194.

Lu, W. and C. Xiong, G. Zhang, Q. Huang, R. Zhang, J.Z. Zhang and C. Li. 2009. Targeted photothermal ablation of murine melanomas with melanocyte-stimulating hormone analog-conjugated hollow gold nanospheres. Clin. Cancer. Res. 15: 876–886.

Madison, K.C. and D.C. Swartzendruber, P.W. Wertz and D.T. Downing. 1987. Presence of intact intercellular lamellae in the upper layers of the *stratum corneum*. J. Invest. Dermatol. 88: 714–718.

Magnusson, B.M. and Y.G. Anissimov, S.E. Cross and M.S. Roberts. 2004. Molecular size as the main determinant of solute maximum flux across the skin. J. Invest. Dermatol. 122: 993–999.

Mahanraj, V.J. 2006. Nanoparticles—A review. Trop. J. Pharm. Res. 5: 561–573.

Marks, R. 2004. The *stratum corneum* barrier: the final frontier. J. Nutr. 134: 2017–2021.

Marquis, B.J. and S.A. Love, K.L. Braun and C.L. Haynes. 2009. Analytical methods to assess nanoparticle toxicity. Analyst. 134: 425–439.

Martanto, W. and S.P. Davis, N.R. Holiday, J. Wang, H.S. Gill and M.R. Prausnitz. 2004. Transdermal delivery of insulin using microneedles *in vivo*. Pharm. Res. 21: 947–952.

McIntosh, T.J. 2003. Organization of skin *stratum corneum* extracellular lamellae: diffraction evidence for asymmetric distribution of cholesterol. Biophys. J. 85: 1675–1681.

Menon, G.K. 2002. New insights into skin structure: scratching the surface. Adv. Drug Deliv. Rev. 54: 3–17.

Monteiro-Riviere, N.A. and A.O. Inman and L.W. Zhang. 2009. Limitations and relative utility of screening assays to assess engineered nanoparticle toxicity in a human cell line. Toxicol. Appl. Pharmacol. 234: 222–235.

Muller, R.H. and A. Dingler. 1998. The next generation after the liposomes: solid lipid nanoparticles (SLN, Lipopearls) as dermal carrier in cosmetics. Eurocosmetics. 7: 18–26.

Murphy, R.J. and D. Pristinski, K. Migler, J.F. Douglas and V.M. Prabhu. 2010. Dynamic light scattering investigations of nanoparticle aggregation following a light-induced pH jump. J. Chem. Phys. 132: 194903.

Nasir, A. 2010. Nanotechnology and dermatology: part I—potential of nanotechnology. Clin. Dermatol. 28: 458–466.

Nohynek, G.J. and J. Lademann, C. Ribaud and M.S. Roberts. 2007. Grey goo on the skin? Nanotechnology, cosmetic and sunscreen safety. Crit. Rev. Toxicol. 37: 251–277.

Oberdorster, G. and A. Maynard, K. Donaldson, V. Castranova, J. Fitzpatrick, K. Ausman, J. Carter, B. Karn, W. Kreyling, D. Lai, S. Olin, N. Monteiro-Riviere, D. Warheit and H. Yang. 2005. Principles for characterizing the potential human health effects from exposure to nanomaterials: elements of a screening strategy. Part. Fibre Toxicol. 2: 8.

Oesch, F. and E. Fabian, B. Oesch-Bartlomowicz, C. Werner and R. Landsiedel. 2007. Drug metabolizing enzymes in the skin of man, rat, and pig. Drug Metab. Rev. 39: 659–698.

Otberg, N. and H. Richter, H. Schaefer, U. Blume-Peytavi, W. Sterry and J. Lademann. 2004. Variations of hair follicle size and distribution in different body sites. J. Invest. Dermatol. 122: 14–19.

Pardeike, J. and A. Hommoss and R.H. Muller. 2009. Lipid nanoparticles (SLN, NLC) in cosmetic and pharmaceutical dermal products. Int. J. Pharm. 366: 170–184.

Patzelt, A. and H. Richter, F. Knorr, U. Schäfer, C.M. Lehr, L. Dähne, W. Sterry and J. Lademann. 2011. Selective follicular targeting by modification of the particle sizes. J. Control. Release. 150: 45–48.

Pearton, M. and S.M. Kang, J.M. Song, Y.C. Kim, F.S. Quan, A. Anstey, M. Ivory, M.R. Prausnitz, R.W. Compans and J.C. Birchall. 2010. Influenza virus-like particles coated onto microneedles can elicit stimulatory effects on Langerhans cells in human skin. Vaccine. 28: 6104–6113.

Polat, B.E. and D. Hart, R. Langer and D. Blankschtein. 2011. Ultrasound-mediated transdermal drug delivery: mechanisms, scope, and emerging trends. J. Control. Release. 152: 330–348.

Potts, R.O. and R.H. Guy. 1995. A predictive algorithm for skin permeability: the effects of molecular size and hydrogen bond activity. Pharm. Res. 12: 1628–1633.

Prausnitz, M.R. 2004. Microneedles for transdermal drug delivery. Adv. Drug Deliv. Rev. 56: 581–587.

Prow, T.W. and X. Chen, N.A. Prow, G.J. Fernando, C.S.E. Tan, A.P. Raphael, D. Chang, M.P. Ruutu, D.W.K. Jenkins, A. Pyke, M.L. Crichton, K. Raphaelli, L.Y.H. Goh, I.H. Frazer, M.S. Roberts, J. Gardner, A.A. Khromykh, A. Suhrbier, R.A. Hall and M.A.F. Kendall. 2010. Nanopatch-targeted skin vaccination against West Nile Virus and Chikungunya virus in mice. Small 6: 1776–1784.

Prow, T.W. and J.E. Grice, L.L. Lin, R. Faye, M. Butler, W. Becker, E.M.T. Wurm, C. Yoong, T.A. Robertson, H.P. Soyer and M.S. Roberts. 2011. Nanoparticles and microparticles for skin drug delivery. Adv. Drug Deliv. Rev. 63: 470–491.

Prow, T.W. and N.A. Monteiro-Riviere, A.O. Inman, J.E. Grice, X. Chen, X. Zhao, W.H. Sanchez, A. Gierden, M.A. Kendall, A.V. Zvyagin, D. Erdmann, J.E. Riviere and M.S. Roberts. 2012. Quantum dot penetration into viable human skin. Nanotoxicology. 6: 173–185.

Reddy, M.B. and R.H. Guy and A.L. Bunge. 2000. Does epidermal turnover reduce percutaneous penetration? Pharm. Res. 17: 1414–1419.

Roberts, M.S. and K.A. Walters. Human skin morphology and dermal absorption. pp. 1–15. *In:* M.S. Roberts and K.A. Walters [eds.]. 2008. Dermal Absorption and Toxicity Assessment. Informa Healthcare, New York, USA.

Robertson, T.A. and W.Y. Sanchez and M.S. Roberts. 2010. Are commercially available nanoparticles safe when applied to the skin? J. Biomed. Nanotech. 6: 452–468.

Rouse, J.G. and J. Yang, J.P. Ryman-Rasmussen, A.R. Barron and N.A. Monteiro-Riviere. 2007. Effects of mechanical flexion on the penetration of fullerene amino acid derivatized peptide nanoparticles through skin. Nano. Lett. 7: 155–160.

Ryman-Rasmussen, J.P. and J.E. Riviere and N.A. Monteiro-Riviere. 2006. Penetration of intact skin by quantum dots with diverse physicochemical properties. Toxicol. Sci. 91: 159–65.

Scheuplein, R.J. 1965. Mechanism of percutaneous adsorption. I. Routes of penetration and the influence of solubility. J. Invest. Dermatol. 45: 334–346.

Schmid-Wendtner, M.H. and H.C. Korting. 2006. The pH of the skin surface and its impact on the barrier function. Skin Pharmacol. Physiol. 19: 296–302.

Seidenari, S. and G. Giusti. 1995. Objective assessment of the skin of children affected by atopic dermatitis: a study of pH, capacitance and TEWL in eczematous and clinically uninvolved skin. Acta Derm. Venereol. 75: 429–433.

Seto, J.E. and B.E. Polat, R.F.V. Lopez, D. Blankschtein and R. Langer. 2010. Effects of ultrasound and sodium laurylsulfate on the transdermal delivery of hydrophilic permeants: comparative *in vitro* studies with full-thickness and split-thickness pig and human skin. J. Control. Release. 145: 26–32.

Shim, J. and H. Seok Kang, W.S. Park, S.H. Han, J. Kim and I.S. Chang. 2004. Transdermal delivery of minoxidil with block copolymer nanoparticles. J. Control. Release. 97: 477–484.

Singh, S. and J. Singh. 1993. Transdermal drug delivery by passive diffusion and iontophoresis: a review. Med. Res. Rev. 13: 569–621.

Song, Y.K. and C.K. Kim. 2006. Topical delivery of low-molecular-weight heparin with surface-charged flexible liposomes. Biomaterials. 27: 271–280.

Soppimath, K.S. and L.H. Liu, W.Y. Seow, S.Q. Liu, R. Powell, P. Chan and Y.Y. Yang. 2007. Multifunctional core/shell nanoparticles self-assembled from pH-induced thermosensitive polymers for targeted intracellular anticancer drug delivery. Adv. Funct. Mat. 17: 355–362.

Tamilvanan, S. and N. Venkateshan and A. Ludwig. 2008. The potential of lipid- and polymer-based drug delivery carriers for eradicating biofilm consortia on device-related nosocomial infections. J. Control. Release. 128: 2–22.

Tanner, T. and R. Marks. 2008. Delivering drugs by the transdermal route: review and comment. Skin Res. Technol. 14: 249–260.

Terreno, E. and A. Sanino, C. Carrera, D.D. Castelli, G.B. Giovenzana, A. Lombardi, R. Mazzon, L. Milone, M. Visigalli and S. Aime. 2008. Determination of water permeability of paramagnetic liposomes of interest in MRI field. J. Inorg. Biochem. 102: 1112–1119.

Tinkle, S.S. and J.M. Antonini, B.A. Rich, J.R. Roberts, R. Salmen, K. DePree and E.J. Adkins. 2003. Skin as a route of exposure and sensitization in chronic beryllium disease. Environ. Health Perspect. 111: 1202–1208.

Tobin, D.J. 2006. Biochemistry of human skin—our brain on the outside. Chem. Soc. Rev. 35: 52–67.

Toll, R. and U. Jacobi, H. Richter, J. Lademann, H. Schaefer and U. Blume-Peytavi. 2004. Penetration profile of microspheres in follicular targeting of terminal hair follicles. J. Invest. Dermatol. 123: 168–176.

van der Merwe, D. and J.D. Brooks, R. Gehring, R.E. Baynes, N.A. Monteiro-Riviere and J.E. Riviere. 2006. A physiologically based pharmacokinetic model of organophosphate dermal absorption. Toxicol. Sci. 89: 188–204.

Venuganti, V.V.K. and O.P. Perumal. Nanosystems for skin drug delivery. pp. 124–153. *In:* Y. Pathak and D. Thassu [eds.]. 2009. Nanoparticulate Delivery Systems II. Formulation and Characterization. Informa Healthcare Inc., New York, USA.

Vogt, A. and B. Combadiere, S. Hadam, K.M. Stieler, J. Lademann, H. Schaefer, B. Autran, W. Sterry and U. Blume-Peytavi. 2006. 40 nm, but not 750 or 1,500 nm, nanoparticles enter epidermal CD1a+ cells after transcutaneous application on human skin. J. Invest. Dermatol. 126: 1316–1322.

White, S.H. and D. Mirejovsky and G.I. King. 1988. Structure of lamellar lipid domains and corneocyte envelopes of murine *stratum corneum*. An X-ray diffraction study. Biochemistry. 27: 3725–3732.

Yao, H. and S.S. Ng, L.F. Huo, B.K.C. Chow, Z. Shen, M. Yang, J. Sze, O. Ko, M. Li, A. Yue, L.W. Lu, X.W. Lu, X.W. Bian, H.F. Kung and M.C. Lin. 2011. Effective melanoma immunotherapy with interleukin-2 delivered by a novel polymeric nanoparticle. Mol. Cancer Ther. 10: 1082–1092.

Zhang, L. and F.X. Gu, J.M. Chan, A.Z. Wang, R.S. Langer and O.C. Farokhzad. 2007. Nanoparticles in medicine: therapeutic applications and developments. Clin. Pharmacol. Ther. 83: 761–769.

Zheng, H. and G. Chen, L.A. DeLouise and Z. Lou. 2010. Detection of the cancer marker CD146 expression in melanoma cells with semiconductor quantum dot label. J. Biomed. Nanotechnol. 6: 303–311.

Zvyagin, A.V. and X. Zhao, A. Gierden, W. Sanchez, J.A. Ross and M.S. Roberts. 2008. Imaging of zinc oxide nanoparticle penetration in human skin *in vitro* and *in vivo*. J. Biomed. Opt. 13: 064031.

CHAPTER 5

Nanotechnology for Pulmonary and Nasal Drug Delivery

Helene L. Dugas[a] and *Robert O. Williams III**

ABSTRACT

The development of nanoparticle engineering processes has increased the possibilities of formulating active pharmaceutical ingredients for pulmonary and nasal delivery. These technologies encompass traditional techniques, such as milling and spray drying, as well as more recently developed techniques, such as cryogenic and supercritical processes. Using these techniques, scientists are able to produce engineered particles exhibiting specific physiochemical properties. Pulmonary and nasal physiologies are correlated to particle deposition and absorption. The physicochemical properties of the particles (e.g., size, viscosity, solubility) as well as the aerosol product performance are essential parameters to ensure delivery of the active material to the targeted areas and efficacy of the treatment. Nanoparticle technologies can improve patient outcomes and broaden the therapeutic options for local and systemic therapy.

Introduction

Almost 40% of the drugs currently marketed and close to 90% of the pipeline drugs exhibit poor water solubility and/or poor permeability, leading to an overall low bioavailability (Merisko-Liversidge and Liversidge 2008). Chemical modification, crystal change, and size reduction have been investigated to improve the solubility of those Biopharmaceutics Classification System (BCS) class II, III, and IV drugs. While these techniques have improved their

Pharmaceutics Division, College of Pharmacy, University of Texas at Austin, 2409 West University Avenue, PHR 4.214, Austin, TX 78712, USA.
[a] Email: hdugas@utexas.edu
* Corresponding author: williro@mail.utexas.edu

solubility, their absorption may still be low and their metabolism clearance high, resulting in a low therapeutic effect and potential serious side effects, as high dose must be administered. *In situ* delivery is known to minimize local and systemic side effects by employing a lower drug amount, to increase patient compliance and to improve the efficacy of the treatment. Nanoparticle (NP) engineering technologies play an important role in the improvement of pulmonary and nasal drug delivery. These technologies encompass traditional techniques, such as milling and spray drying, as well as more recent techniques, such as cryogenic and supercritical processes. Using these techniques, scientists are able to produce engineered particles exhibiting specific physiochemical properties. Since pulmonary and nasal drug delivery requires particles with specific criteria and good aerosolization properties, NP technologies are great tools to produce inhaled and nasal drug formulations with optimum characteristics for lung and nose delivery. Developing such formulations will broaden the therapeutic options used to treat pulmonary, nasal, as well as certain systemic diseases. Pulmonary and nasal physiologies are correlated to particle deposition and absorption, and will be discussed in this chapter. NP technologies used in the pharmaceutical industry in addition to more innovative processes will be detailed. Finally the clinical considerations of pulmonary and nasal delivery of drug NPs will be discussed through several pertinent examples taken from the literature.

Pulmonary Physiology, Nasal Physiology, and Drug Delivery

Physiology of the lung

The primary function of the lung resides in its ability to facilitate gas exchange between the external environment and the systemic circulation, and to maintain a constant systemic pH. The lung can be divided into two main compartments: the conducting zone and the respiratory zone (Altiere and Thompson 2007). The conducting zone includes the trachea branching into intrapulmonary bronchi further dividing into smaller diameter bronchi and bronchioles, and ends with terminal bronchioles. As its name indicates, the conducting zone allows air circulation in and out of the lung during the ventilation process. The respiratory zone consists of the respiratory bronchioles containing the alveolar ducts and sacs participating in the gas exchange function of the lung. In this zone, with a mean alveolar number of 480 million (Ochs et al. 2004), the total cross-sectional area approaches 140 to 160 m². This large surface area, combined with a thin alveolar epithelial layer ranging from 0.57 to 0.69 μm (Hogan et al. 1986), offer a real potential for drug delivery. The alveolar epithelium is primarily constituted of type I and II pneumocytes. Gases diffuse through type I pneumocytes while type II secrete lung surfactant that lines the alveolar luminal surface (Groneberg et al. 2003, Altiere and Thompson 2007).

In the conducting airways, ciliated cells line the surface of the epithelium. A biphasic mucous layer covers the ciliated surface, protecting the epithelium from dehydration and foreign substances (e.g., inhaled particles, virus, bacteria, and drugs). The mucociliary escalator moves the mucous layer and the substances trapped within it toward the oral cavity, where they are either swallowed or coughed up. In the tracheobronchial region, this mucociliary clearance is a major barrier to pulmonary delivery (Groneberg et al. 2003, Labiris and Dolovich 2003). In the respiratory zone, depending on the physicochemical properties of the substance deposited, the clearance process will occur either by dissolution, direct passage and uptake by the vascular system, transport in the lymphatic system, or phagocytosis by circulating alveolar macrophages (Patton and Byron 2007) (Fig. 5.1).

The increasing interest in pulmonary drug delivery over the last 30 years can be attributed to the non-invasive nature of the treatment, delivery directly at the disease site, avoidance of the first-pass metabolism, and decrease in systemic side effects while increasing the onsite drug levels. Lung delivery has been also associated with rapid onset of action and increased bioavailability, over traditional oral dosage forms (Labiris and Dolovich 2003, Patton and Byron 2007).

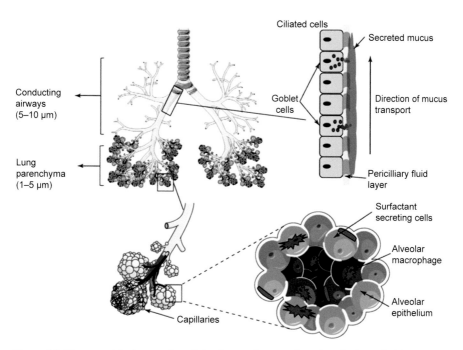

Figure 5.1. Diagram of the lung and particle-size requirements based on the intended deposition region in the respiratory tract. Reprinted with permission from Sou et al. (2011). Copyright Elsevier Ltd. (2011).

Physiology of the nose

The nasal passageways function as a means to warm, humidify, and filter the inhaled air before it reaches the lungs. The nasal cavity has a large surface area ($\approx$ 180 cm^2) and is highly vascularized. It is divided in two by the septum and further segmented into the superior, middle, and inferior concha, also called turbinates. The nares are the keratinized regions of the nose covered with hair and composed of a stratified squamous epithelium. The atrium epithelium is characterized by both squamous and pseudostratified columnar epithelial cells, and the turbinates by ciliated and non-ciliated pseudostratified epithelial cells only (Illum 2003).

Particle clearance in the nasal cavity is governed by the solubility properties of the particles. If insoluble substances deposit on the mucus layer lining, the non-ciliated nasal epithelium, sneezing or nose wiping will remove them. Similar to the tracheobronchial region, substances depositing on the mucus covering the ciliated epithelium, the mucociliary clearance will transport the mucus towards the nasopharynx region where it will be either swallowed or expectorated. If the particles are soluble, they may be absorbed through the mucus and nasal epithelium into systemic circulation (Patton and Byron 2007).

The nasal route offers several advantages for drug delivery: high absorption of small hydrophobic molecules, avoidance of the first-pass metabolism, and ease of administration (Türker et al. 2004, Costantino et al. 2007). It is also effective at stimulating the local and systemic immune system (Almeida and Alpar 1996, Illum 2003), and delivering drugs to the brain (Badhan et al. 2014).

Particles and deposition

In the lung

The objective of pulmonary delivery of drugs is to target the deep lung where maximal bioavailability is expected. Among other physicochemical properties of inhaled aerosols, particle size and flow rate influence the deposition in the different regions of the lung. The literature shows evidence of the importance of the aerodynamic diameter (d_a) of the particles over their geometric diameter (d_v) (Edwards et al. 1998, Courrier et al. 2002). In fact, even particles exhibiting a large d_v have the ability to deposit in the respiratory zone of the lung as soon as their d_a is < 5 μm. The d_a accounts for the d_v of the particles as well as for their shape and density, as shown below (de Boer et al. 2002, Telko and Hickey 2005, Chow et al. 2007):

$$d_a = d_v \sqrt{\frac{\rho}{\chi \cdot \rho_0}} \qquad (1)$$

where ρ is the particle density, χ is the dynamic shape factor (χ = 1 for spherical particles, but changes with the geometric of the particles) and ρ_0 is the reference density (usually ρ_0 = 1). The shape factor χ is the ratio of the resistance force exerted on the actual particles in movement in a fluid, by the resistance force exerted on spherical particles having identical volume. Hinds (1999) has provided an extensive review of the experimental or model based determinations of the dynamic shape factor, which is beyond the scope of this chapter. Depending on the d_a, particles will deposit in different regions of the lung: large particles ($d_a > 5$ µm) will deposit in the oropharyngeal and trachea regions, whereas 1 to 5 µm-sized particles will most likely settle in the respiratory bronchioles and the alveoli. NPs ($d_a < 1$ µm) will reach the alveolar region but ≈ 80% of the inhaled particles will actually be exhaled due to their lack of inertia and gravity.

The mechanisms of deposition can be organized into five categories: inertial impaction, sedimentation, diffusion, interception, and electrostatic precipitation (Gonda 2004, Telko and Hickey 2005). Inertial impaction occurs when the momentum of the particles is such that they move in a straight direction, independently of the airflow. Hence, impaction happens when the particles or droplets collide onto the lung epithelium. The impact is more likely to happen if the particles travel long distances, since they will not stop due to the friction forces between the particles and the air (Cai and Yu 1988, Gonda 2004, Carvalho et al. 2011). The traveled distance is based on the equation below:

$$S = B \cdot m \cdot v \tag{2}$$

where S is the distance, B is the particle mechanical mobility, m is the mass, and v is the particle velocity. The inertial deposition can also be related to the Stokes number (Stk): as it increases, the inertial impaction efficiency increases. Since the Stk is directly proportional to the square of the diameter, the inertial deposition efficiency increases with particle size (Kim et al. 1994, Gonda 2004, Zhang et al. 2005).

$$Stk = \frac{\rho \cdot d^2 \cdot V}{18 \cdot \eta \cdot R} \tag{3}$$

where ρ is the particle density, d is the particle diameter, V is the air velocity, η is the air viscosity, and R is the radius of the airway. Most of the particle deposition models assume a laminar parabolic flow in all airway generations. Therefore, inertial impaction is expected to occur preferentially in the upper airways, at the airway bifurcations (Kim et al. 1994, Gonda 2004, Zhang et al. 2005, Carvalho et al. 2011).

Sedimentation occurs because of the gravity applied to the particles. Stokes law governs the terminal settling velocity (V_{ts}) in the laminar region:

$$V_{ts} = \frac{(\rho - \rho_a) \cdot d^2 \cdot g}{18 \cdot \eta} \tag{4}$$

where ρ_a is the air density and g the gravitational acceleration. However, as the particle size decreases, the Stokes law does not apply by itself and must be corrected with a slip correction factor, C_C, derived by Cunningham. The V_{ts} with the slip factor can be written as (Hinds 1999, Crowder et al. 2002, Gonda 2004, Carvalho et al. 2011):

$$V_{ts}(slip) = V_{ts} \cdot C_C \tag{5}$$

where:

$$C_C = 1 + K_n \left(2.514 + 0.8 \cdot e^{-\frac{0.55}{K_n}} \right) \tag{6}$$

where K_n is the Knudsen number in air.

Another parameter to consider when characterizing particle sedimentation behavior is the Reynolds number: if it indicates laminar flow, Stokes law is applicable. Otherwise, a turbulent drag correction factor must be applied to model the appropriate V_{ts} (Gonda 2004, Carvalho et al. 2011).

The last particle deposition mechanism mentioned in this chapter is diffusion. This phenomenon, also called Brownian motion, occurs when the particle size is so small that the particles undergo random motion due to particle collisions in the fluid. The rate of diffusion is proportional to the diffusion coefficient given by the Stokes-Einstein Equation:

$$Dif = \frac{k \cdot T}{3\pi \cdot \eta \cdot d} \tag{7}$$

where k is the Boltzmann's constant and T is the absolute temperature (Hinds 1999, Gonda 2004, Carvalho et al. 2011).

The diffusion driven deposition is only dependent on particle size and not its density: it will increase as the particle size decreases.

In the nose

The deposition mechanisms in the nose are identical to the ones described earlier. Particle deposition in the nasal cavity highly depends on the particle size as well as airflow velocity. The airflow behavior is intimately related to the breathing rate: while the airflow is laminar for a breathing rate of 15 L/minute, it becomes turbulent at breathing rate ≥ 25 L/minute (Hahn et al. 1993, Schreck et al. 1993). The major part of flow passes through the middle and inferior turbinates, and a smaller portion passes through the upper turbinate, including the meatuses and the olfactory region (Zamankhan et al. 2006), where most of the drug absorption is expected to happen. Particular attention should be paid to the particle size: particles > 10 μm in size will deposit in the nasal cavity. Particle < 10 μm will also start depositing in the airways of the lungs and when the particle size reaches the nano-sized range (< 200 nm), < 20% is anticipated to deposit in the nasal region (Fry and Black 1973, Gradon and Yu 1989, Schwab and Zenkel 1998, Kelly et al. 2004a,b, Zamankhan et al. 2006). Kelly et al. (2004a,b) also reported that the surface quality of the nasal epithelium and small anatomical variations do not affect nasal deposition significantly.

Particle Engineering Technologies

The definition of NP can be ambiguous across fields involved in the nanosciences. A common definition used in research and industry, and accepted by the International Organization for Standardization (2008), considers particles to be in the nanoscale when they are between 1 and 100 nm in every direction. Other governmental and environmental groups consider NPs to have a larger size: between 200 and 300 nm. The Food and Drug Administration, on the other hand, recommends not adopting a strict definition of nanomaterials due to the broad and complex fields employing this term (Watts and Williams 2011). In the pharmaceutical field, the definition is still unclear and the literature suggests that particles < 1 μm in all three dimensions should be considered as NPs given that, in this range, enhancements in membrane permeability and absorption are already observed (Kreuter 2004). For pulmonary delivery, technologies are employed to create NPs with the ultimate goal of improving powder dispersion and aerosol performance to deliver the drug to the deep lung.

NPs can be produced through a wide variety of particle engineering technologies. These particle size reduction technologies can be divided into two general categories: top-down and bottom-up processes. The top-down process is based on size reduction by consecutive fracture, abrasion, or cleavage of the bulk material. The bottom-up process refers to the gradual build-up of the particles until reaching the desired size range.

Top-down approach

Milling techniques

While different milling techniques are available on the market, only a couple of them are capable of producing particles in the nano-sized range (Table 5.1). Here only the milling techniques leading to nanomaterials will be described.

Ball Milling. Ball milling is a wet or dry process capable of reducing the particle size to the nano-sized range. In this technique, the milling cylinder is partially filled with fine milling pearls or balls made of steel, glass, zirconium oxide, tungsten carbide, high cross-linked plastic, such as hard polystyrene, with sizes ranging from 0.1 mm to more than 10 mm (Kwade and Schwedes 2007). The final particle size will depend on the speed of the disk stirrer, the rotation speed of the cylinder, the filling ratio of grinding beads and their sizes, as the impact, pressure and shear forces between the moving balls and the particles will be different. At high speed, the forces created by the balls falling from

Table 5.1. Approximate particle size obtainable by various milling techniques. Adapted with permission from Burcham et al. (2008). Copyright John Wiley & Sons Inc. (2008).

	Size (µm)	Hammer mill	Universal and pin mill	Jet mill	Jet mill with internal classifier	Media mill	Toothed rotor-stator	Colloid mill
Type	–	Dry	Dry	Dry	Dry	Wet	Wet	Wet
Very fine	50–150	×	×		×		×	
Super fine	10–50	×	×	×	×	×	×	×
Ultra fine	< 10		×	×	×	×		×
Colloidal	< 1				×	×		×

the top to the bottom of the cylinder provide coarse dry grinding of the bulk substance. At low speed, very fine grinding is achieved by attrition of the powder between the milling pearls, and the milling pearl and the wall of the milling chamber. Also, as the milling ball size decreases, the surface area increases, offering a large number of contact points with the bulk powder resulting in a slower but finer grinding.

In this type of top-down particle reduction technique, shear forces of the fluid can be considered too low to break the particles. Therefore, the particles can only be broken when stressed in between two grinding pearls or between a grinding pearl and the wall of the milling chamber. The efficiency of the process will depend on the number of particles captured between the grinding elements, the number of stress events and their intensity (Kwade 1999, Hennart et al. 2009). Depending on the number of particles caught in this process, the energy transferred to the particles will vary. First, if only one particle is captured, the entire force will transfer to the particle. Second, if more than one particle is captured between the balls, the first particle to be captured will be the largest one and/or the closest one to the connection point between each ball, hence receiving the largest force. The subsequent particles captured between the two pearls will be stressed but at considerably lower energies of different intensities. Single particle stressing occurs rarely and the number of captured particles depends preferentially on the concentration of the dispersion and on the particle size. Kwade (1999) reported that the ratio between the diameter of active volume between the two grinding balls, d_{act}, and the average distance between two particles in suspension, y, could be a mean of evaluating the number of particle captured. The active volume is the volume in which a particle is captured between two grinding balls. The average distance between the centers of two particles is linked to the solids volume concentration of the dispersion and the size of the particles.

$$\frac{d_{act}}{y} = \sqrt[3]{\frac{6C_v}{\pi}} \cdot \sqrt{2(1-r) \cdot \frac{d_{GM}}{d} + 1 - r^2} \; ; r = \frac{a}{d} \tag{8}$$

where d_{GM} is the diameter of the grinding balls, d is the diameter of a particle, a is the minimum distance between the grinding balls, and C_v is the concentration of the particles in the dispersion.

If the ratio d_{act}/y is greater than 1 and d tends to zero, then multiple particles are expected to be captured between the grinding balls. Moreover, as the size decreases, the fluid flow will drive the smaller particles better than the large ones, increasing the probability of capture between the chamber wall and the grinding balls. Therefore the d_{act}/y ratio increases with decreasing particle size. In addition, the viscosity of a suspension containing particles < 2 µm increases, in comparison to a suspension of the same concentration with larger particles, and the mobility decreases, hence the probability of having a bed of particles captured between the grinding balls increases and the efficacy of the collision decreases, increasing at the same time the process duration to obtain finer particles.

The stress events leading to the capture of particles between the grinding balls, or the grinding balls and the chamber wall can be organized in three possible mechanisms: acceleration of the grinding balls from the disk stirrer geometry to the chamber walls acquiring kinetic energy, centrifugal acceleration causing the grinding balls to press against the chamber wall, and the motion of the grinding elements in tangential direction at high velocity and their collision with other grinding elements with lower velocities. The average number of stress events (SN) for each particle can be estimated as follow (Kwade 1999):

$$SN = \frac{N_C \cdot P_S}{N_P} \tag{9}$$

where N_C is the number of media contacts, P_S is the probability of the particles to be captured and sufficiently stressed when in contact with the grinding balls, and N_P is the number of particles inside the wet mill.

The stress intensities can be described as the results of the force acting on the grinding balls and the kinetic energy of the grinding balls, and depends on the type of stress mechanisms considered. Kwade (1999) provided a detailed study on the estimation of the stress intensities.

While the dry ball mill can decrease the particle size down to ≈ 0.5 µm, wet ball milling, also called media milling, is capable of decreasing the particle size far < 400 nm. In 1992, the NanoCrystal® Technology was the first wet milling nanotechnology to achieve particles in the nano-sized range (Merisko-Liversidge et al. 2003, Merisko-Liversidge and Liversidge 2011) (Fig. 5.2). Wet milling is based on the same technique as the dry ball milling process but employs grinding poorly water-soluble drugs (water solubility < 10 mg/mL) dispersed in an aqueous dispersion containing stabilizers and surfactants. Surfactants and stabilizers are used during the fabrication process

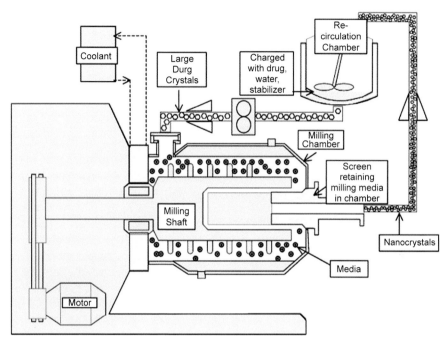

Figure 5.2. NanoCrystal® Technology from Elan Pharmaceuticals. The milling chamber charged with polymeric media is the active component of the mill. The mill can be operated in a batch or re-circulation mode. Crude slurry consisting of drug, water, and stabilizer is fed into the milling chamber and processed into a nanocrystalline dispersion. The typical residence time required to generate a nanometer-sized dispersion with a mean diameter < 200 nm is 30 to 60 minutes. Reprinted with permission from Merisko-Liversidge et al. (2003). Copyright Elsevier BV (2003).

to avoid aggregation of the crystals in the nanodispersion. The amount of surface modifiers can vary between 0.1 and 90% by weight, and the drug concentration in the dispersion is usually ≤ 400 mg/mL. It is a popular technique due to its ease of scalability (from 25 mg to 1 ton) and its relatively short process time (30 to 60 minutes). It also offers thermal control over the process: precooling or cooling the suspending media can control the process temperature enabling the use of heat-sensitive materials. Hence, the chemical degradation, solid phase transition, and melting of the milled substances can be prevented (Merisko-Liversidge et al. 2003). This wet mill technology has expanded the use of NPs for oral, pulmonary, intravenous, intramuscular, subcutaneous, and ocular drug delivery systems (Merisko-Liversidge and Liversidge 2008). Ostrander et al. (1999) reported beclomethasone dipropionate milled to a mean size of 164 nm using the NanoCrystal® technology. Nebulization of beclomethasone dipropionate made by the NanoCrystal® process exhibited a fine particle dose (amount of drug anticipated to deposit deep in the lungs) upon *in vitro* characterization improved by a factor of two in comparison to the commercialized product Vanceril® inhaler.

Fluid Energy Milling. Fluid energy milling technology, also called air jet milling, is based on inter-particle impactions and sometimes even particle-wall collisions to reduce the particle size: the average size range of particles generated is very diverse and depends on the type of air jet mill used. In the industry, fluid energy mills are very popular dry milling techniques due to their efficiency and scalability. One type of fluid energy mill is the spiral jet mill consisting of a horizontal circular grinding chamber into which the drug substance is fed. The particle size generated is < 10 μm (Dobson and Rothwell 1969). The powder to micronize is metered into a feed funnel. Compressed air or gas from the injector draws the feed material in the grinding chamber through a vacuum created by the Venturi tube. The grinding air or gas supplies high pressure air or gas to the grinding chamber in a rotational direction and is forced through the grinding nozzles at high speed. The high velocity air or gas vortex created in the chamber accelerates the feed powder generating particle-particle impaction and leading to particle size reduction. The centrifugal forces maintain the larger particles in the outer area of the grinding chamber where particle collisions occurs, while the finer particles travel towards the center due to centripetal forces and exit the grinding chamber in the draft generated by the vortex finder or inner classification tube. A schematic of the fluid energy mill is shown in Fig. 5.3.

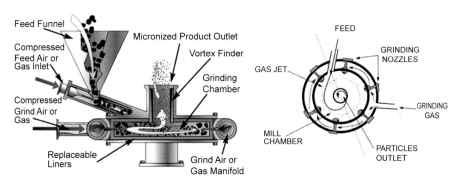

Figure 5.3. Right: Fluid energy mill or jet mill. Sturtevant Jet Mill Micronizer®, courtesy of Sturtevant, Inc. Left: Schematic of a spiral jet mill grinding chamber. Reprinted with permission from Midoux et al. (1999). Copyright Elsevier S.A. (1999).

The parameters affecting the particle size of the final product are the geometric parameters related to the mill design and the operational condition related to the solid feed rate, the injector pressure, the grinding pressure, and the material itself (Midoux et al. 1999), with the most significant variables being the feed rate, the volumetric flow rate of the grinding air or gas, and the height of the vortex finder when grinding at constant pressure (Tuunila and Nystrom 1998). An extensive analysis of process scale-up of the spiral jet mill was provided by Midoux et al. (1999).

During the grinding process, disorder of the crystal structure of the milled drug substance may happen, leading to amorphous or partially amorphous particles. Since the recrystallization phenomenon is random, the particle size growth is generally uncontrolled. Brodka-Pfeiffer et al. (2003a,b) performed thorough studies on the micronization of salbutamol sulfate intended for pulmonary delivery, using the spiral air jet mill. In their first study (Brodka-Pfeiffer et al. 2003a), after milling of salbutamol sulfate, they obtained large loose aggregates of very fine particles that could be easily redispersed. The average particle size obtained was 1.71 μm. The amorphous content varied depending on the grinding pressure. Their subsequent publication (Brodka-Pfeiffer et al. 2003b) focused on the recrystallization phenomena upon storage of the milled salbutamol sulfate in different storage conditions and the associated particle growth. On one hand, no particle growth and crystal structure changes were observed in the dry conditioning, but this type of conditioning is not a feasible approach in the industry. On the other hand, complete recrystallization was observed within 24 hours when the powder was stored at ≤ 55% relative humidity, with the largest particle growth seen at 40°C and 75% relative humidity. Even if crystal growth was observed, the particle size remained < 5 μm, in the respirable range.

Cryogenic Milling. Cryogenic milling or cryomilling involves the mechanical attrition of powders in cryogenic conditions. The process is similar to ball milling where the particles are either milled in a slurry, formed with a cryogenic milling media, or dry milled using a cryogenic liquid to decrease the temperature of the milling chamber. In either case, both fabrication processes control the temperature of the grinding chamber using a cryogenic media while the particle size reduction occurs by attrition (Witkin and Lavernia 2006, Lavernia et al. 2008). Cryomilling offers advantages for the particle size reduction of heat-sensitive compounds, increases the particle brittleness favoring particle fracture upon impaction, but also has certain limitations related to the cryogenic liquid removal such as particle aggregation.

Niwa et al. (2010) developed an ultra cryomilling technique (Fig. 5.4). It is based on media ball milling techniques but uses liquid nitrogen as the dispersing media instead of water, due to the rare solubility of solid particles in this cryogenic liquid. Liquid nitrogen was chosen due to its low viscosity (0.158 mPa·s at –196°C) and low surface tension (8.85 mN/m at –196°C) preventing coaggregation of the particles during the milling process, and because materials become more brittle at cryogenic temperatures (under –150°C). The authors optimized the ultra cryomill process conditions to obtained particles in the nano-sized range: the size of grinding beads, the volume of bead loading, and the agitation speed of the rotation shaft and disks were investigated. Using this technology, NPs of phenytoin, ibuprofen, and salbutamol sulfate were produced and the ultra cryomill technology lead to higher percentages of submicron particles for each drug in comparison to the jet mill technology. However, particle aggregation upon evaporation of liquid nitrogen was a major

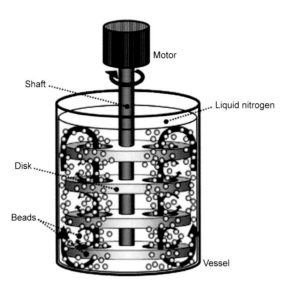

Figure 5.4. Diagram of ultra cryomilling apparatus in liquid nitrogen. The beads, disks, shaft, and inner wall of vessel are made of zirconia. Reprinted with permission from Niwa et al. (2010). Copyright Elsevier BV (2010).

concern. Even though particle reduction increases the specific surface area, the particle size reduction of poorly water-soluble drug has the tendency to form poorly water-soluble aggregates with low wettability capability. Sugimoto et al. (2012) also used the ultra cryomill technology and suggested the use of surfactants and stabilizers to prevent particle agglomeration and improve wetting. Solubility enhancement of phenytoin co-ground with different pharmaceutical excipients using the ultra cryomill was proven.

Cryogenic milling technologies are interesting techniques to reduce particle size. The process parameters can be tailored to achieve a particular particle size range. However, additional scale-up studies are necessary to make this technology appropriate for use in the pharmaceutical industry.

High-pressure homogenization

The homogenization process forms homogeneous or narrowed particle size distributions in suspensions or emulsions. Homogenization techniques can be separated into two categories: low-energy input homogenization specific to emulsions, and high-energy input homogenization used to fabricate suspensions and emulsions. Here only the high-energy homogenization processes and more specifically the different type of high-pressure homogenization techniques as they are the most commonly used in the top-down processes will be highlighted. High-pressure homogenizers utilize three different types of energy transfer mechanisms depending on the process conditions: collision/impaction, shear stress, and cavitation. Homogenization processes are advantageous due to various volume capacities, ranging from milliliters to a few thousand liters, the tailoring of the particle size and the possible modification of the crystalline nature of the substrate, from crystalline to partially amorphous to completely amorphous. These processes are therefore easily scalable and the solubility is improved thanks to particle size reduction and crystal structure modifications.

Piston-Gap Homogenization. Most piston-gap homogenization techniques are based on cavitation forces to reduce the particle size. In this particle engineering technique, the substances are dispersed in water and passed through a very small gap ($\leq$ 25 μm) at high pressure ($\approx$ 1,500 bar) (Fig. 5.5). According to the Bernouilli's principle, the high streaming velocity created by the passage of the particle suspension through the very small gap and the increased dynamic pressure of the fluid lead to the boiling of the dispersant (water) at room temperature. The gas bubbles formed collapse as the fluid exits the piston gap causing cavitation-induced shock waves, therefore fracturing the particles and reducing their size (Muller and Peters 1998, Rabinow 2004, Morales et al. 2012). The particle size range and polydispersity index obtained highly depend on the process pressure and the number of cycle applied (Muller and Peters 1998, Liedtke et al. 2000). Budesonide for pulmonary administration has been successfully produced using the piston-gap homogenization technology (Jacobs and Muller 2002). The suspension was first pre-milled to the micron-size range at increasing pressure and then reduced to the nano-sized range at high pressure during 20 cycles. The stabilizers and surfactants played an important role in the final particle size of the suspension as steric and electrostatic stabilizations were necessary to prevent

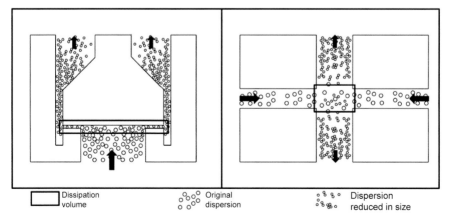

| Dissipation volume | Original dispersion | Dispersion reduced in size |

Figure 5.5. Basic homogenization principles. Left: piston-gap homogenizer arrangement where the macrosuspension is forced through a small gap and particle fracture occurs due to shear forces, cavitation, and impaction. Right: jet-stream homogenizer arrangement where impact forces fracture the particle due to the collision of two high-velocity stream. Reprinted with permission from Morales et al. (2012). Copyright Springer Science+Business Media (2012).

particle agglomeration. After choosing the optimized formulation, scale-up and increase of drug content were performed and did not significantly affect the particle size. The budesonide suspension was shown to be stable over a one-year period.

Other technologies based on the same piston-gap homogenizing technique were developed. DissoCubes™ technology, developed by Müller et al. and acquired by SkyePharma PLC (Junghanns and Muller 2008), increases the saturation solubility and induces structural changes in the particle (the high energy input increases the amorphous fraction). The feasibility of the process was investigated and several poorly water-soluble drugs could be converted into nanosuspension with a mean particle size diameter < 1 µm (Möeschwitzer et al. 2004, Keck and Muller 2006, Teeranachaideekul et al. 2008).

NanoPure® technology, developed by PharmaSol GmbH, uses the piston-gap homogenization approach but utilizes low vapor pressure dispersion media and low homogenization temperature. The boiling of the dispersing media is almost non-existent, hence the particle size reduction is exclusively the result of shear stress, collision, and turbulence, and not cavitation. The low temperatures used in this process allow the use of thermo-labile compounds and because non-aqueous media can be used, degradation of the drug substances via hydrolysis is prevented (Keck and Muller 2006, Möeschwitzer and Müller 2006, Junghanns and Muller 2008). Nanosuspensions of amphoterin B using the NanoPure® technology with a mean diameter of 250 nm and a polydispersity index of 0.3 have been prepared (Keck and Muller 2006).

Jet-Stream Homogenization. Jet-stream homogenizers, also called microfluidizers, use the impaction of jet streams to induce particle size reduction. The concept of jet stream interaction front was invented and patented by Cook and Lagace (1985) to produce solid lipid NP emulsions and owned by Microfluidics Corporation. Later on, the concept was applied to suspension and particle size reduction. The pre-homogenized coarse suspension in the inlet reservoir is passed through an intensifier pump generating pressures up to 40,000 psi and accelerated into the interaction chamber. Inside the interaction chamber, the stream divides into microchannels. The high-pressure streams generated are forced to collide upon themselves at ultrahigh velocity up to 400 m/s. The impaction and shearing forces produced cause particle breakage and size reduction.

The microfluidizer presents disadvantages including the obtaining of a rather large quantity of particles in the larger size range (Illig et al. 1996), the high number of passes necessary to obtain particles within the desired size range (sometimes up to 100 passes), translating into long processing times, and the compatibility of the process with "soft" drugs rather than "hard" drugs (Keck and Muller 2006). These drawbacks have been overcome by the introduction of "Y" multi-slotted interaction chamber resulting in ease of scalability and the obtaining particles in the nano-sized range in as little as two passes.

Bottom-up approach

Spray Drying. Spray drying techniques have been used industrially for well over a century and are therefore well-understood processes. Its simplicity, robustness, and scalability have convinced a variety of industrials to use this technology for a vast panel of products. In the pharmaceutical industry, spray drying has been used to generate bulk active ingredients such as small and large molecules, vitamins, and bulk excipients (Miller and Gil 2012). It has also been used as a process technology to provide unique physical and chemical properties to pharmaceutical powders including increased porosity, crystal changes, and sphericity.

Spray drying technology is a multi-step process (Fig. 5.6) (Chow et al. 2007, Cal and Sollohub 2010, Miller and Gil 2012): the preparation of a feed fluid, which can consist of a solution, suspension, or emulsion, the atomization of that fluid through a nozzle in the drying chamber, the evaporation of solvent droplets after contact with the hot drying gas, which are converted into particles, the separation of those particles from the wet drying gas into the cyclone or filter bag. The final particle size and characteristics rely on the operating parameters chosen, such as the type of atomizer, the atomization pressure, the airflow, and the drying temperature. The atomizer is a key parameter of the spray drying technology, as it will impact the degree of atomization of the feed fluid. Several types of atomizer are available: rotary nozzles, pneumatic two-fluid nozzles, three- and four-fluid nozzles, pressure nozzles, ultrasonic nozzles, and monodispersed nozzles. The atomizer selection is based on the feed fluid properties (e.g., nature of the fluid, viscosity, rheological behavior),

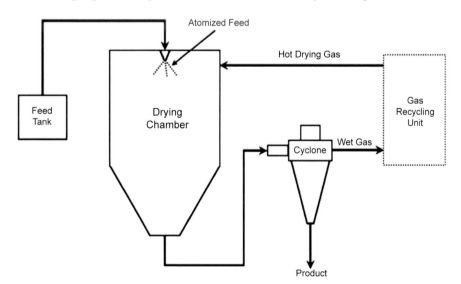

Figure 5.6. Schematic of the spray drying technology. Reprinted with permission from Miller and Gil (2012). Copyright Springer Science+Business Media (2012).

the feed flow capacity, particle size distribution targeted, and the air disperser design of the spray drying unit (Cal and Sollohub 2010, Pilcer and Amighi 2010, Miller and Gil 2012). Then, the drying gas-droplet contact may occur according to two different configurations: co-current, where both the drying gas and the atomized droplets originate from the top of the drying chamber, and counter-current, where the atomized droplets originate from the top of the drying chamber while the drying gas exits through the bottom of the chamber. The collecting systems include cyclones, the common collection system used in the pharmaceutical industry, filter bags, which are usually placed after the cyclones to prevent particles from being carried in the gas recycling system, and electrostatic precipitators that are used to collect NPs and improved recovery efficiencies (Cal and Sollohub 2010, Miller and Gil 2012).

This technology has been very popular for the fabrication of particles for pulmonary and nasal delivery. One of the recent examples is Exubera™ commercialized by Pfizer. It was the first approved pharmaceutical product treating type I and type II diabetes through pulmonary delivery of insulin. The product was formulated as a dry homogeneous powder produced by spray drying (Atkins 2005). Despite its commercial failure, due to a lack of success, this inhaled insulin formulation was a major breakthrough in the systemic drug delivery via the inhalation route.

Drugs to treat pulmonary diseases, such as anti-asthmatics, immunosuppressants, antifungals, anticancer drugs, and potential vaccines have been formulated using the spray drying technology. Also, excipients, such as lactose and mannitol, have been physically modified using this technology to serve as drug carrier for pulmonary delivery. The advantage offered by this process is the production of low density, usually highly porous particles. The geometric of those particles is large but their d_a is small. First, it results in improved aerosolization of the particle due to the smaller surface area to volume ratio, which reduces the risk of aggregation and promotes immediate dispersion of the particles by the airflow shear forces (Edwards et al. 1997); but because of their small d_a, the particles are efficiently deposited in the deep lung with fine particle fraction reaching 65 to 95% (Platz et al. 2002). Second, because of their large diameter, the particles escape the phagocytosis clearance mechanism providing a sustained release in the lungs (Edwards et al. 1997). Finally, those large, porous particles may be used as carriers for systemic delivery of small molecules, and therapeutic proteins and peptides via the lungs and are often referred as Trojan particles (Tsapis et al. 2002, Hadinoto et al. 2007).

Cryogenic technologies

Cryogenic technologies were developed to improve the solubility and dissolution properties of poorly water-soluble drugs by increasing the specific surface area of the particles through nanostructures, and creating amorphous materials (Rogers et al. 2003b, Overhoff et al. 2007). As its name suggests, the cryogenic technology uses cryogenic liquids to rapidly freeze a feed formulation containing the drug and, sometimes, additional pharmaceutical excipients. The commonly used cryogen is liquid nitrogen: it is colorless, odorless, non-flammable, and has a boiling temperature of –195°C. Its alternative is liquid argon with a boiling temperature of –185°C. Liquid argon is however an asphyxiating gas and is more expensive than liquid nitrogen. Other cryogens are used, such as liquid hydrocarbons, but they exhibit a higher boiling point and on a safety stand point, are more dangerous as they are highly combustible. The feed solution containing the drug and the excipients are often dissolved or emulsified in a solvent or co-solvent system, and the frozen matter has to be dried to get the free-flowing powder. Sublimation processes such as lyophilization and atmospheric freeze-drying are used for solvent removal. The sublimation step is critical as the advantageous physicochemical properties imparted during the cryogenic process may be lost if melting occurs.

Spray Freeze-Drying (SFD). This cryogenic method has been used in the pharmaceutical industry for over 60 years. It was first used for proteins and peptides, because unlike spray drying techniques, no heat is required which prevents proteins and peptides denaturation (Benson and Ellis 1948). It was only in the early 1990s that SFD started to be used by pharmaceutical industries to prepare amorphous forms of poorly water-soluble drugs (Mumenthaler and Leuenberger 1991, Zijlstra et al. 2007).

The particle engineering technique is generally described as a three step process comprising the atomization of a feed solution, emulsion, or suspension containing the drug and, potentially, pharmaceutical excipients, rapid freezing of the atomized droplets above the surface of the cryogenic liquid and sublimation of the solvent from the frozen material to obtain a final, usually amorphous, dry powder.

The atomization of the drug solution, emulsion, or suspension is possible using different types of specialized fluid nozzle or vibrating orifice droplet generators. They include two-fluid nozzles, ultrasound, or vibration nozzles, and monodisperse droplet generators. The particle size and the morphology of the particles rely on the physicochemical properties of the feed liquid, i.e., surface tension and viscosity, the type of nozzle used and the atomization parameters, i.e., liquid processing rate, liquid pressure, atomizing gas, etc. Two-fluid nozzles allow the highest processing rate (up to 15 L/minute) but the particle size distribution can easily spread over several orders of magnitude. The physicochemical properties of the liquid formulation, the nozzle geometry, and the velocity of the liquid and atomizing gas control the particle size distribution with this type of nozzle. In addition to generating a wide particle size distribution, the use of the atomizing gas decreases the efficiency and effectiveness of the cryogenic vapor to freeze the atomized droplets by increasing its temperature. Ultrasonic or vibration nozzles offer a lower processing rate than the two-fluid nozzles even though it is considered to be relatively high (up to 100 mL/minute). Its advantages over the two-fluid nozzles are the control of the particle size and its narrow distribution, and the lower cost, as it does not utilize large amounts of atomizing gas. Particle size is controlled by properties of the feed liquid and nozzle, i.e., orifice size and atomizing area, and the frequency of the vibration/sonication. The last type of nozzle, monodisperse droplet generators, utilizes ink jet printing technology. They create highly monodispersed droplets but the processing rates are extremely low (≈ 0.1 mL/minute) and the viscosity of the feed solution limits the technology as they may clog the droplet generators.

The freezing of the atomized droplets occurs in the cryogenic vapors. In many cases, the cryogenic vapor is created over the cryogen reservoir ensuring complete freezing of the atomized droplets as they enter the cryogen. This technology has been used to generate solid dispersions of cyclosporine A (CsA) for pulmonary delivery (Zijlstra et al. 2007). The particles obtained at different drug loadings are characterized by an d_a well within the respirable range. The SFD technology was also used to prepare dry powder of whole inactivated influenza virus for nasal vaccination (Garmise et al. 2007). Here the particle size range was above the respirable range to enhance deposition in the nasal cavity.

Spray Freezing into Liquid (SFL). SFL is a more recently reported particle engineering technology developed and patented by Williams III et al. (2002), and commercialized by The Dow Chemical Company, and more recently Enavail LLC. A feed solution consisting of an aqueous, organic, or aqueous/organic cosolvent system, aqueous/organic emulsion, or suspension containing the drug alone or the drug with pharmaceutical excipients, is sprayed under pressure into cryogenic liquid through an insulated nozzle. The cryogenic liquid includes compressed fluid carbon dioxide, helium, propane, ethane, liquid nitrogen, liquid argon, or hydrofluoroethers (Williams III et al. 2002); but as mentioned earlier, the most common cryogen used is liquid nitrogen. The spray generates frozen atomized droplets of the feed solution upon contact with the cryogen. The frozen material is then dried via sublimation to collect dry flowing drug particles.

The powders processed with the SFL technology are generally characterized by micron-sized aggregates exhibiting primary nanostructures (Hu et al. 2004a, Yu et al. 2006) with an amorphous morphology, high porosity, hence, high surface area; all contributing to improve wettability in water and enhance dissolution properties of the poorly water-soluble drugs processed by SFL (Hu et al. 2002, 2004b, Rogers et al. 2003a). The SFL technology has been used to generate successful formulations for pulmonary delivery (Hoeben et al. 2006, Vaughn et al. 2006, Alvarez et al. 2007). Nanostructures of itraconazole formulations were delivered to mice as prophylaxis against invasive pulmonary aspergillosis (Alvarez et al. 2007). The survival rate of mice treated with the SFL itraconazole formulation was greater in comparison to the group receiving the marketed product via oral gavage.

The SFL process and the SFD process are two similar NP engineering technologies, but the SFL process produces products with better stability. In fact, both the SFL and the SFD processes were shown to produce microparticles of similar porosity when fabricating lysozyme particles (Yu et al. 2006). The degree of protein aggregation and the loss of protein activity were however lower in the SFL process than in the SFD. Also, due to reduced exposure time to the air-water interface in the SFL technology, the product made with the SFL technology was more stable than with the SFD process.

Thin Film Freezing (TFF). The TFF technology is also known as ultra rapid freezing, cold metal block freezing, spray forming, thermal spray coating, splat cooling, slat quenching solidification, powder spray deposition, etc. (Overhoff et al. 2009). Similar to the SFL and the SFD technologies, the TFF process starts with a feed solution containing the drug alone or with pharmaceutical excipients. The feed solution is frozen drop wise on a rotating cryogenic substrate pre-cooled to a given temperature, usually below the lowest freezing temperature of the solvent used to dissolve the drug and the excipients. The frozen thin pellets are then removed from the cryogenic surface by a scraper and maintained in a frozen state in liquid nitrogen. Again, similar to the SFD and SFL technologies, the solvents are removed by sublimation to obtain dry powders. The schematic diagram of the TFF process is depicted in Fig. 5.7 (Beinborn et al. 2012).

This process is utilized to create micro-aggregates containing primary nanostructures of amorphous or crystalline materials. It improves the dissolution of poorly water soluble drugs by increasing the specific surface area of the particles as well as modifying their crystal structure (Overhoff et al.

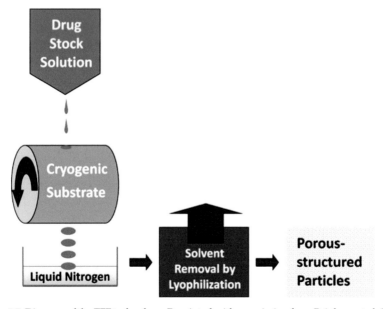

Figure 5.7. Diagram of the TFF technology. Reprinted with permission from Beinborn et al. (2012). Copyright Elsevier BV (2012).

2007). The cooling rate of the TFF process ($\approx 10^2$ K/s) produces rapid nucleation and significantly prevents particle growth, as the particles are immobilized in the frozen state. The size of the primary structures is controlled by the process parameters and the formulation composition: the solvent composition, the percentage of dissolved solids in the feed solution, and the temperature of the cryogenic surface (Engstrom et al. 2008, Beinborn et al. 2012). Several formulations for pulmonary delivery have been developed using the TFF technology (Sinswat et al. 2008, Yang et al. 2008, 2010). However, due to the excipient limitations for use in inhalation therapy, stabilizing the active pharmaceutical ingredient in its amorphous state without compromising on the final product potency can be challenging. The TFF process is also limited by its costs when used at production scale: the maintenance of a low humidity environment and the use of high quantities of liquid nitrogen are major drawbacks.

Controlled precipitation technology

The precipitation technology is one of the earliest processes developed to fabricate NPs and microparticles. They are based on the control of the particle growth mechanisms: nucleation, condensation, and coagulation (Fig. 5.8). The overall process consists of the dissolution of the drug in an appropriate solvent, the addition of that solution to an antisolvent, causing the precipitation of fine drug particles, and finally solvent removal.

Antisolvent Precipitation. The antisolvent precipitation process is one of the most commonly used bottom-up processes to form NPs due to its simplicity, cost effectiveness, and ease of scale-up. The production of hydrolsols

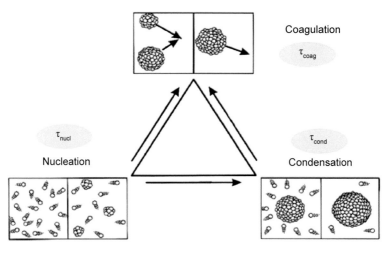

Figure 5.8. Particle growth mechanisms. τ_{cond} is the condensation time, τ_{nucl} is the nucleation time, and τ_{coag} is the coagulation time. Reprinted with permission from Matteucci et al. (2006). Copyright American Chemical Society (2006).

and Nanomorph® products by Novartis and Abbott, respectively, have demonstrated the scalability of this particle engineering technique (Keck and Muller 2006). In the antisolvent precipitation process, the drug is dissolved in an organic solvent, which is then added to an antisolvent, usually water. The drug must be sparingly soluble in the antisolvent, but the solvent and antisolvent must be miscible in the fabrication conditions. During the two-phase mixing, the solubility of the drug drops increasing the degree of supersaturation and subsequently the degree of nucleation. Due to the miscibility of the solvent in the aqueous media, the nuclei are spread apart limiting coagulation. The addition of stabilizers further prevents particle growth by condensation and coagulation: upon precipitation, the hydrophilic portion of the stabilizer extends in the aqueous phase while the hydrophobic portion adsorbs at the surface of the particle, providing steric stabilization and, depending on the chemistry of the stabilizer, electrostatic stabilization (Wu et al. 2011). A schematic diagram of the antisolvent precipitation driving mechanism is given in Fig. 5.9.

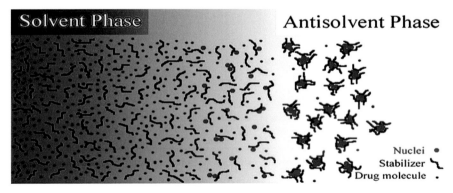

Figure 5.9. Antisolvent precipitation in the presence of amphiphilic stabilizers. Reprinted with permission from Matteucci et al. (2006). Copyright American Chemical Society (2006).

This technique more commonly produces micron-sized particles rather than nano-sized particles. As mentioned earlier, the degree of miscibility of the solvent with the antisolvent is a factor contributing to the formation of drug NPs, as it facilitates supersaturation and adsorption of the stabilizers at the surface of the nucleating particles. Another critical parameter influencing the final size of the particle is the efficiency of mixing of the solvent and antisolvent. The Damkohler number (D_a) measures the influence of mixing on phase separation (Matteucci et al. 2006).

$$D_a = \frac{\tau_{mix}}{\tau_{precip}} \tag{10}$$

where τ_{mix} and τ_{precip} are the mixing and precipitation times, respectively. τ_{precip} is a function of the condensation time τ_{cond} and the coagulation time τ_{coag}

(see Fig. 5.8). A large D_a (> 1) implies a process controlled by mixing (τ_{mix} is large) leading to low and heterogeneously distributed levels of supersaturation, and low nucleation rates relative to particle growth rates. The particles obtained are generally large and polydisperse. In this case, D_a can be reduced by increasing the mixing intensity, which generates greater supersaturation and more rapid nucleation (decrease in τ_{mix}). Also, the addition of stabilizers may extend the coagulation and condensation time, therefore increasing τ_{precip} and bringing D_a closer to 1. A low D_a (< 1) implies a process controlled by precipitation. The nucleation occurs more rapidly, relative to particle growth, as a result of a rapid and more homogeneous supersaturation levels. A large number of nuclei are formed and the particles generated are small and monodispersed.

Matteucci et al. (2006) have thoroughly investigated the critical variables of the antisolvent precipitation process: the rate of drug solvent added, the degree of miscibility of the solvent and antisolvent, the antisolvent to solvent ratio, the type and amount of stabilizers, the degree of mixing, the type of nozzle, the temperature, etc. Several drugs intended for pulmonary administration have been generated using this particle engineering technology: atropine sulfate (Ali et al. 2009), beclomethasone dipropriate (Wang et al. 2007), insulin (Klingler et al. 2009), salbutamol sulfate (Bhavna et al. 2009), CsA (Tam et al. 2008), paclitaxel (El-Gendy and Berkland 2009), progesterone (Ragab et al. 2010), budesonide (Hu et al. 2008). The particles obtained were in the submicron range and well within the respirable size range.

Evaporative Precipitation into Aqueous Solution (EPAS). The EPAS technology has been developed and patented by Johnston et al. (2004) and is owned by The Dow Chemical Company, and more recently Enavail LLC. This technology involves the dissolution of the drug alone or with pharmaceutical excipients in a low boiling temperature organic solvent, the atomization of this solution into an aqueous solution heated above the boiling point of the organic solvent, and the precipitation of the NPs in the aqueous media. Stabilizers and surfactants are incorporated in the aqueous phase, the organic phase, or both. The rapid evaporation of the organic solvent induces supersaturation of the drug and therefore its nucleation. The nucleating surfaces increase the interfacial area generating a strong driving force for the adsorption of the stabilizers at the surface of the newly formed particles. The resulting particles are then dried by one of the following process: filtration, lyophilization, TFF followed by sublimation, spray drying (Rowe and Johnston 2012).

The particle size and its distribution, and the morphology of the particles obtained by this particle engineering technique, rely on the nozzle design, the process temperature, the flow rate, the degree of mixing, the choice of organic solvent, the choice of stabilizers and their concentration, and the final drug loading of the final aqueous suspension. The organic solvent influences the particle size of the product because the degree of miscibility of the solvent with water will control the particle growth via Ostwald ripening and the capability of the stabilizers to adsorb on the surface of the particles and provide steric stabilization. Chen et al. (2002) showed a significant particle size reduction when producing CsA NPs stabilized with Pluronic® F-127 with dichloromethane than diethyl ether. The particles produced when using diethyl ether were about three-fold larger than the one produced with dichloromethane (1,218 nm vs. 423 nm).

The organic solvent is heated to improve the drug solubility and promote rapid evaporation during atomization. The aqueous media is also heated to accelerate the evaporation process even more and enhance the nucleation rates. However, the benefits of increased temperatures of the aqueous media depend on the nature of the stabilizers. In fact, when fabricating polyvinylpyrrolidone-stabilized CsA, Chen et al. (2002) observed a decrease in the particle size when increasing the temperature from 55 to 85°C. On the contrary, when using polysorbate 80, they observed an increasing average particle size as the temperature of the aqueous media increased. This phenomenon can be attributed to the weakening of the hydrogen bonding between the ethylene oxide groups of polysorbate 80 at high temperatures, which interfered with the steric stabilization of the particles (Blankschtein et al. 1986). The choice of stabilizers and their amounts are hence intimately related to the process parameters (Sinswat et al. 2005).

The typical sizes of particles obtained from the EPAS technology range between 1 and 10 μm. However, when the process parameters are chosen well, particles in the nanometer range can be produced. The EPAS process successfully produced itraconazole NPs for the prevention of invasive pulmonary aspergillosis (Hoeben et al. 2006). The particles were within the respirable range and the pulmonary administration of the EPAS itraconazole powder significantly improved survival in comparison to the commercial oral product in a murine model.

Emulsion Templates. The emulsion template process consists in creating a micro- or nano-emulsion followed by solvent evaporation. The solvent evaporation can be performed via vacuum evaporation, lyophilization, spray drying, or one of the cryogenic technologies mentioned previously in this chapter, followed by sublimation.

The key to this technology is first to create a stable emulsion. Emulsions are, by nature, thermodynamically instable system due to their positive free energy of emulsion formation (ΔG_f). The interfacial energy term ($\lambda\Delta A$) is positive and much larger than the entropy of droplet formation (ΔS_f), such that the free energy of emulsion formation can never be entropy driven (Anton et al. 2008).

$$\Delta G = \lambda\Delta A - T\Delta S_f \qquad (11)$$

where λ is the surface tension, ΔA is the surface area gained with emulsification, and T the temperature.

Emulsion destabilization results from the tendency to try to reduce the large interfacial area between the two immiscible phases created during the emulsion formation. The use of surfactants is therefore critical to ensure stability of the emulsion formed as they reduce the surface tension between the two phases.

The emulsification methods may involve high and low energy emulsification processes. Here only the high-energy emulsification methods as they are the most commonly used to produce formulations for inhalation and nasal delivery will be discussed. Three types of devices are mainly reported in the literature to generate nanoscale emulsions: the rotor/stator devices, the ultrasonic devices, and the microfluidizers, being discussed earlier in this chapter. These devices induce mechanical stress disrupting the interface between the two phases, oil and water, followed by the adsorption or arrangement of the surfactants at the oil/water interface ensuring steric and/or electrostatic stabilization of the droplets formed. The rotor/stator devices induce droplet size reduction by shear forces and impaction. Even though they are great tools to generate microemulsions, rotors/stators are not the preferred device to create nanoemulsions as the final emulsions are fairly polydispersed (Walstra 1993, Abismaïl et al. 1999). The energy provided by the mechanical agitation is primarily dissipated as heat and wasted in viscous friction, resulting in an energy transferred to the system not sufficient to create the nanoemulsion. Ultrasound devices are the second type of high-energy devices and use cavitation forces to generate the emulsions. The waves produced by the ultrasonic horn induce a series of mechanical rarefaction and compression, leading to the implosion of the cavitation bubbles generated (Anton et al. 2008). Here again the energy created by the ultrasonic horn is dissipated by heat but the energy remaining is sufficient to increase the interfacial area and create an emulsion. The efficiency of this nanoemulsification process depends both on the power of the sonication as well as the composition of the formulation. This process is very useful at the laboratory level but industrials will preferentially turn themselves toward high-pressure homogenizers as their batch capacities are considerably larger. The high-pressure homogenizers described earlier can be utilized to create nanosuspension as well as nanoemulsion, and the theory behind this technology remains the same for both systems.

In high-energy emulsification methods, the nature of the surfactants, i.e., functional groups responsible for the hydrophilic/hydrophobic interactions, zeta potential, etc., and their amount are factors determining the final droplet and ultimately particle size distribution (Jacobs and Muller 2002). It is important for the stabilizer to adsorb at the oil/water interface and provide sufficient steric and/or electrostatic stabilization of the nanoemulsion. In fact, upon solvent removal, the stabilization of the particle is achieved thanks to the hydrophobic nature of the poorly water soluble drug in the aqueous media, leading to the adsorption of the surfactant hydrophobic portion on the surface of the particles. As the hydrophilic portion of the stabilizer extends from the surface of the particles, the distance between the particles increases such that the van der Walls attraction become ineffective and steric stabilization is provided (Burgess 2005). When the concentration of surfactant is sufficient, the particles repel each other thanks to volume restriction and osmotic pressure effect (Tadros 2009). However, if its concentration is too low, bridging flocculation may occur causing the hydrophilic portion of the surfactant to have multiple points of contact on the surface of the particles and lie along that surface rather than extend away from it (Burgess 2005). Similarly, when using ionic surfactants, the electrostatic charges are created at the oil/water interface and later at the particle/water interface have to be sufficient to provide electrostatic stabilization.

Following spray drying or cryogenic freezing and solvent sublimation, NPs can be produced and used for potential pulmonary and nasal applications (Christensen et al. 2001, Rogers et al. 2003c, Zhang et al. 2008).

Supercritical or compressed fluid technology

The supercritical and compressed fluid technologies are alternatives to the conventional liquid antisolvent precipitation techniques mentioned earlier. Compressed and supercritical fluids (SCFs) are fluids compressed or heated above their critical point (Fig. 5.10). In the SCF region, gases exhibit specific physical properties: their diffusivity increases significantly ($\approx$ 100 times greater than liquid diffusivity) and their viscosity decreases ($\approx$ 100 times lower than liquid viscosity). These properties lead to rapid diffusion of the SCF in the liquid solvent, enabling rapid supersaturation and nucleation and production of small particles. Multiple SCFs may be used but the most prevalent in the pharmaceutical industry is carbon dioxide (CO_2) as it has a mild critical point (31.1°C and 72.6 bar), and it is non-flammable, non-toxic, inexpensive, and safe to use. Early SFC processes showed limitations in the production of particles in the respirable size range but could be useful for nasal delivery. More recent progress in those technologies enabled the production of particles in the nanoscale range. A schematic diagram summarizing two representative SCF

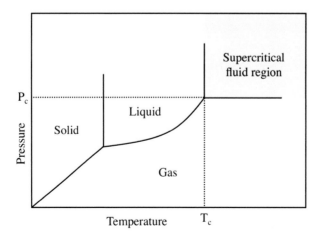

Figure 5.10. Phase diagram showing the supercritical region, being defined by the critical pressure (P_c) and the critical temperature (T_c).

processes (Gaseous Antisolvent Precipitation, GAS, and Rapid Expansion of Supercritical Solutions, RESS) is shown in Fig. 5.11.

Gaseous Antisolvent Precipitation. The GAS technology consists of the addition of a SCF antisolvent, usually CO_2, to an organic solution containing the drug and stabilizers, followed by the solubilization of the SCF in the organic solvent (Rowe and Johnston 2012). As the SCF dissolves in the organic phase, the solubility of the drug in that phase decreases, hence generating supersaturation and nucleation of the drug. To obtain homogeneous supersaturation and high degree of nucleation, corresponding to small monodispersed particles, the SCF and the organic solvent must be highly miscible and the drug must be practically insoluble in the SCF. The use of stabilizers is important, as they will adsorb on the particles surface as the solubility decreases and provide steric and/or electrostatic stabilization preventing the coagulation and condensation phenomena. The major drawback related to this technology is the difficulty to collect the drug particles from the organic solvent while preventing growth and agglomeration: a steep decrease in the drug solubility from a certain SCF concentration must occur to ensure rapid and homogeneous precipitation of small uniform particulates. Many drugs show a slow decrease in solubility as the SCF concentration increases: the typical particle size obtained from the GAS process ranges from 1 to 10 µm.

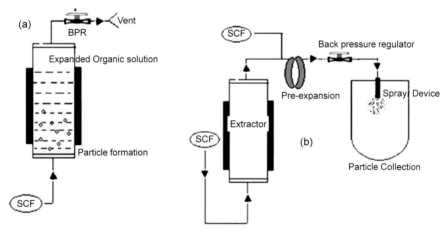

Figure 5.11. Diagram of two representative SCF particle engineering technologies: (a) GAS, and (b) RESS. Adapted with permission from Vemavarapu et al. (2005). Copyright Elsevier BV (2005).

Supercritical or Compressed Fluid Precipitation. The supercritical or compressed fluid precipitation, in contrast to the GAS method, atomizes the drug directly in the SCF antisolvent. The solvent containing the drug and potential stabilizers is first atomized with the SCF, using two-fluid nozzles or ultrasonic dispersion devices, in a chamber pressurized with the compressed gas or the SCF (Rowe and Johnston 2012). More rapid mixing, due to the continuous feed of SCF or compressed gas through the atomization nozzle, and higher pressure maintained in the chamber favor rapid and higher supersaturation than in GAS processes. The atomization facilitates rapid mass transfer between the drug solution and the SCF in every direction: it increases the surface area of the solvent droplets, thereby increasing the contact with the SCF and promoting rapid supersaturation and precipitation of small uniform particles. Upon precipitation, the residual solvents are removed, the pressure in the chamber is returned to atmospheric pressure, and the drug particulates are collected on a filter at the bottom of the chamber.

Most drugs have a limited solubility in carbon dioxide, the preferred SCF used in the pharmaceutical industry, and therefore this particle engineering technique has been quite popular for the fabrication of NPs. Steroids (Steckel et al. 1997), terbutaline sulfate (Rehman et al. 2004), and fluticasone (Steckel and Muller 1998) micronized powders for pulmonary delivery have been produced using this process. This technology has also been compared against the more traditional jet-mill technologies described earlier: the SCF method resulted in particles with a lower mass median d_a in comparison to the jet-milled particle (4 μm vs. 6 μm) (Della Porta et al. 2005).

Rapid Expansion of Supercritical Solutions (RESS). In this technology, the SCF is used as a solvent and not as an antisolvent. The active pharmaceutical ingredient and additional stabilizers are dissolved in the SCF. The mix is preheated and passed through a saturator to then be atomized with a heated nozzle into a collection chamber at atmospheric pressure. The instant vaporization of the SCF resulting from the sudden depressurization promotes rapid nucleation and precipitation of drug particulates. The rapid depressurization generates an intense turbulence, which instantaneously creates evenly distributed supersaturation regions. The intense degree of nucleation produced leads to the production of small monodispersed particles (Rowe and Johnston 2012).

Similar to other techniques, several parameters affect the final characteristics of the particles. The temperatures and pressure of the extraction unit, and the SCF-drug solution are critical. The pathway taken by the process along the pressure-temperature diagram for the SCF may lead to atomized SCF in a different state before being vaporized, resulting in the need of a heated nozzle. Also the geometry of the nozzle may influence the particle size as it is directly linked to the degree of atomization. The typical particle size obtained with this technology typically ranges between 1 and 5 μm, even though particles in the nano-sized range were sometimes generated.

The RESS process has also been investigated to generate drug particles for pulmonary delivery. Charpentier et al. (2008) successfully produced NPs of beclomethasone dipropionate for inhaled therapy. They investigated the influence of the process parameters on the final mean particle size. The type and diameter of the atomization nozzle lead to different particle geometries: larger nozzles produced needle-like particles whereas smaller ones gave spherical particles. Smaller drug concentration, higher pre-expansion pressure, and temperature also lead to smaller and more monodispersed particles.

Modified RESS Process. Rapid Expansion from Supercritical to Aqueous Solution (RESAS) has been developed to overcome particle growth due to particle collisions in the RESS process. The supercritical solution containing the drug is atomized through the nozzle directly in an aqueous solution. Again, to prevent particle growth associated with coagulation and condensation mechanisms, stabilizers may be added to the aqueous media to further stabilize the newly form particles. Because the turbulence created by the expansion of the SCF, the aqueous media containing the surfactants will have the tendency to foam excessively. A stream of nitrogen is therefore blown over the surface of the aqueous media to prevent that phenomenon to occur (Rowe and Johnston 2012).

Young et al. (2000) investigated the use of RESAS to produce CsA NPs in comparison to the traditional RESS technology. The CsA particles obtained were in the submicron range, 500 to 700 nm, whereas those obtained from the RESS process were 3 to 20 µm in diameter (Tandya et al. 2006). RESAS was also used to generate NPs of other drugs: ibuprofen (Pathak et al. 2006, Turk 2009), naproxen (Turk 2009), paclitaxel (Pathak et al. 2007), and raloxifene (Keshavarz et al. 2012).

Clinical Considerations of Pulmonary and Nasal Delivery of Nanoparticles

Nasal and pulmonary delivery of active pharmaceutical ingredients offers advantages because of their physiology, as discussed earlier in this chapter. The *in situ* delivery via these non-invasive routes of administration allows the reduction of the effective dose without compromising efficacy by achieving high local deposition, the significant decrease of the systemic side effects, the avoidance of the first-pass hepatic metabolism, when compared to the oral route, the reduction of drug degradation due to the relatively mild environment and low metabolic activity, and the targeting of the drug to specific compartments.

Through various examples reported in the literature, the local and targeted effects of nasal and pulmonary delivery of NPs produced with the particles engineering technologies detailed earlier will be discussed here. Conventionally, the nasal route has been used to deliver drugs to treat nasal allergy, nasal congestion, and nasal infection locally. No significant work has been done to improve local treatment in the nose as the focus has been towards the use of the nasal route to target the systemic and lymphatic systems. Therefore, for the nasal route, only the targeted delivery will be described.

Topical effects of the inhalation route

The main goal when delivering drugs to the lungs is to achieve high drug concentrations to ensure the therapeutic effect and rapid onset of action. NP targeting to the lungs has been investigated for multiple lung disease states, including asthma, Chronic Obstructive Pulmonary Disease (COPD), tuberculosis, cystic fibrosis, lung cancer, allograft rejection, pulmonary hypertension, etc. It also offers a great potential to treat lower respiratory tract infections often associated with lung diseases: community-acquired pneumonia (*Streptococcus pneumonia, Haemophilus influenzae, Moraxella catarrhalis, Chlamydia pneumoniae, Legionella pneumophila*, and *Mycoplasma pneumoniae*), invasive fungal infections (*Aspergillus* spp.) and bacterium infections (*Staphylococcus aureus, Pseudomonas aeruginosa*, and other opportunistic Gram-negative pathogens) (Guthrie 2001).

The nebulization of itraconazole NPs made by the SFL technique showed significantly improved itraconazole lung concentrations in comparison to the oral administration of the itraconazole marketed product, Sporanox®, in rats (Vaughn et al. 2006). Much lower serum levels were also obtained and the toxic side effects reported after oral administration of Sporanox® were not observed in the rats receiving the inhaled amorphous itraconazole. The safety of the itraconazole formulation for inhalation was also investigated during a repeated dose study (Vaughn et al. 2007). No inflammation or changes in pulmonary histology was reported and uptake of the particle by macrophages was observed, which may improve the host defenses against invasive fungal infections and help its prevention.

Various pulmonary formulations of CsA have been developed for the treatment of respiratory inflammation as well as allograft rejection. An inhalable dry-emulsion formulation of CsA prepared by spray drying was tested for dissolution behavior *in vitro*, plasma concentration, and efficacy in asthma/COPD-model rats after pulmonary administration (Onoue et al. 2012). The dry-emulsion showed improved solubility, when compared to amorphous CsA and the commercialized product Neoral®. The plasma concentration after inhalation was much lower than after oral administration of Neoral®, decreasing the risks of nephrotoxicity or hepatotoxicity generally associated with the oral administration of CsA (Alexander et al. 1992). The dry-emulsion CsA formulation for inhalation also demonstrated attenuated inflammatory symptoms, showing the efficacy of the inhaled treatment. Amorphous CsA nanodispersions have been formulated using the antisolvent precipitation process for the prevention of lung allograft rejection (Tam et al. 2008). The amorphous nanodispersion exhibited supersaturation values 18 times the aqueous solubility of crystalline CsA. The lung administration of the nanodispersion showed high lung deposition and plasma levels below the toxic concentration. Clinical trials using the aerosolized solution of CsA (Sandimmun®, Novartis) showed efficacy among patients suffering from severe chronic graft rejection and refractory rejection (Keenan et al. 1995), and as the nanodispersion exhibited higher lung levels than the solution in the animal model, the nanodispersion was expected to demonstrate improved performance in the prevention of lung allograft rejection.

Hollow and highly porous particles have been designed using the spray drying technology exclusively. They are often used as means to improve the aerosolization properties of the formulation, to deliver NPs that would not deposit in the deep lung otherwise because of their size, and to avoid phagocytosis clearance. PulmoSpheres™ and Trojan particles are the typical examples illustrating these features (Fig. 5.12). Newhouse et al. (2003) administered PulmoSpheres™ containing tobramycin to healthy volunteers and compared the effectiveness of this dry powder formulation against the nebulization of a commercialized nebulized tobramycin product (TOBI, Chiron

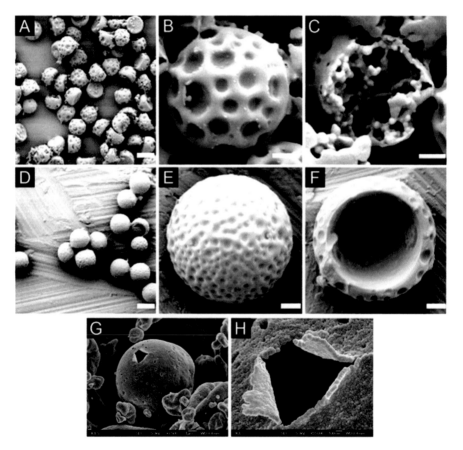

Figure 5.12. SEM images large porous particles using various porogens. (A, B, C) canola oil; (D, E, F) silicon oil. Reprinted with permission from Arnold et al. (2007). Copyright Elsevier BV (2007); (G, H) Trojan or large porous NPs. (A, D) bulk powder, (B, E, G) surface morphology, and (C, F, H) interior morphology. Bar length: 10 μm for A, D, and 2 μm for B, C, E, F. Reprinted with permission from Hadinoto et al. (2007). Copyright Elsevier BV (2007).

Corporation). The results reported significant improvement in lung deposition: 34 ± 6% for the PulmoSpheres™ vs. 5 ± 2% for the nebulized formulation. The PulmoSpheres™ formulation was nine times more efficient than the nebulized tobramycin as its dry powder inhaler loading dose was ≈ 4-fold lower than the nebulized dose (80 mg vs. 300 mg). Another study performed by Duddu et al. (2002) showed the ability of budesonide PulmoSpheres™ to achieve a faster onset of action after lung delivery from a passive dry powder inhaler in comparison to the Pulmicort® Turbohaler (AstraZeneca) (5 minutes vs. 30 minutes) and a higher peak concentration (4.7 ± 2.1 ng/mL vs. 2.2 ± 0.7 ng/mL). Peak Inspiration Flow (PIF) rates must be taken in consideration when developing a formulation for inhalation, as there is a large inter- and intra-patient variability of the aspiration rate depending on the diseased state of the patient. This variability may lead to different deposition profiles depending on the PIF rate generated by the patient. In this study, the plasma concentration profiles at low and high PIF rates were invariant, which showed the ability of the PulmoSphere™ to deposit deep in the lungs independently of the PIF rate.

Trojan particles, also called large porous NP aggregates or porous NP-aggregate particles, incorporate NPs into large, microparticles to associate the advantages of aerosolization and lung deposition of large porous particles to the benefits of NPs. Self-assembled rifampicin-loaded poly(D,L-lactide-*co*-glycolide) (PLGA) NPs were investigated for the treatment of tuberculosis (Sung et al. 2009). The oral, intravenous, and pulmonary administration of the suspension, solution, and large porous NP aggregates, respectively, lead to similar plasma levels of rifampicin. However, the pulmonary delivery of the large porous NP aggregates of rifampicin showed significantly higher and prolonged levels of the drug in the lungs in comparison to the other routes of administration. This system was able to provide both high lung level due to the large porous structures and high plasma levels because of the rapid absorption of the NPs constituting the large particles. This pulmonary formulation was able to provide systemic and local treatment against tuberculosis. Doxorubicin-loaded NPs for chemotherapy were also formulated via the same techniques (Azarmi et al. 2006), as well as salbutamol sulfate, aspirin (Hadinoto et al. 2007), and insulin (Grenha et al. 2005).

Targeted effects

Targeted Delivery via the Pulmonary Route. NPs for pulmonary delivery have been used not only to provide an intense and prolonged active substance concentration in the lungs, but also to target alveolar macrophages and the lymphatic circulation, and to avoid the hepatic first-pass metabolism.

Macrophages located in the lower respiratory tract play a key role in pulmonary clearance responses to inhaled particles. Different types of macrophages have been identified depending on their location within the lung. Alveolar macrophages reside on the epithelial surfaces of the alveolar region, airway macrophages are located in the epithelium of the conducting airways and lung peripheral associated lymphoid tissues, and the interstitial macrophages are found in the perivascular, peribronchiolar, and visceral pleural sites and in the alveoli sub-epithelial region (Lehnert 1992). The phagocytic uptake has been demonstrated to be size and surface properties dependent. While particles in the sub-micron range and particles larger than 5 µm escape the alveolar macrophages uptake resulting in longer residence time or higher lung epithelium permeation, particles between 1 and 5 µm exhibited maximum macrophage uptake (Makino et al. 2003, Champion et al. 2008). Particle uptake by macrophages is very rapid, occuring as early as 15 minutes after pulmonary delivery, and can provide complete particle removal within 24 hours at low substrate concentration (Forsgren et al. 1990, Geiser 2002, Zhou et al. 2005). Since alveolar macrophages play an important role in the host defense mechanism in infectious diseases, autoimmune diseases, and graft rejections, several NP therapies targeting alveolar macrophages have been investigated (Barrow et al. 1998, Anisimova et al. 2000, Pandey et al. 2003, Ito and Makino 2004). In the case of tuberculosis, *Mycobacterium TB* is known to infect alveolar macrophages and multiply in them (Clarkson 1999). Zhou et al. (2005) used the precipitation with compressed antisolvent process to prepare poly(D,L-lactide) (PLA) microparticles of isoniazide methanesulfonate (INH) for prolonged delivery to alveolar macrophages in rats. The use of the compressed antisolvent process technology leads to monodispersed particles between 1 and 3 µm, the optimum size for macrophage uptake. The INH-loaded PLA microparticles after intratracheal administration showed high and sustained concentrations of INH in the broncholavaged alveolar macrophages and very low plasma levels. On the contrary, the intratracheal instillation of INH solution only showed INH levels in the broncholavaged alveolar macrophages 30 minutes after administration and was not detected in the plasma. Finally, low levels of INH in the plasma and in the broncholavaged alveolar macrophages were observed after oral gavage of the INH solution. This example proved the promising use of INH-loaded PLA microparticles to deliver high and sustained levels of INH to alveolar macrophages to treat tuberculosis.

The avoidance of first-pass metabolism offers the advantage of decreasing the loss of bioavailability due to liver metabolism and the potential toxicity due to toxic metabolites generated by hepatic metabolism. In the treatment of tuberculosis, for example, treatment failure is associated with poor patient adherence due to the hepatotoxicity caused by the treatment (Schaberg 1995). The bioavailability of INH is patient dependent because of hepatic acetylator polymorphism leading to fast or slow acetylation of the drug. The liver toxicity has been related to acetylhydrazine, the hydrolyzed form of the main inactive metabolite of INH produced in the liver. In the same study mentioned earlier, Zhou et al. (2005) showed a significant decrease in the acetylhydrazine plasma levels when administering the INH-loaded PLA microparticles to the lung than when administering an INH solution by the oral route. The avoidance of the hepatic first-pass metabolism by delivering the drug directly to the lungs could significantly decrease the amount of the toxic metabolite, hence reducing the hepatotoxicity. In general, the avoidance of the hepatic first-pass metabolism by delivering the active substance to the lung may not only improve the drug bioavailability but also decrease the rate of degradation of the drug, thus providing a prolonged exposure to the therapeutic effect of the drug, and therefore improving the efficacy of the treatment.

Targeted Delivery via the Nasal Route. The challenges to deliver NPs to the nasal cavity include size, since NPs tend to deposit deep in the lung instead of in the nasopharyngeal region, and absorption through the nasal mucosa. While lipophilic drugs are generally readily absorbed through the nasal mucosa, with bioavailabilities near 80%, polar molecules, including low molecular weight drugs and high molecular weight peptides and proteins, exhibit a very low permeability of the nasal mucosa, $\approx 10\%$ and sometimes even down to 1%. This low permeability exposes the drug to mucociliary clearance and enzymatic degradation. The nasal absorption of polar substances is greatly improved by the use of absorption enhancers co-administered with the active substance, such as bile salts, chitosan (CS), cyclodextrins, saponins, phospholipids, etc. The use of mucoadhesives, like CS, *in situ* gels, and swellable particles, have also been investigated to increase the residence time of the active substance on the nasal mucosa and promote absorption. Little has been done on local nasal treatment using particles; nonetheless, extensive work has been performed to deliver drugs to the systemic circulation and the lymphatic system through the nasal route. Among others, anti-migraine, anti-emetics, smoking cessation, acute pain, anti-infective, and calcitonin products have been developed and commercialized. More recently, the nasal route has been used for the delivery of vaccines, such as influenza vaccines.

One of the interesting aspects of the nasal route is its capability to bypass the blood-brain barrier and reach the Central Nervous System (CNS). This concept was first initiated to evaluate the toxicity of environmental pollutants and NPs on the CNS, and was applied later for the delivery of drugs to the CNS. Drug delivery to the CNS via the nasal route has been demonstrated to happen through the blood and predominantly through the olfactory bulbs reaching then the brain and the cerebrospinal fluid (Mistry et al. 2009). Gao et al. (2006) prepared lectin-conjugated poly(ethylene glycol) (PEG)-PLA NPs and showed their capability to avoid the nasal ciliatoxicity and their efficient brain uptake by the use of a fluorescent marker. The NPs were prepared using the nanoemulsion template process and the use of the lectins was based on their specific binding to *N*-acetyl-D-glucosamine and sialic acid, which are present abundantly in the nasal cavity. Another example is the encapsulation of nimodipine in methoxy PEG-PLA NPs (Zhang et al. 2006) using the emulsion template process followed by lyophilization and reconstitution in a biological buffer before nasal administration in rats. The plasma and brain concentrations of the drug after nasal delivery were assessed and compared against the intravenous and intranasal administration of a nimodipine solution. The NPs were able to transport directly into the CNS leading to a greater drug concentration in the brain tissues compared to the nasal and intravenous solution.

Another interesting aspect of the nasal route involves its ability to provide a rapid onset of action and has been therefore investigated for the delivery of analgesics, anti-emetic, and anti-migraine products. Nasal formulations of morphine have been studied to overcome its poor oral bioavailability ($\approx 25\%$) and to provide a rapid therapeutic effect to patients suffering from mild to severe pain. A morphine/CS powder blend and a morphine/CS solution have been administered to human volunteers through the nasal route (Illum et al. 2002). The plasma levels as well as the central effects, such as drowsiness and nausea, were compared to the intravenous administration of the same dose. No significant differences in the plasma concentrations were observed between the nasal formulations and a bioavailability of $\approx 60\%$ was achieved. Nasal formulations of morphine were well tolerated and well accepted, and cancer patients reported some improvements in the treatment of breakthrough pain. Russo et al. (2006) developed a spray dried formulation of amorphous morphine soft agglomerates and compared it to crystalline microparticles of morphine. The idea was to decrease the risk of inhalation by creating large agglomerates, to promote prompt dissolution of the drug in the nasal cavity by administering the amorphous form of the drug, and finally to provide a stable dry powder nasal formulation. The amorphous formulation developed was stable; the *in vitro* tests for insufflation delivery were reproducible with an emitted dose > 90%, and the *in vitro* transport across rabbit nasal mucosa was faster with the agglomerates than with a morphine saturated solution.

The last aspect of nasal delivery that will be discussed here is the use of the nasal route for vaccine delivery. The main reasons for exploiting the nasal route for vaccine delivery are: (i) the nasal mucosa is the first site of contact with the inhaled pathogenic microorganisms; (ii) in humans, mucosal lymphoid tissues are directly located under the nasal mucosa, making *T* and *B* lymphocytes, macrophages, and dendritic cells directly available; (iii) mucosal and systemic immune responses can be created; and, (iv) nasal delivery is non-invasive, making it patient friendly. A schematic overview of the main cellular mechanisms involved in nasal vaccination is shown in Fig. 5.13. There are many publications suggesting the possibility of using NPs for nasal delivery of vaccines and demonstrating real advantages. They are usually functionalized or coated NPs with biocompatible polymers: PLA, PLGA, CS, and PEG. The different nasal vaccine systems described in the literature use either live or attenuated whole cells, split cells, proteins, and polysaccharides, with and without the addition of adjuvants. Nasal vaccines containing CS have been studied extensively. In fact, CS have not only bioadhesive properties but also the ability of transiently opening the tight junctions of the nasal mucosa, which, overall, could lead to improved immune response. There is also some evidence

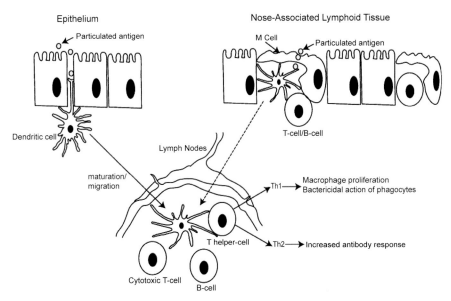

Figure 5.13. Schematic overview of the main cellular mechanisms involved in nasal vaccination. Reprinted with permission from Csaba et al. (2009). Copyright Elsevier BV (2009).

that CS could act as an adjuvant and promote the production of cytokines (Witschi and Mrsny 1999). CS-based influenza, pertussis, and diphteria vaccines have been investigated (Illum et al. 2001). Finally, biodegradable polyesters, PLA and PLGA, have been also investigated as carriers for the delivery of vaccine through the nose. In addition to their controlled release properties, it has been demonstrated that antigen presenting cells may readily engulf them when their particle size ranges between 1 and 5 μm (Lutsiak et al. 2002, Newman et al. 2002, Csaba et al. 2009), enhancing the lymphatic uptake and therefore boosting the immune response (Vila et al. 2005).

Conclusions

Pulmonary and nasal delivery of active substances could significantly improve patient outcomes and broaden the therapeutic options for local and systemic therapy. NP technologies can generate particles tailored to meet the specific criteria necessary to achieve efficient nasal or pulmonary deposition. The physical chemistry of the particles as well as the aerosol product performance are key factors to facilitate targeted delivery and efficacy of the therapy.

Abbreviations

BCS	:	biopharmaceutics classification system
CO_2	:	carbon dioxide
COPD	:	chronic obstructive pulmonary disease

CNS	:	central nervous system
CS	:	chitosan
CsA	:	cyclosporine A
EPAS	:	evaporative precipitation into aqueous solution
d_a	:	aerodynamic diameter
d_v	:	geometric diameter
GAS	:	gaseous antisolvent precipitation
INH	:	isoniazide methanesulfonate
NP	:	nanoparticle
P_c	:	critical pressure
PEG	:	poly(ethylene glycol)
PLA	:	poly(D,L-lactide)
PLGA	:	poly(D,L-lactide-*co*-glycolide)
PIF	:	peak inspiration flow
RESAS	:	rapid expansion from supercritical to aqueous solution
RESS	:	rapid expansion of supercritical solutions
SCF	:	supercritical fluid
SFD	:	spray freeze-drying
SFL	:	spray freezing into liquid
Stk	:	Stokes number
T_c	:	critical temperature
TFF	:	thin film freezing
V_{ts}	:	terminal settling velocity

References

Abismaïl, B. and J.P. Canselier, A.M. Wilhelm, H. Delmas and C. Gourdon. 1999. Emulsification by ultrasound: drop size distribution and stability. Ultrason. Sonochem. 6: 75–83.

Alexander, A.G. and N.C. Barnes and A.B. Kay. 1992. Trial of cyclosporin in corticosteroid-dependent chronic severe asthma. Lancet. 339: 324–328.

Ali, R. and G.K. Jain, Z. Iqbal, S. Talegaonkar, P. Pandit, S. Sule, G. Malhotra, R.K. Khar, A. Bhatnagar and F.J. Ahmad. 2009. Development and clinical trial of nano-atropine sulfate dry powder inhaler as a novel organophosphorous poisoning antidote. Nanomedicine. 5: 55–63.

Almeida, A.J. and H.O. Alpar. 1996. Nasal delivery of vaccines. J. Drug Target. 3: 455–467.

Altiere, R. and D. Thompson. Physiology and pharmacology of the airways. pp. 83–126. *In*: A. Hickey [ed.]. 2007. Inhalation Aerosols: Physical and Biological Basis for Therapy. Informa Healthcare, Hoboken, USA.

Alvarez, C.A. and N.P. Wiederhold, J.T. McConville, J.I. Peters, L.K. Najvar, J.R. Graybill, J.J. Coalson, R.L. Talbert, D.S. Burgess, R. Bocanegra, K.P. Johnston and R.O. Williams III. 2007. Aerosolized nanostructured itraconazole as prophylaxis against invasive pulmonary aspergillosis. J. Infect. 55: 68–74.

Anisimova, Y.V. and S.I. Gelperina, C.A. Peloquin and L.B. Heifets. 2000. Nanoparticles as antituberculosis drugs carriers: effect on activity against mycobacterium tuberculosis in human monocyte-derived macrophages. J. Nanopart. Res. 2: 165–171.

Anton, N. and J.P. Benoit and P. Saulnier. 2008. Design and production of nanoparticles formulated from nano-emulsion templates-a review. J. Control. Release. 128: 185–199.

Arnold, M.M. and E.M. Gorman, L.J. Schieber, E.J. Munson and C. Berkland. 2007. NanoCipro encapsulation in monodisperse large porous PLGA microparticles. J. Control. Release. 121: 100–109.

Atkins, P.J. 2005. Dry powder inhalers: an overview. Respir. Care. 50: 1304–1312.

Azarmi, S. and X. Tao, H. Chen, Z. Wang, W.H. Finlay, R. Löbenberg and W.H. Roa. 2006. Formulation and cytotoxicity of doxorubicin nanoparticles carried by dry powder aerosol particles. Int. J. Pharm. 319: 155–161.

Badhan, R.K. and M. Kaur, S. Lungare and S. Obuobi. 2014. Improving brain drug targeting through exploitation of the nose-to-brain route: a physiological and pharmacokinetic perspective. Curr. Drug Deliv. 11: 458–471.

Barrow, E.L. and G.A. Winchester, J.K. Staas, D.C. Quenelle and W.W. Barrow. 1998. Use of microsphere technology for targeted delivery of rifampin to Mycobacterium tuberculosis-infected macrophages. Antimicrob. Agents Chemother. 42: 2682–2689.

Beinborn, N.A. and H.L. Lirola and R.O. Williams. 2012. Effect of process variables on morphology and aerodynamic properties of voriconazole formulations produced by thin film freezing. Int. J. Pharm. 429: 46–57.

Benson, S.W. and D.A. Ellis. 1948. Surface areas of proteins; surface areas and heats of absorption. J. Am. Chem. Soc. 70: 3563–3569.

Bhavna and F.J. Ahmad, R.K. Khar, S. Sultana and A. Bhatnagar. 2009. Techniques to develop and characterize nanosized formulation for salbutamol sulfate. J. Mater. Sci. Mater. Med. 20: S71–S76.

Blankschtein, D. and G.M. Thurston and G.B. Benedek. 1986. Phenomenological theory of equilibrium thermodynamic properties and phase separation of micellar solutions. J. Chem. Phys. 85: 7268–7288.

Brodka-Pfeiffer, K. and P. Langguth, P. Grass and H. Häusler. 2003a. Influence of mechanical activation on the physical stability of salbutamol sulphate. Eur. J. Pharm. Biopharm. 56: 393–400.

Brodka-Pfeiffer, K. and H. Häusler, P. Grass and P. Langguth. 2003b. Conditioning following powder micronization: influence on particle growth of salbutamol sulfate. Drug Dev. Ind. Pharm. 29: 1077–1084.

Burcham, C.L. and P.C. Collins, D.J. Jarmer and K.D. Seibert. Reduction of particle size of drug substance for low-dose drug products. pp. 205–222. *In*: J. Zheng [ed.]. 2008. Formulation and Analytical Development for Low-Dose Oral Drug Products. John Wiley & Sons, Inc., Hoboken, USA.

Burgess, D. Physical stability of dispersed systems. pp. 1–37. *In*: D. Burgess [ed.]. 2005. Injectable Dispersed Systems: Formulation, Processing, and Performance. Taylor & Francis, Boca Raton, USA.

Cai, F.S. and C.P. Yu. 1988. Inertial and interceptional deposition of spherical particles and fibers in a bifurcating airway. J. Aerosol Sci. 19: 679–688.

Cal, K. and K. Sollohub. 2010. Spray drying technique. I: Hardware and process parameters. J. Pharm. Sci. 99: 575–586.

Carvalho, T.C. and J.I. Peters and R.O. Williams III. 2011. Influence of particle size on regional lung deposition—what evidence is there? Int. J. Pharm. 406: 1–10.

Champion, J.A. and A. Walker and S. Mitragotri. 2008. Role of particle size in phagocytosis of polymeric microspheres. Pharm. Res. 25: 1815–1821.

Charpentier, P. and M. Jia and R.A. Lucky. 2008. Study of the RESS process for producing beclomethasone-17,21-dipropionate particles suitable for pulmonary delivery. AAPS Pharm. Sci. Tech. 9: 39–46.

Chen, X. and T.J. Young, M. Sarkari, R.O. Williams III and K.P. Johnston. 2002. Preparation of cyclosporine A nanoparticles by evaporative precipitation into aqueous solution. Int. J. Pharm. 242: 3–14.

Chow, A.H. and H.H. Tong, P. Chattopadhyay and B.Y. Shekunov. 2007. Particle engineering for pulmonary drug delivery. Pharm. Res. 24: 411–437.

Christensen, K.L. and G.P. Pedersen and H.G. Kristensen. 2001. Preparation of redispersible dry emulsions by spray drying. Int. J. Pharm. 212: 187–194.

Clarkson, E.F. 1999. Tuberculosis. An overview. J. Intraven. Nurs. 22: 216–220.

Cook, E.J. and A.P. Lagace. 1985. Apparatus for forming emulsions. Biotechnology Development Corporation. US4533254.

Costantino, H.R. and L. Illum, G. Brandt, P.H. Johnson and S.C. Quay. 2007. Intranasal delivery: physicochemical and therapeutic aspects. Int. J. Pharm. 337: 1–24.

Courrier, H.M. and N. Butz and T.F. Vandamme. 2002. Pulmonary drug delivery systems: recent developments and prospects. Crit. Rev. Ther. Drug Carrier Syst. 19: 425–498.

Crowder, T.M. and J.A. Rosati, J.D. Schroeter, A.J. Hickey and T.B. Martonen. 2002. Fundamental effects of particle morphology on lung delivery: predictions of Stokes' law and the particular relevance to dry powder inhaler formulation and development. Pharm. Res. 19: 239–245.

Csaba, N. and M. Garcia-Fuentes and M.J. Alonso. 2009. Nanoparticles for nasal vaccination. Adv. Drug Deliv. Rev. 61: 140–157.

de Boer, A.H. and D. Gjaltema, P. Hagedoorn and H.W. Frijlink. 2002. Characterization of inhalation aerosols: a critical evaluation of cascade impactor analysis and laser diffraction technique. Int. J. Pharm. 249: 219–231.

Della Porta, G. and C. De Vittori and E. Reverchon. 2005. Supercritical assisted atomization: a novel technology for microparticles preparation of an asthma-controlling drug. AAPS Pharm. Sci. Tech. 6: E421–E428.

Dobson, B. and E. Rothwell. 1969. Particle size reduction in a fluid energy mill. Powder Technol. 3: 213–217.

Duddu, S.P. and S.A. Sisk, Y.H. Walter, T.E. Tarara, K.R. Trimble, A.R. Clark, M.A. Eldon, R.C. Elton, M. Pickford, P.H. Hirst, S.P. Newman and J.G. Weers. 2002. Improved lung delivery from a passive dry powder inhaler using an Engineered PulmoSphere powder. Pharm. Res. 19: 689–695.

Edwards, D.A. and J. Hanes, G. Caponetti, J. Hrkach, A. Ben-Jebria, M.L. Eskew, J. Mintzes, D. Deaver, N. Lotan and R. Langer. 1997. Large porous particles for pulmonary drug delivery. Science. 276: 1868–1871.

Edwards, D.A. and A. Ben-Jebria and R. Langer. 1998. Recent advances in pulmonary drug delivery using large, porous inhaled particles. J. Appl. Physiol. 85: 379–385.

El-Gendy, N. and C. Berkland. 2009. Combination chemotherapeutic dry powder aerosols via controlled nanoparticle agglomeration. Pharm. Res. 26: 1752–1763.

Engstrom, J.D. and E.S. Lai, B.S. Ludher, B. Chen, T.E. Milner, R.O. Williams 3rd, G.B. Kitto and K.P. Johnston. 2008. Formation of stable submicron protein particles by thin film freezing. Pharm. Res. 25: 1334–1346.

Forsgren, P. and J. Modig, B. Gerdin, B. Axelsson and M. Dahlbäck. 1990. Intrapulmonary deposition of aerosolized Evans blue dye and liposomes in an experimental porcine model of early ARDS. Ups. J. Med. Sci. 95: 117–136.

Fry, F.A. and A. Black. 1973. Regional deposition and clearance of particles in the human nose. J. Aerosol Sci. 4: 113–124.

Gao, X. and W. Tao, W. Lu, Q. Zhang, Y. Zhang, X. Jiang and S. Fu. 2006. Lectin-conjugated PEG-PLA nanoparticles: preparation and brain delivery after intranasal administration. Biomaterials. 27: 3482–3490.

Garmise, R. and H. Staats and A.J. Hickley. 2007. Novel dry powder preparations of whole inactivated influenza virus for nasal vaccination. AAPS Pharm. Sci. Tech. 8: 2–10.

Geiser, M. 2002. Morphological aspects of particle uptake by lung phagocytes. Microsc. Res. Tech. 57: 512–522.

Gonda, I. Targeting by deposition. pp. 65–88. *In*: A. Hickey [ed.]. 2004. Pharmaceutical Aerosol Technology. Marcel Dekker, New York, USA.

Gradon, L. and C.P. Yu. 1989. Diffusional particle deposition in the human nose and mouth. Aerosol Sci. Tech. 11: 213–220.

Grenha, A. and B. Seij and C. Remuñán-López. 2005. Microencapsulated chitosan nanoparticles for lung protein delivery. Eur. J. Pharm. Sci. 25: 427–437.

Groneberg, D.A. and C. Witt, U. Wagner, K.F. Chung and A. Fischer. 2003. Fundamentals of pulmonary drug delivery. Respir. Med. 97: 382–387.

Guthrie, R. 2001. Community-acquired lower respiratory tract infections: etiology and treatment. Chest. 120: 2021–2034.

Hadinoto, K. and K. Zhu and R.B. Tan. 2007. Drug release study of large hollow nanoparticulate aggregates carrier particles for pulmonary delivery. Int. J. Pharm. 341: 195–206.

Hahn, I. and P.W. Scherer and M.M. Mozell. 1993. Velocity profiles measured for airflow through a large-scale model of the human nasal cavity. J. Appl. Physiol. (1985) 75: 2273–2287.

Hennart, S.L.A. and W.J. Wildeboer, P. van Hee and G.M.H. Meesters. 2009. Identification of the grinding mechanisms and their origin in a stirred ball mill using population balances. Chem. Eng. Sci. 64: 4123–4130.

Hinds, W.C. 1999. Aerosol Technology: Properties, Behavior, and Measurement of Airborne Particles. John Wiley & Sons Inc., New York, USA.

Hoeben, B.J. and D.S. Burgess, J.T. McConville, L.K. Najvar, R.L. Talbert, J.I. Peters, N.P. Wiederhold, B.L. Frei, J.R. Graybill, R. Bocanegra, K.A. Overhoff, P. Sinswat, K.P. Johnston and R.O. Williams 3rd. 2006. *In vivo* efficacy of aerosolized nanostructured itraconazole formulations for prevention of invasive pulmonary aspergillosis. Antimicrob. Agents Chemother. 50: 1552–1554.

Hogan, J. and P. Smith, D. Heath and P. Harris. 1986. The thickness of the alveolar capillary wall in the human lung at high and low altitude. Br. J. Dis. Chest. 80: 13–18.

Hu, J. and T.L. Rogers, J. Brown, T. Young, K.P. Johnston and R.O. Williams 3rd. 2002. Improvement of dissolution rates of poorly water soluble APIs using novel spray freezing into liquid technology. Pharm. Res. 19: 1278–1284.

Hu, J. and K.P. Johnston and R.O. Williams 3rd. 2004a. Stable amorphous danazol nanostructured powders with rapid dissolution rates produced by spray freezing into liquid. Drug Dev. Ind. Pharm. 30: 695–704.

Hu, J.H. and K.P. Johnston and R.O. Williams 3rd. 2004b. Rapid dissolving high potency danazol powders produced by spray freezing into liquid process. Int. J. Pharm. 271: 145–154.

Hu, T.T. and H. Zhao, L.C. Jiang, Y. Le, J.F. Chen and J. Yun. 2008. Engineering pharmaceutical fine particles of budesonide for dry powder inhalation (DPI). Ind. Eng. Chem. Res. 47: 9623–9627.

Illig, K.J. and R.L. Mueller, K.D. Ostrander and J.R. Swanson. 1996. Use of microfluidizer processing for preparation of pharmaceutical suspensions. Pharm. Technol. 20: 78–88.

Illum, L. and I. Jabbal-Gill, M. Hinchcliffe, A.N. Fisher and S.S. Davis. 2001. Chitosan as a novel nasal delivery system for vaccines. Adv. Drug Deliv. Rev. 51: 81–96.

Illum, L. and P. Watts, A.N. Fisher, M. Hinchcliffe, H. Norbury, I. Jabbal-Gill, R. Nankervis and S.S. Davis. 2002. Intranasal delivery of morphine. J. Pharmacol. Exp. Ther. 301: 391–400.

Illum, L. 2003. Nasal drug delivery—possibilities, problems and solutions. J. Control. Release. 87: 187–198.

I.S.O. Standards. 2008. Nanotechnologies – Terminology and definitions for nano-objects – Nanoparticle, nanofibre and nanoplate. ISO/TS-27687: 2008.

Ito, F. and K. Makino. 2004. Preparation and properties of monodispersed rifampicin-loaded poly(lactide-co-glycolide) microspheres. Colloids Surf. B Biointerfaces. 39: 17–21.

Jacobs, C. and R.H. Muller. 2002. Production and characterization of a budesonide nanosuspension for pulmonary administration. Pharm. Res. 19: 189–194.

Johnston, K.P. and R.O. Williams, T.J. Young and X. Chen. 2004. Preparation of drug particles using evaporation precipitation into aqueous solutions. Board of Regents University of Texas System. US6756062.

Junghanns, J. and R.H. Muller. 2008. Nanocrystal technology, drug delivery and clinical applications. Int. J. Nanomedicine. 3: 295–309.

Keck, C.M. and R.H. Muller. 2006. Drug nanocrystals of poorly soluble drugs produced by high pressure homogenisation. Eur. J. Pharm. Biopharm. 62: 3–16.

Keenan, R.J. and A. Zeevi, A.T. Iacono, K.J. Spichty, J.Z. Cai, S.A. Yousem, N.P. Ohori, I.L. Paradis, A. Kawai and B.P. Griffith. 1995. Efficacy of inhaled cyclosporine in lung transplant recipients with refractory rejection: correlation of intragraft cytokine gene expression with pulmonary function and histologic characteristics. Surgery. 118: 385–391.

Kelly, J.T. and B. Asgharian, J.S. Kimbell and B.S. Wong. 2004a. Particle deposition in human nasal airway replicas manufactured by different methods. Part I: Inertial regime particles. Aerosol Sci. Technol. 38: 1063–1071.

Kelly, J.T. and B. Asgharian, J.S. Kimbell and B.S. Wong. 2004b. Particle deposition in human nasal airway replicas manufactured by different methods. Part II: Ultrafine particles. Aerosol Sci. Technol. 38: 1072–1079.

Keshavarz, A. and J. Karimi-Sabet, A. Fattahi, A. Golzary, M. Rafiee-Tehrani and F.A. Dorkoosh. 2012. Preparation and characterization of raloxifene nanoparticles using Rapid Expansion of Supercritical Solution (RESS). J. Supercrit. Fluids. 63: 169–179.

Kim, C.S. and D.M. Fisher, D.J. Lutz and T.R. Gerrity. 1994. Particle deposition in bifurcating airway models with varying airway geometry. J. Aerosol Sci. 25: 567–581.

Klingler, C. and B.W. Müller and H. Steckel. 2009. Insulin-micro- and nanoparticles for pulmonary delivery. Int. J. Pharm. 377: 173–179.

Kreuter, J. Nanoparticles as drug delivery systems. pp. 161–180. *In*: H.S. Nalwa [ed.]. 2004. Encyclopedia of Nanoscience and Nanotechnology. American Scientific Publishers, Steveson Ranch, USA.

Kwade, A. 1999. Determination of the most important grinding mechanism in stirred media mills by calculating stress intensity and stress number. Powder Technol. 105: 382–388.

Kwade, A. and J. Schwedes. Wet grinding in stirred media mills. pp. 251–382. *In*: M.G. Agba, D. Salman and J.H. Michael [eds.]. 2007. Handbook of Powder Technology. CRC Press, Hoboken, USA.

Labiris, N.R. and M.B. Dolovich. 2003. Pulmonary drug delivery. Part I: Physiological factors affecting therapeutic effectiveness of aerosolized medications. Br. J. Clin. Pharmacol. 56: 588–599.

Lavernia, E.J. and B.Q. Han and J.M. Schoenung. 2008. Cryomilled nanostructured materials: processing and properties. Mater. Sci. Eng. A 493: 207–214.

Lehnert, B.E. 1992. Pulmonary and thoracic macrophage subpopulations and clearance of particles from the lung. Environ. Health Perspect. 97: 17–46.

Liedtke, S. and S. Wissing, R.H. Müller and K. Mäder. 2000. Influence of high pressure homogenisation equipment on nanodispersions characteristics. Int. J. Pharm. 196: 183–185.

Lutsiak, M.E. and D.R. Robinson, C. Coester, G.S. Kwon and J. Samuel. 2002. Analysis of poly(D,L-lactic-co-glycolic acid) nanosphere uptake by human dendritic cells and macrophages *in vitro*. Pharm. Res. 19: 1480–1487.

Makino, K. and H. Yamamoto, K. Higuchi, N. Harada, H. Oshima and H. Terada. 2003. Phagocytic uptake of polystyrene microspheres by alveolar macrophages: effects of the size and surface properties of the microspheres. Colloids Surf. B Biointerfaces. 27: 33–39.

Matteucci, M.E. and M.A. Hotze, K.P. Johnston and R.O. Williams III. 2006. Drug nanoparticles by antisolvent precipitation: mixing energy versus surfactant stabilization. Langmuir. 22: 8951–8959.

Merisko-Liversidge, E. and G.G. Liversidge and E.R. Cooper. 2003. Nanosizing: a formulation approach for poorly-water-soluble compounds. Eur. J. Pharm. Sci. 18: 113–120.

Merisko-Liversidge, E.M. and G.G. Liversidge. 2008. Drug nanoparticles: formulating poorly water-soluble compounds. Toxicol. Pathol. 36: 43–48.

Merisko-Liversidge, E. and G.G. Liversidge. 2011. Nanosizing for oral and parenteral drug delivery: a perspective on formulating poorly-water soluble compounds using wet media milling technology. Adv. Drug Deliv. Rev. 63: 427–440.

Midoux, N. and P. Hošek, L. Pailleres and J.R. Authelin. 1999. Micronization of pharmaceutical substances in a spiral jet mill. Powder Technol. 104: 113–120.

Miller, D.A. and M. Gil. Spray-drying technology. pp. 363–442. *In*: R.O.O. Williams III, A.B.B. Watts and D.A.A. Miller [eds.]. 2012. Formulating Poorly Water Soluble Drugs. Springer, New York, USA.

Mistry, A. and S. Stolnik and L. Illum. 2009. Nanoparticles for direct nose-to-brain delivery of drugs. Int. J. Pharm. 379: 146–157.

Möeschwitzer, J. and R.H. Müller. 2006. New method for the effective production of ultrafine drug nanocrystals. J. Nanosci. Nanotechnol. 6: 3145–3153.

Möschwitzer, J. and G. Achleitner, H. Pomper and R.H. Müller. 2004. Development of an intravenously injectable chemically stable aqueous omeprazole formulation using nanosuspension technology. Eur. J. Pharm. Biopharm. 58: 615–619.

Morales, J.O. and J.T. McConville and A.B. Watts. Mechanical particle-size reduction techniques. pp. 133–170. *In*: R.O. Williams III, A.B. Watts and D.A. Miller [eds.]. 2012. Formulating Poorly Water Soluble Drugs. Springer, New York, USA.

Muller, R.H. and K. Peters. 1998. Nanosuspensions for the formulation of poorly soluble drugs: I. Preparation by a size-reduction technique. Int. J. Pharm. 160: 229–237.

Mumenthaler, M. and H. Leuenberger. 1991. Atmospheric spray-freeze drying: a suitable alternative in freeze-drying technology. Int. J. Pharm. 72: 97–110.

Newhouse, M.T. and P.H. Hirst, S.P. Duddu, Y.H. Walter, T.E. Tarara, A.R. Clark and J.G. Weers. 2003. Inhalation of a dry powder tobramycin PulmoSphere formulation in healthy volunteers. Chest. 124: 360–366.

Newman, K.D. and P. Elamanchili, G.S. Kwon and J. Samuel. 2002. Uptake of poly(D,L-lactic-co-glycolic acid) microspheres by antigen-presenting cells *in vivo*. J. Biomed. Mater. Res. 60: 480–486.

Niwa, T. and Y. Nakanishi and K. Danjo. 2010. One-step preparation of pharmaceutical nanocrystals using ultra cryo-milling technique in liquid nitrogen. Eur. J. Pharm. Sci. 41: 78–85.

Ochs, M. and J.R. Nyengaard, A. Jung, L. Knudsen, M. Voigt, T. Wahlers, J. Richter and H.J. Gundersen. 2004. The number of alveoli in the human lung. Am. J. Respir. Crit. Care Med. 169: 120–124.

Onoue, S. and H. Sato, K. Ogawa, Y. Kojo, Y. Aoki, Y. Kawabata, K. Wada, T. Mizumoto and S. Yamada. 2012. Inhalable dry-emulsion formulation of cyclosporine A with improved anti-inflammatory effects in experimental asthma/COPD-model rats. Eur. J. Pharm. Biopharm. 80: 54–60.

Ostrander, K.D. and H.W. Bosch and D.M. Bondanza. 1999. An *in-vitro* assessment of a NanoCrystal beclomethasone dipropionate colloidal dispersion via ultrasonic nebulization. Eur. J. Pharm. Biopharm. 48: 207–215.

Overhoff, K.A. and J.D. Engstrom, B. Chen, B.D. Scherzer, T.E. Milner, K.P. Johnston and R.O. Williams 3rd. 2007. Novel ultra-rapid freezing particle engineering process for enhancement of dissolution rates of poorly water-soluble drugs. Eur. J. Pharm. Biopharm. 65: 57–67.

Overhoff, K.A. and K.P. Johnston, J. Tam, J. Engstrom and R.O. Williams 3rd. 2009. Use of thin film freezing to enable drug delivery: a review. J. Drug Deliv. Sci. Technol. 19: 89–98.

Pandey, R. and A. Sharma, A. Zahoor, S. Sharma, G.K. Khuller and B. Prasad. 2003. Poly(DL-lactide-co-glycolide) nanoparticle-based inhalable sustained drug delivery system for experimental tuberculosis. J. Antimicrob. Chemother. 52: 981–986.

Pathak, P. and M.J. Meziani, T. Desai and Y.P. Sun. 2006. Formation and stabilization of ibuprofen nanoparticles in supercritical fluid processing. J. Supercrit. Fluids. 37: 279–286.

Pathak, P. and G.L. Prasad, M.J. Meziani, A.A. Joudeh and Y.P. Sun. 2007. Nanosized paclitaxel particles from supercritical carbon dioxide processing and their biological evaluation. Langmuir. 23: 2674–2679.

Patton, J.S. and P.R. Byron. 2007. Inhaling medicines: delivering drugs to the body through the lungs. Nat. Rev. Drug Discov. 6: 67–74.

Pilcer, G. and K. Amighi. 2010. Formulation strategy and use of excipients in pulmonary drug delivery. Int. J. Pharm. 392: 1–19.

Platz, R.M. and J.S. Patton, L. Foster and M. Eljamal. 2002. Compositions and methods for the pulmonary delivery of aerosolized macromolecules. Nektar Therapeutics. US6797258.

Rabinow, B.E. 2004. Nanosuspensions in drug delivery. Nat. Rev. Drug Discov. 3: 785–796.

Ragab, D. and S. Rohani, M.W. Samaha, F.M. El-Khawas and H.A. El-Maradny. 2010. Crystallization of progesterone for pulmonary drug delivery. J. Pharm. Sci. 99: 1123–1137.

Rehman, M. and B.Y. Shekunov, P. York, D. Lechuga-Ballesteros, D.P. Miller, T. Tan and P. Colthorpe. 2004. Optimisation of powders for pulmonary delivery using supercritical fluid technology. Eur. J. Pharm. Sci. 22: 1–17.

Rogers, T.L. and K.P. Johnston and R.O. Williams 3rd. 2003a. Physical stability of micronized powders produced by spray-freezing into liquid (SFL) to enhance the dissolution of an insoluble drug. Pharm. Dev. Technol. 8: 187–197.

Rogers, T.L. and A.C. Nelsen, M. Sarkari, T.J. Young, K.P. Johnston and R.O. Williams 3rd. 2003b. Enhanced aqueous dissolution of a poorly water soluble drug by novel particle engineering technology: spray-freezing into liquid with atmospheric freeze-drying. Pharm. Res. 20: 485–493.

Rogers, T.L. and K.A. Overhoff, P. Shah, P. Santiago, M.J. Yacaman, K.P. Johnston and R.O. Williams 3rd. 2003c. Micronized powders of a poorly water soluble drug produced by a spray-freezing into liquid-emulsion process. Eur. J. Pharm. Biopharm. 55: 161–172.

Rowe, J. and K. Johnston. Precipitation technologies for nanoparticle production. pp. 501–568. *In*: R.O. Williams III, A.B. Watts and D.A. Miller [eds.]. 2012. Formulating Poorly Water Soluble Drugs. Springer, New York, USA.

Russo, P. and C. Sacchetti, I. Pasquali, R. Bettini, G. Massimo, P. Colombo and A. Rossi. 2006. Primary microparticles and agglomerates of morphine for nasal insufflation. J. Pharm. Sci. 95: 2553–2561.

Schaberg, T. 1995. The dark side of antituberculosis therapy: adverse events involving liver function. Eur. Respir. J. 8: 1247–1249.

Schreck, S. and K.J. Sullivan, C.M. Ho and H.K. Chang. 1993. Correlations between flow resistance and geometry in a model of the human nose. J. Appl. Physiol. (1985) 75: 1767–1775.

Schwab, J.A. and M. Zenkel. 1998. Filtration of particulates in the human nose. Laryngoscope. 108: 120–124.

Sinswat, P. and X. Gao, M.J. Yacaman, R.O. Williams 3rd and K.P. Johnston. 2005. Stabilizer choice for rapid dissolving high potency itraconazole particles formed by evaporative precipitation into aqueous solution. Int. J. Pharm. 302: 113–124.

Sinswat, P. and K.A. Overhoff, J.T. McConville, K.P. Johnston and R.O. Williams 3rd. 2008. Nebulization of nanoparticulate amorphous or crystalline tacrolimus—single-dose pharmacokinetics study in mice. Eur. J. Pharm. Biopharm. 69: 1057–1066.

Sou, T. and E.N. Meeusen, M. de Veer, D.A. Morton, L.M. Kaminskas and M.P. McIntosh. 2011. New developments in dry powder pulmonary vaccine delivery. Trends Biotechnol. 29: 191–198.

Steckel, H. and J. Thies and B.W. Muller. 1997. Micronizing of steroids for pulmonary delivery by supercritical carbon dioxide. Int. J. Pharm. 152: 99–110.

Steckel, H. and B.W. Muller. 1998. Metered-dose inhaler formulation of fluticasone-17-propionate micronized with supercritical carbon dioxide using the alternative propellant HFA-227. Int. J. Pharm. 173: 25–33.

Sugimoto, S. and T. Niwa, Y. Nakanishi and K. Danjo. 2012. Novel ultra-cryo milling and co-grinding technique in liquid nitrogen to produce dissolution-enhanced nanoparticles for poorly water-soluble drugs. Chem. Pharm. Bull. (Tokyo). 60: 325–333.

Sung, J.C. and D.J. Padilla, L. Garcia-Contreras, J.L. Verberkmoes, D. Durbin, C.A. Peloquin, K.J. Elbert, A.J. Hickey and D.A. Edwards. 2009. Formulation and pharmacokinetics of self-assembled rifampicin nanoparticle systems for pulmonary delivery. Pharm. Res. 26: 1847–1855.

Tadros, T. 2009. Polymeric surfactants in disperse systems. Adv. Colloid Interface Sci. 147-148: 281–299.

Tam, J.M. and J.T. McConville, R.O. Williams 3rd and K.P. Johnston. 2008. Amorphous cyclosporin nanodispersions for enhanced pulmonary deposition and dissolution. J. Pharm. Sci. 97: 4915–4933.

Tandya, A. and F. Dehghani and N.R. Foster. 2006. Micronization of cyclosporine using dense gas techniques. J. Supercrit. Fluids. 37: 272–278.

Teeranachaideekul, V. and V.B. Junyaprasert, E.B. Souto and R.H. Müller. 2008. Development of ascorbyl palmitate nanocrystals applying the nanosuspension technology. Int. J. Pharm. 354: 227–234.

Telko, M.J. and A.J. Hickey. 2005. Dry powder inhaler formulation. Respir. Care. 50: 1209–1227.

Tsapis, N. and D. Bennett, B. Jackson, D.A. Weitz and D.A. Edwards. 2002. Trojan particles: large porous carriers of nanoparticles for drug delivery. Proc. Natl. Acad. Sci. U.S.A. 99: 12001–12005.

Turk, M. 2009. Manufacture of submicron drug particles with enhanced dissolution behaviour by rapid expansion processes. J. Supercrit. Fluids. 47: 537–545.

Türker, S. and E. Onur and Y. Ozer. 2004. Nasal route and drug delivery systems. Pharm. World Sci. 26: 137–142.

Tuunila, R. and L. Nystrom. 1998. Effects of grinding parameters on product fineness in jet mill grinding. Miner. Eng. 11: 1089–1094.

Vaughn, J.M. and J.T. McConville, D. Burgess, J.I. Peters, K.P. Johnston, R.L. Talbert and R.O. Williams 3rd. 2006. Single dose and multiple dose studies of itraconazole nanoparticles. Eur. J. Pharm. Biopharm. 63: 95–102.

Vaughn, J.M. and N.P. Wiederhold, J.T. McConville, J.J. Coalson, R.L. Talbert, D.S. Burgess, K.P. Johnston, R.O. Williams 3rd and J.I. Peters. 2007. Murine airway histology and intracellular uptake of inhaled amorphous itraconazole. Int. J. Pharm. 338: 219–224.

Vehring, R. 2008. Pharmaceutical particle engineering via spray drying. Pharm. Res. 25: 999–1022.

Vemavarapu, C. and M.J. Mollan, M. Lodaya and T.E. Needham. 2005. Design and process aspects of laboratory scale SCF particle formation systems. Int. J. Pharm. 292: 1–16.

Vila, A. and A. Sánchez, C. Evora, I. Soriano, O. McCallion and M.J. Alonso. 2005. PLA-PEG particles as nasal protein carriers: the influence of the particle size. Int. J. Pharm. 292: 43–52.

Walstra, P. 1993. Principles of emulsion formation. Chem. Eng. Sci. 48: 333–349.

Wang, Z. and J.F. Chen, Y. Le and Z.G. Shen. 2007. Preparation of ultrafine beclomethasone dipropionate drug powder by antisolvent precipitation. Ind. Eng. Chem. Res. 46: 4839–4845.

Watts, A.B. and R.O. Williams. Nanoparticles for pulmonary delivery. pp. 335–366. In: H.D.C. Smyth and A.J. Hickey [eds.]. 2011. Controlled Pulmonary Drug Delivery. Springer, New York, USA.

Williams III, R.O. and K.P. Johnston, T.J. Young, T.L. Rogers, M.K. Barron, Z. Yu and J. Hu. 2002. Process for production of nanoparticles and microparticles by spray freezing into liquid. Board of Regents, University of Texas System. US6862890.

Witkin, D.B. and E.J. Lavernia. 2006. Synthesis and mechanical behavior of nanostructured materials via cryomilling. Prog. Mater. Sci. 51: 1–60.

Witschi, C. and R.J. Mrsny. 1999. In vitro evaluation of microparticles and polymer gels for use as nasal platforms for protein delivery. Pharm. Res. 16: 382–390.

Wu, L. and J. Zhang and W. Watanabe. 2011. Physical and chemical stability of drug nanoparticles. Adv. Drug Deliv. Rev. 63: 456–469.

Yang, W. and J. Tam, D.A. Miller, J. Zhou, J.T. McConville, K.P. Johnston and R.O. Williams 3rd. 2008. High bioavailability from nebulized itraconazole nanoparticle dispersions with biocompatible stabilizers. Int. J. Pharm. 361: 177–188.

Yang, W. and K.P. Johnston and R.O. Williams 3rd. 2010. Comparison of bioavailability of amorphous versus crystalline itraconazole nanoparticles via pulmonary administration in rats. Eur. J. Pharm. Biopharm. 75: 33–41.

Young, T.J. and S. Mawson, K.P. Johnston, I.B. Henriksen, G.W. Pace and A.K. Mishra. 2000. Rapid expansion from supercritical to aqueous solution to produce submicron suspensions of water-insoluble drugs. Biotechnol. Prog. 16: 402–407.

Yu, Z. and K.P. Johnston and R.O. Williams 3rd. 2006. Spray freezing into liquid versus spray-freeze drying: Influence of atomization on protein aggregation and biological activity. Eur. J. Pharm. Sci. 27: 9–18.

Zamankhan, P. and G. Ahmadi, Z. Wang, P.K. Hopke, Y.S. Cheng, W.C. Su and D. Leonard. 2006. Airflow and deposition of nano-particles in a human nasal cavity. Aerosol Sci. Technol. 40: 463–476.

Zhang, Z. and C. Kleinstreuer, J.F. Donohue and C.S. Kim. 2005. Comparison of micro- and nano-size particle depositions in a human upper airway model. J. Aerosol Sci. 36: 211–233.

Zhang, Q.Z. and L.S. Zha, Y. Zhang, W.M. Jiang, W. Lu, Z.Q. Shi, X.G. Jiang and S.K. Fu. 2006. The brain targeting efficiency following nasally applied MPEG-PLA nanoparticles in rats. J. Drug Target. 14: 281–290.

Zhang, H. and D. Wang, R. Butler, N.L. Campbell, J. Long, B. Tan, D.J. Duncalf, A.J. Foster, A. Hopkinson, D. Taylor, D. Angus, A.I. Cooper and S.P. Rannard. 2008. Formation and enhanced biocidal activity of water-dispersable organic nanoparticles. Nat. Nanotechnol. 3: 506–511.

Zhou, H. and Y. Zhang, D.L. Biggs, M.C. Manning, T.W. Randolph, U. Christians, B.M. Hybertson and K.Y. Ng. 2005. Microparticle-based lung delivery of INH decreases INH metabolism and targets alveolar macrophages. J. Control. Release. 107: 288–299.

Zijlstra, G.S. and M. Rijkeboer, D. Jan van Drooge, M. Sutter, W. Jiskoot, M. van de Weert, W.L. Hinrichs and H.W. Frijlink. 2007. Characterization of a cyclosporine solid dispersion for inhalation. AAPS J. 9: E190–E199.

CHAPTER 6

Lipid Nanoplatforms for Pulmonary Drug Delivery

Bruno M. Ponte,[1,a] *Isis S. Santos,*[1,b] *Ana S. Macedo*[1,c] and
Eliana B. Souto[1,2,*]

ABSTRACT

For drug administration and delivery design, it is important to consider a number of factors, but mainly the drug form and the administration route. The most depends on the characteristics of the target site. Some organs are more exposed than others, being more prone to diseases. The respiratory system is an opening into the human body for aerial detritus that can gain access deliberately by administration of drugs, or involuntarily throughout the inhalation of ambient air. This makes the lungs very exposed to adverse factors. In terms of mortality, incidence, prevalence, and costs, respiratory diseases are in the second place of ranking among most European countries (generally after cardiovascular diseases). It is therefore important to find appropriate therapies to treat and control lung ailments, based on the understanding of the respiratory structure and functioning, and the type of material compatible to the route of administration. Because of its physiology, the respiratory apparatus has an extended exposure to external conditions making it more vulnerable to diseases, e.g., asthma, chronic obstructive pulmonary disease, tuberculosis, and lung cancer. The aerosol therapy has been widely used over the last 50 years to address respiratory diseases. Recently, new approaches

---

[1] Faculty of Health Sciences, Fernando Pessoa University, Rua Carlos da Maia, 296, P-4200-150 Porto, Portugal.
[a] Email: brunop@ufp.edu.pt
[b] Email: isiss@ufp.edu.pt
[c] Email: amacedo@ufp.edu.pt
[2] Institute of Biotechnology and Bioengineering, Centre of Genomics and Biotechnology University of Trás-os-Montes and Alto Douro (CGB-UTAD/IBB), P.O. Box 1013, P-5001-801 Vila Real, Portugal.
[*] Corresponding author: emb.souto@gmail.com; souto.eliana@gmail.com

have been developed, namely Micro/Nanotechnology. They are associated with biocompatible materials that can improve drug targeting and intake, patient compliance, while reducing therapy costs and side effects. The chapter focuses on some common diseases that affect the respiratory apparatus and limit the patients' quality of life, providing new therapeutic strategies based on Micro/Nanotechnology. Commonly used aerosol types composed of lipid microspheres and other lipid nanosystems, e.g., solid lipid nanoparticles and nanostructure lipid carriers, will be addressed, following the anatomical lung particle deposition and the toxicological aspects of these systems.

Introduction

Both respiratory and circulatory systems work together, distributing the oxygen acquired from lung to the cells in exchange for carbon dioxide, which will be exhaled from the lungs, a process known as respiration (Bérubé et al. 2010). The air required to perform vital functions comes from the respiratory system. It passes through the nose to the respiratory apparatus (composed by larynx, trachea, bronchi, lungs), penetrating the bloodstream for its distribution. The lungs function, structure, and environment play a very important role in the deposition of particles and microbes. The lung, because of its large surface area, is constantly exposed to microbes and particles entering by the airways (González-Juarrero and O'Sullivan 2011). As a result, the respiratory apparatus is quite exposed to many external agents being more vulnerable to develop several diseases, some of them with increased prevalence in the population, which deteriorates the life quality and expectancy. Examples of life threatening lung diseases include the Chronic Obstructive Pulmonary Disease (COPD), lung cancer, tuberculosis, and asthma.

COPD is a growing health problem that it is associated with great morbidity worldwide which causes nearly as many deaths as lung cancer, being currently a global health priority whose etymology is not quite defined (Barreiro and Criner 2014). The term COPD is relatively new and it refers to old diseases, i.e., bronchitis, emphysema, asthmatic bronchitis, and chronic bronchitis. This disease is considered as an airflow limitation mutually progressive and linked with an atypical inflammatory response of the lungs to injurious particles or gases, whose progression is not fully reversible (Barreiro and Criner 2014). In summary, COPD is a multicomponent disease with inflammation at its core, in which patients experience progressively worsening lung function, disease symptoms, and quality of life, as well as increasing exacerbations (Hanania et al. 2011). The pharmacological approach of this ailment includes bronchodilators, inhaled corticosteroids, combination therapies, and long-term oxygen therapy (Hanania et al. 2005).

With respect to cancer, this condition is characterized by uncontrolled development and spread of atypical cell that if not detected in time is a major cause of death. Cancer cells consumes a large amount of energy for their proliferation, and the system for producing energy in many cancer cells is different from that in normal cells (Hori et al. 2011). Lung cancer can be the result of external factors (e.g., tobacco, infectious organisms, chemicals, and radiation), internal factors (e.g., inherited mutations, hormones, immune conditions, and mutations that occur from metabolism), or the combination of both (Ridge et al. 2013). Lung cancer is one of the most prevailing diseases in developed countries (Park et al. 2010), which causes more deaths than breast, colorectal, prostate, and pancreatic cancer combined (Ridge et al. 2013). Although being one of the most common types of cancer, people affected with this disease continue to have poor diagnosis, which contributes to its mortality (Hori et al. 2011). The survival of lung cancer affected patients rests on the stage the tumor has extended its detection. However, in most cases, metastases have occurred before the primary tumor is clinically detectable or causes symptoms, which results in an incidence similar to the mortality (Ridge et al. 2013). As a result, it is important to find an effective chemo-preventive therapy or pharmacological therapeutic against lung cancer to reduce its mortality. Conventional pharmacotherapy in lung cancer is the administration of intravenous chemotherapy medicine (e.g., topoisomerase I inhibitors) (Miller et al. 2006).

Another relevant lung disease is tuberculosis. This is an infectious disease caused by the bacillus *Mycobacterium tuberculosis*, which affects preferably the lungs. Tuberculosis is a transmissible ailment whose fate rests on the existence of a sputum-positive case. Given the success of tuberculosis therapy, the mortality is falling globally. This led to a contradictory problem for researchers, since the cases of tuberculosis are insufficient to support the research necessary to maintain and accelerate the decline (Katz et al. 2007). Although the low incidence of tuberculosis in developed countries, *M. tuberculosis* is an obligate human parasite, whose complex life cycle allows persisting indefinitely in human communities as small as a few hundred people (Hunter 2011). *M. tuberculosis* has not been eradicated yet, having some cases of tuberculosis outbreaks all over the world. For the treatment of tuberculosis, the use of appropriate combination of antibiotics is frequent. However, it is important to keep in mind that some strains of *M. tuberculosis* are persistent, presenting some resistance to the treatment (González-Juarrero and O'Sullivan 2011). Thus, it is fundamental to continue the study of effective therapeutic alternatives against the bacterium.

Asthma is a common chronic disease that affects the airways, making them very sensitive and reactive to external factors. Some external factors are triggers to a reduce air intake that it translates as a severe asthma attack, which is recognized by wheezing, coughing, chest tightness, and trouble breathing. This respiratory problem has a negative influence in the quality of life. There is a tendency for the disease to increase in the coming years. Most cases are mild-to-moderate asthma patients that respond to inhaled corticosteroids. However, there are some patients with a severe form of asthma whose symptoms and controls are assumed to be generally insensitive to handling, even with high-dose inhales and systemic corticosteroids

(Wenzel et al. 2007). When not controlled, asthma can have major consequences on morbidity, quality of life, and economic cargo. This highlights the significance of achieving and maintaining an optimal asthma control (Siroux et al. 2009).

Aerosol Therapy

The lungs have a large alveolar surface area, a low thickness epithelial barrier combined with its extensive vascularization that makes the pulmonary route ideal for drug administration (Azarmi et al. 2008). The effective integration of new drugs with devices accomplished the clear distribution of doses to the respiratory apparatus, which has resulted in an established step record for inhalation as a way of administration that limits systemic exposure and offers localized topical delivery (Forbes et al. 2011).

Aerosol therapy has developed the management of numerous ailments comprising obstructive airway diseases. This type of administration is characterized by the drug distribution directly into the lower airways for both topical and systemic effect (Rubin 2006, Khilnani and Banga 2008). A large number of alternatives are currently being developed both for pulmonary and systemic administration via the airway and lung (Rubin 2006). Especially, for the treatment of diseased states within the lung, the inhalation of aerosolized drugs has turn out to be a well-recognized modality (Zeng et al. 1995). Aerosol therapy is now used, not only for asthma and COPD, but also for tuberculosis and lung cancer treatments. Aerosol therapy shows many advantages for drug administration, e.g., aerosol antibiotics can deliver high drug concentrations with low systemic bioavailability, thus reducing toxicity (Rubin 2006).

There are three essential mechanisms, operating in distinctive combinations according to the location of the respiratory apparatus and the drug used, that affects drug delivery of aerosols, i.e., inertial impaction, sedimentation, and diffusion (Khilnani and Banga 2008). Inertial impaction is the process that allows the deposition of a large mass of aerosol particles to be deposited onto a surface in an expected modus in a small period of time (Cooney and Hickey 2011). This mechanism is the main process occurring in the oropharynx and the superior airways for aerosols with fairly large particle dimension (Khilnani and Banga 2008). Diffusion and sedimentation are slow processes and require an extended contact period to deposit substantial doses of particles (Cooney and Hickey 2011). Small size particles (< 0.5 µm) are diffused through Brownian motion (Khilnani and Banga 2008).

However, there are other parameters important in aerosol administration, namely physical characteristics of the aerosol particle (i.e., size and shape, density, electrical charge, hygroscopic character, velocity of the particles) and host factors (inspired volume, inspiratory time, inspiratory flow, breath-hold duration, timing of aerosol delivery during inspiration) (Khilnani and Banga 2008). Generally, aerosol lung deposition is dependent of factors, e.g., aerosol-generating system, particle size distribution of the inhaled aerosol, inhalation pattern, oral or nasal inhalation, properties of the inhaled carrier gas, airflow obstruction, and type and severity of the lung disease (Dolovich and Dhand 2011).

To improve the drug behavior, it is possible to manage some characteristics such as size, shape, or electrical charge, turning drug targeting more effective. The use of nanotechnology can be effective in various pulmonary therapeutic schemes, which may improve the systemic drug bioavailability by offering protection against hostile environmental factors, as well as by displaying controlled release properties (Dailey et al. 2003). The use of biocompatible materials (e.g., lipids similar to the body components) for drug encapsulation is an advantage because of their reduced toxicity. In addition, particle size is determinant in the drug targeting to a specific lung area, the smaller the particle the greater is its ability to reach the inferior lung lobe. However, the finest aerosols (≤ 1 µm) are mostly exhaled lacking deposition (Sakagami et al. 2001). Still it is possible to deliver nanoparticles (NPs) in the lung with the proper carrier system (Azarmi et al. 2008).

In this chapter some types of aerosol available and administration carriers [microspheres, nanospheres, Solid Lipid Nanoparticles (SLNs), and Nanostructured Lipid Carriers (NLCs)] will be analyzed, including their characteristics, applications, and toxicity.

Inhalers and formulation characteristics

Pulmonary drug delivery is an interesting approach which is advantageous in patients suffering from pulmonary diseases, such as cystic fibrosis, asthma, chronic pulmonary infections, and lung cancer. Furthermore, pulmonary drug delivery has reduced systemic side effects and the feasibility of topical drug delivery (Pilcer and Amighi 2010).

Even though inhalation devices and aerosols for pulmonary drug delivery have been widely used since the 19th century, a growing interest has been noted in the systemic drug delivery via the lungs (Pilcer and Amighi 2010). Several drugs (e.g., insulin, human growth hormone, calcitonin, and deslorelin) were incorporated to the bloodstream after pulmonary administration due to lungs anatomical features such as large alveolar surface area, extensive vascularization, and low thickness epithelial barrier. Despite lungs being an efficient port of entry for drugs to the bloodstream due to their characteristics, they also display low local activity and avoidance of first pass metabolism (Pilcer and Amighi 2010).

Most commonly used drug delivery devices for aerosol therapy are nebulizers, pressurized Metered-Dose Inhalers (MDIs), and Dry Powder Inhalers (DPIs). Generally, a delivery device has to produce an aerosol of suitable size (0.5–5 µm), a reproducible dosing, and targeted delivery, while protecting the physicochemical stability of the formulation. Furthermore, the ideal inhalation system must be simple, convenient, inexpensive, and portable (Siekmeier and Scheuch 2008, Pilcer and Amighi 2010).

Nebulizers were the first devices launched in the market for inhalation therapy. Nebulization has low efficiency, great variability and, consequently, great variability. Alongside these advantages, nebulization is very time consuming and requires cleaning. Therefore, an improvement in the efficiency, portability, and administration time of the aerosol delivery system was greatly needed. MDIs were then developed to overcome the nebulization gaps. In MDIs, pharmaceuticals are dissolved or suspended in a propellant, generally chlorofluorocarbons, such as dichlorofluoromethane, dichlorotetrafluoroethane, and trichlorofluoromethane. The propellant should be non-toxic, non-inflammable, and compatible with formulated drugs. MDIs have been used for the last 50 years to treat asthma and COPD. However, MDIs are unsuccessful in drug delivery since only a small portion of the administered drug reaches the patient's lungs, and they are not environmentally friendly. Additionally, they are suited for the delivery of macromolecules (e.g., proteins and peptides) due to impaired stability, agent denaturation, and high particle distribution. Moreover, the deposition of aerosolized drugs on the mouth and oropharyngeal regions can be greater than 70%, and reach 90% depending on the application technique (Siekmeier and Scheuch 2008, Pilcer and Amighi 2010).

To overcome the problems with MDIs, DPI devices were developed that are simple, smaller, and do not use propellants. DPI devices are based on a powder technology that disperses dry particles as an aerosol. Therefore, coordination of actuation and inhalation is not required, resulting in better lung drug delivery compared to MDIs. DPIs are formulated with solid particle blends which contribute to high stability. In addition, DPIs can be divided into two categories: (i) unit-dose or single-dose devices, in which the drug is packaged in individual doses, e.g., capsules; and, (ii) multi-unit and multi-dose devices, in which the doses are in a blister or a reservoir of drug.

A DPI dose depends on the properties of the drug formulation, especially powder flow, particle flow, particle geometry and surface properties, carrier interaction, performance of the inhaler device, correct inhalation technique, and aspiratory flow rate (Pilcer and Amighi 2010). Moreover, these formulations require the use of excipients which are known to interfere with the inhaler device and have limited use for pulmonary drug delivery and tend to agglomerate. The powder must be dispersed into a flow of hair to break the agglomeration, therefore a turbulent airstream must generate inside the inhaler while it also causes particles to split from the carrier. A way to circumvent this problem is the engineering of particles to achieve a narrow particle size and high dispersibility (Labiris and Dolovich 2003, Pilcer and Amighi 2010).

Particle aerodynamic diameter

One of most important characteristics to be taken into account when developing a formulation is the particle geometry, as well as density, electrical charge, and hygroscopic character. The superior airways (nose, mouth larynx, and pharynx) as well as the branching anatomy of the tracheobronchial tree act as selective filters of particles (Pilcer and Amighi 2010).

Mechanisms by which the particles deposit in the respiratory tract are highly dependent on particle sizes. They include impaction (inertial deposition), sedimentation, Brownian diffusion, interception, and electrostatic precipitation. Firstly, impaction occurs near airway bifurcations, especially in extrathoracic and large conducting airway, due to the high flow velocities and rapid changes in the direction of bulk airflow resulting in significant inertial forces. The increase in velocity, breathing rate, and particle size and density, augment the probability of impaction (Pilcer and Amighi 2010).

Given the low air velocity, particles of size 0.5–5 μm deposit in the small conducting airways by gravitational sedimentation. Larger particles are mostly affected by gravity which causes their deposition and a longer residence time, however it also decreases with the increasing in breathing rates (Pilcer and Amighi 2010). On the other hand, smaller particles (< 0.5 μm) have a random motion caused by the collision with surrounding air molecules. This Brownian motion causes particles to diffuse and deposit in small airways and alveoli where bulk airflow is low. As a result, aerosols must have aerodynamic diameters between 0.5 and 5 μm to reach the lower respiratory tract and achieve pulmonary drug deposition. The bigger particles (5 μm) suffer deposition in the oropharynx and are easily cleared, whereas smaller particles (0.5 μm) settle very slowly due to Brownian motion and may not be deposited. The addition of carrier particles have shown to improve flow properties. Particle interaction must be overcome to avoid particle aggregation. In fact, particles can aggregate by several mechanisms: (i) mechanical interlocking due to surface asperities; (ii) capillary forces from the presence of water; (iii) electrostatic arising from insulating nature of the material; and, (iv) van der Waals forces from the fundamental electromagnetic nature of matter (Pilcer and Amighi 2010).

Particle dispersion is prevented by particle surface features or roughness by mechanical interlocking. The forces created are related to the diameter of the pores between particles and interfacial tension resulted from hydrogen bonding of water. Moisture content is intrinsically related to capillary forces. Capillary forces are also related to electrostatic forces, which plays a preponderant role in particle dispersion. Capillary forces are caused by dynamic condensation of water molecules onto the particle surface. These molecules form a meniscus between contact points of adjacent surfaces. Furthermore, moisture uptake is a function of the specific surface area of the material at low relative humidity. As relative humidity increases, water content also increases in crystalline solid particles. Furthermore, the number of excipients approved for pulmonary drug delivery is very restricted which leads to a need of developing an optimized delivery system with superior delivery efficiency (Pilcer and Amighi 2010).

One approach that can increase the benefits one can get from pulmonary drug delivery would be the delivery of the necessary amount of drugs to the site of interest for the required period of time. This strategy requires particle engineering in such a way that: (i) a narrow particle size distribution is attained; (ii) formulation dispersibility and drug stability are improved; (iii) bioavailability is optimized; and, (iv) sustained drug release and specific targeting is assured. The extensive application of dry powder formulations alongside with the aerodynamic behavior of the inhaler devices, the behavior of the respiratory system, and the interparticulate interactions have turned the development of pulmonary drug delivery formulations into one of the most challenging areas (Pilcer and Amighi 2010).

Lipid Microspheres and Nanospheres

Lipid microspheres have a particle size of 0.2 μm and are very stable. They can be stored at room temperature up to two years. Microspheres are mainly composed of soybean oil and lecithin, which are non-toxic lipids. For this reason, no particular adverse side effects have been reported, even at high doses. They are considered to be physicochemically stable, biocompatible, and feasible for scale-up at low cost (Jaspart et al. 2007). Similar to liposomes, microspheres are able to accumulate in inflamed tissues and other lesions. Due to these properties, microspheres have been proposed as drug delivery systems. Microspheres were developed to overcome several limitations of conventional drug delivery. For example, prostaglandins, cytokines, and other peptides have strong physiological activities, give rise to local effect, and are rapidly metabolized. Due to their fast metabolization, high doses must be administered to have an effective response; on the other hand, administering high doses cause severe side effects and toxicity. Additionally, local pain and inflammation have also been observed after administration (Yamaguchi 1996).

Lipid microspheres were first used as drug delivery systems in the 70's: they were used to encapsulate barbituric acid, and later they were applied to nitroglycerin and cyclandelate. Lipid microspheres are able to target passively at a specific diseased site, such as inflammation and arteriosclerotic lesions, and showed clinically promising efficacy (Yamaguchi 1996). Drug delivery microsystems have some advantages when compared to nanosystems. Microparticles can be prepared as dry powder forms, which improves storage stability, and ultimately extends the shelf life avoiding cold chain storage. Moreover, they are able to be administered by standard inhalers, which are more convenient than nebulizers, and they avoid low inertia making them very practical (Wan et al. 2012). Microparticles for drug delivery are mainly porous particles (Siekmeier and Scheuch 2008). Large microparticles have geometric sizes over 5 mm and 0.1 g/cm³ of mass density. Its main advantages are related to the low uptake by macrophages, high dispersibility, and enhanced delivery efficiency. Promising results were obtained regarding insulin administration via the pulmonary route (Edwards et al. 1997). Results have shown that after inhalation of insulin-loaded large porous microparticles, glucose systemic levels were suppressed during 96 hours comparing to the 4 hours effect caused by small non-porous particles. In fact, the existence of voids in particles lower their density, and several strategies include the use of shell forming excipients and gas forming agents to increase porous surfaces. Another strategy proposed was the development of lipid-based microspheres (PulmoSphere™) which showed great potential as a carrier for pulmonary delivery of biopharmaceuticals. PulmoSphere™ is produced by spray drying an emulsion, whose submicron droplets are dispersed in a liquid phase that evaporates slower than the continuous phase. The dispersed phase is stabilized by phospholipids which delay droplets coalescence during the evaporation of the continuous phase. Nanodroplets become closely packed as the droplets shrink forming an interface of foam-like structure which solidifies. The space created by the nanodroplets becomes empty, creating porous microparticles with low density. Microparticles are such versatile systems that can be loaded with NPs and benefit from synergic advantages. So far, their use as Trojan horses have been applied to microparticles loaded with protein-lipid/polymer nanocomplexes and nanoparticulate aggregates (Wan et al. 2012). Other production methods include solvent emulsification-diffusion or supercritical extraction methods (Mezzena et al. 2009).

The delivery of proteins and peptides through the pulmonary route to achieve a systemic effect is technically challenging: (i) powders tend to agglomerate due to the electrostatic forces and van der Waals forces; (ii) mucociliary clearance rapidly clears foreign particles from the pulmonary tract; and, (iii) particles suffer enzymatic degradation and phagocytosis by alveolar macrophages. It was developed as a two-step process for the delivery of a hydrophilic drugs incorporated in lipid microspheres (Cook et al. 2005). These systems dissociate into NPs in an aqueous medium to be therapeutically effective. Therefore, the addition of hydrophilic excipients that binds NPs enables microparticles to be dispersed (Li et al. 2010).

Lipid nanospheres have been prepared as colloidal therapeutic carriers by many researchers (Hu et al. 2008, Chon et al. 2011, Erdal et al. 2012, Mukhopadhyay et al. 2012, Yang et al. 2012). SLNs and NLCs are two main types of lipid carriers. SLNs combine the advantages of emulsions, liposomes, and polymeric NPs. The solid matrix can protect incorporated active ingredients against chemical degradation and provide the highest flexibilities in the modulation of the drug release profiles. Moreover, SLNs are composed of well physiologically tolerated excipients and can be produced on large industrial scale by high pressure homogenization. However, there are also some potential limitations, i.e., limited drug loading capacity, drug expulsion during storage due to the crystallization of lipid matrix. NLCs composed of solid lipid matrix with certain content of liquid lipid are a new generation of lipid NPs (Dong et al. 2011, Han et al. 2011, Hao et al. 2011). The incorporation of liquid lipids into solid lipid matrix generates great imperfections in the crystal lattice of NPs, thus leading to improved drug loading capacity and reduced drug expulsion during storage. The high pressure homogenization is the main method for the preparation of lipid nanospheres given the large scale production ability (Dong et al. 2011, Hao et al. 2011). However, the high temperatures used in the process could affect the stability of the drug and the carriers, and the higher emulsifier concentration was also believed to cause the burst drug release. Due to these reasons, a solvent diffusion method in an aqueous system was developed to prepare the lipid nanospheres. This method does not need emulsifiers and it is a simple preparation procedure (Hu et al. 2008, Chon et al. 2009, 2011, Hariharan et al. 2012). In general, for the preparation of lipid nanospheres, the drug is usually dissolved into 5 mL mixed organic solvent of ethanol/methanol and acetone (1:1, v/v) at 50°C. The resultant organic solution is then quickly dispersed into distilled water or a drug saturated aqueous solution. The drug-loaded lipid nanosphere dispersion is obtained under mechanical stirring (400 rpm, 5 minutes) (Chon et al. 2009, 2011, Erdal et al. 2012, Hariharan et al. 2012).

A large variety of solid lipids and liquid lipids including natural, semi-synthetic, and synthetic lipids with various structures (e.g., triglycerides, partial glycerides, fatty acids, waxes, and steroids) are available as matrix lipids for NLC production. However, the lipids used as matrix lipids need to be carefully selected as they will directly influence the performance of the carrier system (Patlolla and Vobalaboina 2008, Patlolla et al. 2010). Properties directly influenced by the lipids selected are: (i) the toxicity and biocompatibility, by selecting well tolerated physiological and biodegradable lipids (Patlolla and Vobalaboina 2008, Abdelbary and Fahmy 2009, Abdel-Mottaleb et al. 2011, Abbasalipourkabir et al. 2012); (ii) the drug entrapment efficiency, by choosing lipids in which the drug shows a high solubility (Almeida and Souto 2007, Abbasalipourkabir et al. 2012); (iii) drug expulsion during storage which can be minimized or avoided with lipid matrices with a low tendency to crystallize or with a less ordered structure; (iv) controlled drug release properties via the way of drug incorporation into the lipid matrix (Pandey et al. 2005, Qi et al. 2012); and, (v) increased chemical drug stability (photosensitive drugs, and drugs sensitive to hydrolysis or oxidation are incorporated in the matrix) (Almeida and Souto 2007, Chattopadhyay et al. 2007, Muller et al. 2011, Iqbal et al. 2012).

Therapeutic applications

Currently it is quite difficult to find applications of nanospheres for pulmonary therapy. One reason may be the lack of studies, and furthermore current formulations are effective in different treatments. However, some studies report the potential of SLNs for treating lung cancer (Atinkaya et al. 2005, Almeida and Souto 2007, Bustos et al. 2008, Choi et al.

2008, Abbasalipourkabir et al. 2012). For instance, SLNs have been loaded with phosphosulindac, a modified form of sulindac and sulindac sulfone that strongly inhibit lung tumors in mice, reducing lung tumor multiplicities (Al-Jamal et al. 2008, Bustos et al. 2008, Cerchia et al. 2012, Chen et al. 2012, Broza et al. 2013). SLNs have been reported to efficiently improve the pharmacokinetic profile of phosphosulindac (facilitating a targeted drug delivery to tumor sites), while minimizing systemic side effects. Phosphosulindac-loaded SLNs were four-fold more potent than the drug itself in inhibiting the growth of A549 and H510 cells. It was observed that the SLNs enhanced the cellular uptake and facilitated drug accumulation in mitochondria, leading to oxidative stress and apoptosis via the mitochondrial-apoptosis pathway. In addition, phosphosulindac-loaded SLNs were highly effective in suppressing the growth of A549 xenografts (78% inhibition compared to control, $p < 0.01$), while the drug itself had no significant effect. Formulation of phosphosulindac-loaded SLNs resulted in improved pharmacokinetics in mice and an enhanced ($\approx$ 14-fold) accumulation of the drug and its metabolites in A549 xenografts (Marchetti et al. 2009, Brunell et al. 2011, Moschos et al. 2011, Zhu et al. 2012).

Another important example is the lung delivery of itraconazole for the treatment of yeasts infections. Examples of itraconazole sensitive fungi are *Candida* spp., *Aspergillus* spp., *Penicillium* spp., *Histoplasma capsulatum*, and *Blastomyces dermatitidis* (Kasongo et al. 2011, Pardeike et al. 2011). Opportunistic fungal infections such as aspergillosis, histoplasmosis, blastomycosis, or candidiasis can be life-threatening for immuno-compromised patients. The lung as a major port of entry into the body and often as a site of infection plays an important role in these diseases. Therefore, the pulmonary application of itraconazole seems to be a promising therapeutic strategy especially since: (i) the lung epithelium can be directly reached resulting in a faster onset of action; (ii) the necessary drug dose and dosing frequency can be reduced compared to traditional administration routes such as oral application; and, (iii) undesirable side effects of itraconazole such as nausea, abdominal/epigastric pain, and hepatotoxicity can be avoided. Thus, the use of NLCs for pulmonary delivery may allow reaching the lower respiratory tract, as reducing the particle size < 500 nm leads to an increased deposition in all lung regions thanks to an enhanced mobility by diffusion (Pardeike et al. 2009, Pardeike et al. 2011). In addition, bioadhesive properties of NLCs (due to their small particle size as well as their lipophilic character) lead to prolonged residence times in the lung (Pandey et al. 2005, Almeida and Souto 2007, Chattopadhyay et al. 2007, Jaafar-Maalej et al. 2011, Pardeike et al. 2011, Iqbal et al. 2012). Furthermore, controlled release properties of drugs from the solid particle matrix can prolong the therapeutic effect as well as the inhalation interval (Pandey et al. 2005, Patlolla et al. 2010).

Finally, celecoxib has shown a synergistic anticancer activity in combination with other anticancer agents such as docetaxel (Patlolla and Vobalaboina 2008, Patlolla et al. 2010, Kasongo et al. 2011). A celecoxib-loaded NLC formulation was prepared by hot melt homogenization technique (Patlolla et al. 2010), showing a mean particle size of ≈ 220 nm. The cytotoxicity of celecoxib-loaded NLCs was determined against A549 lung carcinoma cells. *In vitro* cytotoxicity results showed a direct relation between celecoxib concentrations vs. exposure time. After 24 hours of exposure, celecoxib solution and celecoxib-NLCs showed the half maximum inhibitory concentration (IC_{50}) values of ≈ 79 and 250 µg/mL, respectively. The differences were associated to the controlled release of celecoxib and/or to cell internalization of the NLCs over time (Patlolla et al. 2010).

Toxicology

One of the major tasks in developing a drug delivery system is to define inhalable drug formulations with sufficient stability and appropriate size. Particularly, inhalation devices as well as the physicochemical characteristics of the formulation could influence the aerodynamic size of the particles and ultimately affect the site of aerosol deposition (Sager and Castranova 2009, Nassimi et al. 2009, 2010). Next to inhalation devices, drug-loaded NPs are equally important for the effectiveness of respiratory delivery. To develop an ideal pulmonary drug delivery system, NPs with suitable properties are required. Particles with average sizes in the nanometer range exhibit some well-defined and delicate characteristics, which have created an attractive and efficient approach for pulmonary delivery of drugs (Chattopadhyay et al. 2007, Harush-Frenkel et al. 2010, Nassimi et al. 2010, Al-Hallak et al. 2011, 2012). SLNs combine the advantages of the safety of lipids (lipids are well tolerated by the body) and the possibility of large-scale production. It could be shown that the degradation velocity depends on the composition of the lipid matrix (Al-Hallak et al. 2011, 2012). For pulmonary administration, SLN dispersions can be nebulized without any significant change in mean particle size, and SLN powders could be used in a DPI (Hureaux et al. 2009, Nassimi et al. 2009, Schleh et al. 2009, Al-Hallak et al. 2011, 2012).

However, the final introduction of SLNs into the clinic requires a complete toxicological risk assessment. Recently, the toxicological and inflammatory potentials of SLNs have been investigated by using *in vitro*, *ex vivo*, and *in vivo* methods (Harush-Frenkel et al. 2010). In this investigation, the *in vitro* cytotoxicity of the nanodispersion in human type II pneumocyte-like cells (A549 cell line) was assessed by 3-(4,5-dimethylthiazole-2-yl)-2,5-diphenyltetrazolium bromide (MTT) and neutral red uptake (NRU) assays, and the inflammatory potential was determined by measuring the interleukin (IL)-8 content in the supernatant. The inflammatory response was assessed by measuring chemokine KC and tumor necrosis factor-alpha (TNF-α) content in the supernatants. To evaluate the *in vivo* situation, a 16-day inhalation toxicity study was performed. The cytotoxic potential was estimated by investigating lactate dehydrogenase and total protein contents in the bronchoalveolar lavage (BAL) fluid. The inflammation status was assessed by counting and differentiation of BAL cells, by determination of chemokine KC and IL-6 levels in BAL fluid, and by histopathological evaluation of the lung, liver, spleen, and kidneys (Nassimi et al. 2009, 2010, Al-Hallak et al. 2011, 2012).

Toxicity of SLNs has been studied for more than 15 years (Weyenberg et al. 2007, Gokce et al. 2008). However, the composition of the SLNs used in the experiments was not uniform, differing in the nature of the lipids used and the total percentage of lipids in the lipid matrix. Due to the poor comparability of toxicity data in the literature, the toxicity of lipid NPs should be investigated first *in vitro*, then *ex vivo*, and finally *in vivo*. In the development of drug delivery systems, toxicological studies *in vitro* are useful prior to *in vivo* tests (Nassimi et al. 2009, 2010). To determine whether cell toxicity occurs, in a first step, different *in vitro* viability and cytotoxicity assays can be applied using human epithelial cells (e.g., A549) and murine lung tissue (precision-cut lung slices) as cellular systems. This *ex vivo* lung model can be used to get closer to the *in vivo* situation. Compared to other *in vitro* models, this model allows both biochemical and pathological evaluations of the toxic potentials of exogenous compounds that cannot be done in single cell-type cultures (You et al. 2007a,b, Yuan et al. 2008). If TNF-α level in *ex vivo* experiments are kept unchanged, it can be concluded that SLNs do not induce TNF-α (Nassimi et al. 2009, 2010). Finally, SLNs must be tested *in vivo* to determine their toxicity as a required part of validation and safety to humans.

Conclusions

New drug delivery systems for inhalation application of drugs have been developed on the basis of NPs, with the aim of providing a specific targeting, thereby improving efficacy and minimizing side effects. These systems are believed to be able to deliver the drug specifically to the targeted tissue, release the drug at a controlled rate, and to be biodegradable. Targeting drug delivery into the lungs has become an important aspect of systemic or local drug delivery systems. Drug inhalation enables rapid deposition in the lungs and induces fewer side effects than administration by other routes. Reports in the literature investigating the toxicological potential of NPs are contradictory, and complete/standardized *in vitro*, *ex vivo*, and *in vivo* studies are encouraged to beat the challenge.

Acknowledgements

The authors wish to acknowledge *Fundação para a Ciência e Tecnologia do Ministério da Ciência e Tecnologia* (FCT, Portugal) under the reference ERA – Eula/002/2009.

Abbreviations

BAL	:	bronchoalveolar lavage
COPD	:	chronic obstructive pulmonary disease
DPI	:	dry powder inhaler
IC_{50}	:	half maximum inhibitory concentration
IL	:	interleukin
MDI	:	metered-dose inhaler
MTT	:	3-(4,5-dimethylthiazole-2-yl)-2,5-diphenyltetrazolium bromide
NLC	:	nanostructured lipid carrier
NP	:	nanoparticle
NRU	:	neutral red uptake
SLN	:	solid lipid nanoparticle
TNF-α	:	tumor necrosis factor-alpha

References

Abbasalipourkabir, R. and A. Salehzadeh and R. Abdullah. 2012. Characterization and stability of nanostructured lipid carriers as drug delivery system. Pak. J. Biol. Sci. 15: 141–146.

Abdelbary, G. and R.H. Fahmy. 2009. Diazepam-loaded solid lipid nanoparticles: design and characterization. AAPS Pharm. Sci. Tech. 10: 211–219.

Abdel-Mottaleb, M.M. and D. Neumann and A. Lamprecht. 2011. Lipid nanocapsules for dermal application: a comparative study of lipid-based versus polymer-based nanocarriers. Eur. J. Pharm. Biopharm. 79: 36–42.

Al-Hallak, M.H. and M.K. Sarfraz, S. Azarmi, W.H. Roa, W.H. Finlay and R. Lobenberg. 2011. Pulmonary delivery of inhalable nanoparticles: dry powder inhalers. Ther. Deliv. 2: 1313–1324.

Al-Hallak, M.H. and M.K. Sarfraz, S. Azarmi, W.H. Roa, W.H. Finlay, C. Rouleau and R. Lobenberg. 2012. Distribution of effervescent inhalable nanoparticles after pulmonary delivery: an *in vivo* study. Ther. Deliv. 3: 725–734.

Al-Jamal, W.T. and K.T. Al-Jamal, B. Tian, L. Lacerda, P.H. Bomans, P.M. Frederik and K. Kostarelos. 2008. Lipid-quantum dot bilayer vesicles enhance tumor cell uptake and retention *in vitro* and *in vivo*. ACS Nano. 2: 408–418.

Almeida, A.J. and E. Souto. 2007. Solid lipid nanoparticles as a drug delivery system for peptides and proteins. Adv. Drug Deliv. Rev. 59: 478–490.

Atinkaya, C. and N. Ozlem Kucuk, H. Koparal, G. Aras, S.D. Sak and N. Ozdemir. 2005. Mediastinal intraoperative radioisotope sentinel lymph node mapping in non-small-cell lung cancer. Nucl. Med. Commun. 26: 717–720.

Attama, A.A. and B.C. Schicke, T. Paepenmüller and C.C. Müller-Goymann. 2007. Solid lipid nanodispersions containing mixed lipid core and a polar heterolipid: characterization. Eur. J. Pharm. Biopharm. 67: 48–57.

Azarmi, S. and W.H. Roa and R. Löbenberg. 2008. Targeted delivery of nanoparticles for the treatment of lung diseases. Adv. Drug Deliv. Rev. 60: 863–875.

Barreiro, E. and G.J. Criner. 2014. Update in chronic obstructive pulmonary disease 2013. Am. J. Respir. Crit. Care Med. 189: 1337–1344.

Bérubé, K. and Z. Prytherch, C. Job and T. Hughes. 2010. Human primary bronchial lung cell constructs: the new respiratory models. Toxicology. 278: 311–318.

Brioschi, A. and F. Zenga, G.P. Zara, M.R. Gasco, A. Ducati and A. Mauro. 2007. Solid lipid nanoparticles: could they help to improve the efficacy of pharmacologic treatments for brain tumors? Neurol. Res. 29: 324–330.

Broza, Y.Y. and R. Kremer, U. Tisch, A. Gevorkyan, A. Shiban, L.A. Best and H. Haick. 2013. A nanomaterial-based breath test for short-term follow-up after lung tumor resection. Nanomedicine. 9: 15–21.

Brunell, D. and D. Sagher, S. Kesaraju, N. Brot and H. Weissbach. 2011. Studies on the metabolism and biological activity of the epimers of sulindac. Drug Metab. Dispos. 39: 1014–1021.

Bustos, M.E. and J.J. Camargo, G. Resin Geyer and C. Feijó Andrade. 2008. Intraoperative detection of sentinel lymph nodes using Patent Blue V in non-small cell lung cancer. Minerva Chir. 63: 29–36.

Cerchia, L. and C.L. Esposito, S. Camorani, A. Rienzo, L. Stasio, L. Insabato, A. Affuso and V. de Franciscis. 2012. Targeting Axl with a high-affinity inhibitory aptamer. Mol. Ther. 20: 2291–2303.

Chattopadhyay, P. and B.Y. Shekunov, D. Yim, D. Cipolla, B. Boyd and S. Farr. 2007. Production of solid lipid nanoparticle suspensions using supercritical fluid extraction of emulsions (SFEE) for pulmonary delivery using the AERx system. Adv. Drug Deliv. Rev. 59: 444–453.

Chen, D.B. and T.Z. Yang, W.L. Lu and Q. Zhang. 2001. *In vitro* and *in vivo* study of two types of long-circulating solid lipid nanoparticles containing paclitaxel. Chem. Pharm. Bull. (Tokyo). 49: 1444–1447.

Chen, Z.Z. and L. Cai, X.M. Dong, H.W. Tang and D.W. Pang. 2012. Covalent conjugation of avidin with dye-doped silica nanoparticles and preparation of high density avidin nanoparticles as photostable bioprobes. Biosens. Bioelectron. 37: 75–81.

Choi, S.H. and S.E. Jin, M.K. Lee, S.J. Lim, J.S. Park, B.G. Kim, W.S. Ahn and C.K. Kim. 2008. Novel cationic solid lipid nanoparticles enhanced p53 gene transfer to lung cancer cells. Eur. J. Pharm. Biopharm. 68: 545–554.

Chon, H. and S. Lee, S.W. Son, C.H. Oh and J. Choo. 2009. Highly sensitive immunoassay of lung cancer marker carcinoembryonic antigen using surface-enhanced Raman scattering of hollow gold nanospheres. Anal. Chem. 81: 3029–3034.

Chon, H. and S. Lee, S.Y. Yoon, S.I. Chang, D.W. Lim and J. Choo. 2011. Simultaneous immunoassay for the detection of two lung cancer markers using functionalized SERS nanoprobes. Chem. Commun. (Camb.). 47: 12515–12517.

Cook, R.O. and R.K. Pannu and I.W. Kellaway. 2005. Novel sustained release microspheres for pulmonary drug delivery. J. Control. Release. 104: 79–90.

Cooney, D.J. and A.J. Hickey. 2011. Cellular response to the deposition of diesel exhaust particle aerosols onto human lung cells grown at the air–liquid interface by inertial impaction. Toxicol. *In Vitro*. 25: 1953–1965.

Dailey, L.A. and T. Schmehl, T. Gessler, M. Wittmar, F. Grimminger, W. Seeger and T. Kissel. 2003. Nebulization of biodegradable nanoparticles: impact of nebulizer technology and nanoparticle characteristics on aerosol features. J. Control. Release. 86: 131–144.

Dolovich, M.B. and R. Dhand. 2011. Aerosol drug delivery: developments in device design and clinical use. Lancet. 377: 1032–1045.

Dong, Z. and S. Xie, L. Zhu, Y. Wang, X. Wang and W. Zhou. 2011. Preparation and *in vitro, in vivo* evaluations of norfloxacin-loaded solid lipid nanopartices for oral delivery. Drug Deliv. 18: 441–450.

Edwards, D. and J. Hanes, G. Caponetti, J. Hrkach, A. Ben-Jebria, M. Eskew, J. Mintzes, D. Deaver, N. Lotan and R. Langer. 1997. Large porous particles for pulmonary drug delivery. Science. 276: 1868–1872.

Erdal, E. and D. Kavaz, M. Sam, M. Demirbilek, M.E. Demirbilek, N. Saglam and E.B. Denkbas. 2012. Preparation and characterization of magnetically responsive bacterial polyester based nanospheres for cancer therapy. J. Biomed. Nanotechnol. 8: 800–808.

Ernsting, M.J. and M. Murakami, E. Undzys, A. Aman, B. Press and S.D. Li. 2012. A docetaxel-carboxymethylcellulose nanoparticle outperforms the approved taxane nanoformulation, Abraxane, in mouse tumor models with significant control of metastases. J. Control. Release. 162: 575–581.

Forbes, B. and B. Asgharian, L.A. Dailey, D. Ferguson, P. Gerde, M. Gumbleton, L. Gustavsson, C. Hardy, D. Hassall, R. Jones, R. Lock, J. Maas, T. McGovern, G.R. Pitcairn, G. Somers and R.K. Wolff. 2011. Challenges in inhaled product development and opportunities for open innovation. Adv. Drug Deliv. Rev. 63: 69–87.

Freitas, C. and R.H. Muller. 1999. Correlation between long-term stability of solid lipid nanoparticles (SLN) and crystallinity of the lipid phase. Eur. J. Pharm. Biopharm. 47: 125–132.

Gokce, E.H. and G. Sandri, M.C. Bonferoni, S. Rossi, F. Ferrari, T. Guneri and C. Caramella. 2008. Cyclosporine A loaded SLN: evaluation of cellular uptake and corneal cytotoxicity. Int. J. Pharm. 364: 76–86.

González-Juarrero, M. and M.P. O'Sullivan. 2011. Optimization of inhaled therapies for tuberculosis: the role of macrophages and dendritic cells. Tuberculosis. 91: 86–92.

Han, B. and Q. Xiu, H. Wang, J. Shen, A. Gu, Y. Luo, C. Bai, S. Guo, W. Liu, Z. Zhuang, Y. Zhang, Y. Zhao, L. Jiang, J. Zhou and X. Jin. 2011. A multicenter, randomized, double-blind, placebo-controlled study to evaluate the efficacy of paclitaxel-carboplatin alone or with endostar for advanced non-small cell lung cancer. J. Thorac. Oncol. 6: 1104–1109.

Hanania, N.A. and N. Ambrosino, P. Calverley, M. Cazzola, C.F. Donner and B. Make. 2005. Treatments for COPD. Respir. Med. 99: S28–S40.

Hanania, N.A. and M.J. King, S.S. Braman, C. Saltoun, R.A. Wise, P. Enright, A.R. Falsey, S.K. Mathur, J.W. Ramsdell, L. Rogers, D.A. Stempel, J.J. Lima, J.E. Fish, S.R. Wilson, C. Boyd, K.V. Patel, C.G. Irvin, B.P. Yawn, E.A. Halm, S.I. Wasserman, M.F. Sands, W.B. Ershler, D.K. Ledford and Asthma in Elderly workshop participants. 2011. Asthma in the elderly: current understanding and future research needs—a report of a National Institute on Aging (NIA) workshop. J. Allergy Clin. Immunol. 128: S4–S24.

Hao, J. and X. Fang, Y. Zhou, J. Wang, F. Guo, F. Li and X. Peng. 2011. Development and optimization of solid lipid nanoparticle formulation for ophthalmic delivery of chloramphenicol using a Box-Behnken design. Int. J. Nanomedicine. 6: 683–692.

Hariharan, R. and S. Senthilkumar, A. Suganthi and M. Rajarajan. 2012. Synthesis and characterization of doxorubicin modified ZnO/PEG nanomaterials and its photodynamic action. J. Photochem. Photobiol. B 116: 56–65.

Harush-Frenkel, O. and M. Bivas-Benita, T. Nassar, C. Springer, Y. Sherman, A. Avital, Y. Altschuler, J. Borlak and S. Benita. 2010. A safety and tolerability study of differently-charged nanoparticles for local pulmonary drug delivery. Toxicol. Appl. Pharmacol. 246: 83–90.

Hori, S. and S. Nishiumi, K. Kobayashi, M. Shinohara, Y. Hatakeyama, Y. Kotani, N. Hatano, Y. Maniwa, W. Nishio, T. Bamba, E. Fukusaki, T. Azuma, T. Takenawa, Y. Nishimura and M. Yoshida. 2011. A metabolomic approach to lung cancer. Lung Cancer. 74: 284–292.

Hu, F.Q. and Y. Zhang, Y.Z. Du and H. Yuan. 2008. Nimodipine loaded lipid nanospheres prepared by solvent diffusion method in a drug saturated aqueous system. Int. J. Pharm. 348: 146–152.

Huang, Z.R. and S.C. Hua, Y.L. Yang and J.Y. Fang. 2008. Development and evaluation of lipid nanoparticles for camptothecin delivery: a comparison of solid lipid nanoparticles, nanostructured lipid carriers, and lipid emulsion. Acta Pharmacol. Sin. 29: 1094–1102.

Hunter, R.L. 2011. Pathology of post primary tuberculosis of the lung: an illustrated critical review. Tuberculosis (Edinb.). 91: 497–509.

Hureaux, J. and F. Lagarce, F. Gagnadoux, L. Vecellio, A. Clavreul, E. Roger, M. Kempf, J.L. Racineux, P. Diot, J.P. Benoit and T. Urban. 2009. Lipid nanocapsules: ready-to-use nanovectors for the aerosol delivery of paclitaxel. Eur. J. Pharm. Biopharm. 73: 239–246.

Iqbal, M.A. and S. Md, J.K. Sahni, S. Baboota, S. Dang and J. Ali. 2012. Nanostructured lipid carriers system: recent advances in drug delivery. J. Drug Target. 20: 813–830.

Ito, M. and Y. Minamiya, H. Kawai, S. Saito, H. Saito, T. Nakagawa, K. Imai, M. Hirokawa and J. Ogawa. 2006. Tumor-derived TGFbeta-1 induces dendritic cell apoptosis in the sentinel lymph node. J. Immunol. 176: 5637–5643.

Jaafar-Maalej, C. and V. Andrieu, A. Elaissari and H. Fessi. 2011. Beclomethasone-loaded lipidic nanocarriers for pulmonary drug delivery: preparation, characterization and *in vitro* drug release. J. Nanosci. Nanotechnol. 11: 1841–1851.

Jaspart, S. and P. Bertholet, G. Piel, J.M. Dogne, L. Delattre and B. Evrard. 2007. Solid lipid microparticles as a sustained release system for pulmonary drug delivery. Eur. J. Pharm. Biopharm. 65: 47–56.

Kasongo, K.W. and J. Pardeike, R.H. Muller and R.B. Walker. 2011. Selection and characterization of suitable lipid excipients for use in the manufacture of didanosine-loaded solid lipid nanoparticles and nanostructured lipid carriers. J. Pharm. Sci. 100: 5185–5196.

Katz, D. and R. Albalak, J.S. Wing, V. Combs and Tuberculosis Epidemiologic Studies Consortium. 2007. Setting the agenda: a new model for collaborative tuberculosis epidemiologic research. Tuberculosis (Edinb.). 87: 1–6.

Kawai, H. and Y. Minamiya, M. Ito, H. Saito and J. Ogawa. 2008. VEGF121 promotes lymphangiogenesis in the sentinel lymph nodes of non-small cell lung carcinoma patients. Lung Cancer. 59: 41–47.

Khilnani, G.C. and A. Banga. 2008. Aerosol therapy. Indian J. Chest Dis. Allied Sci. 50: 209–219.

Labiris, N.R. and M.B. Dolovich. 2003. Pulmonary drug delivery. Part II: the role of inhalant delivery devices and drug formulations in therapeutic effectiveness of aerosolized medications. Br. J. Clin. Pharmacol. 56: 600–612.

Li, Y. and X. Sun, T. Gong, J. Liu, J. Zuo and Z. Zhang. 2010. Inhalable microparticles as carriers for pulmonary delivery of thymopentin-loaded solid lipid nanoparticles. Pharm. Res. 27: 1977–1986.

Marchetti, M. and L. Resnick, E. Gamliel, S. Kesaraju, H. Weissbach and D. Binninger. 2009. Sulindac enhances the killing of cancer cells exposed to oxidative stress. PLoS One. 4: e5804.

Mezzena, M. and S. Scalia, P. Young and D. Traini. 2009. Solid lipid budesonide microparticles for controlled release inhalation therapy. AAPS J. 11: 771–778.

Miller, A.A. and A. Al Omari, D.J. Murry and D. Case. 2006. Phase I and pharmacologic study of sequential topotecan-carboplatin-etoposide in patients with extensive stage small cell lung cancer. Lung Cancer. 54: 379–385.

Moschos, C. and I. Psallidas, T. Cottin, A. Kollintza, S. Papiris, C. Roussos, G.T. Stathopoulos, A. Giannis and I. Kalomenidis. 2011. A sulindac analogue is effective against malignant pleural effusion in mice. Lung Cancer. 73: 171–175.

Mukhopadhyay, A. and C. Grabinski, A.R. Afrooz, N.B. Saleh and S. Hussain. 2012. Effect of gold nanosphere surface chemistry on protein adsorption and cell uptake *in vitro*. Appl. Biochem. Biotechnol. 167: 327–337.

Muller, R.H. and R. Shegokar and C.M. Keck. 2011. 20 years of lipid nanoparticles (SLN and NLC): present state of development and industrial applications. Curr. Drug Discov. Technol. 8: 207–227.

Nassimi, M. and C. Schleh, H.D. Lauenstein, R. Hussein, K. Lubbers, G. Pohlmann, S. Switalla, K. Sewald, M. Muller, N. Krug, C.C. Muller-Goymann and A. Braun. 2009. Low cytotoxicity of solid lipid nanoparticles in *in vitro* and *ex vivo* lung models. Inhal. Toxicol. 21: 104–109.

Nassimi, M. and C. Schleh, H.D. Lauenstein, R. Hussein, H.G. Hoymann, W. Koch, G. Pohlmann, N. Krug, K. Sewald, S. Rittinghausen, A. Braun and C. Muller-Goymann. 2010. A toxicological evaluation of inhaled solid lipid nanoparticles used as a potential drug delivery system for the lung. Eur. J. Pharm. Biopharm. 75: 107–116.

Olbrich, C. and U. Bakowsky, C.M. Lehr, R.H. Muller and C. Kneuer. 2001. Cationic solid-lipid nanoparticles can efficiently bind and transfect plasmid DNA. J. Control. Release. 77: 345–55.

Olbrich, C. and A. Gessner, O. Kayser and R.H. Muller. 2002a. Lipid-drug-conjugate (LDC) nanoparticles as novel carrier system for the hydrophilic antitrypanosomal drug diminazenediaceturate. J. Drug Target. 10: 387–396.

Olbrich, C. and R.H. Muller, K. Tabatt, O. Kayser, C. Schulze and R. Schade. 2002b. Stable biocompatible adjuvants—a new type of adjuvant based on solid lipid nanoparticles: a study on cytotoxicity, compatibility and efficacy in chicken. Altern. Lab. Anim. 30: 443–458.

Olbrich, C. and N. Scholer, K. Tabatt, O. Kayser and R.H. Muller. 2004. Cytotoxicity studies of Dynasan 114 solid lipid nanoparticles (SLN) on RAW 264.7 macrophages-impact of phagocytosis on viability and cytokine production. J. Pharm. Pharmacol. 56: 883–891.

Pandey, R. and S. Sharma and G.K. Khuller. 2005. Oral solid lipid nanoparticle-based antitubercular chemotherapy. Tuberculosis (Edinb.). 85: 415–420.

Pardeike, J. and A. Hommoss and R.H. Muller. 2009. Lipid nanoparticles (SLN, NLC) in cosmetic and pharmaceutical dermal products. Int. J. Pharm. 366: 170–184.

Pardeike, J. and S. Weber, T. Haber, J. Wagner, H.P. Zarfl, H. Plank and A. Zimmer. 2011. Development of an itraconazole-loaded nanostructured lipid carrier (NLC) formulation for pulmonary application. Int. J. Pharm. 419: 329–338.

Park, S.K. and L.Y. Cho, J.J. Yang, B. Park, S.H. Chang, K.S. Lee, H. Kim, K.Y. Yoo and C.T. Lee. 2010. Lung cancer risk and cigarette smoking, lung tuberculosis according to histologic type and gender in a population based case–control study. Lung Cancer. 68: 20–26.

Patlolla, R.R. and V. Vobalaboina. 2008. Folate-targeted etoposide-encapsulated lipid nanospheres. J. Drug Target. 16: 269–275.

Patlolla, R.R. and M. Chougule, A.R. Patel, T. Jackson, P.N. Tata and M. Singh. 2010. Formulation, characterization and pulmonary deposition of nebulized celecoxib encapsulated nanostructured lipid carriers. J. Control. Release. 144: 233–241.

Pilcer, G. and K. Amighi. 2010. Formulation strategy and use of excipients in pulmonary drug delivery. Int. J. Pharm. 392: 1–19.

Qi, J. and Y. Lu and W. Wu. 2012. Absorption, disposition and pharmacokinetics of solid lipid nanoparticles. Curr. Drug Metab. 13: 418–428.

Ridge, C.A. and A.M. McErlean and M.S. Ginsberg. 2013. Epidemiology of lung cancer. Semin. Intervent. Radiol. 30: 93–98.

Rubin, B.K. 2006. Other medications for aerosol delivery. Paediatr. Respir. Rev. 7: S76–S79.

Sager, T.M. and V. Castranova. 2009. Surface area of particle administered versus mass in determining the pulmonary toxicity of ultrafine and fine carbon black: comparison to ultrafine titanium dioxide. Part. Fibre Toxicol. 6: 15.

Sakagami, M. and K. Sakon, W. Kinoshita and Y. Makino. 2001. Enhanced pulmonary absorption following aerosol administration of mucoadhesive powder microspheres. J. Control. Release. 77: 117–129.

Sawant, K.K. and S.S. Dodiya. 2008. Recent advances and patents on solid lipid nanoparticles. Recent Pat. Drug Deliv. Formul. 2: 120–135.

Schleh, C. and C. Mühlfeld, K. Pulskamp, A. Schmiedl, M. Nassimi, H.D. Lauenstein, A. Braun, N. Krug, V.J. Erpenbeck and J.M. Hohlfeld. 2009. The effect of titanium dioxide nanoparticles on pulmonary surfactant function and ultrastructure. Respir. Res. 10: 90.

Siekmeier, R. and G. Scheuch. 2008. Systemic treatment by inhalation of macromolecules—principles, problems, and examples. J. Physiol. Pharmacol. 59: 53–79.

Siroux, V. and A. Boudier, J. Bousquet, J.L. Bresson, J.L. Cracowski, J. Ferran, F. Gormand, J. Just, N. Le Moual, S. Morange, R. Nadif, M.P. Oryszczyn, C. Pison, P. Scheinmann, R. Varraso, D. Vervloet, I. Pin, F. Kauffmann and Epidemiological Study on the Genetics and Environment of Asthma. 2009. Phenotypic determinants of uncontrolled asthma. J. Allergy Clin. Immunol. 124: 681–687.e3.

Smola, M. and T. Vandamme and A. Sokolowski. 2008. Nanocarriers as pulmonary drug delivery systems to treat and to diagnose respiratory and non respiratory diseases. Int. J. Nanomedicine. 3: 1–19.

Souto, E.B. and R.H. Müller. 2010. Lipid nanoparticles: effect on bioavailability and pharmacokinetic changes. Handb. Exp. Pharmacol. (197): 115–141.

Tabatt, K. and M. Sameti, C. Olbrich, R.H. Muller and C.M. Lehr. 2004. Effect of cationic lipid and matrix lipid composition on solid lipid nanoparticle-mediated gene transfer. Eur. J. Pharm. Biopharm. 57: 155–162.

Thakkar, H. and R. Kumar Sharma and R.S. Murthy. 2007. Enhanced retention of celecoxib-loaded solid lipid nanoparticles after intra-articular administration. Drugs R. D. 8: 275–285.

Wan, F. and E.H. Møller, M. Yang and L. Jørgensen. 2012. Formulation technologies to overcome unfavorable properties of peptides and proteins for pulmonary delivery. Drug Discov. Today Technol. 9: e141–e146.

Wenzel, S.E. and W.W. Busse and National Heart, Lung, and Blood Institute's Severe Asthma Research Program. 2007. Severe asthma: lessons from the Severe Asthma Research Program. J. Allergy Clin. Immunol. 119: 14–21.

Weyenberg, W. and P. Filev, D. Van Den Plas, J. Vandervoort, K. De Smet, P. Sollie and A. Ludwig. 2007. Cytotoxicity of submicron emulsions and solid lipid nanoparticles for dermal application. Int. J. Pharm. 337: 291–298.

Yamaguchi, T. 1996. Lipid microspheres as drug carriers: a pharmaceutical point of view. Adv. Drug Deliv. Rev. 20: 117–130.

Yang, M. and H. Yamamoto, H. Kurashima, H. Takeuchi, T. Yokoyama, H. Tsujimoto and Y. Kawashima. 2012. Design and evaluation of poly(DL-lactic-co-glycolic acid) nanocomposite particles containing salmon calcitonin for inhalation. Eur. J. Pharm. Sci. 46: 374–380.

You, J. and F.Q. Hu, Y.Z. Du and H. Yuan. 2007a. Polymeric micelles with glycolipid-like structure and multiple hydrophobic domains for mediating molecular target delivery of paclitaxel. Biomacromolecules. 8: 2450–2456.

You, J. and F.Q. Hu, Y.Z. Du, H. Yuan and B.F. Ye. 2007b. High cytotoxicity and resistant-cell reversal of novel paclitaxel loaded micelles by enhancing the molecular-target delivery of the drug. Nanotechnology. 18: 495101.

Yuan, H. and J. Miao, Y.Z. Du, J. You, F.Q. Hu and S. Zeng. 2008. Cellular uptake of solid lipid nanoparticles and cytotoxicity of encapsulated paclitaxel in A549 cancer cells. Int. J. Pharm. 348: 137–145.

Zeng, X.M. and G.P. Martin and C. Marriott. 1995. The controlled delivery of drugs to the lung. Int. J. Pharm. 124: 149–164.

Zhu, R. and K.W. Cheng, G. Mackenzie, L. Huang, Y. Sun, G. Xie, K. Vrankova, P.P. Constantinides and B. Rigas. 2012. Phospho-sulindac (OXT-328) inhibits the growth of human lung cancer xenografts in mice: enhanced efficacy and mitochondria targeting by its formulation in solid lipid nanoparticles. Pharm. Res. 29: 3090–3101.

CHAPTER 7

Nanotechnology for Ocular and Otic Drug Delivery and Targeting

Anthony A. Attama,* Charles Lovelyn[a] and Ebele B. Onuigbo[b]

ABSTRACT

Nanoparticulate carriers have been widely exploited in the field of drug delivery science as they provide a more selective targeting along with sustained release of molecules at the desired site. The use of nanocarriers in drug delivery is expected to increase the specificity of drugs and thus reduce the side effects by decreasing the drug dose. Application of nanotechnology can be very appealing in the treatment of diseases affecting the eye and the inner ear. Poor bioavailability of drugs from ocular dosage form is mainly due to pre-corneal loss factors which include tear dynamics, non-productive absorption, transient residence time in the cul-de-sac, and relative impermeability of the corneal epithelial membrane. Development of better alternatives to conventional ocular drug formulations that would facilitate the sustained delivery of drug molecules is a major challenge. In this line, the development of pharmaceutical nanoformulations is expected to: enhance drug permeation, control drug release, and/or target the drug to the site of action. As more candidates for the treatment of inner ear disorders are being discovered, it is necessary to develop appropriate strategies for non-invasive administration. Nanotechnology-based delivery systems for otic drugs could provide a platform to address the inherent limitations of conventional ear drops. This chapter focuses on nanoparticulate platforms for ocular and otic drug delivery and targeting, and their current developments and applications in overcoming various static and dynamic barriers associated with these organs.

Drug Delivery Research Unit, Department of Pharmaceutics, Faculty of Pharmaceutical Sciences, University of Nigeria, Nsukka 410001, Enugu State, Nigeria.

[a] Email: charles.lovelyn @unn.edu.ng
[b] Email: ebele.onuigbo@unn.edu.ng
* Corresponding author: anthony.attama@unn.edu.ng; aaattama@yahoo.com

Introduction

The complex nature of the eye makes ocular drug delivery a challenge. Conventional systems like eye drops, suspensions, and ointments are not optimal in the treatment of vision threatening ocular diseases. More than 90% of marketed ophthalmic formulations are in the form of eye drops, which mainly target anterior segment eye diseases. Topical drug delivery is often impaired by innate protective characteristics of the eye against entry of foreign compounds. Due to the removal mechanism (blinking and tears) and complex composition and dynamic character of the lachrymal fluid (Attama et al. 2008), the bioavailability of an instilled formulation is generally low with only a small fraction reaching the target site (< 5%). The major challenge in ocular drug delivery is to get adequate amount of the drug to the target site and maintain contact with the ocular tissue of interest.

Otic drug delivery systems (DDSs) are meant to deliver drugs to the inner ear. Access to the inner ear is limited by the presence of a blood-cochlear barrier (BCB), which is anatomically and functionally similar to the blood-brain barrier. Due to tight junctions between cells, substances in systemic circulation encounter substantial physical barriers to entry, preventing many molecules with potential therapeutic effect from gaining access to their inner ear targets. Additionally, the cochlea is a closed space, and cochlear function is sensitive to small changes in fluid volume. Therefore, delicate approaches are required to avoid possible damage from the delivery method itself (Leary-Swan et al. 2008). Current applications for inner ear drug delivery are grouped into three main categories: otoprotection, sudden sensorineural hearing loss (SSNHL), and acute inflammatory ear diseases. Drugs are used to minimize or reverse hearing loss due to sudden events of unknown nature and to immune reactions within the cochlea. Inner ear drug delivery methods can be divided into two main categories based on the location of entry of the drug. Intratympanic delivery involves depositing the therapeutic agent in the middle ear, relying primarily on diffusion through the round window membrane (RWM) for access to the scala tympani. The second method, intracochlear, depends on a cochleostomy with direct delivery into the inner ear space, completely bypassing the middle ear (Leary-Swan et al. 2008).

Nanoparticles (NPs) are particles with size less than 1 μm. The properties of materials change when prepared as NPs. This is typically because NPs have a greater surface area per weight/volume than larger particles, and this has a lot of implication on drug delivery as the specific surface area of NPs affects the payload capacity and other biophysical properties such as interaction with membranes.

Many novel DDSs have been used to treat eye conditions such as implants, hydrogels, and microspheres. Nano-sized DDSs for ocular and otic infections have recently received some attention. Use of NPs to treat ocular and otic diseases has many potential advantages: decrease peak concentration resulting in decrease in the toxicity, localization of drug delivery, stabilization of the drug, and increased half-life of encapsulated drugs. Particulate systems of adequate size have the advantage of intraocular or otic delivery and targeting by injection. NPs can diffuse rapidly and can be internalized in ocular and otic tissues and cells. A major problem in ocular and otic therapeutics with classical formulations is the maintenance of an effective drug concentration at the site of action for a long period of time. Enhancement of ocular and otic bioavailability with increased dose penetration and longer retention time at desired sites could be achieved with NP formulations.

The most prominent advantage of nano-sized drug carriers over conventional DDSs is the selective delivery of drugs to the site of action, i.e., drug targeting, which can be classified into active and passive targeting. Passive targeting is achieved without a specific targeting moiety incorporated on the particle surface. It occurs through different administration routes, after intravenous application or towards an epithelium (Ulbrich and Lamprecht 2010). Active targeting after systemic administration is achieved by modification of the particles' surface with targeting ligands. Antibodies or other specific adhesion molecules are bound to the surface of particles and antigens or other specific adhesion molecule counterparts on the surface of cells can be recognized (Simone et al. 2009). The drug formulation should specifically be delivered to the site of action followed by potential intracellular uptake.

Using nanotechnology to improve ocular and otic therapeutics could be helpful in the following ways:

- Improving patient compliance compared with injections. Injections are highly invasive but these novel technologies are non-invasive and when properly functionalized they are capable of transporting poorly permeable small molecule drugs and macromolecules (such as proteins and peptides) to the posterior segment of the eye.
- There could be increased drug retention and sustained release. The bioadhesive action of the NPs causes them to be retained on topical delivery with sustained effect and reduction in dosing frequency.
- Functionalized NPs possess the ability to increase permeability and tissue partitioning thus improving drug transport compared with non-functionalized NPs (Kompella et al. 2006). Surface functionalization enhances permeability and specific tissue levels of therapeutics (Attama et al. 2009).
- It is possible to target NPs to a specific area to increase drug localization in the target tissues or reduce drug delivery to non-target tissues associated with drug side effects. This can potentially increase the therapeutic index. For instance, using intravenous administration of NPs functionalized with arginine-glycine-aspartic acid peptide or transferrin, it was demonstrated that the back of the eye delivery of anti-vascular endothelial growth factor (anti-VEGF) intraceptor plasmid-loaded NPs can be enhanced in a choroidal neovascularization (CNV) model (Singh et al. 2009).

- Nanosystems can be used to target subcellular organelles in addition to cell surface receptors. This is relevant for poorly permeable molecules such as proteins, peptides, and nucleic acids. Gene delivery by NPs requires entry of the active agent or the delivery systems carrying the active agent into the nucleus. Intracellular trafficking depends on the constitution of the nanosystem, size of the particle, and other surface effects. Protection of the nanocarrier is necessary as destruction within the cytosol or lysosomes could occur.

Anatomy of the Eye

From anatomical and physiological point of view, the eye (Fig. 7.1) is a unique organ. It contains several highly different structures with specific physiological functions. The eye is divided into anterior and posterior segments, which function both independently and in tandem on application of ocular preparation.

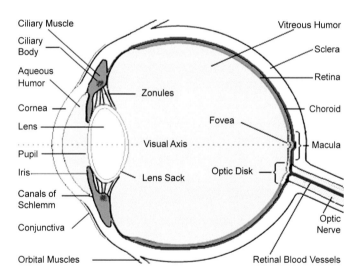

Figure 7.1. Anatomy of the eye (cross section) (http://www.99main.com/~charlief/Blindness. htm#ir. Accessed 29 April 2013).

The eye has three main chambers (anterior, posterior, and vitreous). The anterior chamber is bound in front by the cornea and a small portion of the sclera and posteriorly by the external surface of the iris, a variable area of anterior surface of the lens and a part of the ciliary body. The posterior chamber is limited by the iris and the lens. Both fluid-filled chambers are separated from each other by the iris. The vitreous chamber is filled with the amorphous and some gelatinous material of the vitreous body. The conjunctiva, a thin mucous membrane lining inside of the eyelids and the visible anterior sclera, is a significant barrier against topically applied eye drops. The presence of tight barriers regulating the environment of ocular tissues in the anterior and posterior parts of the eye is essential for normal visual function. The development of strategies to overcome these barriers for the targeted ocular delivery of drugs remains a major challenge (Hornof et al. 2005).

Drug Delivery Barriers of the Eye

Surface removal

Lachrymal secretions wash away topically applied drugs continuously and the excess of the lachrymal fluids flow down the nasolachrymal duct rapidly. Due to the presence of an extensive network of capillaries in the conjunctival sac and the nasal cavity, most of the drugs applied topically are absorbed into the systemic circulation, thereby reducing the ocular bioavailability from 5–10% (Urtti and Salminen 1993). There are two main pathways of drug entry into the anterior segment of the eye: the corneal and the non-corneal (conjunctival-scleral) pathways. There is greater absorption of hydrophilic drugs via the conjunctival route as the conjunctiva is endowed with leakier and more numerous tight junctions than the cornea. Systemic absorption of drugs from ocular surface can cause adverse side effects, especially if the patient has various medication needs. For instance, timolol and other intra-ocular pressure reducing agents can cause cardiac and vascular complications in susceptible patients. Other pre-corneal factors limiting ocular drug absorption are drainage of the instilled solution, tear production (induced lachrymation), drug metabolism, and normal tear turn-over.

Epithelial barrier

The corneal route is the main route through which topically administered drugs reach the aqueous humor (AH). The cornea is a multilayered tissue consisting of the corneal epithelium, basement membrane, Bowman's layer, etc. (Fig. 7.2). The epithelial layer is lipophilic and consists of tight junctions that limit the entry of hydrophilic drugs and macromolecules (Mainardes et al. 2005). This barrier can be breached by an epithelial defect or by subconjunctival injection. In some eye conditions such as glaucoma and conjunctivitis, corneal absorption increases significantly due to morphological changes. This, along with the use of permeation enhancers and mucoadhesives, can be explored to achieve better corneal drug penetration.

Beneath the epithelium is a hydrophilic layer called the stroma constituting a large portion of the corneal endothelium. The epithelium is the main barrier for hydrophilic drugs while the stroma and endothelium limit the entry of lipophilic drugs. The passive permeability of a drug across the cornea is influenced by various factors, such as the lipophilic character, charge, degree of ionization of the drug, and molecular weight. Increasing the molecular

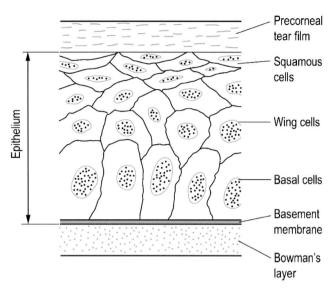

Figure 7.2. Layers of the cornea (http://medical-dictionary.thefreedictionary.com/_/viewer. aspx?path=ElMill&name=F0C-20-S2958.jpg. Accessed 29 April 2013).

size of the permeating drug decreases the rate of paracellular permeation (Hämäläinen et al. 1997). The corneal epithelium pores are negatively charged at physiological pH and negatively charged molecules permeate slower than positively charged and neutral molecules.

Blood-ocular barriers

The establishment and maintenance of therapeutic drug concentrations in the retina and the vitreous humor (VH) usually require either systemic or intravitreal drug administration. Systemic application by oral or intravenous administration has the disadvantage that high doses of the drug are administered, since only a very small fraction of the drug reaches ocular tissues due to the limited blood flow and the blood-ocular barriers (BOBs). The remainder of the drug is distributed in the entire body leading to unwanted side effects. BOBs can be overcome by the intravitreal injection of drugs but this route of administration is associated with several problems, including risk of endophthalmitis, damage to lens or retinal detachment, and low patient compliance (Urtti and Salminen 1993). There are two BOBs: blood-aqueous barrier (BAB) and blood-retinal barrier (BRB), which provide a controlled environment for the internal tissues.

Blood-aqueous barrier

The BAB is located in the anterior part of the eye. It is formed by endothelial cells of the blood vessels in the iris and the non-pigmented cell layer of the ciliary epithelium. Tight junctional complexes are present in both cell layers. These cell layers prevent non-specific passage of solutes into the intraocular milieu that might otherwise negatively influence transparency and chemical equilibrium of the ocular fluids (Cunha-Vaz 1997). It limits the entry of hydrophilic drugs from the systemic circulation into the AH. This barrier gets disrupted sometimes due to inflammation and results in enhanced temporary drug permeation (Urtti and Salminen 1993). Small and lipophilic drugs can enter the uveal blood circulation via the BAB and they are consequently eliminated more rapidly from the anterior chamber than larger and more hydrophilic drugs, which are eliminated by AH turn-over only.

Blood-retinal barrier

The BRB limits the entry of drugs from the systemic circulation to the retina. It is formed by the endothelial cells of retinal blood vessels (inner BRB) and the retinal pigment epithelial cells (outer BRB) (Hornof et al. 2005). The BRB, along with the BAB, protects the eyes from entry of xenobiotics and harmful substances. This physiological defense mechanism limits systemic drug delivery to the retina and VH via the choroid through the systemic circulation.

Ocular Drug Delivery

Current ocular therapeutic options are limited due to the low systemic access owing to the BRB, BAB, and blood-vitreous barrier. Oral therapy for ocular diseases requires high doses of active agent to reach therapeutic concentrations at the site of action, which may cause severe side effects. The most common and well-accepted route is the topical administration generally employed to treat superficial diseases such as infections (e.g., conjunctivitis, blepharitis, keratitis), and to provide intraocular treatment through the cornea for diseases such as glaucoma or uveitis (Başaran and Yazan 2012). For ocular DDSs to be successful, they should: have a small particle size (< 10 µm) with a narrow size range, be non-irritant, be compatible with the ocular tissue, be adequately bioavailable, and cause no blurred vision (Sahoo et al. 2008), while facilitating its delivery to the ocular epithelia or its transport through biological barriers.

Classical attempts for improving the ocular bioavailability of drugs mostly include the use of viscosity enhancers (e.g., cellulose derivatives), mucoadhesive polymers (e.g., polysaccharides), and *in situ* gel-forming systems. However, these strategies are saddled with frequent instillations, which can lead to lack of compliance, toxic side effects, and cellular damage at the ocular surface. Current approaches are to increase the corneal permeability using biocompatible penetration enhancers, which would preferably act reversibly, to prolong the contact time with the ocular surface or to target the ocular tissues. These approaches can be fulfilled by the use of NPs because of their size-dependent bioadhesive properties.

Routes of delivery to the eye

There are several possible routes of drug delivery into the ocular tissues (Fig. 7.3). The route of administration depends on the target tissue. Conventionally, many ocular diseases are treated with either topical or systemic medications. Systemic administration could be oral or by parenteral (injection), with parenteral having many variants. These methods have disadvantages and limitations; hence there is a need to develop novel drug carriers which are safe, convenient, and efficient in crossing potential ocular barriers.

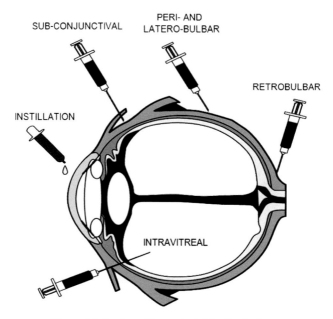

Figure 7.3. Routes of drug administration to the eye.

Topical administration

Topical administration, mostly in the form of eye drops, is employed to treat disorders affecting the anterior segment of the eye. For most of the topically applied drugs, the site of action is usually different layers of the cornea, conjunctiva, sclera, and the other tissues of the anterior segment such as the iris and the ciliary body (anterior uvea). Upon administration, precorneal factors and anatomical barriers negatively affect the bioavailability of topical formulations which are absorbed either by the corneal route (cornea → AH → intraocular tissues) or by the non-corneal route (conjunctiva → sclera → choroid/retinal pigment epithelium). Precorneal loss factors include nasolacrymal drainage, blinking, tear turn-over, induced lacrimation, and drug binding to tear proteins. Human tear volume is estimated to be 7 µL, and the cul-de-sac can transiently contain ≈ 30 μL of the administered eye drop. However, tear film displays a rapid restoration time of 2 to 3 minutes, and most of the topically administered solutions are washed away within just 15 to 30 seconds after instillation. Taking into account all the precorneal loss factors, contact time with the absorptive membranes is lower, which is considered to be the primary reason for < 5% of the applied dose reaching the intraocular tissues. The dose is mostly absorbed to the blood circulation via the conjunctival and nasal blood vessels. For example, at least 70% of timolol dose is systemically absorbed within 5 minutes (del Amo and Urtti 2008).

Systemic administration

Following systemic administration, the BAB and BRB are the major barriers for anterior segment and posterior segment, respectively. BAB prevents the entry of solutes into the intraocular environment (Barar et al. 2008) such as the AH. BRB, which is selectively permeable to more lipophilic molecules, limits the entry of drugs into the posterior segment of the eye. This results in frequent administration of high amounts of drugs leading to systemic side effects.

Although topical and systemic (oral) routes are convenient, lack of adequate bioavailability and failure to deliver therapeutic amounts of drugs to the retina, has led to the search for alternative routes of administration. Periocular route has been considered as the most promising and efficient route for administering drugs to posterior eye segment. It is a broad term, which includes peribulbar, posterior juxtascleral, retrobulbar, subtenon, and subconjunctival routes (Fig. 7.3). Formulations administered by periocular injections can reach the posterior segment by three different pathways: transscleral pathway, systemic circulation through the choroid, and the anterior pathway through the tear film, cornea, AH, and the VH (Ghate and Edelhauser 2006).

Intravitreal injections (Fig. 7.3) have gained considerable momentum during the past two decades. This method involves injection of a drug solution directly into the VH using a 30 G needle. Unlike other routes, an intravitreal injection offers higher drug concentrations in VH and retina as it bypasses the BOB and reduces systemic side effects. However, drug distribution in VH is non-uniform. Small molecules can rapidly distribute through the vitreous, whereas the diffusion of larger molecules is restricted. It is associated with various short-term complications such as retinal detachment, endophthalmitis, intravitreal hemorrhages, and cataract. Repeated injections are frequently required and patients need to be carefully monitored.

The need for drug targeting in ocular disease conditions

Most of the topically applied drugs, in addition to ineffective absorption, are removed by the rapid drainage and tear wash-out within a short time after application (≈ 15 to 30 seconds). This is an innate mechanism of the eye to clear debris and pathogens efficiently so that it can remain clear. The cornea must remain moist or transparency is lost. Nanotechnology-based DDSs are set to address these issues through enhancing penetration, and controlling release and targeting.

Nanotechnology and Ocular Drug Delivery

Many ocular nanoparticulate systems based on self-assembly systems, lipids, or polymers, like polymeric NPs, liposomes, and micelles, are currently under different stages of investigation.

Applications of nanotechnology can be very exciting in the treatment of a range of diseases affecting the anterior and posterior segments of the eye. Delivery of a drug via nanotechnology-based products fulfills mainly three objectives: (i) enhances drug permeation; (ii) controls the drug release; and, (iii) targets the drug to the site of action (Sahoo et al. 2008). Nanomedicines offer promise as viable alternatives to conventional drops, gels, or ointments to improve ocular drug delivery. Because of their small size, they are bioadhesive and are well tolerated, thus preventing washout and increasing bioavailability (Müller-Goymann 2004). The small nature of NPs delivered to the ocular surface may reduce the risk of blurring.

Physicochemical properties such as particle size, surface net charge, shape, solubility, degree of ionization, and lipophilic character influence drug ocular absorption and determine the route of administration (Mainardes et al. 2005). These factors can be tailored using novel nanoparticulate DDSs that enhance the ocular bioavailability of drugs. Nano-sized drug carriers should be biodegradable, transparent, and comfortable. Various biodegradable artificial polymers and natural polymers (e.g., chitosan, albumin) show promise. Solid lipid nanoparticles (SLNs), polymer NPs, niosomes, dendrimers, nanosuspensions, liposomes, and nanoemulsions have been studied for ocular drug delivery. These systems alleviate problems associated with poorly soluble drugs, increase drug bioavailability while decreasing the administered dose and toxicity, overcome BOB and efflux-related issues associated with the parent drug, and provide controlled release of the drug at the target site.

Liposomes

Liposomes (Figs. 7.4 and 7.5) are vesicles consisting of one or more layers of amphiphilic phospholipids, which spontaneously arrange in aqueous solution as bilayers to form closed vesicles. When a single bilayer encloses an aqueous compartment, it is called an unilamellar lipid vesicle, whereas multilamellar vesicles have more than one bilayer present.

There are many methods for the preparation of tailor-made liposomes. Hydrophilic and lipophilic drugs can be encapsulated in the lipid walls or

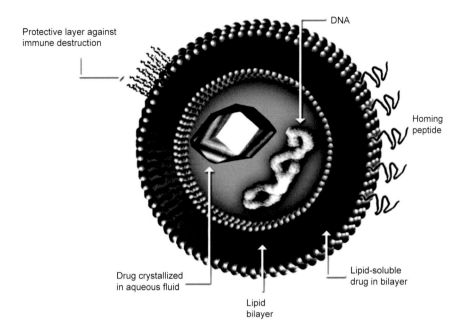

Figure 7.4. General structure of a liposome (http://upload.wikimedia.org/wikipedia/en/2/28/Liposome.jpg. Accessed 29 April 2013).

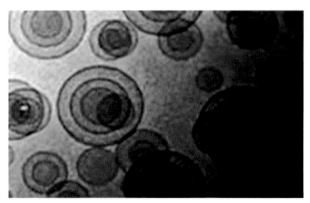

Figure 7.5. Transmission electron microphotograph of liposomes (http://www.phospholipid.jp/?gclid=CO-c34Hv2q8CFQrwzAodxiuLAg. Accessed 29 April 2013).

the aqueous interior of the liposomes, respectively. The liposomes are taken up by phagocytic cells, like the retinal pigment epithelium cells thus enabling intracellular drug delivery. Liposome technology has been used to develop light-induced systems for the treatment of retinal diseases (e.g., Visudyne®, Novartis Pharmaceuticals, USA) (Ruiz-Moreno and Montero 2006). The surface charge may be positive, negative, or neutral depending on the liposome composition. Investigations have shown that drug absorption can be enhanced when encapsulated in liposomes following topical instillation.

Almost every class of topically or subconjunctivally applied ophthalmic drugs have been studied in liposomal form, including antibiotics, antifungals, and steroids (Ghate and Edelhauser 2006) with promising penetration and pharmacokinetics. Topical dexamethasone poorly penetrates the intact ocular surface, however, dexamethasone-loaded liposomes have been formulated and the concentration in the anterior segment of the eye, evaluated. High levels of the drug were found in the conjunctiva, suggesting that liposomes enhance ocular penetration.

Nanoparticles

NPs are defined as particles with a diameter of < 1 μm, comprising of various biodegradable or non-biodegradable polymers, lipids, phospholipids, or metals (Sahoo et al. 2008). They may be a matrix system in which the drug is dissolved, entrapped, encapsulated, and/or to which the drug is adsorbed or attached. It is important that the particle size for ophthalmic application is kept within the nano-sized range to avoid irritation, foreign body sensation, and blurring of vision.

NP formulations of several ophthalmic drugs have been studied, and have demonstrated increased corneal permeability. The proposed mechanism is an enhanced retention time in the cul-de-sac, due to bioadhesion or other properties. SLNs loaded with tobramycin were developed for topical drug delivery. This particulate system was retained for longer duration on the corneal surface and also on the conjunctival sac compared with an aqueous solution of the drug. *In vivo* testing showed sustained drug release over a period of 6 hours compared with the short duration from equal dose of eye drops (Ripal et al. 2009). Among the commonly used biodegradable polymers for ocular NP formulation, which undergo hydrolysis in tears (Gupta et al. 2011), poly(D,L-lactide-*co*-glycolide) (PLGA) is the most suitable candidate because of ease of formulation and its approval for use in drug delivery applications by the Food and Drug Administration. Bourges et al. (2003) showed that NPs are retained within the retinal pigment epithelium cells even four months after a single intravitreal injection. Thus, intravitreal injection may provide steady and continuous delivery of drugs or oligonucleotides. Albumin-based NPs are interesting delivery systems for intravitreal drug administration. *In vivo* studies in rat demonstrated their localization in the vitreous cavity and ciliary body for at least two weeks after a single intravitreal injection (Irache et al. 2005). Some NP preparations evaluated for ocular application have been published as a review (Prow 2010), and several *in vitro* studies have been conducted using bioengineered human cornea (Attama et al. 2008, 2009).

The formation of a coating layer around particles is a novel approach to prolong their corneal residence time. Mucoadhesive polymers that interact with the mucus layer have been developed. Examples of mucoadhesive polymers used in ophthalmic drug delivery include macromolecular hydrocolloids with numerous hydrophilic functional groups, such as polyacrylic acid, carboxymethylcellulose, and hyaluronic acid, which attach to the precorneal mucin layer by means of non-covalent bonds. In the absence of bioadhesion, NP elimination from the precorneal site occurs as rapidly as an aqueous solution.

Hyaluronic acid is a high-molecular-mass biopolymer composed of linear polysaccharides present in the vitreous body of the eye and in low concentrations in the AH. It is a potent mucoadhesive polymer, probably given its topical pseudoplastic properties, which result in improved protection of the cornea (Du Toit et al. 2011). Chitosan is a biodegradable and mucoadhesive polymer that possesses penetration-enhancing properties and low toxicity, making it a unique material for the design of systems for ocular delivery. Chitosan NPs in particular showed great promise because of the mucoadhesive properties of chitosan. Yuan et al. (2006) reported the utility of amphiphilic chitosan self-aggregated NPs as hydrophobic drug carriers for ocular application with increased retention ability at the precorneal area. De Campos et al. (2001) investigated the potential use of chitosan and chitosan-coated NPs for the specific delivery of drugs to the ocular mucosa. They considered the advantages of intimate contact with the corneal and conjunctival surfaces, increasing drug delivery to only external ocular tissues and maintaining long-term drug levels. The systems showed great promise with at least 24 hours corneal and conjunctival residence time. Mucoadhesive chitosan-sodium alginate NPs were investigated as a new vehicle for prolonged ophthalmic delivery of the antibiotic gatifloxacin with promising results (Motwani et al. 2008).

Hydrophobic nanosystems consisting of poly(alkylcyanoacrylates) and polyesters, particularly poly(ε-caprolactone) as well as PLGA, have high affinity for the corneal epithelium owing to an appropriate surface charge. However, they have the tendency of aggregating when in contact with the mucosal surface. To avoid this, hydrophilic materials such as poly(ethylene glycol) and chitosan are used because of their protein-rejecting properties (shielding effect), and mucoadhesive and penetration-enhancing properties and good biocompatibility with ocular structures, respectively (Calvo et al. 1996). Drugs like chloramphenicol, flubiprofen, and diclofenac have been delivered to ocular tissues with the help of PLGA NPs (Gupta et al. 2011).

SLNs containing ion pairs of pilocarpine and an aqueous solution of pilocarpine ion pairs were examined. *In vivo* study using the two different formulations, administered topically to male New Zealand albino rabbits in comparison with reference solutions, showed that the area under the miotic effect vs. time curves increased ≈ 2.5 times for aqueous solution of pilocarpine ion pairs and ≈ 2.8 times for the SLN dispersion (Cavalli et al. 1995). Both formulations were biocompatible, and no irritation of the ocular tissues was observed. SLN-based ocular DDSs for tobramycin were prepared, evaluated, and administered topically to rabbits. The SLN dispersion contained 2.5% of tobramycin as ion pair. Preocular retention of SLNs in rabbit eyes examined using drug-free fluorescent SLNs demonstrated longer retention times on the corneal surface and in the conjunctival sac than a fluorescent aqueous solution (Cavalli et al. 2002). A dispersion of tobramycin (0.3%, w/v)-loaded SLNs was also administered topically to rabbits, and the AH concentration of tobramycin was monitored for up to 6 hours. Compared with an equal dose of tobramycin administered in the form of commercial eye drops, the SLNs produced a significantly higher tobramycin bioavailability in the AH.

Nanostructured lipid carriers were also found to be good vectors for drug delivery to the ocular mucosa (Shen et al. 2010). It combines many features, which include, prolonged release of actives, drug targeting, and an increasing amount of drug penetrating into mucosa, with studies indicating increased ocular bioavailability of lipophilic drugs without inducing discomfort or irritation (Li et al. 2008).

Nanosuspensions

These are sub-micron systems consisting of poorly water-soluble drugs, suspended in a dispersion medium stabilized by surfactants. They help in the enhancement of drug solubility and bioavailability. Drug nanosuspensions have low viscosity that enhances their administration as eye drops, with intimate interaction with the ocular surface and a greater penetration into the deeper layers of the ocular tissues. The possibility of prolonging the release of a drug makes these vehicles very attractive systems for ocular delivery, as they can greatly decrease the frequency of drug administration. Nanosuspensions have been shown to impart stability to the drug in the formulation as exemplified by a cloricromene nanosuspension using Eudragit® RS 100 and RL, wherein the shelf life and bioavailability were enhanced. Nanosuspensions enhanced the ocular absorption of the glucocorticoid and increased the bioavailability of piroxicam in Eudragit® RS 100 (Pignatello et al. 2006).

Dendrimers

Dendrimers are macromolecular compounds made up of a series of branches around a central core. Their nanometer size, ease of preparation, functionalization, and possibility to attach multiple surface groups render them suitable alternative vehicles for ophthalmic drug delivery (Sahoo et al. 2008). Dendrimers, characterized by orderly and symmetrical structures, possess physical properties that are dictated by the functional groups on the molecular surface, which can be synthesized with anionic carboxyl, cationic amine, or non-ionic hydroxyl groups. Their applicability to ocular drug delivery is because of their hydrophobic character and bioadhesive properties. However, in addition to understanding their ocular retention and drug release characteristics, the ocular toxicity of dendrimers needs to be investigated thoroughly. Dendrimeric polyguanidilyated translocators are nano-sized structures that are used to efficiently translocate molecules across barriers such as cell membranes. This generated a four-fold increase in solubility and delivery of gatifloxacin to the posterior segment of rabbit eyes and produced a significant increase in tissue concentrations in the conjunctiva and cornea.

Niosomes

Niosomes are non-ionic surfactant vesicles. Like liposomes, niosomes are vesicular structures that can entrap both hydrophilic and lipophilic drugs. Niosomal formulation of coated (chitosan or Carbopol®) timolol maleate exhibited significant intraocular pressure lowering effect in rabbits as compared to timolol solutions. Cyclopentolate-loaded niosomal formulation was developed, which released the drug independent of the pH value, resulting in significant enhancement of the ocular bioavailability (Ripal et al. 2009).

Nanoemulsions

Nanoemulsions are submicrometric emulsions, adequate for the encapsulation and delivery of both hydrophilic and hydrophobic drugs. The major disadvantage of nanoemulsions is the limited stability and lack of adhesivity. Despite this, some formulations containing the polypeptide cyclosporine A are under clinical evaluation, for example a cationic nanoemulsion for the treatment of the mild dry-eye syndrome (Cationorm®, Novagali Pharma, France), or even on the market, as Restasis® (Allergan, CA, USA), approved for the treatment of kerato-conjunctivitis sicca.

Anatomy of the Ear

The inner ear is a very delicate structure (Fig. 7.6). The outer ear transmits sound to the tympanic membrane. The pinna, made of cartilage covered by skin, collects sound and channels it into the ear canal. The ear canal is ≈ 4 cm long and consists of an outer and inner part. The outer portion is lined with hairy skin containing sweat glands and oily sebaceous glands, which together form ear wax. The ear canal has a slight bend where the outer cartilaginous part joins the bony thin skinned inner portion, so that the outer part runs somewhat backwards and the inner part somewhat forward. This bend also restricts foreign objects from reaching the tympanic membrane.

The tympanic membrane shaped like a loudspeaker cone separates the ear canal from the middle ear. The whole membrane is < 0.1 mm thick. It covers a round opening ≈ 1 cm in diameter into the middle ear cavity. The middle ear is an air filled space connected to the back of the nose by a long, thin tube called the Eustachian tube. The middle ear space houses three little bones [the hammer, the anvil, and the stirrup (malleus, incus, and stapes)], which conduct sound from the tympanic membrane to the inner ear (cochlear). The middle ear is an extension of the respiratory air spaces of the nose and the

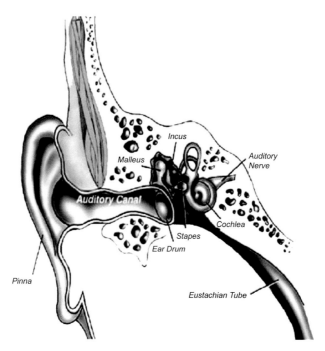

Figure 7.6. Anatomy of the ear (cross section) (http://www.nidcd.nih.gov/health/hearing/pages/innear.aspx. Accessed 29 April 2013).

sinuses and is lined with respiratory membrane, thick near the Eustachian tube and thin as it passes into the mastoid. It has the ability to secrete mucus. The Eustachian tube is bony as it leaves the ear but as it nears the back end of the nose, in the nasopharynx, consists of cartilage and muscle. Contracture of muscle actively opens the tube and allows the air pressure in the middle ear and the nose to equalize.

Drug Delivery to the Inner Ear

The inner ear represents a geometrically complex structure, with characteristic large fluid-filled extracellular spaces (scalae), each with multiple interfaces with other scalae and with outside compartments, such as the systemic blood circulation and the middle ear cavity. Scala tympani and scala vestibuli contain perilymph, a fluid similar in ionic composition to other extracellular fluids, whereas the endolymphatic space contains fluid with a unique, high potassium composition (Salt and Plontke 2005). In contrast to most other body fluids, the inner-ear fluids do not move or flow appreciably and are not actively "stirred". As a result, the spread of locally applied drugs through the ear occurs only slowly and predominantly by passive diffusion. The diffusion coefficient depends on the physical characteristics of the diffusing particles/molecules, with their molecular weight playing a major role (Salt and Plontke 2005).

The principal challenge in the treatment of inner ear diseases remains the inaccessibility of targets for therapy, due largely to the presence of the BCB. Oral medications are typically blocked by the BCB and, therefore, clinicians have resorted to delivering drugs intratympanically for a range of auditory and vestibular conditions (McCall et al. 2010). Intratympanic delivery of compounds for the treatment of inner ear diseases relies on diffusion through the RWM, a structure with widely distinct transport properties depending on the patient and disease state. This variability results in poor dosage control, and coupled with the reliance on passive diffusion mechanisms to transport drugs along the length of the cochlea, has limited the effectiveness of intratympanic drug delivery. Hence, recent efforts have shifted toward intracochlear drug delivery approaches, as a means to directly and controllably deliver medications to specific targets in the inner ear (Borkholder 2008).

Routes of drug delivery to the inner ear

Systemic delivery

Systemic therapy consists of dosing medication via the oral, intravenous, or intramuscular route with the intention of altering inner ear function. Two examples of systemic medications delivered for the control of inner ear disease include systemic antibiotics (e.g., streptomycin for vertigo control) and systemic steroids for SSNHL. Variable penetration of drugs into the inner ear due to the presence of a BCB and the potential for undesirable systemic side effects are the major drawbacks to systemic drug delivery to the ear. Recent technological advancements in emerging fields such as microfluidics and microsystems technologies permit the development of DDSs designed to release drugs directly to the inner ear over a sustained period of time (Pararas et al. 2012).

Unfortunately, there are concerns regarding the clinical efficacy of many systemic medications currently in use for the treatment of inner ear disorders. The primary concern has been the potential side effects associated with the delivery via the systemic route. These side effects can be sometimes life threatening. For instance, use of steroids for systemic therapy of otic conditions has been associated with many side effects including hyperglycemia, hypertension, hypokalemia, peptic ulcer disease, osteoporosis, immunosuppression, and if given over a sustained period of time, adrenal suppression. Other medications given systemically for inner ear disease similarly have side effects associated with their use. These side effects can lead to lack of compliance by patients or serious organ damage.

Other concerns regarding systemic delivery may fall outside the side effects of the drugs. Each medication is subject to a range of pharmacokinetic factors that influence the concentration of that particular drug in the inner ear.

These factors include differing total body volumes of distribution, variability among different medications in their ability to cross the blood-labyrinth barrier, different drug metabolic pathways, and different routes of excretion (Paulson et al. 2008). Even for a single agent, variability in concentration in the inner ear is exacerbated by systemic variability, potentially leading to variable clinical outcomes.

Intratympanic delivery

Intratympanic drug delivery for inner ear therapy avoids some of the problems associated with systemic delivery and has now become a routine strategy for treating inner ear disease. The development of adjunctive devices and carrier mechanisms are active areas of research focused on improving drug delivery via the intratympanic route. Potential drawbacks of intratympanic drug delivery include anatomic barriers to absorption at the RWM, variable or unknown pharmacokinetic profiles of medications currently delivered via this route, and loss of drug down the Eustachian tube. Current strategies in various stages of development and use include transtympanic injection, the Silverstein Microwick® (Silverstein et al. 2004), microcatheter implantation, hydrogels, and NPs.

Transtympanic injection or myringotomy

The simplest form of intratympanic medication delivery is via injection into the middle ear either directly with a needle or through myringotomy with or without a tympanostomy tube. This form of delivery is quick, can be performed in the clinic setting, and is currently in widespread use. Transtympanic injection does require the need for repeat procedures should dosing of medication be necessary beyond a one-time application. Placement of a tympanostomy tube has the risk of persistent perforation of the tympanic membrane upon extrusion of the tube, otorrhea associated with the presence of the tube, and the need to keep the ear dry to avoid a middle ear infection (Licameli et al. 2008). Several types of inner ear-specific DDSs have been developed, most of which use the round window as a route to deliver the agent into the inner ear, because the round window is a unique structure in that the inner ear is not covered with bone but sealed with a RWM (Sakamoto et al. 2010).

Intracochlear delivery

The cochlea resides along with the vestibular organ in the inner ear. It is the small size and remote location of the cochlea that renders direct drug delivery to the organ so difficult. The cochlea, roughly 32 mm in length in humans, comprises three coiled fluid-filled tubes, the scala tympani, the scala vestibule, and the scala media. Methods for intracochlear delivery include use of osmotic pumps, direct injection, micro-injector, infusion with canalostomy, reciprocating system, and cochlear implant-mediated delivery (Borenstein 2011). Some inner ear diseases potentially amenable to intracochlear drug delivery include autoimmune inner ear disease, SSNHL, Meniere's disease, tinnitus, etc.

Nanoparticulate drug delivery systems to the inner ear

NP-based delivery to the inner ear has emerged as a new promising platform for delivering drugs to the cochlea in a sustained and controllable manner. The NPs may be comprised of biodegradable or non-degradable materials, depending upon the application and the desired pharmacokinetic profile.

NPs are particles typically in the size range of 200 nm or less when used for drug delivery to the inner ear. NPs generated from biodegradable/bioresorbable PLGA have the potential to deliver the encapsulated medication in a sustained release fashion. PLGA NPs have been shown to be present within the cochlea either when delivered systemically or when applied topically to the RWM, with an increase in intracochlear concentration when applied locally (Tamura et al. 2005). PLGA NPs applied to the RWM distributed to the following structures: the RWM, perilymph, basilar membrane, stria vascularis, and within the organ of Corti (Ge et al. 2007).

For instance, Zou et al. (1993) investigated lipid nanocapsules as a potential inner ear therapeutic delivery system. When applied to the RWM, the nanocapsules were taken up by spiral ganglion, inner hair cells, pillar cells, outer hair cells, spiral ligament, and stria vascularis. Liposomes represent another NP-based mode for delivery to the inner ear, and these vehicles have been explored as a means for gene therapy. It is a viable approach for intratympanic delivery (Leary-Swan et al. 2008). The liposomes can either be injected or delivered using an osmotic pump. NP-based DDSs such as dendrimers, nanosuspensions, niosomes, and nanoemulsions are also very relevant in otic drug delivery, although the volume of research using these vectors is very low. The approach is to select the appropriate otic active drug and formulate using any of these nanotechnologies. These nano-sized DDSs are capable of entering cells/crossing membranes and barriers by different mechanisms and thereby are appropriate for accessing portions of the inner ear not easily reached by conventional formulations. They are also capable of prolonging the release of the encapsulated drug.

Drug Targeting of Ocular and Otic Tissues

Nano-sized materials containing drugs and diagnostics are being developed to image the distribution of tumor cells in the body, target and attach to cancer cells, destroy unwanted cells via ablation, or interference with cellular functions. Drug targeting might overcome the problem of repeated administration by facilitating the efficacy of the drug administered systemically and attenuating side effects on healthy tissues. Ultimately, NPs represent versatile DDSs, with the ability to overcome physiological barriers and guide the drug to specific cells or intracellular compartments by means of passive targeting or ligand-mediated targeting mechanisms (Sahoo et al. 2008).

At present, there is paucity of research results dealing with targeting of ocular or otic drugs to certain cellular targets in the organs. However, with the knowledge of the pathophysiological/passive targeting approaches used in cancer chemotherapy, it is possible to develop nanocarriers for targeting drug to appropriate cells in the ocular and otic domains. Small molecules administered systemically are easily eliminated through the kidney into the urine and distributed equally not only in the target tissue but also in other healthy tissues, resulting in less efficacy and more possible side effects (Yasukawa et al. 2011). On the other hand, large molecules have longer plasma half-life and tend to be passively delivered to the lesions with highly permeable vessels in neovascularization and inflammation. This tendency is remarkable especially in solid tumors because of high density of neovascular vessels and immature lymph systems, and is termed the Enhanced Permeability and Retention (EPR) effect.

Passive targeting of drugs to the eye

Passive targeting is achieved by modifying the pharmacokinetics of the drug through conjugation to large molecules on the basis of the EPR effect. CNV has an environment similar to that of solid tumors in regard to no lymph systems under the retina and development of highly permeable vessels. Yasukawa et al. (1999) demonstrated that polyvinyl alcohol binding TNP-470, an anti-angiogenic agent, accumulated around the CNV in a rabbit model for a prolonged period after intravenous administration. This conjugate inhibited CNV while free TNP-470 exhibited no inhibitory effect. Also, Yasukawa et al. (2002) demonstrated the possibility of targeted delivery of cytokines by use of metal coordination. Diethylenetriamine-pentaacetic acid, a chelating residue used in metal chelating affinity chromatography, was introduced to dextran, and the resulting complex was able to bind proteins (interferon β) through metal coordination in the presence of zinc or copper ion just by simple mixing. This conjugate of interferon β accumulated around and inhibited the CNV in the rabbit. Ideta et al. (2004) reported that micelles and NPs were successfully targeted to experimental CNV in rats.

Active targeting of drugs to the eye

Active targeting property of formulations can be achieved by addition of specific molecules such as antibodies and magnetic particles. Uveitis is the inflammation of the tissues forming the uveal tract, namely iris, ciliary body, choroids, and contiguous structures. If local application is desired, it is inevitable to use bioadhesive materials for effective retention in the ocular cul-de-sac. However, it is possible to target uveal tissues actively. The effect and localization of poly(D,L-lactide) NPs encapsulating betamethasone phosphate after a single intravenous injection to rats with experimental autoimmune uveoretinitis (EAU) was evaluated by Sakai et al. (2006). Confocal images showed that no NPs were in the normal retina of healthy rats whereas several NPs in the retina and a few NPs in the outer nuclear layer could be observed 3 hours after the injection in EAU rats. These NPs remained in the retina of rats with EAU even seven days post-administration. The prolonged and rapid anti-inflammatory effects achieved were equal to those of a five-times greater dose of free betamethasone phosphate.

Novel sialyl-Lewix-X-conjugated liposomes were loaded with dexamethasone and were injected to EAU mice. Mice which were treated with the liposomes showed double the concentration of dexamethasone in the eyes than those injected with the free drug solution (Hashida et al. 2008). To confirm whether the liposomes target E-selectin, P-selectin, or both, a binding inhibition assay was done which clearly demonstrated that liposomes were able to target *in vivo* both selectin types on the activated vascular endothelial cells.

In the treatment of CNV, proteins expressed preferentially on proliferating endothelial cells can be a potential candidate of antigens for antibody-mediated active targeting, involving integrin $\alpha_v \beta_3$, VEGF receptor, endoglin (CD105), intercellular adhesion molecule (ICAM)-1, and E-selectin, to cite just a few (Yasukawa et al. 2011). Immunoconjugates of these antibodies and small anti-angiogenic agents may be effectively targeted to the CNV lesion on the basis of high affinity to neovascular vessels. It was demonstrated that the immunoconjugate of mitomycin C-binding dextran with molecular weight of 70,000 Da and antibody against CD105, a component of transforming growth factor β receptor, or integrin $\alpha_v \beta_3$, which both are preferentially expressed on proliferating vascular endothelial cells, exhibited inhibitory effect on angiogenesis *in vitro* and *in vivo* (Yasukawa et al. 2002). These immunoconjugates would be effective only when they bind to specific antigens expressed on proliferating endothelial cells, accumulate on angiogenesis, and slowly release the conjugated drug, which could stagnate around new vessels on the basis of the EPR effect.

Targeting of agents to the inner ear

Although, drug targeting to the inner ear has not been extensively studied as ocular targeting, some studies have shown that it is possible to even target genetic materials into the inner ear. The introduction of foreign genes into cells has become an effective means of achieving intracellular expression of foreign proteins, both for therapeutic purposes and for experimental manipulation. Gene therapy, besides being a useful research tool, has significant promise as a potential clinical treatment in otology. The human inner ear is accessible through either the RWM or the stapes footplate. It is possible to choose a variety of vectors to target a variety of tissues. Several animal studies have demonstrated that expression of exogenous genes in the cochlea does not result in loss of hearing function. Protective strategies such as prevention of neuronal degeneration and protection of auditory hair cells from oxidative stress are potential examples where gene therapy may be useful (Staecker et al. 2004). Some therapeutic compounds in development towards a range of diseases of the inner ear, including disease target, state of development, and current status have been reported (Borenstein 2011).

Preliminary data demonstrated the functional capacity of targeting as adenoviral-induced expression of neurotrophic and growth factors protected hair cells and spiral ganglion neurons from ototoxic insults. Subsequent efforts confirmed the feasibility of adenoviral transfection of cells in the auditory neuroepithelium via cochleostomy into the scala media (Hussemann and Raphael 2009). Herpes simplex type-1 and vaccinia virus vectors were both found to infect and elicit transgene expression successfully in many cells in the guinea pig cochlea, including cells in the organ of Corti (Derby et al. 1999). These data demonstrate the feasibility of gene delivery to the inner ear and might be used to develop gene therapy strategies for some forms of hearing loss.

The utility of nerve growth factor-derived peptide-functionalized NPs to target cells of the inner ear has been reported (Roy et al. 2010). These NPs when introduced to organotypic explant cultures of the mouse inner ear and to PC-12 rat pheochromocytoma cells did not show any signs of toxicity, but achieved specific targeting and higher binding affinity to spiral ganglion neurons, Schwann cells, and nerve fibers of the explant cultures through ligand mediated multivalent binding to tyrosine kinase receptors and to p75 neurotrophin receptors. Unspecific uptake of NPs was investigated and results indicated selective cochlear cell targeting by the NPs, which may be a potential tool for cell specific drug and gene delivery to the inner ear.

Conclusions

A major drawback associated with systemic administration of ocular and otic drugs is that only a minor fraction of the administered drug reaches the target. Though topical and systemic routes are convenient, lack of adequate bioavailability and failure to deliver therapeutic amounts of drugs has led to the search for novel nano-sized DDSs. The most relevant and appealing characteristic of NPs is their intrinsic capacity to adhere to the biological surface and interact with the epithelium and traffic cells, in addition to targeting amenability. The performance of a nanocarrier as ocular or otic delivery vehicle and its tolerability can be greatly affected by the material used for their preparation. Therefore, a rational selection of the biomaterials used for the preparation of NPs must be made. Biodegradability would also be a basic requirement to avoid accumulation of these nanocarriers in the ocular or otic tissues. Ocular and otic drug delivery can be revolutionized by the use nano-sized systems which are endowed with many advantages over conventional DDSs. As a result of the variable pharmacokinetic profiles and systemic side effects, investigators have sought alternative means of delivering medications to the posterior eye segment or inner ear. Nanotechnology-based DDSs have shown promise to address such variability due to their targeting capabilities.

Acknowledgement

The authors are very grateful to Prof. E.C. Ibezim of the Department of Pharmaceutics (University of Nigeria) for proof reading this manuscript.

Abbreviations

AH	:	aqueous humor
BAB	:	blood-aqueous barrier
BCB	:	blood-cochlear barrier
BOB	:	blood-ocular barrier
BRB	:	blood-retinal barrier
CNV	:	choroidal neovascularization
DDS	:	drug delivery system
DNA	:	deoxyribonucleic acid
EAU	:	experimental autoimmune uveoretinitis
EPR	:	enhanced permeability and retention
NP	:	nanoparticle
PLGA	:	poly(D,L-lactide-*co*-glycolide)
RWM	:	round window membrane
SLN	:	solid lipid nanoparticle
SSNHL	:	sudden sensorineural hearing loss
VEGF	:	vascular endothelial growth factor
VH	:	vitreous humor

References

Attama, A.A. and S. Reichl and C.C. Müller-Goymann. 2008. Diclofenac sodium delivery to the eye: *in vitro* evaluation of novel solid lipid nanoparticle formulation using human cornea construct. Int. J. Pharm. 355: 307–313.

Attama, A.A. and S. Reichl and C.C. Müller-Goymann. 2009. Sustained release and permeation of timolol from surface modified solid lipid nanoparticles through bio-engineered human cornea. Curr. Eye Res. 34: 698–705.

Barar, J. and A.R. Javadzadeh and Y. Omidi. 2008. Ocular novel drug delivery: impacts of membranes and barriers. Expert Opin. Drug Deliv. 5: 567–581.

Başaran, E. and Y. Yazan. 2012. Ocular application of chitosan. Expert Opin. Drug Deliv. 9: 701–712.

Borenstein, J.T. 2011. Intracochlear drug delivery systems. Expert Opin. Drug Deliv. 8: 1161–1174.

Borkholder, D.A. 2008. State-of-the-art mechanisms of intracochlear drug delivery. Curr. Opin. Otolaryngol. Head Neck Surg. 16: 472–477.

Bourges, J.L. and S.E. Gautier, F. Delie, R.A. Bejjani, J.C. Jeanny, R. Gurny, D. BenEzra and F.F. Behar-Cohen. 2003. Ocular drug delivery targeting the retina and retinal pigment epithelium using polylactide nanoparticles. Invest. Ophthalmol. Vis. Sci. 44: 3562–3569.

Calvo, P. and A. Sanchez and J. Martinez. 1996. Polyester nanocapsules as new topical ocular delivery systems for cyclosporin A. Pharm. Res. 13: 311–315.

Cavalli, R. and S. Morel, M.R. Gasco, P. Chetoni and M.F. Saettone. 1995. Preparation and evaluation *in vitro* of colloidal lipospheres containing pilocarpine as ion-pair. Int. J. Pharm. 117: 243–246.

Cavalli, R. and M.R. Gasco, P. Chetoni, S. Burgalassi and M.F. Saettone. 2002. Solid lipid nanoparticles (SLN) as ocular delivery system for tobramycin. Int. J. Pharm. 238: 241–245.

Cunha-Vaz, J.G. 1997. The blood-ocular barriers: past, present and future. Doc. Ophthalmol. 93: 149–157.

De Campos, A.M. and A. Sanchez and M.J. Alonso. 2001. Chitosan nanoparticles: a new vehicle for the improvement of the delivery of drugs to the ocular surface. Application to cyclosporin A. Int. J. Pharm. 224: 159–168.

Del Amo, E.M. and A. Urtti. 2008. Current and future ophthalmic drug delivery systems. A shift to the posterior segment. Drug Discov. Today. 13: 135–143.

Derby, M.L. and M. Sena-Esteves, X.O. Breakefield and D.P. Corey. 1999. Gene transfer into the mammalian inner ear using HSV-1 and vaccinia virus vectors. Hear. Res. 134: 1–8.

Du Toit, L.C. and V. Pillay, Y.E. Choonara, T. Govender and T. Carmichael. 2011. Ocular drug delivery-a look towards nanobioadhesives. Expert Opin. Drug Deliv. 8: 71–94.

Ge, X. and R.L. Jackson and J. Liu. 2007. Distribution of PLGA nanoparticles in chinchilla cochleae. Otolaryngol. Head Neck Surg. 137: 619–623.

Ghate, D. and H.F. Edelhauser. 2006. Ocular drug delivery. Expert Opin. Drug Deliv. 3: 275–287.

Gupta, H. and M. Aqill, R.K. Khar1, A. Ali, A. Bhatnagar and G. Mittal. 2011. Biodegradable levofloxacin nanoparticles for sustained ocular drug delivery. J. Drug Target. 19: 409–417.

Hämäläinen, K.M. and K. Kananen, S. Auriola, K. Kontturi and A. Urtti. 1997. Characterization of paracellular and aqueous penetration routes in cornea, conjunctiva, and sclera. Invest. Ophthalmol. Vis. Sci. 38: 627–634.

Hashida, N. and N. Ohguro, N. Yamazaki, Y. Arakawa, E. Oiki, H. Mashimo, N. Kurokawa and Y. Tano. 2008. High efficacy site-directed drug delivery system using sialyl-Lewis X conjugated liposome. Exp. Eye Res. 86: 138–149.

Hornof, M. and E. Toropainen and A. Urtti. 2005. Cell culture models of the ocular barriers. Eur. J. Pharm. Biopharm. 60: 207–225.

Husseman, J. and Y. Raphael. 2009. Gene therapy in the inner ear using adenovirus vectors. Adv. Otorhinolaryngol. 66: 37–51.

Ideta, R. and Y. Yanagi, Y. Tamaki, F. Tasaka, A. Harada and K. Kataoka. 2004. Effective accumulation of polyion complex micelle to experimental choroidal neovascularization in rats. FEBS Lett. 557: 21–25.

Irache, J.M. and M. Merodio and M.S. Espuelas Millán. 2005. Albumin nanoparticles for the intravitreal delivery of anticytomegaloviral drugs. Mini Rev. Med. Chem. 5: 293–305.

Kompella, U.B. and S. Sundaram, S. Raghava and E.R. Escobar. 2006. Luteinizing hormone-releasing hormone agonist and transferrin functionalizations enhance nanoparticle delivery in a novel bovine *ex vivo* eye model. Mol. Vision. 12: 1185–1198.

Leary-Swan, E.E. and M.J. Mescher, W.F. Sewell, S.L. Tao and J.T. Borenstein. 2008. Inner ear drug delivery for auditory applications. Adv. Drug Deliv. Rev. 60: 1583–1599.

Li, X. and S.F. Nie, J. Kong, N. Li, C.Y. Ju and W.S. Pan. 2008. A controlled-release ocular delivery system for ibuprofen based on nanostructured lipid carriers. Int. J. Pharm. 363: 177–182.

Licameli, G. and P. Johnston, J. Luz, J. Daley and M. Kenna. 2008. Phosphorylcholine-coated antibiotic tympanostomy tubes: are post tube placement complications reduced? Int. J. Pediatr. Otorhinolaryngol. 72: 1323–1328.

Mainardes, R.M. and M.C.C. Urban, P.O. Cinto, N.M. Khalil, M.V. Chaud, R.C. Evangelista and M.P. Daflon Gremiao. 2005. Colloidal carriers for ophthalmic drug delivery. Curr. Drug Target. 6: 363–371.

Marmor, M.F. and A. Negi and D.M. Maurice. 1985. Kinetics of macromolecules injected into the subretinal space. Exp. Eye Res. 40: 687–696.

McCall, A.A. and E.E. Swan and J.T. Borenstein. 2010. Drug delivery for treatment of inner ear disease: current state of knowledge. Ear Hear. 31: 156–165.

Meisner, D. and M. Mezei. 1995. Liposome ocular delivery systems. Adv. Drug Deliv. Rev. 16: 75–93.

Motwani, S.K. and S. Chopra, S. Talegaonkar, K. Kohli, F.J. Ahmad and R.K. Khar. 2008. Chitosan-sodium alginate nanoparticles as submicroscopic reservoirs for ocular delivery: formulation, optimisation and *in vitro* characterisation. Eur. J. Pharm. Biopharm. 68: 513–525.

Müller-Goymann, C.C. 2004. Physicochemical characterization of colloidal drug delivery systems such as reverse micelles, vesicles, liquid crystals and nanoparticles for topical administration. Eur. J. Pharm. Biopharm. 58: 343–356.

Pararas, E.E. and D.A. Borkholder and J.T. Borenstein. 2012. Microsystems technologies for drug delivery to the inner ear. Adv. Drug Deliv. Rev. 64: 1650–1660.

Paulson, D.P. and W. Abuzeid, H. Jiang, T. Oe, B.W. O'Malley and D. Li. 2008. A novel controlled local drug delivery system for inner ear disease. Laryngoscope. 118: 706–711.

Pignatello, R. and N. Ricupero, C. Bucolo, F. Maugeri, A. Maltese and G. Puglisi. 2006. Preparation and characterization of Eudragit retard nanosuspensions for the ocular delivery of cloricromene. AAPS Pharm. Sci. Tech. 7: E1–E7.

Prow, T.W. 2010. Toxicity of nanomaterials to the eye. Wiley Interdiscip Rev. Nanomed. Nanobiotechnol. 2: 317–333.

Ripal, G. and J. Jwala, S.H.S. Boddu and A.K. Mitra. 2009. Recent perspectives in ocular drug delivery. Pharm. Res. 26: 1191–1216.

Roy, S. and A.H. Johnston, T.A. Newman, R. Glueckert, J. Dudas, M. Bitsche, E. Corbacella, G. Rieger, A. Martini and A. Schrott-Fischer. 2010. Cell-specific targeting in the mouse inner ear using nanoparticles conjugated with a neurotrophin-derived peptide ligand: potential tool for drug delivery. Int. J. Pharm. 390: 214–224.

Ruiz-Moreno, J.M. and J.A. Montero. 2006. Photodynamic therapy in macular diseases. Expert Rev. Ophthalmol. 1: 97–112.

Sahoo, S.K. and F. Dilnawaz and S. Krishnakumar. 2008. Nanotechnology in ocular drug delivery. Drug Discov. Today. 13: 144–151.

Sakai, T. and H. Kohno, T. Ishihara, M. Higaki, S. Saito, M. Matsushima, Y. Mizushima and K. Kitahara. 2006. Treatment of experimental autoimmune uveoretinitis with poly(lactic acid) nanoparticles encapsulating betamethasone phosphate. Exp. Eye Res. 82: 657–663.

Sakamoto, T. and T. Nakagawa, R.T. Hoire, H. Hiraumi, N. Yamamoto, Y. Kikkawa and J. Ito. 2010. Inner ear drug delivery system from the clinical point of view. Acta Otolaryngol. 130: 101–104.

Salt, A.N. and S.K.R. Plontke. 2005. Local inner-ear drug delivery and pharmacokinetics. Drug Discov. Today. 10: 1299–1306.

Shen, J. and Y. Deng, X. Jin, Q. Ping, Z. Su and L. Li. 2010. Thiolated nanostructured lipid carriers as a potential ocular drug delivery system for cyclosporine A: improving *in vivo* ocular distribution. Int. J. Pharm. 402: 248–253.

Silverstein, H. and J. Thompson, S.I. Rosenberg, N. Brown and J. Light. 2004. Otolaryngol. Clin. North Am. 37: 1019–1034.

Simone, E. and B.S. Ding and V. Muzykantov. 2009. Targeted delivery of therapeutics to endothelium. Cell Tissue Res. 335: 283–300.

Singh, S.R. and H.E. Grossniklaus, S.J. Kang, H.F. Edelhauser, B.K. Ambati and U.B. Kompella. 2009. Intravenous transferrin, RGD peptide and dual-targeted nanoparticles enhance anti-VEGF intraceptor gene delivery to laser-induced CNV. Gene Ther. 16: 645–659.

Staecker, H. and D.E. Brough, M. Praetorius and K. Baker. 2004. Drug delivery to the inner ear using gene therapy. Otolaryngol. Clin. North Am. 37: 1091–1108.

Tamura, T. and T. Kita and T. Nakagawa. 2005. Drug delivery to the cochlea using PLGA nanoparticles. Laryngoscope. 115: 2000–2005.

Ulbrich, W. and A. Lamprecht. 2010. Targeted drug-delivery approaches by nanoparticulate carriers in the therapy of inflammatory diseases. J. R. Soc. Interface. 7: S55–S66.

Urtti, A. and L. Salminen. 1993. Minimizing systemic absorption of topically administered ophthalmic drugs. Surv. Ophthalmol. 37: 435–456.

Yasukawa, T. and H. Kimura, Y. Tabata, H. Kamizuru, H. Miyamoto, Y. Honda and Y. Ogura. 1999. Targeted delivery of anti-angiogenic agent TNP-470 using water-soluble polymer in the treatment of choroidal neovascularization. Invest. Ophthalmol. Vis. Sci. 40: 2690–2696.

Yasukawa, T. and H. Kimura, Y. Tabata, H. Kamizuru, H. Miyamoto, Y. Honda and Y. Ogura. 2002. Targeting of interferon to choroidal neovascularization by use of dextran and metal coordination. Invest. Ophthalmol. Vis. Sci. 43: 842–848.

Yasukawa, T. and Y. Tabata, H. Kimura and Y. Ogura. 2011. Recent advances in intraocular drug delivery systems. Recent Pat. Drug Deliv. Formul. 5: 1–10.

Yuan, X. and H. Li and Y. Yuan. 2006. Preparation of cholesterol-modified chitosan self-aggregated nanoparticles for delivery of drugs to ocular surface. Carbohydr. Polym. 65: 337–345.

Zou, N. and D. Liggitt, Y. Liu and R. Debs. 1993. Systemic gene expression after intravenous DNA delivery into adult mice. Science 261: 209–211.

CHAPTER 8

Nanotechnology for Vaginal Drug Delivery and Targeting

Mazen M. El-Hammadi[1,2,a] and *José L. Arias*[1,3,4,]*

ABSTRACT

Nanotechnology-based engineering approaches in drug carrier development are facilitating the formulation of efficient, safe, and stable vaginal drug dosage forms. Major considerations on the anatomy and physiology of the vagina, and barriers to vaginal drug delivery are compiled in this chapter. The possibilities given by nanocarriers in the vaginal delivery of drug molecules, nucleic materials, and peptides/proteins, are analyzed. In addition, the most significant aspects to be taken into account when formulating vaginal nanomedicines are discussed, giving special attention to the unique features exhibited by the vagina to be considered during their development and preclinical evaluation. Finally, an updated analysis of the recent advancements in these (nano)technologies and their potential progress into the clinic is also compiled.

Introduction

Nanoplatforms are revolutionizing biomedicine by their application as drug carriers. In fact, numerous investigations describing the variety of therapeutic applications from the use of nano-sized systems as efficient means

[1] Department of Pharmacy and Pharmaceutical Technology, Faculty of Pharmacy, University of Granada, Campus Universitario de Cartuja s/n, 18071 Granada, Spain.
[a] Email: mazenhammadi@yahoo.co.uk
[2] Department of Pharmaceutics and Pharmaceutical Technology, Faculty of Pharmacy, Damascus University, Damascus, Syria.
[3] Institute of Biopathology and Regenerative Medicine (IBIMER), University of Granada, 18100 Granada, Spain.
[4] Biosanitary Institute of Granada (ibs.GRANADA), Andalusian Health Service (SAS) – University of Granada, 18012 Granada, Spain.
* Corresponding author: jlarias@ugr.es

for delivering both small molecules and macromolecules, such as peptides, proteins, and deoxyribonucleic acid (DNA)/ribonucleic acid (RNA), to the site of interest. In fact, nanoplatforms as advanced drug delivery carriers offer distinctive features including high stability, capability to protect their payload, feasibility of incorporating of both polar and apolar active agents, improved pharmacokinetics and increased biodistribution of encapsulated drugs, low toxicity when biocompatible and biodegradable materials are used, and the advantage of use by different routes of administration. Furthermore, the versatility of nanosystems enables easy tuning of their physical chemistry for enhanced drug delivery ability. Such modifications can involve: (i) controlling particle size to enhance permeability and localization at the site of action; (ii) altering the surface charge to optimize solubility, *in vivo* fate (interaction with the reticuloendothelial system), or electrostatic conjugation with ionic drugs; and, (iii) surface functionalization to increase biological circulation time and achieve active/specific drug targeting.

Over the last decade, the level of interest in developing nanocarriers for vaginal drug delivery has grown noticeably. This chapter is dedicated to provide a detailed description of current advancements in nanoparticulate-based drug delivery systems, giving special attention to both polymer-based nanoparticles (NPs) and liposomes, for vaginal drug delivery. Anatomy and physiology of the vagina, advantages of vaginal route of drug administration, and barriers to vaginal drug delivery are also discussed.

Vaginal Drug Delivery

Vaginal drug delivery refers to the delivery of drugs within the vaginal cavity or across the vaginal mucosa to produce local or systemic pharmacological effects. Classically, the vaginal route of drug administration has been used for female-related conditions mainly involving contraception and therapy of local infections. Diverse active agents have been used for local delivery via the vaginal route, e.g., antiprotozoals, antivirals, antibacterials, antifungals, spermicidal agents, and sexual hormones (Acartürk 2009). Although it has been demonstrated that the intravaginal administration of drugs can lead to systemic absorption (Gupta et al. 2011), the potential of the vaginal route for systemic delivery has not been under focus until recently, primarily because of cultural sensitivity and gender specificity. Currently, serious efforts are being made to rediscover this route for the systemic delivery of active agents.

The vaginal route has potential for non-invasive (and controlled) delivery of drugs intended for both local and systemic effect. In fact, the vagina comprises a dense network of blood vessels which provides a large surface area leading to rapid drug absorption and quick onset of action. Moreover, the rich vascularization between the vagina and uterus leads to a "first-pass uterine effect" (preferential distribution to the uterus) enabling uterine targeting of therapeutic agents, such as progesterone and danazol

(Vermani and Garg 2000, Gupta et al. 2011). More importantly, the vaginal route offers a potential alternative to both oral and parenteral administration due to (Vermani and Garg 2000, das Neves and Bahia 2006): (i) bypass of hepatic first-pass metabolism as absorbed drugs enter, via the inferior vena cava, directly to the systemic circulation; (ii) a reduction in hepatic toxicity of drugs, e.g., steroids; (iii) avoidance of gastrointestinal enzymatic degradation and interferences with drug absorption, and reduction in the incidence and severity of adverse effects resulting from the oral route; and, (iv) overcoming the inconvenience caused by pain, tissue damage, and possible infection associated with parenteral routes, and possible self-insertion and removal of the dosage form.

Vaginal physiological and anatomical factors can significantly influence drug performance in the vaginal cavity. Therefore, a comprehensive understanding of these factors is essential in designing a suitable system for intravaginal drug delivery (Gupta et al. 2011).

Physiology/anatomy of the vagina

The vagina is a fibromuscular tube which extends from the body exterior to the uterus, measuring 7 to 10 cm in length (das Neves and Bahia 2006). The vagina is composed of three distinct regions: the outer adventitia, the middle muscular layer, and the innermost mucosal layer (Rohan and Sassi 2009). The latter layer is also sub-composed of lamina propria covered by a non-keratinized, stratified epithelium (Gupta et al. 2011). The mucosal layer varies in thickness depending on the sexual cycle and age (Rohan and Sassi 2009). It forms a series of transverse folds known as rugae and microridges, which significantly multiply the surface area of the vagina and allows the vagina to expand, permitting the placement of vaginal formulations and improving drug absorption (Vermani and Garg 2000). More importantly, the vagina exhibits unique features in terms of secretions, pH, enzyme activity, microflora, and cyclic changes (Table 8.1), which must be considered during the development of a vaginal drug delivery system (Vermani and Garg 2000, das Neves and Bahia 2006, Acartürk 2009, Rohan and Sassi 2009, El-Hammadi and Arias 2015).

Barriers to the vaginal route of drug administration

The therapeutic effect of any given active agent upon intravaginal administration relies on a number of factors associated with formulation issues, drug properties, and vaginal physiological conditions. Despite extensive investigation that has been ongoing to explore numerous possibilities, traditional vaginal dosage forms have certain limitations, e.g., leakage, messiness, and relatively short residence time due to the vaginal self-cleansing action (Acartürk 2009). Furthermore, upon administration of vaginal dosage forms (e.g., capsules, tablets, pessaries, creams, ointments, gels, foams, films, tampons, and douches) undesirable systemic drug absorption has been

Table 8.1. Idiosyncratic attributes of the vagina to be considered during engineering of a vaginal drug delivery system.

Feature	Description	Significance to drug delivery
Vaginal secretions	Mixture of multiple secretions including plasma transudates, and discharges from the upper reproductive tract, e.g., cervical mucus, secretions of the Bartholin's and Skene's glands, exfoliating epithelial cells, and leukocytes	They can either assist or hinder drug delivery. Vaginal fluids can facilitate drug dissolution and diffusion, thus aiding its arrival to the site of action. On the other hand, components of the vaginal secretions may interact with the drug, leading to a reduced efficacy. They can also alter medicine bioadhesion and residence time
Vaginal pH	pH is maintained by *Lactobacilli* spp. which produces lactic acid using glucose, a product of glycogen metabolism by exfoliated epithelial cells. Healthy women of reproductive age have a pH value ≈ 3.5–4.5, protecting against pathogens	pH changes with age, stage of menstrual cycle, infections, estrogen levels, levels of cervical and uterine secretions, and sexual arousal. Such variations can influence the vaginal delivery of drugs. Thus, controlling the vaginal pH is vital for successful therapy
Vaginal microflora	It is influenced by a number of factors, e.g., age, pH, stage of menstrual cycle, hormonal levels, pregnancy, menopause, infection and antimicrobial treatment, and douching practices. Anaerobic and aerobic organisms of both gram positive and gram negative species are naturally present in the vaginal environment, *Lactobacilli* spp. being the most prevalent component	Healthy vaginal environment is generally favorable to aerobic organisms. However, conditions leading to tissue damage can facilitate anaerobic bacteria proliferation, and may result in infections
Enzyme activity	Enzyme activity of the vaginal fluids can cause protein and peptide degradation, thus reducing their effectiveness. The most abundant type of enzymes present in human vaginal mucosa are aminopeptidases and, to a less extent, endopeptidases	Enzymatic activity relatively lower than that of the gastrointestinal tract, thus intravaginal delivery leads to less drug degradation
Cyclic changes	As hormone levels (especially estrogen) change with age, phase of the menstrual cycle, and pregnancy, several alterations in vaginal conditions are induced involving the thickness of the epithelial cell layer, the width of intercellular channels, pH, and secretions	Drug release from the dosage form and drug absorption may be affected. Hormonal changes induce alterations to physiological conditions leading to a large inter- and intra-individual variability in the performance of vaginal drug delivery systems

described (Pavelić et al. 2001). As a consequence, these conventional dosage forms can easily lead to poor patient compliance and may not fulfill clinical requirements.

Formulation considerations are critical for the development of a safe, stable, effective, and acceptable vaginal dosage form. Physicochemical characteristics of drug molecules, e.g., polarity and partition properties, solubility, dissolution rate, molecular weight (M_w), pKa, and chemical stability, are also of substantial significance for intravaginal drug delivery (Gupta et al. 2011). Finally, vaginal physiological factors including vaginal fluids, pH, enzyme activity, microflora, and thickness and permeability of the vaginal epithelium may significantly impact drug absorption and efficacy (Acartürk 2009, Rohan and Sassi 2009).

Beside general formulation requirements, i.e., being stable, non-toxic, cost-effective, easy to apply (administer), and safe for continuous administration, patient's acceptability and convenience must be considered. Several studies have suggested that patients prefer vaginal dosage forms that are odorless and colorless, showing negligible leakage, messiness or feeling of fullness, and do not cause irritation, itching, burning, or swelling (Hardy et al. 2003, Mattsson et al. 2013). Additionally, the drug delivery system should not interfere, or have a minimal interference, with vaginal normal functions and physiological conditions and daily life, be able to provide a sustained drug release to reduce dosing frequency, and in the case of systemic drug delivery, maintain therapeutic drug blood levels over a long period of time (das Neves and Bahia 2006). In search for an ideal vaginal drug delivery system, drug nanocarriers have been under extensive investigation.

Nanostructures for Vaginal Drug Delivery

Vaginal nanocarriers have shown great potential in addressing challenges faced by vaginal delivery of drug molecules and limitations of traditional vaginal dosage forms. The main advantages offered by nano-sized systems over conventional vaginal drug dosage forms are: (i) enhanced patient compliance, thanks to a sustained drug release that prolongs the residence time (and effect) of the drug, and to a significant reduction of the drug toxicity; (ii) drug efficacy is not limited by vaginal physiological conditions, which can even be intelligently used to generate a stimuli-responsive (selective) drug release (i.e., pH); (iii) physical chemistry of the active agent does not affect drug absorption and efficacy, e.g., the nanoplatform can facilitate the dissolution of hydrophobic drugs, while additionally improving drug stability by protecting the drug from hydrolysis and enzymatic degradation; and, (iv) specific drug delivery is possible by surface functionalization of nanocarriers with targeting ligands.

A variety of vaginal drug-loaded nanoplatforms have been designed (El-Hammadi and Arias 2015), including carbon-based nanostructures (fullerenes and carbon nanotubes), polymer-based NPs (das Neves et al. 2012a), cyclodextrins (Demirel et al. 2011, Zhou et al. 2013, Cevher et al. 2014), dendrimers (Vacas Córdoba et al. 2013, Sepúlveda-Crespo et al. 2014), liposomes (Pavelić et al. 2001), solid lipid NPs (Alukda et al. 2011), and oil-in-water (o/w) nanoemulsions, often referred to as microemulsions (Bachhav and Patravale 2009, Mirza et al. 2013).

Polymer-based nanoparticles

NPs for vaginal drug delivery are generally prepared with a variety of materials including biodegradable and biocompatible polymers (Table 8.2), e.g., poly(D,L-lactide) and poly(D,L-lactide-*co*-glycolide) (PLGA). These materials must proportionate sustained drug release properties, mucoadhesive characteristics, and/or diffusive ability to quickly go through the vaginal mucus (and reach the underlying tissues), hence avoiding clearance mechanisms of the mucus (Ballou et al. 2012, El-Hammadi and Arias 2015).

A recent investigation defined the influence of formulation variables, i.e., polymer concentration, sodium triphosphate pentabasic ($Na_5O_{10}P_3$)/polymer weight ratio, and drug/polymer weight ratio, on particle size, drug encapsulation efficiency, and mucoadhesion using chitosan NPs loaded with tenofovir, a nucleotide analog Human Immunodeficiency Virus (HIV) type 1 reverse transcriptase inhibitor and anti-HIV microbicide (Meng et al. 2011). The NPs were prepared following a gelation method by the addition of $Na_5O_{10}P_3$. The optimal formulation had a low encapsulation efficiency of $\approx 6\%$ and a mean particle size of ≈ 210 nm. The particles demonstrated no cytotoxicity and increased mucoadhesive ability from 6 to 12%, as their diameters decrease from ≈ 900 to ≈ 180 nm.

Surface electrical charge can influence the cellular uptake, drug activity, cytotoxicity, and diffusive properties of NPs (das Neves et al. 2012b). NPs loaded with the microbicidal agent dapivirine were formulated using PCL and a different surface modifiers to generate either negative (poloxamer 338 NF, and SLS) or positive (CTAB) surface charges. In general, all NPs had diameters of ≈ 180 nm, with high drug entrapment efficiencies. The formulations proved

Table 8.2. Illustrative examples of polymer-based vaginal nanomedicines.

Polymer composition	Active agent	Mean diameter (nm)	Functionalization	References
Chitosan	Tenofovir	180–900	–	Meng et al. 2011
Poly(ε-caprolactone) (PCL)	Dapivirine	≈ 180–200	Surface modification with poloxamer 338 NF, sodium lauryl sulfate (SLS), or cetyltrimethylammonium bromide (CTAB)	das Neves et al. 2012a,b
PLGA	Raltegravir and efavirenz	≈ 80	–	Date et al. 2012
PLGA	Small interfering ribonucleic acid (*si*RNA)	≈ 200	–	Woodrow et al. 2009
Eudragit® S-100 and PLGA	Tenofovir	300–500	pH-sensitive nanostructure	Zhang et al. 2011

similar or improved antiviral activities compared to the free drug, and were readily taken up by different cell types. However, differences were observed in cytotoxicity: SLS-PCL NPs and poloxamer-PCL NPs showed low cytotoxic effect, while CTAB-PCL NPs were significantly cytotoxic (das Neves et al. 2012a). In addition, it was observed that water negatively charged NPs transported faster than positively charged ones in simulated vaginal fluid. When the effects of pH were examined, diffusion differences augmented as the pH value of this fluid was increased from 4.2 to 7.0 (das Neves et al. 2012b).

Surface functionalization of NPs with poly(ethylene glycol) (PEG) chains (PEGylation) has been proposed to improve particle transport through the vaginal mucosa. This approach imitates the "stealth" migration of viruses that infect mucosal tissues (virus-like diffusion). Small and neutral PEGylated particles can avoid entrapment by size-occlusion or ionic interactions with mucus constituents, leading to fast penetration through the mucus gel and thus enhancing the uptake by the underlining epithelial cells. For instance, intravaginal delivery (mice model) of PEGylated PLGA NPs generated significantly greater concentrations in the tissue of the reproductive tract (5×) up to 6 hours after administration, and higher diffusion through cervical mucus (3×–10×), as compared with unmodified PLGA NPs (Cu et al. 2011). Other surface functionalizing strategies have also been explored, e.g., surface decoration of PLGA NPs surface with avidin, for mucoadhesion, can lead to five-fold greater vaginal retention than unmodified NPs (Cu et al. 2011).

Stimuli-sensitive nanostructures can be considered to be a complementary approach to surface functionalized NPs in the search for a controlled/optimized and selective drug effect (El-Hammadi and Arias 2015). Since healthy human vagina has a pH value ≈ 4–5, pH-sensitive NPs with the ability to retain their cargo at acidic conditions and release it at neutral have been suggested for semen-triggered drug delivery (typical human semen pH is ≈ 7.5), or for treatment of vagina disorders characterized by an increase in pH value. For example, pH-sensitive NPs have been prepared using Eudragit® S-100, a copolymer composed of methacrylic acid and methyl methacrylate (molar ratio 1:2) with $M_w \approx 135,000\ Da$, in combination with PLGA (25:75, 50:50, and 75:25, w/w) (Zhang et al. 2011). It was observed that the NPs presented higher loading efficiency of hydrophobic compounds in comparison with hydrophilic ones. Furthermore, they were internalized by vaginal cells and showed no cytotoxicity. Drug release studies revealed that these pH-sensitive NPs exhibited slow drug release in acidic pH (≈ 4.0) while they rapidly released their content upon increase of pH (≈ 7.5). Finally, increased drug release rate was measured with greater ratios of Eudragit® S-100 in NP composition (Zhang et al. 2011).

Date et al. (2012) developed a thermosensitive vaginal gel containing PLGA NPs for easy application and sustained delivery of active agents. The gel was formulated using a combination of Pluronic® F-127 (20%, w/v) and Pluronic® F-68 (1%, w/v) with thermogelation at 32.5°C. NPs formulated using a modified double emulsion/solvent evaporation (DE/SEV) method (mean size ≈ 80 nm) were loaded with efavirenz, a non-nucleoside reverse transcriptase inhibitor, and raltegravir, a HIV type 1 integrase inhibitor. Upon *in vitro* incubation with HeLa cells, the nanoparticulate-based gel formulation exhibited no cytotoxicity and offered sustained intracellular drug levels for up to 14 days.

Polymer-based NPs have further been reported to be a good tool for the protection and efficient delivery of nucleic materials and proteins/peptides via the vaginal route. For instance, *si*RNA-loaded PLGA NPs have been synthesized for protection against challenge from infectious disease through intravaginal administration (Woodrow et al. 2009). It is well-established that *si*RNA targeting specific viruses and bacteria can produce immunity against these pathogens by activating ribonucleic acid interference (RNA*i*) pathway (Palliser et al. 2006). NPs were formulated using a DE/SEV technique, and *si*RNA molecules were first pre-complexed with a low M_w polyamine (spermidine or protamine) before loading into PLGA NPs. This procedure yielded particles < 200 nm diameter with encapsulation efficiencies of ≈ 40%. Cytotoxicity evaluations in HepG2 hepatocytes or HeLa cervical carcinoma cells revealed that *si*RNA NPs were not cytotoxic at concentrations as high as 10 mg/mL. NPs provided sustained release of *si*RNA which was chemically intact and functional when NPs were incubated at pH 5. It was also found that the intravaginal administration of a single dose of *si*RNA-loaded PLGA NPs to the female mouse induced efficient and sustained gene silencing over the two week-long experiment. A reduction in gene expression was observed throughout the examined regions of the reproductive tract, including vaginal tract, cervix, and uterine horns. Finally, it was also found that NPs penetrated as deep as 120 μm below the lumenal surface.

Liposomes

Liposomes are spherical structures generated by self-assembly of phospholipids into a bilayer membrane confining an aqueous core. As a result, polar drugs can be incorporated inside the liposomal cavity while apolar drugs are trapped within the phospholipid bilayer. Liposomes can be either unilamellar (one bilayer) or multilamellar (many concentric bilayers) with a diameter from ≈ 20 to ≈ 3,000 nm. They have demonstrated their promise as drug carriers for the treatment of vaginal infections (Pavelić et al. 2001, 2005, Ning et al. 2005, Kang et al. 2010), inflammation (Basnet et al. 2012, Li et al. 2012), as well as the induction of mucosal vaccination (Gupta et al. 2012), due to their ability to sustain release and improve tissue distribution of entrapped drugs.

Early work in this area investigated the feasibility of liposomes for enhanced vaginal delivery of commonly used anti-infection agents, e.g., clotrimazole and chloramphenicol, to cite just some illustrative examples (Pavelić et al. 2005). In these studies it was demonstrated that methods such as polyol dilution and pro-liposome techniques can be used to produce nano-sized liposomes ranging (200 to 400 nm in diameter) with adequate drug entrapment efficiencies. It was also proved that the drug entrapment efficiency is significantly influenced by the physical chemistry of the therapeutic agent. For instance, while high entrapment efficiency up to 95% was observed with the hydrophobic substance clotrimazole, less than 10% was entrapped in the case of metronidazole, a drug known for its low water- and lipid-solubility (Pavelić et al. 2005). Moreover, the liposomes demonstrated good *in vitro* stability at pH values simulating vaginal pH. Finally, *in vivo* experiments in female rats revealed that clotrimazole-loaded vaginal liposomes could prolong drug release, thus leading to improved efficacy in comparison with commercial ointment and free drug (Ning et al. 2005).

The incorporation of liposomes into bioadhesive gels to provide liposomal preparations with suitable viscosity for human administration as well as to improve their physical stability has been proposed. Liposomal gels fabricated using Carbopol® hydrogels, known for their polar nature and bioadhesive characteristics, were found to preserve the original size distribution of incorporated liposomes and to improve the retention of encapsulated drugs, leading to a desirable sustained drug release (Pavelić et al. 2001, 2005). Thermosensitive gels composed of poloxamers that can be easily administered and retained in the vagina for an extended time without leakage have also been explored. For example, thermosensitive gels were prepared using a combination of poloxamer 407 and poloxamer 188 (15:15, w/w) which forms a gel at 37°C (Kang et al. 2010). Amphotericin B-loaded cationic liposomes with particle size, zeta potential, and drug encapsulation efficiency of ≈ 450 nm, ≈ 50 mV, and ≈ 55%, respectively, were incorporated into a thermosensitive poloxamer gel. Drug encapsulation in the liposome gel resulted in increased stability and reduced toxicity as compared with amphotericin B-loaded in non-gelled liposomes. More recently, a similar thermosensitive gel (composed of poloxamer 407 and poloxamer 188) was incorporated with pH-sensitive liposomes to generate a pH and temperature dual-sensitive liposomal gel for vaginal administration (Chen et al. 2012). pH-sensitive liposomes were formulated with the addition of the methoxy poly(ethylene glycol) 2000-hydrazone-cholesteryl hemisuccinate (mPEG-Hz-CHEMS) polymer, which contains hydrazone as the pH-sensitive moiety, and loaded with arctigenin, a natural material that exhibits antioxidant, antihuman immunodeficiency virus, antitumor, and anti-inflammatory effects (Kang et al. 2010). It was demonstrated that arctigenin loaded into the dual-sensitive liposome gel was more stable and less toxic than when incorporated into pH-sensitive liposomes. Additionally, drug release studies indicated that dual-sensitive liposomal gels produced a sustained drug release profile at pH 5 over a period of three days, whereas very little arctigenin release was observed at pHs 7.4 and 9.0.

New engineering approaches aiming at increased liposome stability and enhanced drug delivery efficiency have generated more sophisticated systems. In this line, propylene glycol (PG)-embodying liposomes have been loaded with matrine, a component of *Sophora flavescens* root extract with anti-inflammation and immunity-regulation activity (Li et al. 2012). PG-embodying liposomes were incorporated into a post-expansible hydrogel foam aerosol system composed of hydroxyethylcellulose (HEC, as gel forming material), difluoroethane propellants, and sodium dodecylsulfate (to create a flaggingly swelling behavior), leading to enhanced uniformly drug spread over the vaginal mucus. The liposome-based system produced a mucoadhesive swelling gel with prolonged residence time at the site of administration and sustained drug release. In another study, a liposomal gel formulation was prepared in which antigen-loaded liposomes were incorporated into a HEC aqueous gel and subsequently lyophilized to produce a rod-shaped solid dosage form for vaginal immunization against HIV type 1 infection (Gupta et al. 2012). The liposome-HEC-based freeze-dried rods, designed to revert into gel form following intravaginal administration, were found to have appropriate mucoadhesive strength. These freeze-dried formulations can offer several benefits including improved stability, mucoadhesion, and ease of administration.

Conclusions

Nano-sized systems have shown promise for efficient vaginal drug delivery providing sustained drug release and enhanced permeation. In parallel with advancements in drug discovery of new vaginal therapeutic agents, such as peptides, proteins, *si*RNA/DNA, antigens, hormones, and microbicides, nanoplatforms are gaining momentum as prospective vectors for these agents. Thus far, extensive research in this arena has focused on local delivery to the mucus vagina. However, our improved understanding of vaginal route, advantages offered by the vaginal route including being non-invasive and bypassing hepatic first-effect metabolism, and recent success achieved by vaginal drug nanocarriers may open the door for extensive nanotechnology-based research to explore the viability of systemic administration via this route. *In vitro* experiments and preclinical studies addressing existing challenges posed by the vaginal route have provided a concrete rational for the use of drug nanocarriers. It is anticipated that many nanotechnology-based vaginal delivery products will enter clinical trials in the near future, for which concerns, such as *in vivo* toxicity and efficiency, stability, and feasibility of commercialization, are yet to be unfolded.

Acknowledgement

The financial support of the Erasmus Mundus—JOSYLEEM Program is acknowledged as is the post-doctoral fellowship to Mazen M. El-Hammadi.

Abbreviations

CTAB	:	cetyltrimethylammonium bromide
DE/SEV	:	double emulsion/solvent evaporation
DNA	:	deoxyribonucleic acid
HEC	:	hydroxyethylcellulose
HIV	:	human immunodeficiency virus
mPEG-Hz-	:	methoxy poly(ethylene glycol) 2000-hydrazone-
CHEMS		cholesteryl hemisuccinate
M_W	:	molecular weight
$Na_5O_{10}P_3$	:	sodium triphosphate pentabasic
NP	:	nanoparticle
o/w	:	oil-in-water
PCL	:	poly(ε-caprolactone)
PEG	:	poly(ethylene glycol)
PG	:	propylene glycol
PLGA	:	poly(D,L-lactide-*co*-glycolide)
RNA	:	ribonucleic acid
RNA*i*	:	ribonucleic acid interference
SA	:	stearylamine
*si*RNA	:	small interfering ribonucleic acid
SLS	:	sodium lauryl sulfate

References

Acartürk, F. 2009. Mucoadhesive vaginal drug delivery systems. Recent Pat. Drug Deliv. Formul. 3: 193–205.

Alukda, D. and T. Sturgis and B.B. Youan. 2011. Formulation of tenofovir-loaded functionalized solid lipid nanoparticles intended for HIV prevention. J. Pharm. Sci. 100: 3345–3356.

Bachhav, Y.G. and V.B. Patravale. 2009. Microemulsion-based vaginal gel of clotrimazole: formulation, *in vitro* evaluation, and stability studies. AAPS Pharm. Sci. Tech. 10: 476–481.

Ballou, B. and S.K. Andreko, E. Osuna-Highley, M. McRaven, T. Catalone, M.P. Bruchez, T.L. Hope and M.E. Labib. 2012. Nanoparticle transport from mouse vagina to adjacent lymph nodes. PLoS One. 7: e51995.

Basnet, P. and H. Hussain, I. Tho and N. Skalko-Basnet. 2012. Liposomal delivery system enhances anti-inflammatory properties of curcumin. J. Pharm. Sci. 101: 598–609.

Cevher, E. and A. Açma, G. Sinani, B. Aksu, M. Zloh and L. Mülazımoğlu. 2014. Bioadhesive tablets containing cyclodextrin complex of itraconazole for the treatment of vaginal candidiasis. Int. J. Biol. Macromol. 69: 124–136.

Chen, D. and K. Sun, H. Mu, M. Tang, R. Liang, A. Wang, S. Zhou, H. Sun, F. Zhao, J. Yao and W. Liu. 2012. pH and temperature dual-sensitive liposome gel based on novel cleavable mPEG-Hz-CHEMS polymeric vaginal delivery system. Int. J. Nanomedicine. 7: 2621–2630.

Cu, Y. and C.J. Booth and W.M. Saltzman. 2011. *In vivo* distribution of surface-modified PLGA nanoparticles following intravaginal delivery. J. Control. Release. 156: 258–264.

das Neves, J. and M.F. Bahia. 2006. Gels as vaginal drug delivery systems. Int. J. Pharm. 318: 1–14.

das Neves, J. and J. Michiels, K.K. Ariën, G. Vanham, M. Amiji, M.F. Bahia and B. Sarmento. 2012a. Polymeric nanoparticles affect the intracellular delivery, antiretroviral activity and cytotoxicity of the microbicide drug candidate dapivirine. Pharm. Res. 29: 1468–1484.

das Neves, J. and C.M. Rocha, M.P. Gonçalves, R.L. Carrier, M. Amiji, M.F. Bahia and B. Sarmento. 2012b. Interactions of microbicide nanoparticles with a simulated vaginal fluid. Mol. Pharm. 9: 3347–3356.

Date, A.A. and A. Shibata, M. Goede, B. Sanford, K. La Bruzzo, M. Belshan and C.J. Destache. 2012. Development and evaluation of a thermosensitive vaginal gel containing raltegravir+efavirenz loaded nanoparticles for HIV prophylaxis. Antiviral Res. 96: 430–436.

Demirel, M. and G. Yurtdaş and L. Genç. 2011. Inclusion complexes of ketoconazole with beta-cyclodextrin: physicochemical characterization and *in vitro* dissolution behaviour of its vaginal suppositories. J. Incl. Phenom. Macro. 70: 437–445.

El-Hammadi, M.M. and J.L. Arias. 2015. Nano-sized platforms for vaginal drug delivery. Curr. Pharm. Des. 21: 1633–1644.

Gupta, S. and R. Gabrani, J. Ali and S. Dang. 2011. Exploring novel approaches to vaginal drug delivery. Recent Pat. Drug Deliv. Formul. 5: 82–94.

Gupta, P.N. and A. Pattani, R.M. Curran, V.L. Kett, G.P. Andrews, R.J. Morrow, A.D. Woolfson and R.K. Malcolm. 2012. Development of liposome gel based formulations for intravaginal delivery of the recombinant HIV-1 envelope protein CN54gp140. Eur. J. Pharm. Sci. 46: 315–322.

Hardy, E. and K.S. de Pádua, E.M. Hebling, M.J. Osis and L.J. Zaneveld. 2003. Women's preferences for vaginal antimicrobial contraceptives. V: attitudes of Brazilian women to the insertion of vaginal products. Contraception. 67: 391–395.

Kang, J.W. and E. Davaa, Y.T. Kim and J.S. Park. 2010. A new vaginal delivery system of amphotericin B: a dispersion of cationic liposomes in a thermosensitive gel. J. Drug Target. 18: 637–644.

Li, W.Z. and N. Zhao, Y.Q. Zhou, L.B. Yang, W. Xiao-Ning, H. Bao-Hua, K. Peng and Z. Chun-Feng. 2012. Post-expansile hydrogel foam aerosol of PG-liposomes: a novel delivery system for vaginal drug delivery applications. Eur. J. Pharm. Sci. 47: 162–169.

Mattsson, L.A. and A. Ericsson, M. Bøgelund and R. Maamari. 2013. Women's preferences toward attributes of local estrogen therapy for the treatment of vaginal atrophy. Maturitas. 74: 259–263.

Meng, J. and T.F. Sturgis and B.B. Youan. 2011. Engineering tenofovir loaded chitosan nanoparticles to maximize microbicide mucoadhesion. Eur. J. Pharm. Sci. 44: 57–67.

Mirza, M.A. and S. Ahmad, M.N. Mallick, N. Manzoor, S. Talegaonkar and Z. Iqbal. 2013. Development of a novel synergistic thermosensitive gel for vaginal candidiasis: an *in vitro*, *in vivo* evaluation. Colloids Surf. B Biointerfaces. 103: 275–282.

Ning, M.Y. and Y.Z. Guo, H.Z. Pan, H.M. Yu and Z.W. Gu. 2005. Preparation and evaluation of proliposomes containing clotrimazole. Chem. Pharm. Bull. (Tokyo). 53: 620–624.

Palliser, D. and D. Chowdhury, Q.Y. Wang, S.J. Lee, R.T. Bronson, D.M. Knipe and J. Lieberman. 2006. An siRNA-based microbicide protects mice from lethal herpes simplex virus 2 infection. Nature. 439: 89–94.

Pavelić, Z. and N. Skalko-Basnet and R. Schubert. 2001. Liposomal gels for vaginal drug delivery. Int. J. Pharm. 219: 139–149.

Pavelić, Z. and N. Skalko-Basnet and I. Jalsenjak. 2005. Characterisation and *in vitro* evaluation of bioadhesive liposome gels for local therapy of vaginitis. Int. J. Pharm. 301: 140–148.

Rohan, L.C. and A.B. Sassi. 2009. Vaginal drug delivery systems for HIV prevention. AAPS J. 11: 78–87.

Sepúlveda-Crespo, D. and R. Lorente, M. Leal, R. Gómez, F.J. De la Mata, J.L. Jiménez and M.A. Muñoz-Fernández. 2014. Synergistic activity profile of carbosilane dendrimer G2-STE16 in combination with other dendrimers and antiretrovirals as topical anti-HIV-1 microbicide. Nanomedicine. 10: 609–618.

Vacas Córdoba, E. and E. Arnaiz, M. Relloso, C. Sánchez-Torres, F. García, L. Pérez-Álvarez, R. Gómez, F.J. de la Mata, M. Pion and M.Á. Muñoz-Fernández. 2013. Development of sulphated and naphthylsulphonated carbosilane dendrimers as topical microbicides to prevent HIV-1 sexual transmission. AIDS. 27: 1219–1229.

Vermani, K. and S. Garg. 2000. The scope and potential of vaginal drug delivery. Pharm. Sci. Technolo. Today. 3: 359–364.

Woodrow, K.A. and Y. Cu, C.J. Booth, J.K. Saucier-Sawyer, M.J. Wood and W.M. Saltzman. 2009. Intravaginal gene silencing using biodegradable polymer nanoparticles densely loaded with small-interfering RNA. Nat. Mater. 8: 526–533.

Zhang, T. and T.F. Sturgis and B.B. Youan. 2011. pH-responsive nanoparticles releasing tenofovir intended for the prevention of HIV transmission. Eur. J. Pharm. Biopharm. 79: 526–536.

Zhou, Q. and L. Zhong, X. Wei, W. Dou, G. Chou and Z. Wang. 2013. Baicalein and hydroxypropyl-γ-cyclodextrin complex in poloxamer thermal sensitive hydrogel for vaginal administration. Int. J. Pharm. 454: 125–134.

CHAPTER 9

Potential Nanocarriers for Brain Drug Delivery

Mª Ángeles Holgado,[1,*] José L. Venero,[2]
Josefa Álvarez-Fuentes,[1,a] Mercedes Fernández-Arévalo[1,b]
and Lucía Martín-Banderas[1,c]

ABSTRACT

This chapter summarizes recent approaches in drug delivery to the central nervous system. An overview of the blood-brain barrier and the representative pathologies related to its dysfunction is included. Treatment of these disorders is based on strategies aiming to deliver therapeutic agents into the brain by circumvention or disruption of the blood-brain barrier. Particular attention is given to the formulation of drug delivery nanosystems and, more specifically, polymer-based nanoparticles which can be considered to be the most promising tool/strategy for drug delivery to the brain. Nanomedicine development generates revolutionary results in the treatment of brain tumors and neurodegenerative diseases, e.g., Alzheimer's disease, multiple sclerosis, or Parkinson's disease.

[1] Department of Pharmacy and Pharmaceutical Technology, Faculty of Pharmacy, University of Seville, C/Prof. García González n° 2, 41012, Seville, Spain.
[a] Email: ffjalvarez@us.es
[b] Email: mfarevalo@us.es
[c] Email: luciamartin@us.es
[2] Department of Biochemistry and Molecular Biology, Faculty of Pharmacy, University of Seville, C/Prof. García González n° 2, 41012, Seville, Spain.
Email: jlvenero@us.es
* Corresponding author: holgado@us.es

Introduction

The Central Nervous System (CNS) is well protected by the Blood-Brain Barrier (BBB) which maintains its homeostasis. Changes in the BBB functionalities have been reported in cancer and numerous neurological disorders, including Amyotrophic Lateral Sclerosis (ALS), Multiple Sclerosis (MS), Alzheimer's Disease (AD), and Parkinson's Disease (PD) (Zlokovic 2008, Carvey et al. 2009, Weiss et al. 2009, Nag et al. 2011). Recently published investigations have demonstrated that disruption of the BBB in the absence of neuronal damage may trigger different neurodegenerative events, thus emphasizing the role of the BBB as a potential inducer rather than a consequence of the damage.

Regarding drug delivery to the brain, the upload of therapeutic agents is seriously hindered by the BBB, thus being responsible for pharmacotherapy failure (even at the greatest drug doses). To beat the challenge, different strategies have been investigated to deliver therapeutic agents into the brain, e.g., disruption of the BBB, chemical delivery, biological transporters, molecular Trojan horses, and alternative routes of drug administration. Recent advances in molecular neuroscience and nanotechnology have contributed to the evolution of brain imaging and disease diagnosis, and to the efficient delivery of drugs into the brain.

The Blood-Brain Barrier

The adequate functionality of neurons relies on the maintenance of their microenvironment under a tight homeostatic control. To this aim, they are sealed off from the rest of the organism by the BBB. This specialized barrier is formed by different cell phenotypes arranged in a single organization (the neurovascular unit). First elements of the neurovascular unit are the brain microvascular Endothelial Cells (ECs), which interact closely with pericytes, glial cells, and the basement membrane (BM) (Fig. 9.1) (Pardridge 1999).

Endothelial cells

ECs comprise a heterogeneous population completely covering the inner surface of blood vessels, and forming the basic anatomic structure of the BBB (Redzic et al. 2005). ECs are tethered to the BM through focal adhesions, which mainly consist of transmembrane proteins, including selectins and integrins (Golias et al. 2011). The capillary endothelium is 50 to 100 times tighter than peripheral microvessels, thus determining a severe restriction of the paracellular pathway for diffusion of hydrophilic solutes (Cardoso et al. 2010). In addition, brain microvascular ECs have uniform thickness with very few pinocytic vesicles along with absence of fenestrations, a feature closely related to the presence of Tight Junctions (TJs) thereby reducing the diffusion

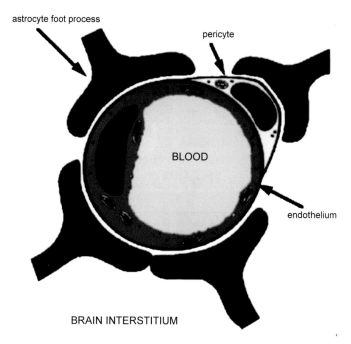

Figure 9.1. The "three cell model" of the brain microvasculature: endothelium, pericyte, and astrocyte foot process. Reprinted with permission from Pardridge (1999). Copyright Informa Healthcare (1999).

of molecules across the vessel (Ballabh et al. 2004, Cardoso et al. 2010). Other features include the small number of caveolae at the luminal surface of the cell (Nag et al. 2011), and a high number of mitochondria associated with a strong metabolic activity (Persidsky et al. 2006). Thanks to all of these characteristics, the ECs can be considered as central mediators between blood and brain. In fact, they regulate the selective transport (and metabolism) of substances from blood to brain, as well as in the opposite way (from the parenchyma back to the systemic circulation) (Cardoso et al. 2010).

Astrocytes

Astrocytes are the most abundant cells in the brain. They display important roles in metabolic support (K⁺ buffering and regulation of immune responses) (Fuller et al. 2010), while they have an important role in maintaining the BBB integrity. From the ≈ 11 phenotypes ascribed to astrocytes, eight correlate with blood vessels (Bernacki et al. 2008). An anatomical examination of the brain microvasculature shows that the endfeet of astrocytic glia form a lacework of fine lamellae closely opposed to the outer surface of the brain endothelium (Abbott 2002).

Different roles have been attributed to astrocytes in the neurovascular unit. A major role of astrocytic endfeet is the regulation of homeostasis to ensure an appropriate neuronal environment. Thus, neuronal activity is accompanied by a substantial efflux of K^+, which gives rise to an osmotic gradient that will induce water redistribution (Sykova 1991). Since K^+ clearance is accompanied by water flux, the polarized expression of the aquaporin-4 water channel determines the significant role played by the astrocytic endfeet in K^+ clearance from the brain parenchyma to the vascular space (Venero et al. 2001). In keeping with this role, neuronal activity triggers the release of vasoactive substances by astrocytes (e.g., prostanoids) that enable the dynamic coupling of the cerebral blood flow with the local demand of energy (Allaman et al. 2011). Astrocytes at the perivascular space are also important in the generation of TJs between ECs of the brain microvasculature (Carvey et al. 2009). Astrocytes further play a critical role in neuronal metabolism, nutrition, and discharge of substrates (Bernacki et al. 2008).

Pericytes

Pericytes are contractile actin-expressing cells that surround capillaries, venules, and arterioles. They wrap around ECs in the brain at high density, and have a number of vasoactive signaling receptors. Hence, it has been proposed that control of blood flow is probably done by pericytes located at the walls of capillaries (the place where the metabolic demand occurs and can be rapidly detected) (Fernandez-Klett et al. 2010). However, during ischemia, the contracting capacity of pericytes may obstruct the capillary blood flow (Yemisci et al. 2009). The average ratio of pericytes to ECs in the human brain is $\approx$ 1:3 to 1:4 (Dore-Duffy and Cleary 2011). Pericytes share the same BM with the ECs (Kim et al. 2006). In fact, pericytes synthesizes the majority of the components of the BM, including proteoglycans (Dore-Duffy and Cleary 2011).

The close association of pericytes to blood vessels may play a key role in EC proliferation, migration, and differentiation (Persidskly et al. 2006). As well, they promote the stabilization of vessels by assuring the integrity of the structure and quiescence of ECs. It has also been suggested that pericytes may play a role in angiogenesis (Dore-Duffy 2008), thus giving the idea that pericytes may exhibit stem cell morphology. A recent study in adult viable pericyte-deficient mice has demonstrated that pericyte loss can determine brain vascular damage by a reduction in the cerebral blood flow and by BBB breakdown, the latter being associated to secondary neuronal degenerative changes (Bell et al. 2010). Additional investigations demonstrated the critical role of pericytes in the integration of endothelial and astrocyte functions at the neurovascular unit, and in the regulation of the BBB (Armulik et al. 2010), including the formation of TJs and vesicle trafficking in ECs (Daneman et al. 2010).

Basement membrane

The BM is an essential part of the BBB consisting of a highly specialized extracellular matrix that surrounds the brain microvascular vessels and engulfs ECs and pericytes, anchoring the cells in place and establishing the connections with the surrounding brain cells (Cardoso et al. 2010). It is composed of more than 50 different macromolecular components, and despite its small thickness (≈ 100 nm), is a mechanically strong structure dominated by a scaffolding of cross-linked type IV collagen molecules co-intertwined with a network of polymeric laminin (Farkas and Luiten 2001). The basic structure of the BM is built by two independent networks of type IV collagen and laminin. The BM is made of three layers: one generated by ECs that contains laminin-4 and laminin-5, another derived from astrocytes that contains laminin-1 and laminin-2, and finally the collagen IV-containing middle layer made of ECs and astrocytes (Weiss et al. 2009). At the precapillary arterioles and postcapillary venules, the BM is separated from the astroglial limiting membrane by the perivascular space, also known as the Virchow-Robin space.

The BM is more than a simple accumulation of extracellular matrix proteins. In fact, significant roles have been attributed to the BM, including angiogenesis, stability/maturation of vessels, and a barrier function (impeding the movement of large charged molecules, and the migration of cells like leukocytes and malignant cells) (Hallmann et al. 2005). Matrix metalloproteinases, particularly metalloproteinase-9, are known to significantly digest the BM, hence contributing to the alteration of the barrier integrity. Therefore, matrix metalloproteinases are thought to play a deleterious role in the etiopathology of brain diseases, including stroke, MS, infection, AD, and PD (Rosenberg 2009).

Tight junctions

TJs are organized as an intricate complex of transmembrane and cytoplasmatic proteins, significantly reducing the permeation of polar molecules from the blood to the brain extracellular fluid, through paracellular diffusion pathways between ECs (Kniesel and Wolburg 2000, Abbott et al. 2010). TJs are structurally characterized by specialized membrane microdomains, and are located on the apical region of ECs (Ueno 2007). TJ proteins span the apical intercellular space, and regulate the passive diffusion of ions and small non-charged solutes via the paracellular space. Consequently, TJs limit the paracellular permeability, and act as a seal that regulates lateral diffusion between the apical and the basolateral plasma membrane domains, which enables the maintenance of asymmetrically distributed integral membrane proteins and lipids (Cardoso et al. 2010). Transmembrane proteins found in the TJs are occludins, claudins, and junctional adhesion molecules, which are attached to the cytoskeleton thereby linking cell-cell and cell-substratum adhesion sites (Ueno 2007, Wolburg et al. 2009). These transmembrane proteins interact with intracellular scaffolding proteins (e.g., zonula occludens, and cingulin) which are involved in the connection of TJs to the actin cytoskeleton (Wolburg et al. 2009).

Adherens junctions

Adherens junctions are tightening structures between ECs in which transmembrane proteins are principally cadherins. Below the TJs, in the basal region of lateral plasma membrane, there are adherens junctions that contribute to the BBB function, being closely connected to the actin (Petty and Lo 2002, Cardoso et al. 2010). Cadherins are transmembrane glycoproteins with extracellular domains that mediate cell-cell adhesion and cytoplasmic tails that directly bind the cytoplasmic protein β-catenin. The capacity to interact with cytoplasmic proteins is crucial to the molecular action of cadherins. β-catenin serves as a scaffold to anchor α-catenin, and p120 catenin associates directly with the membrane-proximal region of the cadherin cytoplasmic tail (Ratheesh and Yap 2012), which locally regulate the organization of the actin cytoskeleton, cadherin stability, and intracellular signaling pathways that control gene transcription (Hartsock and Nelson 2008).

Neurological Disorders

Alterations in the BBB functionalities have been described in neurological disorders, including PD, AD, ALS, and MS (Zlokovic 2008, Carvey et al. 2009, Weiss et al. 2009, Nag et al. 2011). These pathologies are briefly discussed here.

Parkinson's disease

PD is characterized by a clinical syndrome of hypokinesia, rigidity, and tremor, and affects $\approx$ 1 to 3% of the population. Motor dysfunction can be attributed to the progressive degeneration of dopaminergic neurons in the substantia nigra (Obeso et al. 2000). Although PD correlates with mutations of genes encoding several proteins, including α-synuclein, parkin, and ubiquitin C terminal hydrolase-L1 (Mouradian 2002), the etiology of idiopathic PD, which accounts for > 90% of PDs, is still not completely understood (Obeso et al. 2000). James Parkinson hypothesized a link between head trauma and development of PD, an idea that was corroborated in different investigations (Tsai et al. 2002, Bower et al. 2003). These findings raise the possibility that a dysfunctional BBB may be involved in the physiopatology of some forms of PD. In fact, it has been suggested that an impaired BBB function may provoke or at least accelerate the progression of the disease (Kortekaas et al. 2005).

Vascular Endothelial Growth Factor (VEGF) is the most potent angiogenic factor that highly increases the BBB permeability (Ferrara 2000). Augmented levels of VEGF have been found in PD patients (Yasuda et al. 2007). In addition, it has been described that a significant disruption of the BBB is accompanied by a selective death of nigral dopaminergic neurons, and by a prominent microglial inflammatory response (Rite et al. 2007). An increase in the capillary density in the substantia nigra following an augment in the VEGF levels has been shown (Rite et al. 2007). Consequently, it was hypothesized that vascular changes leading to angiogenesis and to a greater permeability in the BBB may play a key role in the death of nigral dopaminergic neurons in PD.

Alzheimer's disease

AD is the most common cause of dementia in the elderly, affecting $\approx$ 10% of the population over 65 years (Jorm and Jolley 1998). The main pathological features are extracellular deposition of the β-amyloid (Aβ) peptide in the neuropil (senile plaques) and cerebral vasculature (cerebral amyloid angiopathy), neuritic cytoskeletal lesions, progressive loss of synapses and cortical neurons, and activation of microglia and astrocytes (Jellinger 2002). Altered cholinergic and glutamatergic neurotransmission, apoptosis, oxidative stress, calcium homeostasis dysfunction, and neuroinflammation are implicated in AD pathogenesis (Selkoe and Schenk 2003). However, the existence of vascular anatomical defects in AD supports the importance of the BBB integrity in AD pathogenesis (Bell and Zlokovic 2009).

The Aβ peptide is transported across the BBB via receptor-mediated transcytosis, thanks to the receptor for advanced glycation endproducts (when the peptide migrates from blood into the brain) and to the low density lipoprotein receptor-related protein-1 (when Aβ pass from the brain to the blood) (Deane et al. 2003). Alterations in the functionalities of these receptors are associated to Aβ peptide accumulation into the brain (Bell and Zlokovic 2009). Apolipoprotein E4 (ApoE4) has been associated with AD (Genin et al. 2011), a protein that is involved in the clearance of the Aβ peptide from the brain (Castellano et al. 2011). ApoE4 can contribute to the disruption of the BBB and to a reduction in the number of blood vessels (and blood flow in some regions of the brain), to further cause neurodegeneration (Bell et al. 2012). In addition, the low expression of the vascular-restricted mesenchyme homeobox 2 gene in AD patients mediates aberrant angiogenesis, thus leading to a leaky BBB, and suppresses the expression of the low density lipoprotein receptor-related protein-1 at the BBB (Wu et al. 2005).

Amyotrophic lateral sclerosis

ALS is a fatal disease characterized by progressive motor neuron degeneration in the brain and spinal cord, leading to muscle atrophy, paralysis, and death typically within three to five years from diagnosis. Only 5 to 10% of ALS cases are genetically linked. Alterations to the permeability of the blood-cerebrospinal fluid barrier (BCSFB) have been described in ALS (Garbuzova-Davis et al. 2011), while abnormally high levels of immunoglobulin G, albumin, and C3a complement component have been further detected in the cerebrospinal fluid of ALS patients. Furthermore, damage to the vasculature has been described to play a key role in the initiation of ALS (Zhong et al. 2008, Henkel et al. 2009). In fact, in these investigations a significant reduction in TJ proteins was detected (ZO-1, occludin, and claudin-5) between ECs along with a substantial BCSFB breakdown to serum proteins prior to motor neuron loss. Deposits of hemosiderin within (and outside) motor neurons suggest microhemorrhages in mice models of ALS.

Multiple sclerosis

Disruption of the BBB is a typical feature of MS, thus allowing the entry of leukocytes into the brain. In this disease, the immune system recognizes CNS myelin as a foreign entity, thus destroying it. Therefore, the pathological hallmark of MS is an inflammatory focal demyelination and axonal loss with limited remyelination, resulting in chronic multifocal sclerotic plaques (Sanders and De Keyser 2007). A deregulation of the TJ adaptor protein ZO-1 in MS tissues from both primary and secondary disease states has been identified (Kirk et al. 2003, Leech et al. 2007). Additionally, metalloproteinases are involved in the ethiopathology of MS, since: i) increase levels of metalloproteinase 1, 2, 3, 7, 9, and 12, have been detected in MS patients, thus allowing degradation of the BM, entry of leukocytes, and degradation of myelin; and, ii) metalloproteinase 8 (also known as neutrophil collagenase) has been identified as a therapeutic target for MS patients, thus highlighting the relevance of these enzymes in the evolution of the disease (Alexander et al. 2010).

Strategies to Optimize Drug Delivery to the Brain

Different routes of drug administration have been evaluated to improve drug accumulation into the brain, e.g., intravenous, oral, inhalation or intratracheal instillation, intranasal, convection-enhanced diffusion, and intrathecal/intraventricular administration. In fact, it has been hypothesized that the route of drug administration can help in circumventing physiological barriers of the brain.

Drug transport across the BBB has been described to be the consequence of one or more mechanisms (Fig. 9.2). Unfortunately, cerebral ECs are responsible for the high degree of impermeability of the BBB to drug molecules, and limited drug penetration into the brain is a rule rather than an exception. In this line, molecular size of the active agent is not the only problem to be faced. In fact, ≈ 98% of small molecules are not able to cross the BBB (Patel et al. 2012). To beat the challenge, numerous strategies have been investigated to optimize drug delivery to the brain (Table 9.1) (Martín-Banderas et al. 2011).

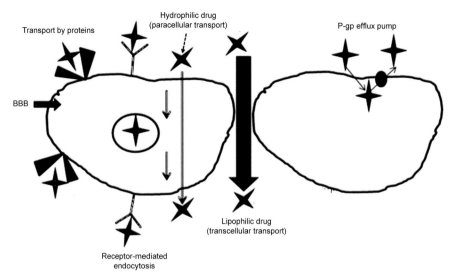

Figure 9.2. Mechanisms for drug transport across the BBB. P-gp: P-glycoprotein. Reprinted with permission from Agarwal et al. (2009). Copyright Bentham Science Publishers (2009).

Nanocarriers for Drug Delivery to the Brain

Nanocarriers provide an alternative approach to drug transport through the BBB. To this aim particulate systems must fulfill some requisites: (i) small size (nano-sized); adequate vehiculization of peptides, proteins, and nucleic acids); (ii) stability in blood (avoiding opsonization processes); (iii) special functionalization for a satisfactory interaction with the BBB (e.g., location of ligands onto the particle surface for receptor-mediated endocytosis); (iv) null immunogenicity, platelet aggregation, and induction of inflammatory responses; (v) minimized interaction with the reticuloendothelial system (and plasma clearance), thus extended plasma half-life; and, (vi) easy scale-up and cost-effective production process (Lockman et al. 2002). The most significant advantages and disadvantages of nanoparticle (NP)-based drug delivery systems are shown in Table 9.2, special emphasis is given here to polymer-based NPs.

Cyclodextrins

The chemical structure of CDs is relatively complex (basket-shaped), with three different forms α, β, and γ. In any case, two areas are basically defined in CDs: a lipophilic core inside an external hydrophilic structure. As a consequence, both hydrophilic/polar and lipophilic/apolar drug molecules can be loaded to CDs. They can further form inclusion complexes for a better drug delivery to the site of action (Brewster and Loftsson 2002).

Table 9.1. Representative strategies to optimize drug delivery to the brain.

Strategy	Method	Description
BBB disruption	Osmotic disruption or hyperosmotic shock	Intra-arterial infusion of hypertonic substances. Shrinkage of cerebral ECs and expansion of the blood volume enhance paracellular diffusion of water-soluble drugs into the brain
	Biochemical disruption	By endogenous vasoactive substances which may have a narrow therapeutic window and dose-limiting side effects
	Disruption by alkylglycerols	Monoacetylglycerols and diacetylglycerols are generally used. Non-toxic strategy
	Disruption by ultrasounds	They induce the breakdown of TJs in absence of cell damage
Chemical delivery	Lipidization	Apolar compounds with a molecular weight < 600 Da can cross the BBB by diffusion
	Prodrugs	Drug in an inactive form, e.g., linked to glucose, being able to target the specific tissue, e.g., by interaction with glucose transporters expressed in the BBB
Biological transporters	Carrier-mediated transport	Some transporters can enhance drug delivery to the CNS, e.g., glucose transporter 1 (GLUT1), large neutral amino acid transporter 1 (LAT1), cationic amino acid transporter 1 (CAT1), monocarboxylic acid transporter 1 (MCT1), concentrative nucleoside transporter 2 (CNT2), and choline transporter
	Receptor-mediated transport	It can be exploited to increase NP migration across the BBB. Choline and transferrin (Tf) transporters are generally used
	Active efflux transport	Efflux transport in the brain is unidirectional. P-gp is one of the most relevant efflux transporters
	Peptide vector strategies	Use of small linear synthetic peptides via a chemical linker. These peptides are habitually derived from protegrin 1, a natural antimicrobial peptide
	Adsorptive-mediated transcytosis	Movement of molecules within endocytic vesicles and across the cerebral ECs. Cationic molecules coupled with proteins are generally used
Molecular Trojan horses		Therapeutic peptide/protein conjugated to a monoclonal antibody (mAb) that binds to a specific receptor in the BBB, e.g., Tf and insulin receptors
Other routes	Nose to brain	NPs directly delivered from the nasal mucosa to the brain by transcellular absorption or endocytosis
	Intracerebral delivery	It involves drug administration directly into the parenchymal space of the brain, e.g., by direct injection, intrathecal catheters, intracerebral implants
	Intrathecal delivery	Injection of therapeutic agents, e.g., for anesthesia or pain treatment, into the subarachnoid space of the spinal cord

Table 9.2. Principal advantages and disadvantages of drug nanocarriers.

Nanocarrier	Advantages	Disadvantages
Cyclodextrin (CD)	Optimization of drug solubility and bioavailability, while minimizing drug biotransformation processes	Expensive
Dendrimer	Low polydispersity, multiple surface functional groups, and engineered for specific applications	Multi-step and tedious synthesis
Nanogel	High drug loading capacity, and low toxicity	To be defined
Polymeric micelle	Optimization of drug solubility, and multiple surface functional groups	Stability in a relatively narrow pH range
Liposome	Loading of both polar and apolar drugs, biocompatible, biodegradable, non-immunogenic, non-toxic, easy administration, and easy to prepare and easy surface functionalization	Expensive, and phospholipids may undergo oxidation and hydrolysis
Lipid NP	Easy surface functionalization, loading of both polar and apolar drugs, biocompatible, no need to use organic solvents, easy to scale-up and sterilize, components of relative low cost, and physically stable in both aqueous and non-aqueous media	Drug loading limited by the drug solubility in the lipid melt, and drug release may occur during storage
Inorganic NP	Stable structure, and adequate diagnostic tool	Potential toxicity, and limited efficiency
Polymeric NP	Biocompatible, approved by the Food and Drug Administration (FDA), non-toxic, formulation under mild conditions, controlled drug release, long residence time at the targeted site, and delivery of multiple therapeutic agents	Some polymers are expensive, complicated surface functionalization, some NP structures may be exceptionally complex, and possibility of NP aggregation in aqueous media

The use of CDs in drug delivery to the brain has been investigated. For instance, galanin-like peptides have been loaded to CDs in order to obtain a greater accumulation in the brain microenvironment. In this study it was found that the route of CD administration influenced the localization of the nanocarrier, i.e., the cerebellum can be reached after intravenous administration, while CD accumulation in the hypothalamus was possible upon intranasal administration (Nonaka et al. 2008). Unfortunately, controversy does exist on the toxicity associated to CD accumulation in the brain (Monnaert et al. 2004, Tilloy et al. 2006).

Dendrimers

The architecture of dendrimers generally consists of a central hydrophobic/apolar core that grows sequentially with a stepwise repetitive reaction sequence. This increased growth is defined by a "generation" number, and each generation of dendrimer is characterized by the geometry, molecular weight, and number of hydrophilic surface functional groups. Additional properties for drug delivery purposes are: a low polydispersity, a well-defined three-dimensional structure, the great number of functional groups located at the surface, and the capability to mimic biomolecules such as proteins and lipids (Najlah and D'Emanuele 2006).

Dendrimers can facilitate the delivery of therapeutic agents, e.g., deoxyribonucleic acid (DNA) (Huang et al. 2007) and methotrexate (Dhanikula et al. 2008), across the BBB. However, an adequate surface functionalization of the dendrimer structure with targeting moieties is needed to reach this aim, e.g., Tf (Huang et al. 2007, Li et al. 2012), lactoferrin (Huang et al. 2008), or angiopep-2 (Ke et al. 2009).

Polymeric micelles

Micelles are aggregates (5 to 20 nm in size) typically formed by 50 to 100 amphiphilic molecules dispersed in a liquid phase (Kabanov and Alakhov 2002). In an aqueous solution, these amphiphilic molecules aggregate exposing their polar head groups outside while hiding their hydrophobic segments in their inner core. This structure facilitates the incorporation/solubilization of hydrophobic drugs within the core.

Pluronic® micelles have been shown *in vitro* and *in vivo* to be highly effective in drug transport across the BBB. For example, Pluronic® P-85 micelles have increased drug permeability up to ≈ 19-fold in a bovine brain microvessel EC monolayer model. Such permeability enhancement was particularly considerable for P-gp substrates, such as paclitaxel, vinblastine, and ritonavir (Zhang and Wu 2009). Multifunctional micelles can be engineered for simultaneous drug delivery and imaging (Gaucher et al. 2005). Again, a proper surface functionalization (e.g., with Tf or peptides) can benefit drug delivery to brain locations, i.e., brain tumors (Daniels et al. 2012). For instance, Tf-modified paclitaxel-loaded polyphosphoester hybrid micelles (drug entrapment efficiency ≈ 90%) have demonstrated a strong antiglioma activity *in vivo*, i.e., mean survival time of mice was greater than Taxol®: ≈ 40 days vs. ≈ 34 days, respectively (Zhang et al. 2012). In this line, angiopep-2-modified micelles efficiently delivered amphotericin B across the BBB (Shao et al. 2010). These micelles further demonstrated *in vitro* a reduced cytotoxicity and hemolysis compared with Fungizone®.

Polymeric nanoparticles

Polymeric NPs have shown very promising possibilities in drug delivery to the CNS (Patel et al. 2012). To this aim, they should be characterized by an adequate geometry (spherical shape and size < 100 nm); they should be made of no-toxic, non-immunogenic, biodegradable and biocompatible polymer(s);

and, should be properly functionalized to assure long plasma half-lives and selective targeting to BBB (receptor-mediated endocytosis) (Martín-Banderas et al. 2011, Chen and Liu 2012). Poly(D,L-lactide-*co*-glycolide) (PLGA), poly(alkylcyanoacrylates), chitosan (CS), and poly(ε-caprolactone) (PCL) are representative polymers being used in the formulation of polymeric NPs for drug delivery to the brain.

Poly(D,L-lactide-co-glycolide) nanoparticles

Poly(D,L-lactide), poly(glycolide), and their copolymers (PLGA) have been approved by the FDA for the preparation of therapeutic nanodevices. PLGA is a biodegradable and biocompatible copolymer being degraded by hydrolysis of its ester linkages in water (Anderson and Shive 1997). Numerous methodologies have been developed to formulate PLGA NPs, e.g., nanoprecipitation, solvent evaporation, coacervation, spray drying. PLGA NPs can be properly modified to assure long-circulating times in blood and the selective targeting to the non-healthy site (Astete and Sabliov 2006).

For instance, PLGA NPs coated with hydrophilic Tween® 80 can successfully cross the BBB (Mittal et al. 2011, Ling et al. 2012). This nanoformulation was very effective in the oral delivery of estradiol to rat brain in a model of AD. In another investigation, PLGA NPs formulated by emulsion solvent diffusion, and surface modified with polysorbate 80, selectively accumulated in the brain of rats upon administration via the carotid artery (thus bypassing the BBB) (Tahara et al. 2011). In this line, the use of CS as a coating material for PLGA NPs has been suggested to enhance transcytosis processes across the BBB (Jaruszewski et al. 2012).

Surface functionalization with cell-penetrating peptides and proteins has been reported to optimize NP delivery through the BBB (Bhaskar et al. 2010). For example, covalent conjugation of PEGylated PLGA NPs to Pep TGN, a 12 amino acid peptide obtained from the bacteriophage clone 12-2, reported an enhanced brain accumulation and low levels in the liver and spleen, compared to plain NPs (Li et al. 2011). Curcumin-loaded PLGA NPs surface conjugated with Tet-1 peptides by a carbodiimide strategy have been tested *in vitro* for the treatment of AD (Mathew et al. 2012). This peptide demonstrated a promising neuronal targeting efficiency.

Similarly, surface coating with proteins, e.g., Tf and lactoferrin, can direct PLGA NPs across the BBB (Chang et al. 2009, 2012, Hu et al. 2011, Kuo et al. 2011). Such functionalization has been further reported to stabilize the nanoparticulate system (avoiding the use of toxic polyvinyl alcohol or Tween®).

Poly(alkylcyanoacrylate) nanoparticles

Poly(alkylcyanoacrylate) nanoparticulate systems can be prepared in the form of nanospheres, nanocapsules, hybrid magnetic NPs, long-circulating

NPs, as well as NPs functionalized with targeting ligands (Yordanov 2012). They have been successfully investigated *in vivo* for drug delivery to the brain. Representative examples of therapeutic molecules loaded to these NPs with this aim are: gemcitabine (Wang et al. 2009), doxorubicin (Petri et al. 2007), dalargin (Kreuter et al. 2003, Das and Lin 2005), methotrexate (Gao and Jiang 2006), rivastigmine (Wilson et al. 2008), and the nerve growth factor (Kurakhmaeva et al. 2009).

Interestingly, poly(butylcyanoacrylate) NPs coated with Tween® 80 can incorporate ApoE onto their surface. Then, the ApoE protein can mimic low density lipoproteins, facilitating the NP transport into the brain via low density lipoprotein receptors (Wagner et al. 2012, Yordanov 2012).

Chitosan nanoparticles

CS is a hydrophilic, biocompatible, and biodegradable polymer that has demonstrated some potential in the form of a nanoparticulate system for neuroprotection against PD and AD. For example, CS NPs loaded with subfragments of the Aβ peptide (which acts as a vaccine providing protection for neurons) can efficiently permeate across the BBB, thus leading to a significant immunogenicity by the production of antibodies against the Aβ peptide (Songjiang and Lixiang 2009).

The caspase-3 enzyme is induced in global brain ischemia and is associated to apoptotic cell death. PEGylated CS NPs have been synthesized and loaded with the peptide z-DEVD-fmk, a caspase-3 inhibitor with neuroprotective effects. The NPs were further functionalized with mAb OX26 moieties with affinity for the Tf receptor located at the BBB, thus facilitating NP endocytosis and uptake into the brain (Aktaş et al. 2005). Similarly, the anti-mouse Tf receptor mAb R17217 was used to surface functionalize PLGA NPs (Karatas et al. 2009).

Poly(ε-caprolactone) nanoparticles

PCL is an apolar biodegradable polyester approved by the FDA for human use, and widely used in drug delivery. PCL NPs have exhibited excellent drug delivery capabilities against brain tumors. For instance, indomethacin-loaded PCL NPs (mean size ≈ 240 nm, zeta potential ≈ –7 mV) have demonstrated a selective and efficient cytotoxic activity in a rat glioma model compared to controls (Bernardi et al. 2009). PEGylated PCL NPs have been further formulated for paclitaxel delivery across the BBB (Xin et al. 2010). Active drug targeting to glioblastomas can be possible by surface functionalization of PEGylated PCL NPs with targeting moieties, e.g., TGN peptide, AS1411 aptamer, and/or GMT8 aptamer (Gao et al. 2012a).

Liposomes

Liposomes are small vesicles of unilamellar or multilamellar phospholipid/ lipid bilayers surrounding central aqueous compartments. They can be advantageously formulated for drug delivery to the brain (Du et al. 2009, Markoutsa et al. 2011, Xie et al. 2012). In this line, PEGylated liposomes can optimize the biodistribution and pharmacokinetics of doxorubicin in patients bearing recurrent high-grade gliomas (Hau et al. 2004).

mAb (to Tf receptors, and insulin receptors), cationized proteins (e.g., cationized human serum albumin), endogenous peptides, and plasma proteins have been conjugated onto the liposome surface for ligand-mediated targeting to the brain (Allhenn et al. 2012). With this advanced functionalization, they can easily cross the BBB through absorptive-mediated transcytosis or by receptor-mediated transcytosis (Alam et al. 2010). *In vitro* and *in vivo* investigations have demonstrated the possibilities of liposomes in drug delivery to the brain. For example, palmitoyl ascorbate-based liposomes can increase the anticancer activity of paclitaxel (Sawant et al. 2010). Liposomes surface functionalized with *p*-aminophenyl-*α*-D-mannopyranoside and Tf moieties can significantly increase the accumulation of daunorubicin in gliomas (Ying et al. 2010).

Lipid nanoparticles

Lipid NPs for drug delivery to the brain consist of a monolayer of lipids as a shell to enclose a hydrophobic drug (Mulder et al. 2006). The incorporation of lipids with a functional moiety (i.e., phosphatidylethanolamine) to the NP structure facilitated the specific interaction of the drug nanocarrier with molecular markers, thus selectively accumulating at the disease site. Several proteins and peptides can be conjugated to the NP structure using different coupling strategies (Mulder et al. 2006).

Lipid NPs are classified into: Solid Lipid NPs (SLNs) and lipid nanocapsules. SLNs consist of a nano-sized spherical solid lipid matrix stabilized by surfactants, and the lipids included in their composition (e.g., triglycerides, complex glyceride mixtures, and waxes) have the particularity of being in a solid form at both room and physiological temperatures (Béduneau et al. 2007). SLNs are generally made of a solid hydrophobic core (where hydrophobic drugs can be found dissolved or dispersed) coated by a monolayer of phospholipids with the polar head groups oriented out of the NP structure (in which hydrophilic drugs may be incorporated) (Kaura et al. 2008, Humtsoe et al. 2011). They can be easily dispersed in water or in an aqueous surfactant solution. It is considered that the physical chemistry of SLNs are particularly suitable for drug delivery to the brain (Ekambaram et al. 2012). SLNs can further take advantage of surface functionalization strategies to facilitate the bypass of the BBB, i.e., lipoproteins have been postulated to target SLNs to brain capillary ECs (Humtsoe et al.

2011). In another study, it was described how SLNs grafted with the anti-Epithelial Growth Factor Receptor (anti-EGFR) can optimize the delivery of doxorubicin to malignant U87MG cells (Kuo and Liang 2011).

Regarding lipid nanocapsules, they are composed of a liquid, oily core (medium-chain triglycerides) surrounded by hydrophilic (PEG 660-hydroxystearate) and lipophilic (phosphatidylethanolamine and phosphatidylcholine) surfactants (Béduneau et al. 2007). They are characterized by high drug loading efficiencies (Venturini et al. 2011). For example, lipid nanocapsules were produced by a phase inversion-based method for the administration of 7-ethyl-10-hydroxy-camptothecin to the brain by the oral route (Roger et al. 2011). Surface decoration with adequate ligands is considered a useful drug targeting strategy to the brain, e.g., with peptides that interact with tubulin-binding sites, or mAbs targeting Tf receptors (Laine et al. 2012).

Inorganic nanoparticles

Inorganic NPs, e.g., iron oxides, can cross the BBB acting as drug delivery or diagnostic nanosystems for numerous pathologies associated to the CNS (Su et al. 2011). The penetration across the BBB and distribution into the brain parenchyma of PEGylated fluorescein-doped magnetic silica NPs into the BBB have been satisfactorily characterized at the cellular level (by confocal laser scanning microscopy) and at the subcellular level (by transmission electron microscopy) (Ku et al. 2010). Gum Arabic-coated magnetic iron oxide NPs ($\approx$ 100 nm in size) can specifically accumulate at the tumor site following intravenous administration to rats harboring 9L glioma tumors, with the help of an external magnetic field (Zhang et al. 2009).

Gold NPs are also a promising tool for the treatment and diagnosis of brain pathologies, especially if they are surface modified to augment its lipophilic character and to reduce its negative electrical surface charge (Guerrero et al. 2010). Conjugating the NPs with the amphipathic peptide CLPFFD, increased the Au concentration by four-fold and simultaneously reduced its retention by the spleen 1 and 2 hours after the injection. Additionally, the NPs did not alter the integrity of the BBB and had no effect on cell viability. In another study (Sousa et al. 2010), the biodistribution of polyelectrolyte multilayer-coated gold NPs in mice was analyzed up to seven days after the injection. The peak concentration in the brain was detected between 19 and 24 hours. *Ex vivo* studies determined that gold NPs mainly accumulate in the hippocampus, thalamus, hypothalamus, and the cerebral cortex.

Conclusions

The development of nanocarriers able to take advantage of any disruption of the BBB is one of the most promising strategies to deliver therapeutic agents to the brain. In this line, an ideal drug nanocarrier should: (i) selectively bypass the BBB; (ii) carry a large drug payload; (iii) transport drug molecules across the cerebral vasculature and deliver them into the site of action; and, (iv) display an extended plasma half-life.

However, some questions need to be better understood to facilitate the complete introduction into the clinic of nanotechnology-based drug delivery to the brain. Challenges yet to be overcome include identification of disease-associated changes in the characteristics of the BBB, and the proper modification of drug molecules or drug nanocarriers with targeting and transport-enhancing agents, e.g., mAbs, peptides, and proteins. Nevertheless, further in-depth studies in the field are needed, given the high complexity of the CNS. In the near future, there will be plenty of possibilities to be explored to optimize drug (nano) delivery to the brain.

Abbreviations

AD	:	Alzheimer's disease
Aβ	:	β-amyloid
ALS	:	amyotrophic lateral sclerosis
anti-EGFR	:	anti-epithelial growth factor receptor
ApoE	:	apolipoprotein E
BBB	:	blood-brain barrier
BM	:	basement membrane
BCSFB	:	blood-cerebrospinal fluid barrier
CAT1	:	cationic amino acid transporter 1
CD	:	cyclodextrin
CNS	:	central nervous system
CNT2	:	concentrative nucleoside transporter 2
CS	:	chitosan
DNA	:	deoxyribonucleic acid
EC	:	endothelial cell
FDA	:	Food and Drug Administration
GLUT1	:	glucose transporter 1
LAT1	:	large neutral amino acid transporter 1
mAb	:	monoclonal antibody
MCT1	:	monocarboxylic acid transporter 1
MS	:	multiple sclerosis
NP	:	nanoparticle
PD	:	Parkinson's disease
PLGA	:	poly(D,L-lactide-*co*-glycolide)
P-gp	:	P-glycoprotein
SLN	:	solid lipid nanoparticle
TJ	:	tight junction
Tf	:	transferrin
VEGF	:	vascular endothelial growth factor

References

Abbott, N.J. 2002. Astrocyte-endothelial interactions and blood-brain barrier permeability. J. Anat. 200: 629–638.

Abbott, N.J. and A.A. Patabendige, D.E. Dolman, S.R. Yusof and D.J. Begley. 2010. Structure and function of the blood-brain barrier. Neurobiol. Dis. 37: 13–25.

Agarwal, A. and N. Lariya, G. Saraogi, N. Dubey, H. Agrawal and G.P. Agrawal. 2009. Nanoparticles as novel carrier for brain delivery: a review. Curr. Pharm. Design. 15: 917–925.

Aktaş, Y. and K. Andrieux, M.J. Alonso, P. Calvo, R.N. Gürsoy, P. Couvreur and Y. Capan. 2005. Preparation and *in vitro* evaluation of chitosan nanoparticles containing a caspase inhibitor. Int. J. Pharm. 298: 378–383.

Alam, M.I. and S. Beg, A. Samad, S. Baboota, K. Kohli, J. Ali, A. Ahuja and M. Akbar. 2010. Strategy for effective brain drug delivery. Eur. J. Pharm. Sci. 40: 385–403.

Alexander, J.S. and M.K. Harris, S.R. Wells, G. Mills, K. Chalamidas, V.C. Ganta, J. McGee, M.H. Jennings, E. Gonzalez-Toledo and A. Minagar. 2010. Alterations in serum MMP-8, MMP-9, IL-12p40 and IL-23 in multiple sclerosis patients treated with interferon-beta1b. Mult. Scler. 16: 801–809.

Allaman, I. and M. Belanger and P.J. Magistretti. 2011. Astrocyte-neuron metabolic relationships: for better and for worse. Trends Neurosci. 34: 76–87.

Allhenn, D. and M.A.S. Boushehri and A. Lamprecht. 2012. Drug delivery strategies for the treatment of malignant gliomas. Int. J. Pharm. 436: 299–310.

Anderson, J.M. and M.S. Shive. 1997. Biodegradation and biocompatibility of PLA and PLGA microspheres. Adv. Drug Deliv. Rev. 28: 5–24.

Armulik, A. and G. Genové, M. Mäe, M.H. Nisancioglu, E. Wallgard, C. Niaudet, L. He, J. Norlin, P. Lindblom, K. Strittmatter, B.R. Johansson and C. Betsholtz. 2010. Pericytes regulate the blood-brain barrier. Nature. 468: 557–561.

Astete, C.E. and C.M. Sabliov. 2006. Synthesis and characterization of PLGA nanoparticles. J. Biomat. Sci. Polym. 17: 247–289.

Ballabh, P. and A. Braun and M. Nedergaard. 2004. The blood-brain barrier: an overview: structure, regulation, and clinical implications. Neurobiol. Dis. 16: 1–13.

Béduneau, A. and P. Saulniera and J.P. Benoit. 2007. Active targeting of brain tumors using nanocarriers. Biomaterials. 28: 4947–4967.

Bell, R.D. and B.V. Zlokovic. 2009. Neurovascular mechanisms and blood-brain barrier disorder in Alzheimer's disease. Acta Neuropathol. 118: 103–113.

Bell, R.D. and E.A. Winkler, A.P. Sagare, I. Singh, B. LaRue, R. Deane and B.V. Zlokovic. 2010. Pericytes control key neurovascular functions and neuronal phenotype in the adult brain and during brain aging. Neuron. 68: 409–427.

Bell, R.D. and E.A. Winkler, I. Singh, A.P. Sagare, R. Deane, Z. Wu, D.M. Holtzman, C. Betsholtz, A. Armulik, J. Sallstrom, B.C. Berk and B.V. Zlokovic. 2012. Apolipoprotein E controls cerebrovascular integrity via cyclophilin A. Nature. 485: 512–516.

Bernacki, J. and A. Dobrowolska, K. Nierwinska and A. Malecki. 2008. Physiology and pharmacological role of the blood-brain barrier. Pharmacol. Rep. 60: 600–622.

Bernardi, A. and E. Braganhol, E. Jäger, F. Figueiró, M.I. Edelweiss, A.R. Pohlmann, S.S. Guterres and A. Battastini. 2009. Indomethacin-loaded nanocapsules treatment reduces *in vivo* glioblastoma growth in a rat glioma model. Cancer Lett. 281: 53–63.

Bhaskar, S. and F. Tian, T. Stoeger, W. Kreyling, J.M. de la Fuente, V. Grazú, P. Borm, G. Estrada, V. Ntziachristos and D. Razansky. 2010. Multifunctional nanocarriers for diagnostics, drug delivery and targeted treatment across blood-brain barrier: perspectives on tracking and neuroimaging. Part. Fibre Toxicol. 7: 3.

Bower, J.H. and D.M. Maraganore, B.J. Peterson, S.K. McDonnell, J.E. Ahlskog and W.A. Rocca. 2003. Head trauma preceding PD: a case-control study. Neurology. 60: 1610–1615.

Brewster, M.E. and T. Loftsson. 2002. The use of chemically modified cyclodextrins in the development of formulations for chemical delivery systems. Pharmazie. 57: 94–101.

Cardoso, F.L. and D. Brites and M.A. Brito. 2010. Looking at the blood-brain barrier: molecular anatomy and possible investigation approaches. Brain Res. Rev. 64: 328–363.

Carvey, P.M. and B. Hendey and A.J. Monahan. 2009. The blood-brain barrier in neurodegenerative disease: a rhetorical perspective. J. Neurochem. 111: 291–314.

Castellano, J.M. and J. Kim, F.R. Stewart, H. Jiang, R.B. DeMattos, B.W. Patterson, A.M. Fagan, J.C. Morris, K.G. Mawuenyega, C. Cruchaga, A.M. Goate, K.R. Bales, S.M. Paul, R.J. Bateman and D.M. Holtzman. 2011. Human apoE isoforms differentially regulate brain amyloid-β peptide clearance. Sci. Transl. Med. 3: 89ra57.

Chang, J. and Y. Jallouli, M. Kroubi, X. Yuan, W. Feng, C. Kang, P. Pu and D. Betbeder. 2009. Characterization of endocytosis of Tf-coated PLGA nanoparticles by the blood-brain barrier. Int. J. Pharm. 379: 285–292.

Chang, J. and A. Paillard, C. Passirani, M. Morille, J.P. Benoit, D. Betbeder and E. Garcion. 2012. Transferrin adsorption onto PLGA nanoparticles governs their interaction with biological systems from blood circulation to brain cancer cells. Pharm. Res. 29: 1495–1505.

Chen, Y. and L. Liu. 2012. Modern methods for delivery of drugs across the blood-brain barrier. Adv. Drug Deliv. Rev. 64: 640–665.

Daneman, R. and L. Zhou, A.A. Kebede and B.A. Barres. 2010. Pericytes are required for blood-brain barrier integrity during embryogenesis. Nature. 468: 562–566.

Daniels, T.R. and E. Bernabeu, J.A. Rodríguez, S. Patel, M. Kozman, D.A. Chiappetta, E. Holler, J.Y. Ljubimova, G. Helguera and M.L. Penichet. 2012. The transferrin receptor and the targeted delivery of therapeutic agents against cancer. Biochim. Biophys. Acta. 1820: 291–317.

Das, D. and S. Lin. 2005. Double-coated poly (butylcyanoacrylate) nanoparticulate delivery systems forbrain targeting of dalargin via oral administration. J. Pharm. Sci. 94: 1343–1353.

Deane, R. and S. Du Yan, R.K. Submamaryan, B. LaRue, S. Jovanovic, E. Hogg, D. Welch, L. Manness, C. Lin, J. Yu, H. Zhu, J. Ghiso, B. Frangione, A. Stern, A.M. Schmidt, D.L. Armstrong, B. Arnold, B. Liliensiek, P. Nawroth, F. Hofman, M. Kindy, D. Stern and B. Zlokovic. 2003. RAGE mediates amyloid-beta peptide transport across the blood-brain barrier and accumulation in brain. Nat. Med. 9: 907–913.

Dhanikula, R.S. and A. Argaw, J.F. Bouchard and P. Hildgen. 2008. Methotrexate loaded polyether-copolyester dendrimers for the treatment of gliomas: enhanced efficacy and intratumoral transport capability. Mol. Pharm. 5: 105–116.

Dore-Duffy, P. 2008. Pericytes: pluripotent cells of the blood brain barrier. Curr. Pharm. Des. 14: 1581–1593.

Dore-Duffy, P. and K. Cleary. 2011. Morphology and properties of pericytes. Methods Mol. Biol. 686: 49–68.

Du, J. and W.L. Lu, X. Ying, Y. Liu, P. Du, W. Tian, Y. Men, J. Guo, Y. Zhang, R.J. Li, J. Zhou, J.N. Lou, J.C. Wang, X. Zhang and Q. Zhang. 2009. Dual-targeting topotecan liposomes modified with tamoxifen and wheat germ agglutinin significantly improve drug transport across the blood-brain barrier and survival of brain tumor-bearing animals. Mol. Pharm. 6: 905–917.

Ekambaram, P. and A.A.H. Sathali and K. Priyanka. 2012. Solid nanoparticle: a review. Sci. Revs. Chem. Commun. 2: 80–102.

Farkas, E. and P.G. Luiten. 2001. Cerebral microvascular pathology in aging and Alzheimer's disease. Prog. Neurobiol. 64: 575–611.

Fernández-Klett, F. and N. Offenhauser, U. Dirnagl, J. Priller and U. Lindauer. 2010. Pericytes in capillaries are contractile *in vivo*, but arterioles mediate functional hyperemia in the mouse brain. Proc. Natl. Acad. Sci. U.S.A. 107: 22290–22295.

Ferrara, N. 2000. Vascular endothelial growth factor and the regulation of angiogenesis. Recent Prog. Horm. Res. 55: 15–35.

Fuller, S. and M. Steele and G. Munch. 2010. Activated astroglia during chronic inflammation in Alzheimer's disease—do they neglect their neurosupportive roles? Mutat. Res. 690: 40–49.

Gao, K. and X. Jiang. 2006. Influence of particle size on transport of methotrexate across blood brainbarrier by polysorbate 80-coated polybutylcyanoacrylate nanoparticles. Int. J. Pharm. 310: 213–219.

Gao, H. and J. Qian, S. Cao, Z. Yang, Z. Pang, S. Pan, S. Fan, Z. Xi, X. Jiang and Q. Zhang. 2012a. Precise glioma targeting of and penetration by aptamer and peptide dual-functioned nanoparticles. Biomaterials. 33: 5115–5123.

Gao, H. and J. Qian, Z. Yang, Z. Pang, Z. Xi, S. Cao, Y. Wang, S. Pan, S. Zhang, W. Wang, X. Jiang and Q. Zhang. 2012b. Whole-cell SELEX aptamer-functionalised poly (ethyleneglycol)-poly(ε-caprolactone) nanoparticles for enhanced targeted glioblastoma therapy. Biomaterials. 33: 6264–6273.

Garbuzova-Davis, S. and M.C. Rodrigues, D.G. Hernandez-Ontiveros, M.K. Louis, A.E. Willing, C.V. Borlongan and P.R. Sanberg. 2011. Amyotrophic lateral sclerosis: a neurovascular disease. Brain Res. 29: 113–125.

Gaucher, G. and M.H. Dufresne, V.P. Sant, N. Kang, D. Maysinger and J.C. Leroux. 2005. Block copolymer micelles: preparation, characterization and application in drug delivery. J. Control. Release. 109: 169–188.

Genin, E. and D. Hannequin, D. Wallon, K. Sleegers, M. Hiltunen, O. Combarros, M.J. Bullido, S. Engelborghs, P. De Deyn, C. Berr, F. Pasquier, B. Dubois, G. Tognoni, N. Fiévet, N. Brouwers, K. Bettens, B. Arosio, E. Coto, M. Del Zompo, I. Mateo, J. Epelbaum, A. Frank-Garcia, S. Helisalmi, E. Porcellini, A. Pilotto, P. Forti, R. Ferri, E. Scarpini, G. Siciliano, V. Solfrizzi, S. Sorbi, G. Spalletta, F. Valdivieso, S. Vepsäläinen, V. Alvarez, P. Bosco, M. Mancuso, F. Panza, B. Nacmias, P. Bossù, O. Hanon, P. Piccardi, G. Annoni, D. Seripa, D. Galimberti, F. Licastro, H. Soininen, J.F. Dartigues, M.I. Kamboh, C. Van Broeckhoven, J.C. Lambert, P. Amouyel and D. Campion. 2011. APOE and Alzheimer's disease: a major gene with semi-dominant inheritance. Mol. Psychiatry. 16: 903–907.

Golias, C. and A. Batistatou, G. Bablekos, A. Charalabopoulos, D. Peschos, P. Mitsopoulos and K. Charalabopoulos. 2011. Physiology and pathophysiology of selectins, integrins, and IgSF cell adhesion molecules focusing on inflammation. A paradigm model on infectious endocarditis. Cell Commun. Adhes. 18: 19–32.

Guerrero, S. and E. Araya, J.L. Fiedler, J.I. Arias, C. Adura, F. Albericio, E. Giralt, J.L. Arias, M.S. Fernández and M.J. Kogan. 2010. Improving the brain delivery of gold nanoparticles by conjugation with an amphipathic peptide. Nanomedicine (Lond.). 5: 897–913.

Hallmann, R. and N. Horn, M. Selg, O. Wendler, F. Pausch and L.M. Sorokin. 2005. Expression and function of laminins in the embryonic and mature vasculature. Physiol. Rev. 85: 979–1000.

Hartsock, A. and W.J. Nelson. 2008. Adherens and tight junctions: structure, function and connections to the actin cytoskeleton. Biochim. Biophys. Acta. 1778: 660–669.

Hau, P. and K. Fabel, U. Baumgart, P. Rummele, O. Grauer, A. Bock, C. Dietmaier, W. Dietmaier, J. Dietrich, C. Dudel, F. Hübner, T. Jauch, E. Drechsel, I. Kleiter, C. Wismeth, A. Zellner, A. Brawanski, A. Steinbrecher, J. Marienhagen and U. Bogdahn. 2004. Pegylated liposomal doxorubicin-efficacy in patients with recurrent high-grade glioma. Cancer. 100: 1199–1207.

Henkel, J.S. and D.R. Beers, S. Wen, R. Bowser and S.H. Appel. 2009. Decreased mRNA expression of tight junction proteins in lumbar spinal cords of patients with ALS. Neurology. 72: 1614–1616.

Hu, K. and Y. Shi, W. Jiang, J. Han, S. Huang and X. Jiang. 2011. Lactoferrin conjugated PEG-PLGA nanoparticles for brain delivery: preparation, characterization and efficacy in Parkinson's disease. Int. J. Pharm. 415: 273–283.

Huang, R. and Y.H. Qu, W. Ke, J.H. Zhu, Y. Pei and C. Jiang. 2007. Efficient gene delivery targeted to the brain using a transferrin-conjugated polyethylene glycol-modified polyamidoamine dendrimer. FASEB J. 21: 1117–1125.

Huang, R. and W. Ke, Y. Liu, C. Jiang and Y. Pei. 2008. The use of lactoferrin as a ligand for targeting the polyamidoamine-based gene delivery system to the brain. Biomaterials. 29: 238–246.

Humtsoe, L.C. and N. Jawahar, K. Gowthamarajan, S.N. Meyyanathan and S. Sood. 2011. Brain delivery by solid lipid nanoparticles for CNS drugs. Int. J. Pharm. Res. Dev. 3: 206–216.

Jaruszewski, K.M. and S. Ramakrishnan, J.F. Poduslo and K.K. Kandimalla. 2012. Chitosan enhances the stability and targeting of immuno-nanovehicles to cerebro-vascular deposits of Alzheimer's disease amyloid protein. Nanomedicine. 8: 250–260.

Jellinger, K.A. 2002. Alzheimer's disease and cerebrovascular pathology: an update. J. Neural. Transm. 109: 813–836.

Jorm, A.F. and D. Jolley. 1998. The incidence of dementia: a meta-analysis. Neurology. 728–733.

Kabanov, A.V. and V.Y. Alakhov. 2002. Pluronic block copolymers in drug delivery: from micellar nanocontainers to biological response modifiers. Crit. Rev. Ther. Drug Carrier Syst. 19: 1–72.

Karatas, H. and Y. Aktas, Y. Gursoy-Ozdemir, E. Bodur, M. Yemisci, S. Caban, A. Vural, O. Pinarbasli, Y. Capan, E. Fernandez-Megia, R. Novoa-Carballal, R. Riguera, K. Andrieux, P.

Couvreur and T. Dalkara. 2009. A nanomedicine transports a peptide caspase-3 inhibitor across the blood-brain barrier and provides neuroprotection. J. Neurosci. 29: 13761–13769.

Kaura, I.P. and R. Bhandarib, S. Bhandarib and V. Kakkara. 2008. Potential of solid lipid nanoparticles in brain targeting. J. Control. Release. 127: 97–109.

Ke, W. and K. Shao, R. Huang, L. Han, Y. Liu, J. Li, Y. Kuang, L. Ye, J. Lou and C. Jiang. 2009. Gene delivery targeted to the brain using an Angiopep-conjugated polyethyleneglycol-modified polyamidoamine dendrimer. Biomaterials. 30: 6976–6985.

Kim, J.A. and N.D. Tran, Z. Li, F. Yang, W. Zhou and M.J. Fisher. 2006. Brain endothelial hemostasis regulation by pericytes. J. Cereb. Blood Flow Metab. 26: 209–217.

Kirk, J. and J. Plumb, M. Mirakhur and S. McQuaid. 2003. Tight junctional abnormality in multiple sclerosis white matter affects all calibres of vessel and is associated with blood-brain barrier leakage and active demyelination. J. Pathol. 201: 319–327.

Kniesel, U. and H. Wolburg. 2000. Tight junctions of the blood-brain barrier. Cell. Mol. Neurobiol. 20: 57–76.

Kortekaas, R. and K.L. Leenders, J.C. van Oostrom, W. Vaalburg, J. Bart, A.T. Willemsen and N.H. Hendrikse. 2005. Blood-brain barrier dysfunction in parkinsonian midbrain *in vivo*. Ann. Neurol. 57: 176–179.

Kreuter, J. and P. Ramge, V. Petrov, S. Hamm, S.E. Gelperina, B. Engelhardt, R. Alyautdin, H. von Briesen, and D.J. Begley. 2003. Direct evidence that polysorbate-80-coated poly(butylcyanoacrylate) nanoparticles deliver drugs to the CNS via specific mechanisms requiring prior binding of drug to the nanoparticles. Pharm. Res. 20: 409–416.

Ku, S.T. and F. Yan, Y. Wang, Y.L. Sun, N. Yang and L. Ye. 2010. The blood-brain barrier penetration and distribution of PEGylated fluorescein-doped magnetic silica nanoparticles in rat brain. Biochem. Biophys. Res. Commun. 394: 871–876.

Kuo, Y. and C. Liang. 2011. Cationic solid lipid nanoparticles carrying doxorubicin for inhibiting the growth of U87MG cells. Colloid Surf. B Biointerfaces. 85: 131–137.

Kuo, Y. and P. Lin and C. Wang. 2011. Targeting nevirapine delivery across human brain microvascular endothelial cells using transferrin-grafted poly(lactide-co-glycolide) nanoparticles. Nanomedicine (Lond.). 6: 1011–1026.

Kurakhmaeva, K.B. and I.A. Djindjikhashvili, V.E. Petrov, V.U. Balabanyan, T.A. Voronina, S.S. Trofimov, J. Kreuter, S. Gelperina, D. Begley and R.N. Alyautdin. 2009. Brain targeting of nerve growth factor using poly(butyl cyanoacrylate) nanoparticles. J. Drug Target. 17: 564–574.

Laine, A.L. and N.T. Huynh, A. Clavreul, J. Balzeau, J. Béjaud, A. Vessieres, J.P. Benoit, J. Eyer and C. Passirani. 2012. Brain tumour targeting strategies via coted ferrociphenol lipid nanocapsules. Eur. J. Pharm. Biopharm. 81: 690–693.

Leech, S. and J. Kirk, J. Plumb and S. McQuaid. 2007. Persistent endothelial abnormalities and blood-brain barrier leak in primary and secondary progressive multiple sclerosis. Neuropathol. Appl. Neurobiol. 33: 86–98.

Li, J. and L. Feng, L. Fan, Y. Zha, L. Guo, Q. Zhang, J. Chen, Z. Pang, Y. Wang, Y. Jiang, Y. Xinguo, V.C. Yang and L. Wen. 2011. Targeting the brain with PEG-PLGA nanoparticles modified with phage-displayed peptides. Biomaterials. 32: 4943–4950.

Li, Y. and H. He, X. Jia, W.L. Lu, J. Lou and Y. Wei. 2012. A dual-targeting nanocarrier based on poly(amidoamine) dendrimers conjugated with transferrin and tamoxifen for treating brain gliomas. Biomaterials. 33: 3899–3908.

Ling, Y. and K. Wei, F. Zou and S. Zhong. 2012. Temozolomide loaded PLGA-based superparamagnetic nanoparticles for magnetic resonance imaging and treatment of malignant glioma. Int. J. Pharm. 430: 266–275.

Lockman, P.R. and R.J. Mumper, M.A. Khan and D.D. Allen. 2002. Nanoparticle technology for drug delivery across blood-brain barrier. Drug Dev. Ind. Pharm. 28: 749–771.

Markoutsa, E. and G. Pampalakis, A. Niarakis, I.A. Romero, B. Weksler, P. Couraud and S.G. Antimisiaris. 2011. Uptake and permeability studies of BBB-targeting immunoliposomes using the hCMEC/D3 cell line. Eur. J. Pharm. Biopharm. 77: 265–274.

Martín-Banderas, L. and M.A. Holgado, J.L. Venero, J. Álvarez-Fuentes and M. Fernández-Arévalo. 2011. Nanostructures for drug delivery to the brain. Curr. Med. Chem. 18: 5303–5321.

Mathew, A. and T. Fukuda, Y. Nagaoka, T. Hasumura, H. Morimoto, Y. Yoshida, T. Maekawa, K. Venugopal and D. Sakthi. 2012. Curcumin loaded-PLGA nanoparticles conjugated with tet-1 peptide for potential use in Alzheimer's disease. PLoS One. 7: e32616.

Mittal, G. and H. Carswell, R. Brett, S. Currie and M.N.V. Kumar. 2011. Development and evaluation of polymer nanoparticles for oral delivery of estradiol to rat brain in a model of Alzheimer's pathology. J. Control. Release. 150: 220–228.

Monnaert, V. and S. Tilloy, H. Bricout, L. Fenart, R. Cecchelli and E. Monflier. 2004. Behavior of alpha-, beta-, and gamma-cyclodextrins and their derivatives on an *in vitro* model of blood-brain barrier, J. Pharmacol. Exp. Ther. 310: 745–751.

Mouradian, M.M. 2002. Recent advances in the genetics and pathogenesis of Parkinson's disease. Neurology. 58: 179–185.

Mulder, W.J.M. and G.J. Strijkers, G.A.F. Tilborg, A.W. Griffioen and K. Nicolay. 2006. Lipid-based nanoparticles for contrast-enhanced MRI and molecular imaging. NMR Biomed. 19: 142–164.

Nag, S. and A. Kapadia and D.J. Stewart. 2011. Review: molecular pathogenesis of blood-brain barrier breakdown in acute brain injury. Neuropathol. Appl. Neurobiol. 37: 3–23.

Najlah, M. and A. D'Emanuele. 2006. Crossing cellular barriers using dendrimer nanotechnologies. Curr. Opin. Pharm. 6: 522–527.

Nonaka, N. and S.A. Farr, H. Kageyama, S. Shioda and W.A. Banks. 2008. Delivery of galaninlike peptide to the brain: targeting with intranasal delivery and cyclodextrins. J. Pharmacol. Exp. Ther. 325: 513–519.

Obeso, J.A. and M.C. Rodriguez-Oroz, M. Rodriguez, J.L. Lanciego, J. Artieda, N. Gonzalo and C.W. Olanow. 2000. Pathophysiology of the basal ganglia in Parkinson's disease. Trends Neurosci. 23: S8–S19.

Pardridge, W.M. 1999. Blood-brain barrier biology and methodology. J. Neurovirol. 5: 556–569.

Patel, M.M. and B.R. Goyal, S.V. Bhadada, J.S. Bhatt and A.F. Amin. 2009. Getting into the brain: approaches to enhance brain drug delivery. CNS Drugs. 23: 35–58.

Patel, T. and J. Zhou, J.M. Piepmeier and W.M. Saltzman. 2012. Polymeric nanoparticles for drug delivery to the central nervous system. Adv. Drug Deliv. Rev. 64: 701–705.

Persidsky, Y. and S.H. Ramirez, J. Haorah and G.D. Kanmogne. 2006. Blood-brain barrier: structural components and function under physiologic and pathologic conditions. J. Neuroimmune Pharmacol. 1: 223–236.

Petri, B. and A. Bootz, A. Khalansky, T. Hekmatara, R. Müller, R. Uhl, J. Kreuter and S. Gelperina. 2007. Chemotherapy of brain tumour using doxorubicin bound to surfactant-coated poly(butyl cyanoacrylate) nanoparticles: revisiting the role of surfactants. J. Control. Release. 117: 51–58.

Petty, M.A. and E.H. Lo. 2002. Junctional complexes of the blood-brain barrier: permeability changes in neuroinflammation. Prog. Neurobiol. 68: 311–323.

Ratheesh, A. and A.S. Yap. 2012. A bigger picture: classical cadherins and the dynamic actin cytoskeleton. Nat. Rev. Mol. Cell Biol. 13: 673–679.

Redzic, Z.B. and J.E. Preston, J.A. Duncan, A. Chodobski and J. Szmydynger-Chodobska. 2005. The choroid plexus-cerebrospinal fluid system: from development to aging. Curr. Top. Dev. Biol. 71: 1–52.

Rite, I. and A. Machado, J. Cano and J.L. Venero. 2007. Blood-brain barrier disruption induces *in vivo* degeneration of nigral dopaminergic neurons. J. Neurochem. 101: 1567–1582.

Roger, E. and F. Lagarce and J.P. Benoit. 2011. Development and characterization of a novel lipid nanocapsule formulation of Sn38 for oral administration. Eur. J. Pharm. Biopharm. 79: 181–188.

Rosenberg, G.A. 2009. Matrix metalloproteinases and their multiple roles in neurodegenerative diseases. Lancet Neurol. 8: 205–216.

Sanders, P. and J. De Keyser. 2007. Janus faces of microglia in multiple sclerosis. Brain Res. Rev. 54: 274–285.

Sawant, R.R. and O.S. Vaze, K. Rockwell and V.P. Torchilin. 2010. Palmitoyl ascorbate-modified liposomes as nanoparticle platform for ascorbate-mediated cytotoxicity and paclitaxel co-delivery. Eur. J. Pharm. Biopharm. 75: 321–326.

Selkoe, D.J. and D. Schenk. 2003. Alzheimer's disease: molecular understanding predicts amyloid-based therapeutics. Annu. Rev. Pharmacol. Toxicol. 43: 545–584.

Shao, K. and R. Huang, J. Li, L. Han, L. Ye, J. Lou and C. Jiang. 2010. Angiopep-2 modified PE-PEG based polymeric micelles for amphotericin B delivery targeted to the brain. J. Control. Release. 147: 118–126.

Songjiang, Z. and W. Lixiang. 2009. Amyloid-beta associated with chitosan nano-carrier has favorable immunogenicity and permeates the BBB. AAPS Pharm. Sci. Tech. 10: 900–905.

Sousa, F. and S. Mandal, C. Garrovo, A. Astolfo, A. Bonifacio, D. Latawiec, R.H. Menk, F. Arfelli, S. Huewel, G. Legname, H.J. Galla and S. Krol. 2010. Functionalized gold nanoparticles: a detailed *in vivo* ultimodal microscopic brain distribution study. Nanoscale. 2: 2826–2834.

Su, X. and X. Zhan, F. Tang, J.Y. Yao and J. Wu. 2011. Magnetic nanoparticles in brain disease diagnosis and targeting drug delivery. Curr. Nanosci. 7: 37–46.

Sykova, E. 1991. Ionic and volume changes in neuronal microenvironment. Physiol. Res. 40: 213–222.

Tahara, K. and Y. Miyazaki, Y. Kawashima, J. Kreuter and H. Yamamoto. 2011. Brain targeting with surface-modified poly(D,L-lactic-co-glycolic acid) nanoparticles delivered via carotid artery administration. Eur. J. Pharm. Biopharm. 77: 84–88.

Tilloy, S. and V. Monnaert, L. Fenart, H. Bricout, R. Cecchelli and E. Monflier. 2006. Methylated beta-cyclodextrin as P-gp modulators for deliverance of doxorubicin across an *in vitro* model of blood–brain barrier. Bioorg. Med. Chem. Lett. 16: 2154–2157.

Tsai, C.H. and S.K. Lo, L.C. See, H.Z. Chen, R.S. Chen, Y.H. Weng, F.C. Chang and C.S. Lu. 2002. Environmental risk factors of young onset Parkinson's disease: a case-control study. Clin. Neurol. Neurosurg. 104: 328–333.

Ueno, M. 2007. Molecular anatomy of the brain endothelial barrier: an overview of the distributional features. Curr. Med. Chem. 14: 1199–1206.

Venero, J.L. and M.L. Vizuete, A. Machado and J. Cano. 2001. Aquaporins in the central nervous system. Prog. Neurobiol. 63: 321–336.

Venturini, C.G. and E. Jäger, C.P. Oliveira, A. Bernardi, A.M.O. Battastini, S.S. Guterres and A.R. Pohlmann. 2011. Formulation of lipid core nanocapsules. Colloids Surf. A Physicochem. Eng. Aspects. 375: 200–208.

Wagner, S. and A. Zensi, S.L. Wien, S.E. Tschickardt, W. Maier, T. Vogel, F. Worek, C.U. Pietrzik, J. Kreuter and H. Briesen. 2012. Uptake mechanism of ApoE-modified nanoparticles on brain capillary endothelial cells as a blood-brain barrier model. PLoS One. 7: e32568.

Wang, C.X. and L.S. Huang, L.B. Hou, L. Jiang, Z.T. Yan, Y.L. Wang and Z.L. Chen. 2009. Antitumor effects of polysorbate-80 coated gemcitabine polybutylcyanoacrylate nanoparticles *in vitro* and its pharmacodynamics *in vivo* on C6 glioma cells of a brain tumor model. Brain Res. 1261: 91–99.

Weiss, N. and F. Miller, S. Cazaubon and P.O. Couraud. 2009. The blood-brain barrier in brain homeostasis and neurological diseases. Biochim. Biophys. Acta. 1788: 842–857.

Wilson, B. and M.K. Samanta, K. Santhi, K.P. Kumar, N. Paramakrishnan and B. Suresh. 2008. Poly(n-butylcyanoacrylate) nanoparticles coated with polysorbate 80 for the targeted delivery of rivastigmine into the brain to treat Alzheimer's disease. Brain Res. 1200: 159–168.

Wolburg, H. and S. Noell, A. Mack, K. Wolburg-Buchholz and P. Fallier-Becker. 2009. Brain endothelial cells and the glio-vascular complex. Cell Tissue Res. 335: 75–96.

Wu, Z. and H. Guo, N. Chow, J. Sallstrom, R.D. Bell, R. Deane, A.I. Brooks, S. Kanagala, A. Rubio, A. Sagare, D. Liu, F. Li, D. Armstrong, T. Gasiewicz, R. Zidovetzki, X. Song, F. Hofman and B.V. Zlokovic. 2005. Role of the MEOX2 homeobox gene in neurovascular dysfunction in Alzheimer's disease. Nat. Med. 11: 959–965.

Xie, F. and N. Yao, Y. Qin, Q. Zhang, H. Chen, M. Yuan, J. Tang, X. Li, W. Fan, Q. Zhang, Y. Wu, L. Hai and Q. He. 2012. Investigation of glucose-modified liposomes using polyethylene glycols with different chain lengths as the linkers for brain targeting. Int. J. Nanomedicine. 7: 163–175.

Xin, H. and L. Chen, J. Gu, X. Ren, Z. Wei, J. Luo, Y. Chen, X. Jiang, X. Sha and X. Fang. 2010. Enhanced anti-glioblastoma efficacy by PTX-loaded PEGylated poly(ε-caprolactone) nanoparticles: *in vitro* and *in vivo* evaluation. Int. J. Pharm. 402: 238–247.

Yasuda, T. and M. Fukuda-Tani, T. Nihira, K. Wada, N. Hattori, Y. Mizuno and H. Mochizuki. 2007. Correlation between levels of pigment epithelium-derived factor and vascular endothelial growth factor in the striatum of patients with Parkinson's disease. Exp. Neurol. 206: 308–317.

Yemisci, M. and Y. Gursoy-Ozdemir, A. Vural, A. Can, K. Topalkara and T. Dalkara. 2009. Pericyte contraction induced by oxidative-nitrative stress impairs capillary reflow despite successful opening of an occluded cerebral artery. Nat. Med. 15: 1031–1037.

Ying, X. and H. Wen, W.L. Lu, J. Du, J. Guo, W. Tian, Y. Men, Y. Zhang, R.J. Li, T.Y. Yang, D.W. Shang, J.N. Lou, L.R. Zhang and Q. Zhang. 2010. Dual-targeting daunorubicin liposomes improve the therapeutic efficacy of brain glioma in animals. J. Control. Release. 141: 183–192.

Yordanov, G. 2012. Poly(alkyl cyanoacrylate) nanoparticles as drug carriers: 33 years later. Bulg. J. Chem. 1: 61–73.

Zhang, S. and L. Wu. 2009. Amyloid-beta associated with chitosan nano-carrier has favourable immunogenicity and permeates BBB. AAPS Pharm. Sci. Tech. 10: 900–905.

Zhang, L. and F.Q. Yu, A.J. Cole, B. Chertok, A.E. David, J.K. Wang and V.C. Yang. 2009. Gum arabic-coated magnetic nanoparticles for potential application in simultaneous magnetic targeting and tumor imaging. AAPS J. 11: 693–699.

Zhang, P. and L. Hu, Q. Yin, Z. Zhang, L. Feng and Y. Li. 2012. Transferrin-conjugated polyphosphoester hybrid micelle loading paclitaxel for brain-targeting delivery: synthesis, preparation and *in vivo* evaluation. J. Control. Release. 159: 429–434.

Zhong, Z. and R. Deane, Z. Ali, M. Parisi, Y. Shapovalov, M.K. O'Banion, K. Stojanovic, A. Sagare, S. Boillee, D.W. Cleveland and B. Zlokovic. 2008. ALS-causing SOD1 mutants generate vascular changes prior to motor neuron degeneration. Nat. Neurosci. 11: 420–422.

Zlokovic, B.V. 2008. The blood-brain barrier in health and chronic neurodegenerative disorders. Neuron. 57: 178–201.

CHAPTER 10

Nanomaterials and Cancer Therapy

Laura Cabeza,[1,a,†] Gloria Perazzoli,[1,b,†] Raúl Ortiz,[2,c] Octavio Caba,[2,d] Pablo A. Álvarez,[1,e] Consolación Melguizo,[1,f] José C. Prados[1,*] and Antonia Aránega[1,g]

ABSTRACT

Nanotechnology plays an important role in developing a new generation of cancer therapies designed to overcome the numerous biological, biophysical, and biomedical obstacles to conventional treatments. A wide range of nanomedicines have been investigated for this purpose, including polymeric micelles and nanoparticles, dendrimers, and liposomes. The targeted delivery of drug molecules to the tumor tissue is one of the most important and challenging endeavors in pharmaceutics. Significant progress has been made over recent years in the ability to concentrate the drug at its site of action, leading to a significant improvement in the effects of chemotherapy while minimizing the associated toxicity. The chapter describes the different types of nanomaterials explored to date for cancer therapy, and outlines the significant advances achieved in improving drug delivery to tumor cells by an advanced functionalization of the nanoplatforms.

[1] Institute of Biopathology and Regenerative Medicine (IBIMER), Department of Anatomy and Embryology, School of Medicine, University of Granada, 18071 Granada, Spain.
[a] Email: lautea@correo.ugr.es
[b] Email: wannea@correo.ugr.es
[e] Email: pabrolancia@hotmail.com
[f] Email: melguizo@ugr.es
[g] Email: aranega@ugr.es
[2] Department of Health Sciences, University of Jaén, Jaén, Spain.
[c] Email: roquesa@ugr.es
[d] Email: ocaba@ugr.es
[†] Equally contributed to the Chapter.
[*] Corresponding author: jcprados@ugr.es

Introduction

According to the World Health Organization, cancer is a major cause of death worldwide, $\approx 13\%$ of all deaths. Deaths by cancer are expected to rise to > 13.1 million in the next two decades, being $\approx 70\%$ of all cancer deaths in low- and middle-income countries. Among women, the most frequent type is breast cancer, with an age-standardized rate per 100,000 of ≈ 66, while it is lung cancer among men, with an age-standardized rate of ≈ 62 (Jemal et al. 2011). The main objective of research in this field is to develop therapeutic strategies that cure the disease, or significantly prolong the life of the patient and improve its quality of life.

At present, the three pillars of cancer treatment are surgery, radiotherapy, and chemotherapy, applied individually or in combination. The first line of action in cancer is surgery, with the aim of eliminating part or most of the tumor. Surgical resection is the standard of care for early-stage cancers of different types, e.g., breast, lung, and carries only a low risk of hospital death and complications (Schroedl and Kalhan 2012). Radiation therapy can now be delivered with great precision, destroying tumors while limiting damage to nearby healthy tissues (Lawrence et al. 2008). Irradiation kills cancer cells by directly damaging their deoxyribonucleic acid (DNA) or by creating DNA-damaging free radicals within the cells. For its part, chemotherapy can kill cells that divide rapidly, one of the main properties of most malignant cells, but it also damages cells that divide rapidly in normal tissues, such as hair follicles, bone marrow, or the digestive tract. Currently, these techniques are typically used in treatment schedules that combine the effects of radiation therapy, and / or surgery, and / or chemotherapy. This approach has yielded good outcomes in breast cancer (Vilaprinyo et al. 2012) and brain cancer (Scoccianti et al. 2012) among others, but most advanced or recurrent cancers remain incurable by conventional treatments in any combination. In this context, the introduction of nanoparticles (NPs) in classical cancer treatments may confer several advantages of significant benefit for the prognosis of the patients.

Cancer and Tumor Cells

The term cancer refers to more than 100 diseases in which the body produces an excess of malignant cells. The main characteristics of these cells are their uncontrolled growth and their capacity to spread to other tissues (metastasis) (DeBerardinis and Thompson 2012). Further features of the cells include their ability to evade growth suppressors, sustain proliferative signaling, resist cell death, induce angiogenesis, and reprogram energy metabolism (Fig. 10.1).

Altered cell proliferation in cancer cells is related to tumor suppressor genes, among others. The main tumor suppressors encode the TP53 protein, which can arrest the cell cycle if damage to the genome is excessive or if levels of nucleotide pools, growth-promoting signals, glucose, or oxygenation

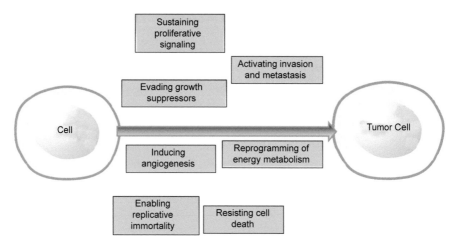

Figure 10.1. Major characteristics that enable tumor growth and metastatic dissemination.

are suboptimal (Suzuki and Matsubara 2011). Another suppressor is the retinoblastoma-associated protein, which controls whether or not a cell can advance through its growth and division cycle (Burkhart and Sage 2008). When either genes, retinoblastoma-associated or TP53, are altered, adequate cell cycle regulation fails and cell proliferation becomes persistent (Hanahan and Weinberg 2011). However, other mechanisms may underlie the immortality of tumor cells. Telomerase is a specialized DNA polymerase that adds telomere repeat segments to the ends of telomeric DNA (Blasco 2005), countering the progressive erosion of the telomere and thereby permitting replicative immortality in tumor cells (Hanahan and Weinberg 2011). Tumor cells can also achieve continuous proliferation by resisting cell death through the inhibition of apoptosis. Thus, the loss of TP53 tumor suppressor function not only modulates cell proliferation, but also eliminates a critical damage sensor for apoptosis. Cells can also avoid apoptosis by short-circuiting the extrinsic ligand-induced death pathway, by increasing the expression of anti-apoptotic regulators, e.g., Bcl-2 and Bcl-xL, or by down-regulating pro-apoptotic factors, e.g., Bax, Bim, and Puma (Adams and Cory 2007).

In order to grow, the tumor mass requires nutrients and oxygen (Hanahan and Weinberg 2011). Cancer cells sustain proliferation by sending signals to stimulate normal cells within the supporting tumor-associated stroma or by producing growth factor ligands that result in autocrine proliferative stimulation (Witsch et al. 2010). Angiogenesis is essential for all of these activities, and a continuous process of neoangiogenesis allows expansion of the tumor in cancer progression (Hanahan and Folkman 1996, Hanahan and Weinberg 2011).

The ability of tumor cells to metastasize remains an enigma. Local invasion and distant metastasis are known to be related to alterations in the shape of tumor cells, and to their adhesion to other cells and to the extracellular matrix.

Changes that have been linked to tumor cell mobility include the reduced expression or the alteration (by mutation) of E-cadherin, a key cell adhesion molecule (Berx and Van Roy 2009, Hanahan and Weinberg 2011). However, although some progress has been made in understanding these mechanisms, they are not well understood and require considerable further research.

Finally, energy metabolism reprogramming has emerged as a characteristic of tumor cells. One of the most striking discoveries was the cells' ability to reprogram their glucose metabolism by the so-called "aerobic glycolysis for energy production" (Jones and Thompson 2009, Hanahan and Weinberg 2011).

Multidrug resistance

Multidrug resistance (MDR) is one of the main causes of chemotherapy failure in most types of cancer. Some cells in the tumor are sensitive to chemotherapeutic drugs but others are intrinsically resistant, and chemotherapy destroys the sensitive cells but not the resistant cells, allowing the tumor to grow despite the treatment (Fig. 10.2). Different and unrelated mechanisms that may produce resistance to chemotherapy include enhancement of DNA repair or alterations to the drug metabolism, transmembrane drug transport, or drug target (Fig. 10.3).

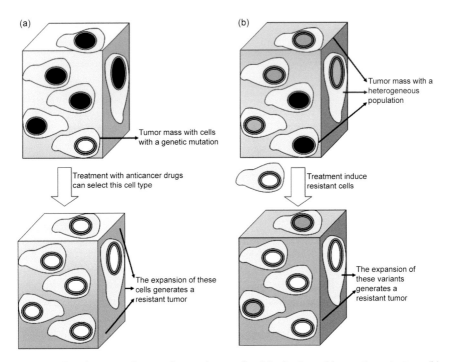

Figure 10.2. Development of cancer drug resistances by: (a) selection with genetic mutants, or (b) induction of a phenotypically resistant subpopulation.

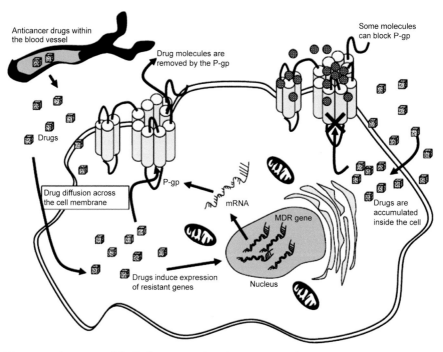

Figure 10.3. Activation of the P-glycoprotein (P-gp) resistance mechanism. Drug diffusion through the cell membrane induces expression of resistance genes that can be previously overexpressed in the cell. P-gp acts as an efflux pump that removes the drug from the cell cytoplasm. When the mechanism is blocked by P-gp inhibitors, drug accumulation occurs inside the cell. *m*RNA: messenger ribonucleic acid.

Numerous authors have reported that resistant tumors overexpress multi-specific adenosine triphosphate (ATP) binding cassette (ABC) transporters, which are the main molecular MDR mechanism. These pumps (anchored to the cell membrane) can modify the accumulation of the drug within the cell (Wesolowska 2011), and 12 of the 48 ABC transporters that have been identified in humans are known to be drug transporters. However, it appears that clinically relevant resistance is only related to three of these proteins: P-gp (ABCB1), multidrug resistance-associated protein 1 (MRP1, ABCC1), and breast cancer resistance protein (BCRP, ABCG2) (Choudhuri and Klaassen 2006).

P-gp is a member of a superfamily of ATP-dependent membrane transport proteins. It pumps substrates out of tumor cells via an ATP-dependent mechanism in a unidirectional manner. P-gp expression on a tumor cell membrane results in a reduced intracellular drug concentration, decreasing the cytotoxicity of a broad spectrum of antitumor drugs, including anthracyclines (e.g., doxorubicin, Dox), vinca alkaloids (e.g., vincristine), podophyllotoxins (e.g., etoposide), and taxanes (e.g., paclitaxel, Ptx) (Wesolowska 2011). MRP1 is a member of the ABC family that it is also expressed in normal human tissues (e.g., muscle, lung, spleen, bladder, adrenal gland, and gall bladder), being capable of transporting organic anion drug conjugates as well as intact anticancer drugs. Anthracyclines such as Dox, vinca alkaloids, and etoposide are substrates of MRP1, which reduces the intracellular accumulation of drugs by pumping them out of the tumor cells, thus making the cells resistant (Gradilone et al. 2011). BRCP is a dimer or multimer molecule located in the cell membrane that confers resistance to anthracyclines (e.g., mitoxantrone) and topoisomerase inhibitors, although it does not appear to affect taxanes, vinca alkaloids, or cisplatin. BRCP is mainly located in the epithelial layer, seromucous glands, and capillary endothelium, and its expression has been detected in acute leukemia and some solid tumors, including lung cancer. Very little data are available on the clinical significance of this new MDR protein (Sève and Dumontet 2005).

Nanotechnology in Cancer Treatment

Nanobiotechnology is an interdisciplinary field that is revolutionizing the development of drug delivery systems. It combines biology, medicine, engineering, physics, and chemistry to create new materials that permit the controlled release of new or classic therapeutic agents, including drugs, proteins, nucleic acids, etc. (Kayser et al. 2005, Hanahan and Weinberg 2011). The potential benefits of nano-sized drug delivery systems include enhancement of the therapeutic index of any given active agent, minimization of its toxic side effects, and regulation of its biodistribution (Goldberg et al. 2007). NPs have a number of key properties that make them well suited for application to cancer (Heidel and Davis 2011).

Relevant properties of nanoparticles in drug delivery to cancer

The most important characteristics of NPs are the size and distribution capacity, which determine their biological fate, targeting capacity, toxicity, and biodistribution, and influence the stability of NPs, and their drug loading and release capacities (Singh and Lillard 2009). The size is comparable to that of biological macromolecules such as peptides, proteins, and nucleic acids (Goldberg et al. 2007), making the NPs excellent candidates for targeted drug delivery to cancer. Nanomedicines against cancer should be in the 10 to 100 nm size range, as experimentally established (Davis et al. 2008). The lower size limit (10 nm) is determined by the removal (filtration) of material from plasma through pores within the glomerular capillary wall of the kidney. In this case, the goal is the retention in the circulation, given that materials with diameters < 5 nm are subject to rapid kidney clearance, unlike particles with diameters > 10 nm. The 100 nm upper size limit is less well defined, and is based on the leaky nascent vasculature known to exist within tumors, whose poor lymphatic system can lead macromolecules to leak from the fenestrated vasculature (Heidel and Davis 2011). This is the mechanism behind the Enhanced Permeability and Retention (EPR) effect.

NPs are made of biodegradable materials, and the loaded drug molecules can be released in a sustained manner over a period of days or even weeks. Examples include poly(D,L-lactide-*co*-glycolide) (PLGA), poly(D,L-lactide) (PLA), and poly(ε-caprolactone) (PCL) (Singh and Lillard 2009).

Enhanced permeability and retention effect and size

As noted above, the tendency for molecules of a certain size (liposomes, NPs, and macromolecular drugs) to accumulate much more in the tumor tissue than in healthy tissues is known to be the consequence of the EPR effect. The effect is based on the stimulation of a faster growth of blood vessels in the tumor interstitium. The abnormal vascular architecture (hyper-vasculature) of the tumor plays a major role in its excessive vascular permeability. Besides a defective vascular architecture, e.g., large openings and fenestration, this excessive permeability is attributable to: (i) poor lymphatic clearance, which increases the retention of macromolecular drugs and lipid particles in the tumor interstitium; (ii) a greater leakage from tumor vessels in hypertension; and, (iii) a slow venous return, which facilitates the accumulation of macromolecular drugs and lipid particles in the tumor interstitium.

The EPR effect allows the NP to remain in contact with the tumor site during an extended period of time, allowing the sustained drug release. This has proved to be a vital mechanism for the passive targeting of drug delivery nanosystems to tumor tissues (Talekar et al. 2011). Thanks to the EPR effect, passively targeted NPs can deliver anticancer drugs to tumor tissues, but the drugs must be internalized from the tumor interstitium into the tumor cell to properly exert their chemotherapeutic effect. This can be achieved by using actively targeted NPs, which carry a specific component attached onto their surface. Such a nanostructure is capable of recognizing a specific target within the tumor tissue/cell, thus attaching to it and then generally undergoing receptor-mediated endocytosis and accumulation within the cancer cell.

Cancer targeting

The selective targeting of chemotherapy is one of the main aims of current cancer therapy strategies, and the utilization of NPs has brought this achievement methodologically closer (Brown et al. 2010). As mentioned above, there are two types of drug targeting approaches: passive and/or active. Active drug targeting is possible with specific ligands (Table 10.1), such as monoclonal antibodies (mAbs) or peptides, located on the NP surface, and improves the effectiveness of chemotherapy by ensuring the accumulation of the active agent at specific sites in the cell. Active targeting can further be the consequence of

Table 10.1. Ligands that can be advantageously used in NP engineering (surface conjugated) to optimize the accumulation of the nanomedicine into malignant cells.

Ligand	Characteristics	Size (nm)	Tumor	Target
mAbs	High affinity, divalent, many clinically approved examples, contains biologically active constant region, long circulation	15–20	Prostate tumor	Prostate specific antigen (PSA) total and free
				Prostate specific membrane antigen (PSMA)
			Breast tumor	Cancer antigens 15-3, 27, and 29
			Epithelial ovarian tumor (90% of all ovarian cancer)	Cancer antigen 125
Small molecules	Chemical synthesis, simple modification and coupling chemistries, can be biologically active, highly variable affinities	0.5–2	Oral carcinoma, metastatic breast cancer, colorectal tumor	Folate receptor
			Liver	Asialoglycoprotein receptor (PK2)
Peptides	Easy synthesis and modification, diverse libraries and screening technologies, susceptible to peptidases, renal retention	Variable	Brain tumors, liver tumors	Apolipoprotein E (ApoE)
Aptamers [DNA, ribonucleic acid (RNA)]	Rapid clearance, automated chemical synthesis, susceptible to nucleases without chemical modification	2–3	Aptamers have not yet been approved for cancer treatment	

NP engineering with stimuli-sensitive materials, where drug release can be selectively triggered in the site of action when these nanostructures are under the influence of an adequate stimulus, e.g., pH, redox potential, enzymatic activity, magnetic or electric fields, ultrasounds, temperature (hyperthermia), or light (Singh and Lillard 2009). Passive drug targeting, takes advantage of physical interactions between the NPs and the tumor microenvironment (Fig. 10.4), e.g., blood flow, lymphatic drainage, and/or the leaky (permeable) blood vasculature (Scheinberg et al. 2010).

NP targeting can be divided into two steps, i.e., primary targeting and secondary targeting. In the first, NPs are targeted to a specific organ in accordance with their particle size, surface electrical charge, mechanical properties, physical chemistry, and/or route of administration. In secondary targeting (e.g., actively assured by surface functionalization of the NPs with targeting moieties, Fig. 10.5), the particles interact precisely with a specific cell type or even with a particular subcellular localization. For instance, cancer

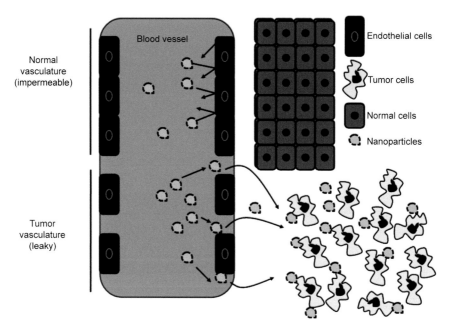

Figure 10.4. Passive targeting of NPs. In the tumor tissue there is an increase of gaps between vascular endothelial cells which facilitates the passive NP accumulation, while healthy vascular endothelial cells are impermeable to NPs.

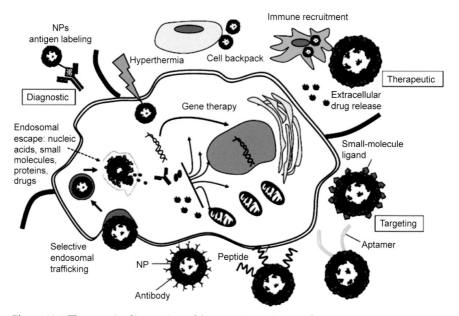

Figure 10.5. Therapeutic, diagnostic, and/or targeting activities of NPs in cancer cells.

cells can express proteins that are usually revealed only during embryonic development, or that can up-regulate the expression of certain biomolecules onto the cell surface.

Drug loading and delivery

To be effective against cancer, the chemotherapeutic drug must reach and destroy its final target in a safe and effective manner. However, a large proportion of the drug dose administered to a patient may be removed by the liver and kidneys, or may even be cytotoxic in healthy tissues. Nanotechnology offers a solution to these problems, because NPs can specifically target the drug and control its release into the malignant tissue. Therefore, an important goal is to optimize drug loading to the nanosystem, which often requires modification of the composition and structure of the NPs.

The drug of interest is usually dissolved, entrapped, adsorbed, attached to and/or encapsulated within a nanomatrix. According to the method selected for NP preparation, nanospheres or nanocapsules can be designed to possess different properties and characteristics for an optimized drug release (Barratt 2000). There are two methods of drug loading: surface adsorption, and entrapment into the NP matrix. In the first method, the therapeutic agent is incorporated after NP synthesis, by incubating the particles with a concentrated drug solution. The efficiency of the process depends on the solubility of the therapeutic agent and the chemical composition of the NP. In the entrapment method, the drug is incorporated during the NP synthesis, thus being found into the matrix (Govender et al. 2000).

Drug release largely depends on the solubility and diffusion of the drug across the NP matrix, on the biodegradation of the NP, on the method by which the therapeutic agent was loaded, and/or on the coating of the NP. Drug-loaded NPs must travel through the bloodstream until they reach the tumor site, where they should remain as long as possible without being degraded. They must also evade the immune system, avoiding their recognition as foreign bodies and phagocytosis by macrophages or neutrophils. Some NPs are hydrophobic and require the incorporation of a hydrophilic shell to maximize their permanence in the bloodstream, because certain blood components can bind to the NP surface and inhibit their arrival to the target site. In this line, NPs can be functionalized with shells of hydrophilic polymers or surfactants, or they can be linked to biodegradable hydrophilic copolymers (Singh and Lillard 2009). Once the NP reaches the tumor tissue, it can be internalized into the tumor cells by endocytosis. The NP is then biodegraded within the cell, in the phagolysosome, and the active agent is released to exert its therapeutic effect. In the case of active targeting, the drug-loaded NP can penetrate the cell by receptor-mediated endocytosis. For example, Dox-loaded polysorbate 80-coated poly(butylcyanoacrylate) NPs have been engineered against brain cancer cells (glioblastome multiforme). They can incorporate onto their surface plasma proteins such as ApoE, which can interact with its specific receptor at the endothelial cells of the blood-brain barrier. As a consequence of a receptor-mediated endocytosis process, the drug-loaded NPs can enter into the brain (Kreuter et al. 2003, Petri et al. 2007, Pereverzeva et al. 2008).

Toxicity

Many of the components used in the synthesis of nanoplatforms for cancer treatment have been extensively studied in humans, demonstrating their safety and efficacy, e.g., mAbs, lipid components, and poly(ethylene glycol) (PEG). However, the development of novel nanosystems to carry drugs requires the tolerability and therapeutic index to be tested, given the numerous interactions of the nanomedicine (plus drug and other components) in a living organism (Scheinberg et al. 2010).

NPs may also induce changes in several cellular structures and functions by the formation of a cell-NP interphase that can influence their toxicity. NP administration may lead to the production of intra and extracellular Reactive Oxygen Species (ROS), such as superoxide and hydroxyl radicals, which affect the integrity of the cell membrane by lipid peroxidation, therefore compromising cell survival. When relatively large-sized NPs are internalized by the cell, they can produce irreversible mechanical damage to the cell membrane. Once inside the cell, the NP may be degraded, leading to mechanic damage in cell organelles, e.g., lisosomes, endoplasmatic reticule, and nucleus. Degraded NPs may also alter cell functionality through the chemical interaction of functional groups and electronic structures with the biological environment (Suh et al. 2009). The (spherical or non-spherical) shape of NPs can determine their persistence in the bloodstream and their excretion time, thus affecting their toxicity (Geng et al. 2007).

Nanomaterials for Use in Cancer Treatment

Diverse nanomaterials can be used in the engineering of nanomedicines against cancer, all for the same purpose, i.e., the development of a biodegradable carrier that can transport a drug, protein, and/or nucleic acid to the tumor interstitium/cell, where its load is released in a sustained manner (ideally triggered by a specific stimulus), thus optimizing the therapeutic effect while reducing non-specific toxicity (Singh and Lillard 2009) (Table 10.2). Nanomaterials can further help in the solubilization of drugs that are insoluble in water (Lu et al. 2007). Recently, cell-like structures (nanocells, average diameter ≈ 400 nm, derived from bacteria) have been formulated as drug delivery nanosystems against cancer (MacDiarmid et al. 2007).

Table 10.2. Representative nanostructures for cancer diagnosis and/or therapy.

Type	Main properties
Solid lipid NPs (SLNs)	They are biodegradable and can protect the therapeutic agent from (bio)degradation
Liposomes	Vesicles formed by one or more lipid bilayers. They can transport hydrophobic and hydrophilic drugs
Micelles	Vesicles formed by layers of amphiphilic copolymers. They can transport hydrophobic and hydrophilic drugs
Hydrogel NPs	They are made of hydrophobic polysaccharides
Nanoshells	Silica NPs with optical functionalities. They can be used for disease imaging, and treatment applications if it is used a near-infrared region (NIR) laser
Dendrimers	Tree-like polymeric nanostructures typically used in disease imaging, i.e., in magnetic resonance imaging (MRI), and also in disease therapy
Carbon nanotubes	Cylindrical NPs that generate or modify an electrical signal upon binding to a specific target
Polymersomes	Liposome-like structures in which the vesicle is made of amphiphilic block copolymers. They can be used in the engineering of multifunctional NPs
Quantum dots (QDs)	Semiconductor and fluorescent NPs which are used in disease imaging, also combined with photothermal therapy
Gold (Au) NPs	Interesting optical properties that can be used in disease imaging and therapy
Magnetic NPs	Metallic NPs that can be used in disease imaging, and as drug delivery systems
Nanowires	Non-spherical nanostructures used in arrays to detect cancer biomarkers
Nanorods	Non-spherical NPs mainly used in thermal ablation of tumors

Solid lipid nanoparticles

SLNs have been the most widely studied nanocarriers for cancer treatment due to their physical stability, biocompatibility, biodegradability, and capacity to protect labile drugs from (bio)degradation. SLNs are colloidal solid systems composed of solid lipids (triglycerides, PEGylated lipids, steroids, and/or fatty acids), emulsifiers (polysorbates, lecithin, poloxamer, and/or bile acids), and water. Typical NP size is < 200 nm, given the small diameter of blood capillaries and cellular structures that may interact with them (Kreuter et al. 2003, Suh et al. 2009). Satisfactory results have been obtained when using SLN-based nanomedicines against the liver, breast, colorectal, lung, brain, stomach, and intestinal cancers (Mathur et al. 2010).

SLNs have been shown to reduce *in vivo* the adverse effects of numerous anticancer drugs. For instance, the cardiotoxicity of Dox can be reduced in mice when loaded to these NPs, because the SLNs can modify the drug biodistribution, which becomes more focalized to tumor tissues (Pereverzeva et al. 2008).

Liposomes

Liposomes are spherical vesicles formed by one or more lipid bilayers, with a core and surface region that are water-soluble, and an inner lipophilic membrane. They can be loaded with hydrophilic drugs in the core, and with hydrophobic drugs in the inner lipid membrane. Liposomes can carry numerous drug molecules, and they are generally considered to be biocompatible, rarely producing allergic, antigenic, and toxic reactions. In fact, they are typically made of naturally-derived phospholipids. Special attention should be given to their final size to avoid an easy recognition by the reticuloendothelial system and plasma clearance. PEGylation is a typical solution to this problem (Mok et al. 2009). Because of their biocompatibility, liposomes are among the most widely studied nanocarriers, along with SLNs. *In vitro* and *in vivo* studies, and clinical trials have demonstrated their potential in the treatment of breast cancer, ovarian cancer, multiple myeloma, acquired immune deficiency syndrome-related Kaposi's sarcoma, lymphomas, and leukemias. Liposomes are usually loaded with Dox, cisplatin, oxaliplatin, irinotecan, Ptx, daunorubicin, cytarabine, and vincristine (Slingerland et al. 2012).

Liposomes have also been formulated to protect and deliver small interfering ribonucleic acid (*si*RNA) in cancer treatment, along with SLNs, carbon nanotubes, and dendrimers (Kesharwani et al. 2012). *si*RNA is a double-strand RNA processed into short RNAs (19 to 23 nucleotides in length) that recognize and down-regulate its complementary *m*RNA. Hence, *si*RNA can modulate gene expression after transcription in a specific sequence manner (Dykxhoorn and Lieberman 2006). *si*RNAs have demonstrated several shortcomings *in vivo*, including: rapid degradation by extracellular nucleases, low concentration into non-healthy cells, and degradation by endosomes within these cells (Whitehead et al. 2009). Liposomes must be cationic materials to neutralize the negative charge of *si*RNA and to overcome the electrostatic repulsion of the cell membrane (Höbel et al. 2010). Liposomes are widely developed to transport nucleic acids, because they can be easily loaded with large molecules, can protect them from enzymatic degradation, and can release them only within the non-healthy cells (Spagnou et al. 2004). Liposomes loaded with *si*RNA targeted to endothelial genes (CD31 and Tie2) have been tested in mice. Biodistribution studies demonstrated that they mainly accumulated in the vascular endothelium of the liver, heart, and lungs, where these genes are mainly localized (Santel et al. 2006). *si*RNA-loaded cationic liposome formulations are commercially available, e.g., Lipofectamine™ and

Oligofectamine™. They can increase the transfection efficiency of plasmid DNA, *m*RNA and *si*RNA into *in vitro* cell cultures by lipofection. Finally, surface functionalization of *si*RNA-loaded liposomes with mAbs can help in the selective delivery to malignant cells. For instance, *si*RNA-loaded liposomes surface decorated with antitransferrin mAbs have demonstrated *in vivo* a promising inhibition of pancreatic tumor growth. Such encouraging results were suggested to be the consequence of the selective targeting of the Epidermal Growth Factor Receptor (EGFR), highly expressed in pancreatic cancers (Pirollo and Chang 2008).

Micelles

Micelles are spherical assemblies of amphiphilic copolymers (Singh and Lillard 2009). Micelles have a monolayer structure divided into two compartments: a hydrophobic core, which can accommodate apolar drugs; and a hydrophilic brush-like corona (shell) that allows the micelle to dissolve in water. The shell can protect the encapsulated drug from degradation by enzymes and macrophage activities. However, despite these benefits, the weak *in vivo* stability of micelles limited their clinical use. In fact, they have been described to dissociate in blood, then being excreted via the kidney (Burt et al. 1999).

Hydrogel nanoparticles

Hydrogel NPs are synthesized by covalent bonding of hydrophobic polysaccharides. They have been loaded with numerous antitumor drugs, e.g., curcumin, an active agent that can induce apoptosis, blockade of nuclear factor kappa B activation, and down-regulation of inflammatory cytokines. However, experiments in animal models and clinical trials have demonstrated that curcumin has a low absorption, poor accumulation in non-healthy tissues, and a very fast metabolism that limits the duration of its therapeutic effect (Anand et al. 2007). It has been demonstrated that encapsulating curcumin in hydrogel NPs can overcome these limitations (Bisht et al. 2007).

Nanoshells

They are typically based on a silica core and a thin metal shell (West and Halas 2000). Nanoshells possess optical properties at any wavelength of interest. Changes in shape of nanoshells in NIR determine that they could be used as excellent contrast agents for diagnostic imaging, and also for the treatment of cancer. For example, nanoshells injected *in vivo* and irradiated with a NIR laser have been found to induce photothermal tumor ablation (Morton et al. 2010). Most of the research done on nanoshells has been done in breast cancer. In this line, Au nanoshells have been tested against SKBr3 human breast epithelial carcinoma cells by using NIR irradiation

(Hirsch et al. 2003a,b). It was demonstrated that the nanoshell/laser treatment reported greater cell membrane destruction in comparison to control cells treated only with laser. Hyperthermia of SKBr3 cells demonstrated high cytotoxicity levels exclusively when NIR laser was applied to the nanoshells. In addition, the use of nanoshells for tumor photothermal ablation reported very good results in numerous animal models of human cancer. For example, after 10 days of treatment with PEGylated nanoshells, tumors in mice subcutaneously inoculated with CT26 colon cancer cells were completely reabsorbed (O'Neal et al. 2004). It has been described that nanoshells may passively accumulate into tumors due to the EPR effect, but it is also possible to formulate nanoshells for active drug targeting applications by attaching mAbs or other ligands onto their surface in order to improve their access to (and treatment of) hypoxic tumor areas (Lal et al. 2008).

Dendrimers

Dendrimers are polymers synthesized from branched monomers, displaying a characteristic tree-like structure (Chetan et al. 2010). They have been proposed as nanocarriers for contrast agents in imaging techniques, such as MRI, and they can also be specifically targeted to cancer cells, e.g., by incorporating onto their surface folic acid moieties, mAbs, or Epidermal Growth Factors (EGFs) (Hussain et al. 2004, Patri et al. 2004, Licciardi et al. 2009). The structure of dendrimers allows transporting drugs of different chemical natures, thus enabling a combined therapy with a single nanocarrier (Lee and Nan 2012). In this line, dendrimers have been simultaneously loaded with Dox and *si*RNA against glioblastoma multiforme *in vitro* (Kaneshiro and Lu 2009), and with Ptx and alendronate against metastatic bone cancer *in vivo* (Clementi et al. 2011). Dendrimers can be further wisely formulated for photodynamic therapy, boron neutron capture therapy, and gene therapy applications (Baker 2009).

Carbon nanotubes

Carbon nanotubes are nano-sized cylinders with two characteristic structures: single-walled carbon nanotubes and multi-walled carbon nanotubes. They are mainly used to detect cancer biomarkers (see Nanotechnology Applications for Cancer Detection) (Kierny et al. 2012).

Polymersomes

The structure of a polymersome is comparable to that of a liposome. They are formulated employing amphiphilic synthetic block copolymers to obtain a vesicle membrane. Polymersomes can be disrupted in acidic environments (Singh and Lillard 2009). They have demonstrated very promising results as nanocarriers for imaging contrast agents in cancer diagnosis (Ghoroghchian et al. 2007) (see Imaging applications of nanotechnology in cancer). Similar to liposomes, they have the capacity to transport large amounts of hydrophilic or hydrophobic entities, thus they may simultaneously carry anticancer drugs and contrast agents. Furthermore, specific ligands can be bound to their surface for active drug targeting functionalizations (Levine et al. 2008). Dox and Ptx are the anticancer drugs most frequently associated to polymersomes, either individually or in combination, both characterized by low water solubilities (Ahmed et al. 2006a,b, Li et al. 2007). For example, poly(ethylene oxide) (PEO)-block-PCL polymersomes have been loaded with Dox, and PEO-block-poly(butadiene) polymersomes have been loaded with Ptx, displaying very promising anticancer activities (Levine et al. 2008).

Quantum dots

QDs are made of semiconductor and fluorescent materials, and their absorption and emission properties can be precisely controlled by modifying their geometry. They can be used in the detection and diagnosis of cancer because they give rise to long term, high sensitivity, and multicontrast imaging (Chetan et al. 2010). Different investigations explored their potential use in the diagnosis, follow up, and treatment of cancer (Azzazy et al. 2007). Cancer treatment is based on laser irradiation of QDs, which transform the light energy into heat (photothermal treatment), that kills tumor cells by generating ROS (Chu et al. 2012).

Gold nanoparticles

Au NPs exhibit many properties making them suitable for applications in the treatment and diagnosis of cancer, including: (i) excellent optical properties, due to localized surface plasmon resonance; (ii) controllable surface chemistry; (iii) negligible toxicity; and, (iv) easy manipulation of particle geometry during synthesis. Hence, they can be considered to be multifunctional (Lim et al. 2011, Jain et al. 2012). In addition, attachment of PEG chains to the surface of Au NPs facilitates their accumulation into the tumor site (passive targeting) (Huang et al. 2008). Au NPs have been loaded with cetuximab (a mAb targeting the EGFR) and gemcitabine for the treatment of pancreatic cancer (Patra et al. 2010). *In vivo* studies in mice with orthotopic pancreatic cancer demonstrated a reduction of $\approx 80\%$ in tumor growth in comparison to controls, while both active agents in free form allowed a decrease of $\approx 30\%$ vs. controls (Patra et al. 2008).

Magnetic nanoparticles

Magnetic NPs have found promising applications in the diagnosis and treatment of cancer. They generally contain magnetic elements such iron (iron oxide), nickel, or cobalt, and they can be manipulated by the use of magnetic fields (Prados et al. 2012). The drug delivery ability of magnetic NPs, their distribution into the site of action, and their therapeutic effects on disease progression can be followed up in real time (Medarova et al. 2006). The most frequently used magnetic NPs are iron oxides, mainly magnetite NPs and maghemite NPs. The magnetic cores are usually coated with a polymer shell to improve its biocompatibility, and further functionalities can be introduced to the nanostructure by incorporation of therapeutic agents (drugs, genes, etc.), targeting molecules (for active drug targeting purposes), and/or organic fluorophores (disease imaging).

Iron oxide NPs coated with oleic acid and stabilized with a Pluronic® chains were loaded with both Dox and Ptx. The NPs improved by 78% the IC_{50} value in comparison to the combined use of free Dox and Ptx, thus evidencing a strong synergic antiproliferative effect (Jain et al. 2008). MRI was satisfactorily used to follow the biodistribution of the NPs in mice.

Nanowires

Nanowires are one-dimensional nanomaterials that have a very small diameter with respect to their length. Nanowire sensor arrays have shown promising results in the real time electrical detection of cancer biomarkers with ultrahigh sensitivity (Zheng et al. 2005). Nanowires have been proposed as a powerful diagnostic tool for cancer when functionalized with mAbs against tumor biomarkers. They may also be used to detect cancer metastasis and to induce the photothermal destruction of tumor cells circulating in blood (Park et al. 2012) (see Nanotechnology Applications for Cancer Detection).

Nanorods

Nanorods are another type of one-dimensional, non-spherical NPs. Au nanorods are characterized by a large light absorption cross-section and two distinct surface plasmon oscillations: a longitudinal band, with a strong band in the NIR; and a transverse band, with a weak band in the visible region. They can be used to induce hyperthermia, which is a non-invasive technique in which the non-healthy tissue is subjected to high temperatures (41–47°C) to promote the selective destruction of abnormal cells. Hyperthermia induces irreversible damage to the tumor cell membrane by denaturing proteins, thus the cell is destroyed or becomes more sensitive to cancer chemotherapy. In an *in vitro* study, Au nanorods were incubated with glioblastoma cells and exposed to laser irradiation (for 20 minutes), adsorbing the light on their surface and transforming it into heat, thereby killing glioblastoma cells in a very effective manner. Optical microscopy, flow cytometry, and lactate dehydrogenase determinations confirmed that cell death was significantly greater when combining the use of Au nanorods and laser, in comparison to the use of the laser alone which does not induce the hyperthermia effect (Fernández et al. 2012).

Nanoparticles in Market and Clinical Trials

Over 150 new anticancer medicines are based on nanotechnology. Some are already approved (Table 10.3) (Wagner et al. 2006, Jain 2010), while the rest are under development (Table 10.4) (Chetan et al. 2010, Jain et al. 2010). The majority of these NPs are based on liposomes, given their excellent capacity to transport both hydrophilic and lipophilic drugs, and their biocompatibility. Iron oxide NPs are principally used in MRI of liver tumors (Suzuki et al. 2008).

Nanotechnology Applications for Cancer Detection

The most widely studied nanosystems in cancer diagnosis are QDs and Au NPs. QDs are inorganic fluorophores that offer numerous advantages over fluorescent labels given their very broad spectrum of emission (from ultraviolet to red), which can be adjusted by controlling their size and composition (Ghoroghchian et al. 2009, Walker et al. 2012). As an illustrative example of the possibilities offered by QDs, it is well-known that aberrant DNA hypermethylation contributes to carcinogenesis by "silencing" the expression of tumor suppressor genes, which appears to be an early epigenetic event that precedes genetic mutations and thus the origin of tumor cells. In order to detect DNA hypermethylation, an ultrasensitive and safe method based on methylation-specific QD fluorescence resonance energy transfer has been developed, which combines the high specificity of the methylation-specific polymerase chain reaction with the high sensitivity and simplicity of the QD fluorescence resonance energy transfer technology. Hence, QDs can bind to methylated DNA strands and light up, the fluorescence can be detected by spectrophotometry. It has been demonstrated that this technique is adequate for early cancer diagnosis, tumor progression follow-up, and cancer therapy (Bailey et al. 2009). In addition, it has been hypothesized that QDs may be of value in the development of personalized oncology, given the capacity to precisely localize the tumor in high-quality high-definition images (Gao et al. 2004, Chen et al. 2012).

Au NPs can also be used in cancer diagnosis. For instance, Au NPs surface functionalized with anti-EGFR mAbs have shown an optimized affinity for tumor cell surfaces. This binding generates a sharper absorption band in surface plasmon resonance images, and shows a maximum red shift when the Au NPs are bound to a tumor cell. Therefore, surface plasmon resonance absorption spectroscopy or scattering imaging of these mAb-conjugated Au NPs represent a highly promising approach in cancer diagnosis, thanks to the high affinity and non-toxicity of the nanoformulation, the ability to obtain instant results, and the fact that expensive high-powered microscopes or lasers are not required (El-Sayed et al. 2006).

Table 10.3. Marketed nanomedicines in cancer diagnosis and therapy (Wagner et al. 2006, Jain 2010).

Name	Composition	Clinical use	Company
Abraxane®	Ptx-loaded albumin NPs	Breast and lung cancer	Abraxis BioScience, USA. AstraZeneca, UK
Caelyx®	Dox-loaded liposomes	Breast and ovarian cancer, and Kaposi's sarcoma	Schering-Plough Corporation, USA
DaunoXome®	Daunorubicin citrate-loaded liposomes	Kaposi's sarcoma	Gilead Sciences Inc., USA
DepoCyt®	Cytarabine-loaded liposomes	Solid tumors, lymphoma or leukemia. Lymphomatous meningitis	SkyePharma, UK. Enzon Pharmaceuticals Inc., USA
Doxil®	Dox-loaded liposomes	Ovarian cancer and Kaposi's sarcoma	Schering-Plough Corporation, USA
Genexol-PM®	Ptx-loaded micellar diblock copolymers	Breast, lung, ovarian, and pancreatic cancer	Samyang Pharma, Korea
Myocet®	Dox-loaded liposomes	Breast cancer	Zeneus Pharma/Cephalon Inc., USA
Oncaspar®	L-asparaginase-loaded polymeric NPs	Acute lymphoblastic leukemia	Enzon Pharmaceuticals Inc., USA
Resovist®	Iron oxide NPs	MRI of liver tumors	Schering, Germany
Endorem®	Iron oxide NPs	MRI of liver tumors	Guerbet, France
Feridex®	Iron oxide NPs	MRI of liver tumors	Advanced Magnetics Inc., USA

Table 10.4. Representative examples of nanomedicines under development for cancer diagnosis and therapy (Matsumura et al. 2004a,b, Matei et al. 2009, Chetan et al. 2010, Jain 2010, Valle et al. 2010).

	Name	Composition	Clinical use	Trial phase
Diagnosis	Magnevist®	Polyamidoamine dendrimer	MRI contrast agent	Preclinical
	Combidex® / Ferumoxtran-10®	Iron oxide NPs	MRI contrast agent	3 (clinical trial NCI-2009-00600)
Treatment	Aurolase™	Au nanoshells	Head and neck cancer	Preclinical
	CPX-1	Liposomes loaded with irinotecan and floxuridine	Solid tumors	2
	IT-101	Conjugation of Cyclosert™ (β-cyclodextrin) and camptothecin	Solid tumors	2
	INGN 401	Lipid-based NPs loaded with the tumor suppression gene FUS1	Lung cancer	1
	LE-SN38	Irinotecan-loaded liposomes	Colorectal cancer	2 (clinical trial NCT00046540)
	MCC-465	Dox-loaded PEGylated immunoliposomes	Gastric cancer	1
	NC-6004	Cisplatin-loaded micelles	Gastric cancer	2 (clinical trial NCT00910741)
	NK-105	Ptx-loaded micelles	Gastric cancer	2 (clinical trial NCT01644890)
	NK-911	Dox-loaded micelles	Solid tumors	1
	Panzem® NCD	2-methoxyestradiol NanoCrystal® dispersion	Glioblastoma	2
	PK1	Dox-loaded copolymers of *N*-(2-hydroxypropyl) methacrylamide	Breast, lung, and colorectal cancer	3
	SP1049C	Dox-loaded Pluronic® micelles	Esophagus and gastroesophageal cancer	3
	Targeted Nano-Therapeutics™ (TNT™)	Immunomagnetic NPs	Solid tumors	Preclinical

Nanotechnology can also be used to detect cancer biomarkers (Wang et al. 2004, Jain 2010). Their detection is crucial to assure an early cancer diagnosis, and for monitoring this disease during therapy. Numerous nanostructures have been investigated as candidates for the detection of biomarkers, including Au NPs, QDs, carbon nanotubes, nanowires, metal NPs, magnetic NPs, and silica NPs (Zhang et al. 2009, Choi et al. 2010, Lerner et al. 2012). For instance, nanowire arrays have been developed for the detection of PSA and carcinoembryonic antigens, demonstrating ultrahigh sensitivity and selectivity to detect 0.9 pg/mL of tumor markers in serum (Zheng et al. 2005). The technique has been used to detect very low concentrations (< 100 pM) of Vascular Endothelial Growth Factor (VEGF), an angiogenic substance essential for tumor growth serving as an early diagnostic marker of cancer (Lee et al. 2009a). Carbon nanotubes have been developed as a nanotool to detect up to four antigens associated to prostate cancer: PSA, interleukin 6, platelet factor 4, and PSMA (Rusling et al. 2009). Carbon nanotubes have been further surface functionalized with mAbs for the detection of head and neck squamous cell carcinoma (Rusling et al. 2010), carcinoembryonic antigens (Park et al. 2006), and neuroendocrine tumor biomarkers (Wang et al. 2007), markedly lowering the limit of detection.

Nanotechnology may also be useful to detect tumor metastases (Ross et al. 2011, Wang et al. 2012). The existence of tumor cells in blood indicates the spread of tumor cells in the organism. In this line, magnetic NPs have been satisfactorily tested in mice, demonstrating a promising capacity to capture tumor cells in the bloodstream (Galanzha et al. 2009). Silicon nanowires coated with Au nanoclusters and surface functionalized with mAbs that recognizes breast cancer cells have also been developed with this aim (Park et al. 2012). Interestingly, the nanoformulation was capable of capturing ≈ 90% of circulating breast cancer cells after 40 minutes of incubation. Once tumor cells were attached to the nanowire, a near-infrared laser was applied to kill them by photothermal therapy.

Future Directions in the Development of Nanoplatforms for Cancer Diagnosis and Treatment

There appear to be two main directions in current and future research on the use of nanotechnology to optimize cancer diagnosis and treatment (Fig. 10.6) (Chetan et al. 2010). The first one is the formulation of multifunctional nanosystems that can develop two or more activities (Arias 2011, Bae et al. 2011). Briefly, multifunctional NPs (so-called theranostic nanotools) basically consists of a nanostructure containing a magnetic domain for MRI applications and/or an optical probe for microscopy, and properly loaded with therapeutic agents (drug molecules, genes, nucleic acids, *si*RNA) (Derfus et al. 2007, Lee et al. 2009b, Suh et al. 2009). The multifunctional NP can be further

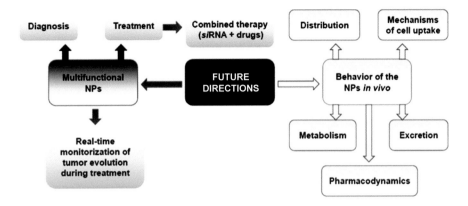

Figure 10.6. Future directions in the investigation of nanoparticulate systems for cancer diagnosis and treatment.

functionalized for passive and/or active targeting (Arias 2011). The second direction in nanotechnology is the complete elucidation of the *in vivo* behavior of the nanoplatforms, including biodistribution, cell uptake mechanisms, metabolism, excretion, and pharmacodynamics.

Research efforts are also devoted to the co-delivery of multiple therapeutic agents (combined therapy), either by using more than one nanocarriers (each one loaded with a different drug) or by employing a single multifunctional nanosystem that can simultaneously deliver different therapeutic molecules (Hu et al. 2010). In this line, liposomes have been synthesized for the co-delivery of Dox and *si*RNAs targeting MRP1 and BCL2 *m*RNA. This multifunctional nanocarrier can induce cell death and overcome MDRs in H69AR lung cancer cells, reporting superior results to controls (Saad et al. 2008).

Conclusion

Nanotechnology is changing the way in which cancer is diagnosed, treated, and perceived. Applications in the field of oncology are growing in parallel to our increasing knowledge of the molecular biology of cancer. Most of the NPs currently used to treat tumors are biocompatible and are metabolized by conventional biochemical pathways. The delivery of drugs to the tumor tissue is becoming more effective with new modifications introduced to these NPs, including the attachment of tumor cell specific ligands onto the particle surface. Surgery, radiotherapy, and chemotherapy are irreplaceable in cancer therapy but can be considerably optimized by the introduction of nanotechnology. For instance, it is hypothesized that nanotechnology may support the precise localization of surgical margins and the detection of lymph nodes and hindered metastatic zones. In addition, nanoplatforms can be formulated to act on residual tumor metastasis without collateral damage, and they can improve the activity of chemotherapeutic agents. Therefore, the introduction of nanotechnology in the tumor arena is expected to optimize the prognosis of cancer.

Acknowledgments

Instituto de Salud Carlos III (FIS, Project PI11/01862, Spain) and Consejería de Salud de la Junta de Andalucía (Project PI-0338, Spain).

Abbreviations

Au	:	gold
ABC	:	adenosine triphosphate binding cassette
ApoE	:	apolipoprotein E
ATP	:	adenosine triphosphate
BCRP	:	breast cancer resistance protein
DNA	:	deoxyribonucleic acid
Dox	:	doxorubicin
EGF	:	epidermal growth factor
EGFR	:	epidermal growth factor receptor
EPR	:	enhanced permeability and retention
IC_{50}	:	percentage of 50 inhibitory concentration
mAb	:	monoclonal antibody
MDR	:	multidrug resistance
*m*RNA	:	messenger ribonucleic acid
MPEG	:	monomethoxy-poly(ethylene glycol)
MRI	:	magnetic resonance imaging
MRP1	:	multidrug resistance-associated protein 1
NIR	:	near-infrared region
NP	:	nanoparticle
PCL	:	poly(ε-caprolactone)
PEG	:	poly(ethylene glycol)
PEO	:	poly(ethylene oxide)
P-gp	:	P-glycoprotein
PK2	:	asialoglycoprotein receptor
PLA	:	poly(D,L-lactide)
PLGA	:	poly(D,L-lactide-*co*-glycolide)
PSA	:	prostate specific antigen
PSMA	:	prostate specific membrane antigen
Ptx	:	paclitaxel
QD	:	quantum dot
RNA	:	ribonucleic acid
ROS	:	reactive oxygen species

*si*RNA	:	small interfering ribonucleic acid
SLN	:	solid lipid nanoparticle
VEGF	:	vascular endothelial growth factor

References

Adams, J.M. and S. Cory. 2007. The Bcl-2 apoptotic switch in cancer development and therapy. Oncogene. 26: 1324–1337.

Ahmed, F. and R.I. Pakunlu, A. Branan, F. Bates, T. Minko and D.E. Discher. 2006a. Biodegradable polymersomes loaded with both paclitaxel and doxorubicin permeate and shrink tumors, inducing apoptosis in proportion to accumulated drug. J. Control. Release. 28: 150–158.

Ahmed, F. and R.I. Pakunlu, F. Srinivas, A. Brannan, F. Bates, M.L. Klein, T. Minko and D.E. Discher. 2006b. Shrinkage of a rapidly growing tumor by drug-loaded polymersomes: pH-triggered release through copolymer degradation. Mol. Pharm. 3: 340–350.

Anand, P. and A.B. Kunnumakkara, R.A. Newman and B.B. Aggarwal. 2007. Bioavailability of curcumin: problems and promises. Mol. Pharm. 4: 807–818.

Arias, J.L. 2011. Advanced methodologies to formulate nanotheragnostic agents for combined drug delivery and imaging. Expert Opin. Drug Deliv. 8: 1589–608.

Azzazy, H.M. and M.M. Mansour and S.C. Kazmierczak. 2007. From diagnostics to therapy: prospects of quantum dots. Clin. Biochem. 40: 917–927.

Bae, K.H. and H.J. Chung and T.G. Park. 2011. Nanomaterials for cancer therapy and imaging. Mol. Cells. 31: 295–302.

Bailey, V.J. and H. Easwaran, Y. Zhang, E. Griffiths, S.A. Belinsky, J.G. Herman, S.B. Baylin, H.E. Carraway and T.H. Wang. 2009. MS-qFRET: a quantum dot-based method for analysis of DNA methylation. Genome Res. 19: 1455–1461.

Baker, J.R., Jr. 2009. Dendrimer-based nanoparticles for cancer therapy. Hematology Am. Soc. Hematol. Educ. Program. 2009: 708–719.

Barrat, G.M. 2000. Therapeutic applications of colloidal drug carriers. Pharm. Sci. Technolo. Today. 3: 163–171.

Berx, G. and F. van Roy. 2009. Involvement of members of the cadherin superfamily in cancer. Cold. Spring. Harb. Perspect. Biol. 1: 1–27.

Bisht, S. and G. Feldman, S. Soni, R. Ravi, C. Karikar, A. Maitra and A. Maitra. 2007. Polymeric nanoparticle-encapsulated curcumin ("nanocurcumin"): a novel strategy for human cancer therapy. J. Nanobiotechnology. 5: 1–18.

Blasco, M.A. 2005. Telomeres and human disease: ageing, cancer and beyond. Nat. Rev. Genet. 6: 611–622.

Brown, S.C. and M. Palazuelos, P. Sharma, K.W. Powers, S.M. Roberts, S.R. Grobmyer and B.M. Moudgil. 2010. Nanoparticle characterization for cancer nanotechnology and other biological applications. Methods Mol. Biol. 624: 39–65.

Burkhart, D.L. and J. Sage. 2008. Cellular mechanisms of tumour suppression by the retinoblastoma gene. Nat. Rev. Cancer. 8: 671–682.

Burt, H.M. and X. Zhang, P. Toleikis, L. Embree and W.L. Hunter. 1999. Development of copolymers of poly(D,L-lactide) and methoxypolyethylene glycol as micellar carriers of paclitaxel. Colloids Surf. B Biointerfaces. 16: 161–171.

Chen, C. and J. Peng, S.R. Sun, C.W. Peng, Y. Li and D.W. Pang. 2012. Tapping the potential of quantum dots for personalized oncology: current status and future perspectives. Nanomedicine (Lond.). 7: 411–428.

Chetan, C.A. and K.J. Girish and S.M.V. Swamy. 2010. Current trends of nanotechnology for cancer therapy. Int. J. Pharm. Sci. Nanotechnol. 3: 1043–1056.

Choi, Y.E. and J.W. Kwak and J.W. Park. 2010. Nanotechnology for early cancer detection. Sensors. 10: 428–455.

Choudhuri, S. and C.D. Klaassen. 2006. Structure, function, expression, genomic organization, and single nucleotide polymorphisms of human ABCB1 (MDR1), ABCC (MRP), and ABCG2 (BCRP) efflux transporters. Int. J. Toxicol. 25: 231–259.

Chu, M. and X. Pan, D. Zhang, Q. Wu, J. Peng and W. Hai. 2012. The therapeutic efficacy of CdTe and CdSe quantum dots for photothermal cancer therapy. Biomaterials. 33: 7071–7083.

Clementi, C. and K. Miller, A. Mero, R. Satchi-Fainaro and G. Pasut. 2011. Dendritic poly(ethylene glycol) bearing paclitaxel and alendronate for targeting bone neoplasm. Mol. Pharm. 8: 1063–1072.

Dantchev, D. and G. Vakchev. 2012. Surface integration approach: a new technique for evaluating geometry dependent forces between objects of various geometry and a plate. J. Colloid Interface Sci. 372: 148–163.

Davis, M.E. and Z.G. Chen and D.M. Shin. 2008. Nanoparticle therapeutics: an emerging treatment modality for cancer. Nat. Rev. Drug. Discov. 7: 771–782.

DeBerardinis, R.J. and C.B. Thompson. 2012. Cellular metabolism and disease: what do metabolic outliers teach us? Cell. 148: 1132–1144.

Derfus, A.M. and A.A. Chen, D. Min, E. Ruoslahti and S.N. Bhatia. 2007. Targeted quantum dot conjugated for siRNA delivery. Bioconjug. Chem. 18: 1391–1396.

Dykxhoorn, D.M. and J. Lieberman. 2006. Knocking down disease with siRNAs. Cell. 126: 231–235.

El-Sayed, I.H. and X. Huang and M. El-Sayed. 2006. Selective laser photo-thermal therapy of epithelial carcinoma using anti-EGFR antibody conjugated gold nanoparticles. Cancer Lett. 239: 129–135.

Fernández, T. and C. Sánchez, A. Martínez, F. del Pozo, J.J. Serrano and M. Ramos. 2012. Induction of cell death in a glioblastoma line by hyperthermic therapy based on gold nanorods. Int. J. Nanomedicine. 7: 1511–1523.

Galanzha, E.I. and E.V. Shashkov, T. Kelly, J.W. Kim, L. Yang and V.P. Zharov. 2009. *In vivo* magnetic enrichment and multiplex photoacoustic detection of circulating tumour cells. Nat. Nanotechnol. 4: 855–860.

Gao, X. and R.M. Levenson, L.W. Chung and S. Nie. 2004. *In vivo* cancer targeting and imaging with semiconductor quantum dots. Nat. Biotechnol. 22: 969–976.

Geng, Y. and P. Dalhaimer, S. Cai, R. Tsai, M. Tewari, T. Minko and D.E. Discher. 2007. Shape effects of filaments versus spherical particles in flow and drug delivery. Nat. Nanotechnol. 2: 249–255.

Ghoroghchian, P.P. and P.R. Frail, G. Li, J.A. Zupancich, F.S. Bates, D.A. Hammer and M.J. Therien. 2007. Controlling bulk optical properties of emissive polymersomes through intramembranous polymer-fluorophore interactions. Chem. Mater. 20: 1309–1318.

Ghoroghchian, P.P. and J.T. Michael and D.A. Hammer. 2009. *In vivo* fluorescence imaging: a personal perspective. Nanomed. Nanotech. 1: 156–167.

Goldberg, M. and R. Langer and X. Jia. 2007. Nanostructured materials for applications in drug delivery and tissue engineering. J. Biomater. Sci. Polym. Ed. 18: 241–268.

Govender, T. and T. Riley, T. Ehtazazi, M.C. Garnett, S. Stolnik, L. Illum and S.S. Davis. 2000. Defining the drug incorporation properties of PLA-PEG nanoparticles. Int. J. Pharm. 199: 95–110.

Gradilone, A. and C. Raimondi, G. Naso, I. Silvestri, L. Repetto, A. Palazzo, W. Gianni, L. Frati, E. Cortesi and P. Gazzaniga. 2011. How circulating tumor cells escape from multidrug resistance: translating molecular mechanisms in metastatic breast cancer treatment. Am. J. Clin. Oncol. 34: 625–627.

Hanahan, D. and J. Folkman. 1996. Patterns and emerging mechanisms of the angiogenic switch during tumorigenesis. Cell. 86: 353–364.

Hanahan, D. and R.A. Weinberg. 2011. Hallmarks of cancer: the next generation. Cell. 144: 646–674.

Heidel, J.D. and M.E. Davis. 2011. Clinical developments in nanotechnology for cancer therapy. Pharm. Res. 28: 187–199.

Hirsch, L.R. and J.B. Jackson, A. Lee, N.J. Halas and J.L. West. 2003a. A whole blood immunoassay using gold nanoshells. Anal. Chem. 75: 2377–2381.

Hirsck, L.R. and R.J. Stafford, J.A. Bankson, S.R. Sershen, B. Riverva, R.E. Price, J.D. Hazle, N.J. Halas and J.L. West. 2003b. Nanoshell-mediated near-infrared thermal therapy of tumors undermagnetic resonance guidance. Proc. Natl. Acad. Sci. U.S.A. 100: 13549–13554.

Höbel, S. and I. Koburger, M. John, F. Czubayko, P. Hadwiger, H. Vomlocher and A. Aigner. 2010. Polyethylenimine/small interfering RNA-mediated knockdown of vascular endothelial growth factor *in vivo* exerts anti-tumor effecs synergistically with Bevacizumab. J. Gene Med. 12: 287–300.

Hu, C.M.J. and S. Aryal and L. Zhang. 2010. Nanoparticle-assisted combination therapies for effective cancer treatment. Ther. Deliv. 1: 323–334.

Huang, W.X. and Z.L. Jiang and A.H. Liang. 2008. Immunonanogold catalytic spectrophotometric determination of trace complement 3. Guang Pu Xue Yu Guang Pu Fen Xi. 28: 2653–2655.

Hussain, M. and M. Shchepinov and M. Sohail. 2004. A novel anionic dendrimer for improved cellular delivery of antisense oligonucleotides. J. Control. Release. 99: 139–155.

Jain, T.K. and J. Richey, M. Strand, D.L. Leslie-Pelecky, C.A. Flask and V. Labhasetwar. 2008. Magnetic nanoparticles with dual functional properties: drug delivery and magnetic resonance imaging. Biomaterials. 29: 4012–4021.

Jain, K.K. 2010. Advances in the field of nanooncology. BMC Med. 8: 1–11.

Jain, S. and D.G. Hirst and J.M. O'Sullivan. 2012. Gold nanoparticles as novel agents for cancer therapy. Br. J. Radiol. 85: 101–113.

Jemal, A. and F. Bray, M.M. Center, J. Ferlay, E. Ward and D. Forman. 2011. Global cancer statistics. CA Cancer J. Clin. 61: 69–90.

Jones, R.G. and C.B. Thompson. 2009. Tumor suppressors and cell metabolism: a recipe for cancer growth. Genes Dev. 23: 537–548.

Kaneshiro, T.L. and R. Lu. 2009. Targeted intra cellular codelivery of chemotherapeutics and nucleic acid with well defined dendrimer-based nanoglobular carrier. Biomaterials. 30: 5660–5666.

Kayser, O. and A. Lemke and N. Hernandez-Trejo. 2005. The impact of nanobiotechnology on the development of new drug delivery systems. Curr. Pharm. Biotechnol. 6: 3–5.

Kesharwani, P. and V. Gajbhiye and N.K. Jain. 2012. A review of nanocarriers for the delivery of small interfering RNA. Biomaterials. 33: 7138–7150.

Kierny, M.R. and T.D. Cunningham and B.K. Kay. 2012. Detection of biomarkers using recombinant antibodies coupled to nanostructured platforms. Nano. Rev. 3: 1–24.

Kreuter, J. and P. Ramge, V. Petrov, S. Hamm, S.E. Gelperina, B. Engelhardt, R. Alyautdin, H.V. Briesen, and D.J. Begle. 2003. Direct evidence that polysorbate-80-coated-poly(butylcyanoacrylate) nanoparticles deliver drugs to the CNS via specific mechanism requiring prior binding of drug to the nanoparticles. Phamacol. Res. 20: 409–416.

Lal, S. and S.E. Clare and N.J. Halas. 2008. Nanoshell-enables phototermal cancer therapy: impending clinical impact. Acc. Chem. Res. 41: 1842–1851.

Lawrence, T.S. and R.K. Ten Haken and A. Giaccia. Principles of radiation oncology. pp. 307–336. *In*: V.T. DeVita, T.S. Lawrence and S.A. Rosenberg [eds.]. 2008. Cancer Principles and Practice of Oncology. 8th ed. Lippincott Williams and Wilkins, Philadelphia, USA.

Lee, H. and K. Kim, C. Kim, S. Hahn and M. Jo. 2009a. Electrical detection of VEGFs for cancer diagnosis using anti-vascular endothelial growth factor aptamer-modified Si nanowire FETs. Biosens. Bioelectron. 24: 1801–1805.

Lee, J. and K. Lee, S.H. Moon, Y. Lee, T.G. Park and J. Cheon. 2009b. All-in-one target cell-specific magnetic nanoparticles for simultaneous molecular imaging and siRNA delivery. Angew. Chem. Int. Ed. Engl. 48: 4174–4179.

Lee, J.H. and A. Nan. 2012. Combination drug delivery approaches in metastatic breast cancer. J. Drug Deliv. 2012: 1–17.

Lerner, M.B. and J. D'Souza, T. Pazina, J. Dailey, B.R. Goldsmith, M.K. Robinson and A.T. Johnson. 2012. Hybrids of a genetically engineered antibody and a carbon nanotube transistor for detection of prostate cancer biomarkers. ACS Nano. 26: 5143–5149.

Levine, D.H. and P.P. Ghoroghchian, J. Freudenberg, G. Zhang, M.J. Therien, M.I. Greene, D.A. Hammer and R. Murali. 2008. Polymersomes: a new multi-functional tool for cancer diagnosis and therapy. Methods. 46: 25–32.

Li, S. and B. Byrne, J. Welsh and A.F. Palmer. 2007. Self-assembled poly(butadiene)-b-poly(ethylene oxide) polymersomes as paclitaxel carriers. Biotechnol. Prog. 23: 278–285.

Licciardi, M. and G. Giammona, J. Du, P. Armes, Y. Tand and A.L. Lewis. 2006. New folate-functionalized biocompatible block copolymer micelles as potential anti-cancer drug delivery systems. Polymer. 47: 2946–2955.

Lim, Z.Z. and J.E. Li, C.T. Ng, L.Y. Yung and B.H. Bay. 2011. Gold nanoparticles in cancer therapy. Acta Pharmacol. 32: 983–990.

Lu, J. and M. Liong, J.L. Zink and F. Tamanoi. 2007. Mesoporous silica nanoparticles as a delivery system for hydrophobic anticancer drugs. Small. 3: 1341–1346.

MacDiarmid, J.A. and N.B. Mugridge, J.C. Weiss, L. Phillips, A.L. Burn, R.P. Paulin, J.E. Haasdyk, K.A. Dickson, V.N. Brahmbhatt, S.T. Pattinson, A.C. James, G. Bakri, R.C. Straw, B. Stillman, R.M. Graham and H. Brahmbnatt. 2007. Bacterially derived 400 nm particles for encapsulation and cancer cell targeting of chemotherapeutics. Cancer Cell. 11: 431–445.

Maeda, H. and G.Y. Bharate and J. Daruwalla. 2009. Polymeric drugs for efficient tumor-targeted drug delivery based on EPR-effect. Eur. J. Pharm. Biopharm. 71: 409–419.

Matei, D. and J. Schilder, G. Sutton, S. Perkins, T. Breen, C. Quon and C. Sidor. 2009. Activity of 2methoxyestradiol (Panzem NCD) in advanced, platinum-resistant ovarian cancer and primary peritoneal carcinomatosis: a Hoosier Oncology Group trial. Gynecol. Oncol. 115: 90–96.

Mathur, V. and Y. Satrawala, M.S. Rajput, P. Kumar, P. Shrivastava and A. Vishvakarma. 2010. Solid lipid nanoparticles in cancer therapy. Int. J. Drug Deliv. 2: 192–199.

Matsumura, Y. and T. Hamaguchi, T. Ura, K. Muro, Y. Yamada, Y. Shimada, K. Shirao, T. Okusaka, H. Ueno, M. Ikeda and N. Watanabe. 2004a. Phase I clinical trial and pharmacokinetic evaluation of NK911, a micelle-encapsulated doxorubicin. Brit. J. Cancer. 91: 1775–1781.

Matsumura, Y. and M. Gotoh, K. Muro, Y. Yamada, K. Shirao, Y. Shimada, M. Okuwa, S. Matsumoto, Y. Miyata, H. Ohkura, K. Chin, S. Baba, T. Yamao, A. Kannami, Y. Takamatsu, K. Ito and K. Takahashi. 2004b. Phase I and pharmacokinetic study of MCC-465, a doxorubicin (DXR) encapsulated in PEG immunoliposome, in patients with metastatic stomach cancer. Ann. Oncol. 15: 517–525.

McDevitt, M.R. and D. Chattopadhyay, B.J. Kappel, J.S. Jaggi, S.R. Schiffman, C. Antczak, J.T. Njardarson, R. Brentjens and D.A. Scheinberg. 2007. Tumor targeting with antibody-functionalized radiolabeled carbon nanotubes. J. Nucl. Med. 48: 1180–1189.

Medarova, Z. and W. Pham, Y. Kim, G. Dai and A. Moore. 2006. *In vitro* imaging of tumor response to therapy using a dual-modality imaging strategy. Int. J. Cancer. 118: 2796–2802.

Mok, H. and K.H. Bae, C.H. Ahn and T.G. Park. 2009. PEGylated and MMP-2 specifically dePEGylated quantum dots: comparative evaluation of cellular uptake. Langmuir. 25: 1645–1650.

Morton, J.G. and E.S. Day, N.J. Halas and J.L. West. 2010. Nanoshells for photothermal cancer therapy. Methods. Mol. Biol. 624: 101–117.

O'Neal, D.P. and L.R. Hirsch, N.J. Halas, J.D Payne and J.L. West. 2004. Photo-thermal tumor ablation in mice using near infrared-absorbing nanoparticles. Cancer Lett. 209: 171–176.

Park, D.W. and Y.H. Kim, B.S. Kim, H.M. So, K. Won, J.O. Lee, K.J. Kong and H. Chang. 2006. Detection of tumor markers using single-walled carbon nanotube field effect transistors. J. Nanosci. Nanotechnol. 6: 3499–3502.

Park, G.S. and H. Kwon, D.W. Kwak, S.Y. Park, M. Kim, J.H. Lee, H. Han, S. Heo, X.S. Li, J.H. Lee, Y.H. Kim, J.G. Lee, W. Yang, H.Y. Cho, S.K. Kim and K. Kim. 2012. Full surface embedding of gold clusters on silicon nanowires for efficient capture and photothermal therapy of circulating tumor cells. Nano. Lett. 12: 1638–1642.

Patra, C.R. and R. Bhattacharya, E. Wang, A. Katarya, J.S. Lau, S. Dutta, M. Muders, S. Wang, S.A. Buhrow, S.L. Safgren, M.J. Yaszemski, J.M. Reid, M.M. Ames, P. Mukheriee and D. Mukhopadhvay. 2008. Targeted delivery of gemcitabine to pancreatic adenocarcinoma using cetuximab as a targeting agent. Cancer Res. 68: 1970–1978.

Patra, C.R. and R. Bhattacharya, D. Mukhopadhayay and P. Mukherjee. 2010. Fabrication of gold nanoparticles for targeted therapy in pancreatic cancer. Adv. Drug. Deliv. Rev. 62: 346–361.

Patri, A.K. and A. Myc, J. Beals, T.P. Thomas, N.H. Bander and J.R. Baker, Jr. 2004. Synthesis and *in vitro* testing of J591 antibody dendrimer conjugates for targeted prostate cancer therapy. Bioconjug. Chem. 15: 1174–1181.

Pereverzeva, E. and I. Treschalin, D. Bodyagin, O. Maksimenki, J. Kreurer and S. Gelperina. 2008. Intravenous tolerance of a nanoparticle-based formulation of doxorubicin in healthy rats. Toxicol. Lett. 178: 9–19.

Petri, B. and A. Bootz, A. Khalansky, T. Hekmatara, R. Müller, R. Uhl, J. Kreuter and S. Gelperina. 2007. Chemotherapy of brain tumour using doxorubicin bound to surfactant-coated poly(butyl-cyanoacrylate) nanoparticles: revisiting the role of surfactants. J. Control. Release. 117: 51–58.

Pirollo, K.F. and E.H. Chang. 2008. Targeted delivery of small interfering RNA: approaching effective cancer therapies. Cancer Res. 68: 1247–1250.

Porter, J.R. and A. Henson and K.C. Popat. 2009. Biodegradable poly(ε-caprolactone) nanowires for bone tissue engineering applications. Biomaterials. 30: 780–788.

Prados, J. and C. Melguizo, R. Ortiz, C. Vélez, P.J. Alvarez, J.L. Arias, M.A. Ruíz, V. Gallardo and A. Aranega. 2012. Doxorubicin-loaded nanoparticles: new advances in breast cancer therapy. Anticancer Agents Med. Chem. 12: 1058–1070.

Ross, R.W. and A.L. Zietman, W. Xie, J.J. Coen, D.M. Dahl, W.U. Shipley, D.S. Kaufman, T. Islam, A.R. Guimaraes, R. Weissleder and M. Harisinghani. 2011. Lymphotropic nanoparticle-enhanced magnetic resonance imaging (LNMRI) identifies occult lymph node metastases in prostate cancer patients prior to salvage radiation therapy. Clin. Imaging. 33: 301–305.

Rusling, J.F. and B.V. Chikkaveeraiah, A. Bhirde, R. Malhotra, V. Patel and J.S. Gutkind. 2009. Single-wall carbon nanotube forest arrays for immunoelectrochemical measurement of four protein biomarkers for prostate cancer. Anal. Chem. 81: 9129–9134.

Rusling, J.F. and R. Malhotra, V. Patel, J.P. Vaque and J.S. Gutkind. 2010. Ultrasensitive electrochemical immunosensor for oral cancer biomarker IL-6 using carbon nanotube forest electrodes and multilabel amplification. Anal. Chem. 82: 3118–3123.

Saad, M. and O.B. Garbuzenko and T. Minko. 2008. Co-delivery of siRNA and an anticancer drug for treatment of multidrug resistant cancer. Nanomedicine (Lond.). 3: 761–776.

Santel, A. and M. Aleku, O. Keil, J. Endurschat, V. Esche, G. Fisch, S. Dames, K. Löffer, M. Fechtner, W. Arnold, K. Giese, A. Klippel and J. Kaufmann. 2006. A novel siRNA-lipoplex technology for RNA interference in the mouse vascular endothelium. Gene Ther. 13: 1222–1234.

Scheinberg, D.A. and C.H. Villa, F.E. Escorcia and M.R. McDevitt. 2010. Conscript of the infinite armada: systemic cancer therapy using nanomaterials. Nat. Rev. Clin. Oncol. 7: 266–276.

Schroeder, A. and D.A. Heller, M.M. Winslow, J.E. Dahlman, G.W. Pratt, R. Langer, T. Jacks and D.G. Anderson. 2012. Treating metastatic cancer with nanotechnology. Nat. Rev. Cancer. 12: 39–50.

Schroedl, C. and R. Kalhan. 2012. Incidence, treatment options, and outcomes of lung cancer in patients with chronic obstructive pulmonary disease. Curr. Opin. Pulm. Med. 18: 131–137.

Scoccianti, S. and S.M. Magrini, U. Ricardi, B. Detti, M. Krengli, S. Parisi, F. Bertoni, G. Sotti, S. Cipressi, V. Tombolini, S. Dall'oglio, M. Lioce, C. Saieva, M. Buglione, C. Mantovani, G. Rubino, P. Muto, V. Fusco, L. Fariselli, C. de Renzis, L. Masini, R. Santoni, L. Pirtoli and G. Biti. 2012. Radiotherapy and temozolomide in anaplastic astrocytoma: a retrospective multicenter study by the central nervous system study group of AIRO (Italian Association of Radiation Oncology). Neuro. Oncol. 14: 798–807.

Sève, P. and C. Dumontet. 2005. Chemoresistance in non-small cell lung cancer. Curr. Med. Chem. Anticancer Agents. 5: 73–88.

Singh, R. and J.W. Lillard. 2009. Nanoparticle-based targeted drug delivery. Exp. Mol. Pathol. 86: 215–223.

Slingerland, M. and H.J. Guchelaar and H. Gelderblom. 2012. Liposomal drug formulations in cancer therapy: 15 years along the road. Drug Discov. Today. 17: 160–166.

Spagnou, S. and A.D. Miller and M. Keller. 2004. Lipidic carriers of siRNA: differences in the formulation, cellular uptake, and delivery with plasmid DNA. Biochemistry. 43: 13348–13356.

Suh, W.H. and K.S. Suslick, G.D. Stucky and Y.H. Suh. 2009. Nanotechnology, nanotoxicology and neuroscience. Prog. Neurobiol. 87: 133–170.

Suzuki, H. and G. Tsurita, S. Ishilara, M. Akahane, J. Kitayama and H. Nagawa. 2008. Resovist-enhanced MRI for preoperative assessment of colorectal hepatic metastases: a case of multiple bile duct hamartomas associated with colon cancer. Case Rep. Gastroenterol. 2: 509–516.

Suzuki, K. and H. Matsubara. 2011. Recent advances in P53 research and cancer treatment. J. Biomed. Biotechnol. 2011: 978312.

Talekar, M. and J. Kendall, W. Denny and S. Garg. 2011. Targeting of nanoparticles in cancer: drug delivery and diagnostics. Anticancer Drugs. 22: 949–962.

Valle, J.W. and A. Armstrong, C. Newman, V. Alakhov, G. Pietrzynski, J. Brever, S. Campbell, P. Corrie, E.K. Rowinsky and M. Ranson. 2010. A phase 2 study of SP1049C, doxorubicin in P-glycoprotein-targeting pluronics, in patients with advanced adenocarcinoma of the esophagus and gastroesophageal junction. Invest. New Drugs. 29: 1029–1037.

Vilaprinyo, E. and T. Puig and M. Rue. 2012. Contribution of early detection and adjuvant treatments to breast cancer mortality reduction in Catalonia, Spain. PLoS One. 7: 1–8.

Wagner, V. and A. Dullaart, A.K. Bock and A. Zweck. 2006. The emerging nanomedicine landscape. Nat. Biotechnol. 24: 1211–1217.

Walker, K.A. and C. Morgan, S.H. Doak and P.R. Dunstan. 2012. Quantum dots for multiplexed detection and characterisation of prostate cancer cells using a scanning near-field optical microscope. PLoS One. 7: 1–17.

Wang, H.Z. and H.Y. Wang, R.Q. Liang and K.C. Ruan. 2004. Detection of tumor marker CA 125 in ovarian carcinoma using quantum dots. Acta Bioch. Biophys. Sin. 36: 681–686.

Wang, C.W. and C.Y. Pan, H.C. Wu, P.Y. Shih, C.C. Tsai, K.T. Liao, L.L. Lu, W.H. Hsieh, C.D. Chen and Y.T. Chen. 2007. *In situ* detection of chromogranin a released from living neurons with a single-walled carbon-nanotube field-effect transistor. Small 3: 1357–1355.

Wang, Y. and Y. Zhang, Z. Du, M. Wu and G. Zhang. 2012. Detection of micrometastases in lung cancer with magnetic nanoparticles and quantum dots. Int. J. Nanomedicine. 7: 2315–2324.

Wesolowska, O. 2011. Interaction of phenothiazines, stilbenes and flavonoids with multidrug resistance-associated transporters, P-Glycoprotein and MRP1. Acta Biochim. Pol. 58: 433–448.

West, J.L. and N.J. Halas. 2000. Applications of nanotechnology to biotechnology commentary. Curr. Opin. Biotechnol. 11: 215–217.

Whitehead, K.A. and R. Langer and D.G. Anderson. 2009. Knocking down barriers: advantages in siRNA delivery. Nat. Rev. Drug Discov. 8: 129–138.

Witsch, E. and M. Sela and Y. Yarden. 2010. Roles for growth factors in cancer progression. Physiology (Bethesda). 25: 85–101.

Zhang, G. and J. Chua, R. Chee, A. Agarwal and S. Wong. 2009. Label-free direct detection of miRNAs with silicon nanowire biosensiors. Biosens. Bioelectron. 24: 2504–2508.

Zheng, G. and F. Patolsky, Y. Cui, W.U. Wang and C.M. Lieber. 2005. Multiplexed electrical detection of cancer markers with nanowire sensor arrays. Nat. Biotechnol. 23: 1294–1301.

Zhou, W. and F. Meng, G.H.M. Engbers and J. Feijen. 2006. Biodegradable polymersomes for targeted ultrasound imaging. J. Control. Release. 116: 62–64.

CHAPTER 11

Nanomedicine in Cardiovascular Disease

Costas Psarros,[1] *Regent Lee,*[2,a] *Alexios Antonopoulos,*[2,b]
Marios Margaritis[2,c] and *Charalambos Antoniades*[2,]*

ABSTRACT

Cardiovascular disease is the leading cause of morbidity and mortality worldwide. It claims the lives of more than 18 million people each year and at an ever increasing rate due to an aging population. Despite the efforts and recent advances in medical therapies, there is still room for significant improvement in both prevention and treatment of this disease. Atherosclerosis is the main cause of cardiovascular diseases worldwide, and it is distinguished by a chronic inflammatory process involving the arterial wall. The complex cascade of pathologies leading to the formation of atherosclerotic plaques and subsequent plaque related complications presents potential targets for therapeutic modulation.

Recent advances in nanotechnology have led to its application in the field of medical research. The ability to synthesize and manipulate novel materials in the nanometer scale which exhibits intriguing properties *in vivo* has led to the spectacular rise of the new entity of nanomedicine. Nanotechnology is emerging as a unique tool in the management of cardiovascular diseases as it offers significant advantages over other traditional treatment modalities.

[1] Department of Experimental Physiology, School of Medicine, National and Kapodistrian University of Athens, Mikras Asias 75 Goudi, Box 14563, Athens, Greece.
Email: cpsarros85@gmail.com
[2] Department of Cardiovascular Medicine, University of Oxford, West Wing, John Radcliffe Hospital, Headington, Level 6, OX39DU, Oxford, UK.
[a] Email: regent.lee@cardiov.ox.ac.uk
[b] Email: alexios.antonopoulos@cardiov.ox.ac.uk
[c] Email: marios.margaritis@cardiov.ox.ac.uk
* Corresponding author: antoniad@well.ox.ac.uk; charalambos.antoniades@cardiov.ox.ac.uk

Nanotechnology can be utilized to the full spectrum of cardiovascular disease management, ranging from early detection and identification of atherosclerosis, to the treatment of acute vascular syndromes, such as cerebral ischemia and acute myocardial infarction.

This chapter summarizes the latest advances in the field of nanomedicine relevant to the treatment of atherosclerosis, followed by an overview of the unresolved issues restricting the routine application of these novel nanomaterials.

Introduction

Cardiovascular (CV) disease is the leading cause of mortality and morbidity worldwide, especially in industrialized and developing countries. Amongst the various causes of CV diseases, atherosclerosis is the most prevalent pathology. Atherosclerosis affects all vascular beds of the body and can manifest as cardiac, cerebral, visceral, or peripheral vascular diseases. Atherosclerosis is a chronic inflammation affecting the vascular wall, leading through a multistep process to the formation of atherosclerotic plaques (Libby et al. 2009).

Atherosclerosis affects the innermost vessel layer (intima) and is characterized by cholesterol and lipid deposition in addition to inflammatory cell infiltration. The theory for atherogenesis has evolved overtime with improved understanding of the underlying pathophysiology (Fig. 11.1). Endothelial injury triggers a compensatory response, which leads to inflammatory cell infiltration (Lee et al. 2012). In addition, Low Density Lipoprotein (LDL) retention and matrix interaction in the subendothelial space is another hallmark event in atherogenesis. Oxidative stress is a critical feature of atherogenesis. Reactive Oxygen Species (ROS) are responsible for direct damage of cellular structures within the vascular wall, while they also trigger a number of redox sensitive transcriptional pathways, shifting towards a pro-atherogenic transcriptomic profile. ROS are further responsible for the oxidation of LDLs to oxidized Low Density Lipoproteins (oxLDLs) in the subendothelial space, which is then taken up by macrophages and leads to the formation of foam cells (Stocker and Keaney Jr. 2004). Over time mature lesions accumulate and form atherosclerotic plaques which may manifest clinically due to plaque related complications. Expansion of atherosclerotic plaques may lead to gradual narrowing of the lumen and eventually occlusion of the vessel.

Clinical symptoms related to such chronic progression are due to the organs affected by restricted blood circulation. For example, patients with stable coronary artery disease typically complain of angina triggered by physical exertion. Atherosclerotic plaques may also become progressively unstable due to local reaction to pro-inflammatory cytokines and proteinases, leading to plaque ulceration or rupture. The exposed lipid core is highly procoagulant and predispose to acute thrombosis of the vessel lumen. This

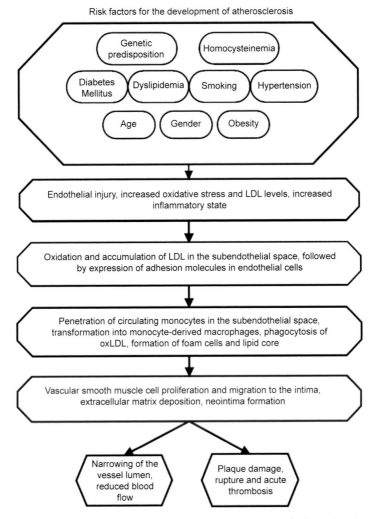

Risk factors for the development of atherosclerosis

Figure 11.1. A model for the development and progression of atherosclerosis.

manifests clinically as acute vascular syndromes, such as acute myocardial infarction or stroke, depending on the vascular territory affected by the disease (Naghavi et al. 2003).

Overview of Nanoparticle Properties

Nanoparticles (NPs) are molecular assemblies belonging to the nanometer scale although sizes ranging from 10 to 100 nm are more appealing for use as Drug Delivery Systems (DDSs) NPs can be organic or inorganic in nature, derived from natural or synthetic materials (Psarros et al. 2012). Due to the availability of several candidate materials for the construction of NPs, they are usually classified according to their shape (linear, block, spheres, etc.), composition [iron oxide (IO), gold (Au), synthetic, natural, etc.], and physical chemistry (magnetic, fluorescent, biodegradable).

Due to their nanometer size, they exhibit unique physicochemical, mechanical, and optical properties completely different to larger counterparts. Their small size still allows interactions with cellular components (such as, membranes, receptors, and proteins), and they can alter the cell physiology. Meanwhile, NPs can avoid detection by the immune system, thus minimizing immune responses and renal clearance. Furthermore, as a result of their high surface area to volume ratio, NPs can be equipped with a wide spectrum of targeting ligands such as proteins, antibodies, peptides, peptide mimics, aptamers, and sugars, as well as diagnostic molecules to enhance their targeting ability, while allowing them to be monitored in order to evaluate their pharmacological activity. Selection from a vast array of materials along with the possibility for extensive modifications (through covalent binding, electrostatic interactions, and adsorption), allows NPs to be engineered specifically for a given application (Goldberg et al. 2007).

In general, NPs applicable to the treatment of CV diseases should have some of the following properties (Lewis et al. 2011): (i) ability to increase the plasma half-life of poorly soluble therapeutic or imaging agents (bioavailability); (ii) delivery of greater payloads, thus lowering the dose and drug toxicity; (iii) ability to accumulate into the site of action via passive or active targeting; (iv) they can be simultaneously used for multiple applications, such as imaging of atherosclerotic plaques and drug delivery; and, (v) production of biodegradable by-products easily expelled via normal metabolic pathways.

Nanoparticles for the Imaging of Cardiovascular Diseases

Medical imaging is a critical part of modern medical practice. The ability to visualize human internal organs using various imaging techniques has given rise not only to diagnostic tools but also to enhanced therapeutic options. Contrast agents are routinely used in medical imaging to enhance the resolution between different types of tissues. The unique optical, electrical, magnetic, and/or fluorescent properties of NPs quickly made them appealing candidates for medical imaging research. The use of NPs as a contrast agent was the first successful application of nanomedicine.

CV disease mechanisms are complex in nature. The myriad cellular pathways involved in the pathophysiology draws the need of specific imaging tools being able to capture information at high resolution. Several cellular and molecular imaging techniques exist nowadays in the field of CV imaging, e.g., ultrasounds, Magnetic Resonance Imaging (MRI), Computed Tomography (CT), Single Photon Emission Computed Tomography (SPECT), Fluorescence Tomography (FT), and Positron Emission Tomography (PET). Furthermore, the development of Atomic Force Microscopy (AFM) for bio-particle and cell imaging has provided new opportunities for imaging in the nanometer scale with ultrahigh resolutions (Parot et al. 2007) (Table 11.1).

Several cells and molecules compose interesting target groups for imaging purposes. These include macrophages and foam cells, which are formed as a result of macrophage lipid accumulation, endothelial and smooth muscle cells, adhesion molecules (Vascular Cell Adhesion Molecule-1, VCAM-1, and Intracellular Adhesion Molecule-1, ICAM-1), integrins, collagen, and matrix metalloproteinases (MMPs) (Sanz and Fayad 2008). The ideal imaging nanosystem should: (i) be selectively activated by a specific biochemical or enzymatic process; (ii) have a selective spectrum for activation; (iii) provide low background signal when circulating in low concentrations and high signal upon accumulation in target areas; and, (iv) have low toxicity (Wickline et al. 2007).

Given the fact that most materials used for imaging purposes have very low *in vivo* stability, low circulation time, and high toxicity, coating materials are of great importance. Poly(ethylene glycol) (PEG), phospholipids, and dextran are some of the coatings used to render the NPs more biocompatible and to improve their efficacy.

Types of nanoparticles and applications in cardiovascular imaging

Atherosclerotic lesions can occur throughout the entire vascular tree. This determines a challenge due to the fact that imaging in different locations of the body often has specific limitations which mandate different imaging strategies. Several NP types have been developed to account for these problems. The most frequently formulated are described below.

Iron oxide and metal nanoparticles

IO NPs are very useful tools in CV imaging. They are usually employed alone or embedded in polymeric matrixes. Given their magnetic property, they are almost exclusively applied as contrast agents in MRI. IO NPs can be coated with receptors or chemically modified, facilitating an efficient delivery to the target thus increasing their efficacy.

Several IO nanosystems are created to achieve the desired imaging results. Sulfated dextran-coated IO NPs ($\approx$ 60 nm in size) were successfully employed as MRI contrast agents for the imaging of macrophage laden plaques in cells and mice (Tu et al. 2011). Since dextran sulfate is a ligand of the macrophage scavenger receptor type A, imaging was much more efficient in comparison with conventional IO NPs. Another interesting category is that of ultrasmall superparamagnetic iron oxides (USPIOs). USPIOs, with sizes $\approx$ 5 to 50 nm, have been coated with numerous materials (e.g., liposomes, dextran, peptides, and antibodies) to improve their biocompatibility. They have been

Table 11.1. Most important imaging methods in the field of CV medicine.

Imaging technique	Plaque components identified/ visualized	Advantages	Disadvantages	Contrast agents
Non-Invasive				
MRI	Lipid composition	Uses non-ionizing radiation, can be performed safely multiple times	Cardiac motion artifact, less spatial resolution, electromagnetic interference	Paramagnetic iron NPs. Gadolinium (Gd^{3+}) NPs
FT	Macrophage contents in plaques	Superior imaging quality, adequate quantification	Mostly *ex vivo* and *in vitro* applications	Magnetofluorescent cross-linked IO NPs. Quantum dots (QDs)
PET	Macrophage contents in plaques	Information about cardiac viability, can monitor glucose metabolism in heart	Limited applications, not yet established	Tracer labeled NPs, i.e., copper-64 (^{64}Cu), fluorine-18 (^{18}F)
CT	Lipid and fibrous components, quantifiable calcium burden	Vulnerable plaque identification	Limited by artifacts, inadequate for visualizing plaque components	Au NPs
Invasive				
Optical coherence tomography	Enables visualization of plaque micro-architecture, measurement of cap thickness	Greater spatial resolution (2 to 30 μm) and data acquisition rate, excellent contrast between lipid and non-lipid components, better analysis capability	Blood displacement required as blood obscures signal, low depth penetration capability	–
Coronary angioscopy	Plaque surface	Able to directly visualize coronary lumen	Blood displacement required as blood obscures signal	–
Intravascular ultrasounds	Plaque volume, vessel and lumen dimensions, visualization of plaque calcification	Better penetration depth	Low spatial resolution (> 100 μm). Cannot fully distinguish intramural thrombus and fibrous cap	–

extensively used in cells, animals, and humans, targeting different components of the atherogenic progress, such as oxLDL, macrophages, and platelets (Te Boekhorst et al. 2012).

Apart from IOs, other metals have drawn the attention of researchers in the field of CV imaging. One of these is Gd^{3+}, thanks to its highly paramagnetic nature. It is mostly used in organic chelate complexes, as it is rapidly cleared from the body through the kidneys before it can be accumulated giving toxic concentrations. Gd^{3+} NPs combined with several materials, such as phospholipids and polymers, have been reported to generate better MRI contrast, thus providing a valid choice for imaging applications. For example, there are reports of successful application of perfluorinated Gd^{3+} NPs (5 to 6 nm in size) in New Zealand rabbits that achieved greater signal to nose ratio, as well as of the use of Gd^{3+} paramagnetic micelles specifically targeting membrane-bound macrophage scavenger receptor type A which were found to increase the signal intensity after accumulation in aortic plaques of apoE$^{-/-}$ mice.

Finally, Au NPs represent a unique category in the field of imaging, thanks to their distinct physical, optical, and electronic properties. Their synthesis can be tightly controlled, enabling to tune most of their aspects in the 1 to 100 nm size range. Au NPs are utilized mostly in CT given their high absorption coefficient, and less interference from bone and soft tissue absorption. An example of Au NP usage is the successful application of Au NPs functionalized with High Density Lipoprotein (HDL) to assess the macrophage burden of atherosclerotic plaques in mice (Cormode et al. 2010). Another group reported the employment of Au NPs surface functionalized with a peptide (acting as a MMP substrate) and a fluorescent cyanine 5.5 (Cy5.5) dye. The nanosystem satisfactorily improved *in vitro* and in mice the near-infrared fluorescence intensity, proving to be a very useful tool when MMPs are expressed (e.g., myocardial infarction, atherosclerosis) (Lee et al. 2008).

Liposomes

Liposomes are made of amphiphilic natural derived materials. They are able to form aggregates, i.e., micelles which consist of a lipid outer layer that encapsulates an aqueous core. Their sizes can vary, ranging from the nanometer to the micrometer scale. When using liposomes for imaging purposes, the contrast agents are generally incorporated in the aqueous phase (Strijkers et al. 2010). It is accepted that liposomes were the first materials to be used for imaging.

An interesting example is the use of liposomes covalently coupled with anti-lipooxygenase-1 antibodies and the fluorescent dye 1,1'-dioctadecyl-3,3,3',3'-tetra-methyl-indocarbocyanine. Lipooxygenase-1 is a receptor for oxLDL which induces apoptosis, MMP release, and expression of adhesion molecules. The liposomes were able to be loaded either with Gd^{3+} ions intended for MRI or with indium-111 (^{111}In) for SPECT or the aforementioned fluorescent dye. When applied to LDL-R$^{-/-}$ and apoE$^{-/-}$ mice fed with an atherogenic diet, they proved to be valuable imaging tools as they were co-localized with apoptotic cells, macrophages, and MMP type 9, all components of rupture prone atherosclerotic plaques (Strijkers et al. 2010).

Quantum dots

QDs are inorganic semiconductor crystals with fluorescent properties far exceeding those of other materials. They have a wide absorbance spectrum, combined with narrow, fully tunable emission spectra, and a high quantum yield. In contrast to other small fluorophores, they do not photobleach, thus keeping their fluorescence intensity intact after exposure. A limiting factor to their applications is the high toxicity of the materials from which they are synthesized, i.e., cadmium. To overcome toxicity issues, QDs are usually embedded in or attached to other materials like polymeric micelles and PEG to increase their biocompatibility and to avoid the accumulation of toxic metals in tissues. Another promising approach to minimize their toxicity is the synthesis of cadmium-free QDs or the use of carbon-based materials like silicon carbide, carbon nanotubes, and nanodiamonds (Douma et al. 2011). Application of QDs in the area of atherosclerosis included an *ex vivo* imaging method of leukocytes and T lymphocytes, both present in atherosclerotic plaques by using spectrally distinct QDs. These were coated with maurocalcine, a cell penetrating peptide, and they were reported to label both cell types without loss of cell function (Jayagopal et al. 2009).

Nanoparticles for Drug Delivery

Another highly attractive area of NP application is that of drug and gene delivery. Given the fact that as aforementioned, many cells and molecules are implicated in the development of atherosclerosis, there are many potential targets for therapeutic intervention. Despite recent advances in drug discovery and CV science, treatment remains suboptimal mostly due to poor drug pharmacokinetics and high toxicity. Therefore, one approach is to combine classical treatment methods with highly efficient, state of the art NPs, or by implementing completely new therapeutic approaches that show significant promise in the field of CV medicine. Numerous DDSs have been created to this aim, each offering distinct advantages for the treatment of a specific area of the CV disease.

Polymeric nanocarriers

Synthetic polymers represent a vast category of macromolecular assemblies that range from polymeric micelles to polymer-protein conjugates. Polymeric micelles represent a very interesting category of DDSs. They are usually made of block copolymers, polymers with two or more different polymeric chains covalently attached to each other, dissolved into a selective solvent, i.e., water, and at solution concentrations above the critical micelle concentration (Antoniades et al. 2010). In an aqueous environment, the hydrophilic components form a corona, while the hydrophobic components tend to gather in the center of the micelle, thus forming the core. Different copolymers can generate micelles with distinctive properties, making them a versatile DDS. Other architectures include linear, graft, dendrimer, and star-shaped designs.

Apart from the variety of materials utilized, other parameters like polymer micro-architecture, hydrophilic/hydrophobic block copolymer ratio, polydispersity, and existence of functional groups can have a catalytic effect on altering the properties of the nanomicelle, offering almost unlimited diversity. These modifications can affect drug loading capacity, targeting ability, bioavailability, water solubility, and toxicity of degradation products. Common polymers used for creating polymeric DDSs include PEG, poly(N-vinylpyrrolidone) (PVP), poly(aspartamides), poly(D,L-lactide-co-glycolide) (PLGA), poly(L-lysine) (PLL), polyamidoamines (PAMAMs), poly(L-glutamic acid), poly(malic acid), to cite just a few. Drugs can either be physically encapsulated into the nanocarrier or covalently attached to the polymer surface.

Drug administration can be systemically or locally, with the second being the generally preferred approach. Techniques of targeting moieties similar to those utilized for NP imaging has been applied for the successful local delivery of NPs. Depending on the NP size, drug release can be outside or inside the target cell. Smaller NPs despite the fact that they carry lower drug payloads compared to their larger counterparts, they can be directly endocytosed thus increasing their overall efficiency (Goldberg et al. 2007). When intended for clinical applications, NPs must be able to avoid macrophage opsonization and recognition by the immune system. In this line, attachment of PEG chains onto the nanocarrier surface (PEGylation) has proved to be the most effective way to assure longer plasma half-lives.

An example is the use of anionic micellar nanocarriers made of four aliphatic chains attached to mucic acid. Combined with the linear PEG segment for improved bioavailability, they were able to successfully retain LDL. Given the detrimental role of LDL in the progression of atherosclerosis and the occurrence of CV diseases, its retention is crucial to inhibit the atherogenic process (Chnari et al. 2005). A somewhat different approach is the incorporation of low molecular weight (M_w) heparin to a third generation PAMAM dendrimer covalently attached to a PEG chain. Heparin is a widely used antithrombotic agent. When applied to a rodent model, this DDS proved to have the same antithrombotic effect (to that of oral heparin administration) with half heparin dose while exhibiting double circulation time (Bai and Ahsan 2009).

Liposomes

Apart from their use in CV imaging, liposomes present favorable possibilities in drug delivery. Thanks to their composition of natural materials, liposomes are highly biocompatible, hence conferring low immunogenicity. However, they are somewhat larger compared to their polymeric counterparts, and their natural composition limits them to lower circulation half-lives (usually a few hours) which is a result of macrophage phagocytosis. In order to overcome bioavailability issues, PEGylation of liposomes is again the preferred method for creating "stealth" liposomes. These are able to avoid recognition and interaction with elements of the immune system, thus increasing the circulation half-life and achieving a more effective drug delivery. In addition, under specific environmental stimuli, drug release can occur via cleavage of the PEG-lipid bonds.

Glucocorticoids represent a category of steroid hormones with potent anti-inflammatory activity, making them a potential therapeutic agent for atherosclerosis. However, their clinical use is limited due to poor pharmacokinetics and low plasma half-lives, requiring greater and more frequent drug doses which can cause systemic side effects. The construction of a PEGylated 3,5-dipentadecyloxybenzamidine hydrochloride liposomes loaded with prednisolone phosphate has proved to be very efficient. The nanoformulation achieved significant suppression of in-stent neointimal growth in atherosclerotic rabbits. Liposomes were formulated to bind to chondroitin sulfate proteoglycans, expressed in the subendothelial matrix but not in vascular endothelial cells, and drug release was possible via endocytosis of the liposome. As a result, lower drug doses were required, thus limiting the systemic toxicity (Joner et al. 2008).

The role of macrophages in the pathophysiology and progression of atherosclerosis is undisputed and therefore they represent another appealing target for the formulation of DDSs. Liposomes have been engineered with egg yolk phosphatidylcholine, cholesterol, and dicetylphosphate (7:2:1 molar ratio) loaded with dexamethasone. They were applied to an atherogenic mouse model and satisfactorily demonstrated anti-atherogenic effects. Interestingly, it was found that the liposome efficacy was correlated with the size. In fact, three liposomal formulations (average sizes: 70, 200, and 500 nm) were investigated. The 200 nm-sized liposomes proved to have the greatest anti-atherogenic effect (Chono et al. 2005).

Nanoparticle-protein conjugates

Synthetic peptides, proteins, and antibodies have emerged as a new class of therapeutic agents over the last few years. While very potent, a common limiting factor is their low plasma half-life and occasionally their high immunogenicity. Nanotechnology can overcome these problems. Probably, a very effective strategy is the conjugation of polymers to proteins or antibodies, thus maximizing their therapeutic potential. The well-known method of PEGylation can be applied to these conjugates, as well as aiming to increase their bioavailability and biocompatibility. Furthermore, newer methods in PEGylation techniques include selective glutamine PEGylation in proteins with the aid of the enzyme transglutaminase and utilizing degradable PEG-protein linkages to increase the efficacy of the protein being delivered (Sato 2002).

The range of therapeutic targets offers many possibilities to the use of NP-protein conjugates in the field of CV medicine. Examples include the use of the enzyme catalase coupled to immunoglobulin (Ig) G targeting ICAM-1 and platelet endothelial cell adhesion molecule-1 (PECAM-1) (Christofidou-Solomidou et al. 2003). These transmembrane glycoproteins are overexpressed in atherosclerotic plaques as a result of cytokine production and macrophage accumulation. Catalase is an enzyme which catalyzes the reaction of hydrogen peroxide to water and oxygen. Hydrogen peroxide, as all peroxides, is considered to be a ROS. As mentioned, ROS have been identified to be a critical element in endothelial injury, leading to edema, atherosclerosis, or even thrombosis.

Another approach is the administration of apolipoprotein (Apo) B-100 antibodies covalently attached to biocompatible and biodegradable poly(D,L-lactide) (PLA) NPs (Maximov et al. 2010). Apo B-100 is a major component of LDL and Apo B-100 antibodies were used to actively target LDLs. The aim of this study was to enhance the delivery of LDL to the liver, where it is metabolized. The NP-antibody conjugates rapidly bind to LDLs and are also quickly uptaken by liver Küpffer cells, thus optimizing the delivery of LDLs to the liver and removing them from circulation. *In vitro* experiments demonstrated a six-fold decrease in the levels of LDL, while maintaining cell viability, thus providing a promising solution for the treatment of hyperlipidemia, a critical factor in the progression of atherosclerosis.

Fullerenes

The discovery of fullerenes three decades ago was a key trigger to the development of a new class of materials which were composed solely of carbon. Fullerenes can be found in various shapes (hollow spheres, ellipsoids, and cylinders) and sizes, and they can undergo almost unlimited chemical modifications. Cylindrical-shaped fullerenes are widely known as carbon nanotubes. These new allotropes of carbon have unique optical, mechanical, and electrical properties, hence the growing interest in nanomedicine.

Oxidative stress and LDL are both critical factors for the progression of CV diseases. In an interesting study the use of a chemically modified highly hydroxylated fullerene was reported to attenuate levels of oxidative stress and inflammation in an adipose tissue equivalent (Xiao et al. 2011). The biomimetic nature of this compound facilitated the endocytosis and localization near to cytoplasmic proteins. One of these was vimentin, a protein responsible for controlling the transportation of LDL from the cells into the bloodstream.

In a similar approach a water-soluble hexasulfobutyl fullerene was found to have significant antioxidant activities, as it protected plasma lipids from peroxidation and reduced their binding capability to other lipoproteins (Hsu et al. 2000). Another approach is the use of sulfonated porous carbon nanotubes and activated carbon composite beards as LDL adsorbent materials for hemoperfusion. Hemoperfusion is recently applied to clinical practice as a straightforward method for effectively removing LDL from circulation. The sulfonic acid groups present in the nanosystem were able to retain larger amounts of LDLs by electrostatic interactions between the adsorbent and the LDL (Lu et al. 2011).

Despite the theoretical advantages of fullerenes, further rigorous investigations are required to establish the safety of its application as DDSs, as there may be unwanted side effects related to their use. For example, a study of carbon nanotubes as an inhalation agent demonstrated that it promoted vascular oxidative stress via activation of the gene heme oxygenase, which directly affects mitochondrial function (Walker et al. 2009).

Nanoparticles for Gene Therapy

An interesting approach for combating CV diseases is gene therapy. Ability to effectively control the local delivery of genes can yield very promising therapeutic results. Gene vectors are deoxyribonucleic acid (DNA) vesicles intended for gene delivery. They are made of the insert and a larger DNA sequence serving as the backbone of the vector. Typical vector examples include plasmids, viruses, and artificial chromosomes. Nanotechnology can again provide new alternatives to gene therapy by the introduction of polymeric nanovectors. Similar to DDSs, these nanosystems need to have high gene transfer output, being biocompatible with negligible cytotoxicity.

Non-viral vectors for gene delivery

Recent advances in materials science and polymer chemistry have provided several alternatives to employ as vectors in gene delivery. The most widely used are described below.

Polyethyleneimine

Polyethyleneimine (PEI) is a polycation containing only secondary amine groups and it was one of the first polymers applied to gene delivery. Due to its high cationic electrical charge it can bind with DNA molecules via electrostatic interactions, forming small PEI-DNA complexes (polyplexes), as well as it can bind to anionic cell membrane components, facilitating its endocytosis. Once inside the cell, protonation of the amines causes osmotic swelling and DNA release which in turn diffuses into the nucleus. Cell penetration can be enhanced by utilizing cell penetrating peptides. However, PEI is very toxic to cells so in most occasions it is conjugated to PEG chains to minimize the toxic side effects.

Dendrimers

Dendrimers are hyperbranched polymers with a symmetric structure around the core geometry. They are defined by their generation number, e.g., G2, a number that indicates the amount of branching cycles repeated during its synthesis. G2/G3PAMAM dendrimers form neutral complexes with DNA and ribonucleic acid (RNA), being easily released thus yielding a high transfection rate.

Chitosan

Chitosan is a linear polysaccharide naturally synthesized from randomly distributed β-(1-4)-linked D-glucosamine and N-acetyl-D-glucosamine. Commercially, it is produced via deacetylation of chintin naturally encountered in the exoskeleton of crustaceans as well as in the cell walls of fungi. Its high biocompatibility, low toxicity, and cost, make up for the low transfection rate achieved. Control of the ratio of nitrogen molecules present in chitosan to the phosphate ones in genes as well as the M_W and degree of deacetylation, can be advantageously used in the engineering of efficient chitosan nanovectors for gene delivery.

Applications in cardiovascular science

Polyplex micelles made from cationic block copolymers have been reported to be effective non-viral vectors. In a study, a PEG segment attached to a cationic polyaspartamide segment with an ethylenediamine unit at the side chain formed a very stable and biocompatible polyplex micelle with a plasmid DNA tightly packed into its core. Results demonstrated effective transfer of the gene to Vascular Smooth Muscle Cells (VSMCs) both *in vitro* and in injured rabbit carotid arteries (Akagi et al. 2007). In addition, the polymeric vector had no cytotoxicity and thrombus formation, upon interacting with blood components.

Small interfering ribonucleic acids (*si*RNAs) are a class of double stranded ribonucleic acid (*ds*RNA) molecules. They are usually 20 to 25 nucleotides long and their most important role is the ability to regulate gene expression. While firstly thought only to down-regulate gene expression, they can also activate it as well via small RNA-induced gene activation. Neointimal formation is very common after arterial interventions. It is accompanied with up-regulation of nicotinamide adenine dinucleotide phosphate oxidase isoform 2 (NOX2). The enzyme produces ROS. In a murine model of accelerated atherosclerosis by a high fat diet, neointimal formation was induced using carotid balloon angioplasty. By using PLL NPs loaded with *si*RNA for the NOX2 Cybb gene, local delivery to the arterial wall after balloon angioplasty was achieved. The *si*RNA delivery was successful as NOX2 Cybb gene expression was down-regulated, greatly reducing neointimal formation (Li et al. 2010).

VSMCs are intimately involved in the development of atherosclerosis and vascular remodeling after arterial injury. Migration of VSMCs is governed by the interplay of signaling pathways involving cytokines and proteases. MMP type 2 is a member of the protease enzymes that play a key role in several biological functions, including embryonic development and tissue remodeling. With the aid of an amphipathic polyplex micelle, composed of deoxycholic acid and modified low M_W PEI, *si*RNA for the MMP type 2 gene was satisfactorily delivered (Kim et al. 2012). The polyplex micelle reported a considerable increase in its uptake by the VSMCs, thus improving *si*RNA delivery *in vitro*. It results in attenuation of MMP type 2 gene expression and subsequently inhibition of VSMC migration to target areas.

Theranostic Nanoparticles

With increasing research in nanotechnology throughout the scientific fields of chemistry, physics, medicine, and biology, advanced tools have been developed to create nanosystems for multiple applications (multifunctional NPs). Of particular interest are those that can be applied for both imaging and drug delivery purposes. They are termed theranostic (therapeutic + diagnostic) NPs. More complex systems can also be formulated by sequential growth and coating of NPs. The addition of biofunctional molecules through such a process can further improve the value of a nanosystem. They can be antibodies, fluorescent dyes, magnetic particles, DNA strands, to cite just a few (Fig. 11.2). The development of such nanosystems is of great importance for combating CV diseases as it offers the opportunity for guiding and evaluating the efficacy of the therapeutic agent being delivered.

Intergrins are receptors responsible for the attachment of a cell with its surrounding environment (other cells or the extracellular matrix). Of particular interest is the $\alpha_v\beta_3$ integrin, expressed in the vasa vasorum, which plays a key role in the angiogenic process. Fumagillin is an anti angiogenic drug that when used at high doses can cause severe toxicity like brain injury. It is hypothesized that when loaded to a DDS, a local drug delivery is possible allowing for lower drug doses and limiting the side effects. A theranostic NP consisting of perfluorocarbon NPs loaded with fumagillin and Gd^{3+} and surface decorated with $\alpha_v\beta_3$ integrin was created for this purpose (Winter et al. 2006). Particle size ranged from 175 to 220 nm, incorporating $\approx$ 9,000 Gd^{3+} ions and carrying a fumagillin payload of 30 µg. In a model of New Zealand rabbits that were fed with atherogenic diet for 80 days, administration of the

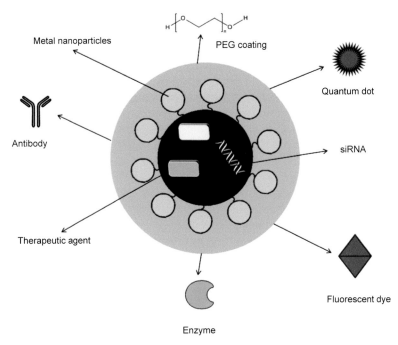

Figure 11.2. Representation of a multifunctional NP. Its properties come from the numerous functional groups that it can be equipped with.

non-toxic DDS was very efficient in reducing cholesterol levels. The presence of the Gd^{3+} coating allowed for the detection of early stage of angiogenesis in the aortic wall by MRI.

Macrophages, observed in abundance in atherosclerotic lesions, are a primary target for drug delivery. A theranostic magnetofluorescent NP was engineered to selectively interact with these macrophages (McCarthy et al. 2006). The nanosystem was characterized by a 10 kDa dextran coating, as well as a 5 nm-sized iron core consisting of ≈ 8,000 iron atoms with a final diameter in water of ≈ 30 nm. The dextran coating allowed for increased uptake in atherosclerotic plaques by macrophages. Furthermore, the photosensitizer 5-(4-carboxyphenyl)-10,15,20-triphenyl-2,3-dihydroxychlorin (TPC) was covalently attached to the NPs. When excited by light at an appropriate wavelength (646 nm), it produces singlet oxygen ($^1O_2$) as a result of the interaction between the excited porphyrinic group and molecular oxygen. $^1O_2$ is highly cytotoxic and can be applied to induce cell apoptosis. Thus, the magnetofluorescent NP allowed for the simultaneous selective delivery of the TCP, effectively killing murine and human macrophages *in vitro*, and *in vivo* imaging with MRI or near-infrared fluorescence for the evaluation of the efficacy of the phototherapy.

Nanoparticles for Detection of Biomarkers

Biomarkers are biomolecules (enzymes, proteins, hormones, genes) whose concentration when measured and quantified can provide crucial prognostic and diagnostic information about the current state of a disease (Vasan 2006). Biomarkers can be measured in numerous biological samples, e.g., blood, tissues, and urine. A biomarker needs to meet the following characteristics: (i) ability for accurate and reproducible measurements; (ii) high specificity for the application desired; (iii) easy interpretation by clinicians; and, (iv) a relatively low cost.

Biomarkers in cardiovascular disease

In the field of CV medicine, several biomarkers have been identified as useful tools for assessing the status of patients suffering from CV diseases. Examples include homocysteine, troponin, and B type-natriuretic peptide (BNP) (Table 11.2).

Table 11.2. Biomarkers during the progression of the CV disease.

Disease stage	Biomarkers expressed
Plaque formation	LDL, oxLDL, C-reactive protein (CRP), interleukins (IL-6, IL-10, and IL-18)
Unstable plaque	MMP type 9, myeloperoxidase, ICAM-1, VCAM-1
Plaque rupture	Soluble CD40 ligand (sCD40L), VCAM-1, placental growth factor (PlGF)
Thrombosis	von Willebrand factor (vWF), D-dimer, sCD40L, plasminogen activator inhibitor type 1 (PAI-1)
Ischemia	BNP, choline, plasma free fatty acid, ischaemia modified albumin (IMA)
Necrosis	cardiac troponin T (cTnT), cardiac troponin I (cTnI), creatine kinase form MB, myoglobin
Left ventricular remodeling	BNP, N-terminal prohormone brain natriuretic peptide (NT-proBNP), MMP

However, few of these cardiac biomarkers are yet to be considered as standard tools in risk assessment, even when used in combination. In addition, biomarker measurements by standardized assays are typically performed in a laboratory and are time consuming. While their detection limits are within the pg/mL area, their application as a diagnostic is challenging since their measurement is often times critical in patients suffering from acute vascular syndromes, where an early treatment is required to maximize the outcome benefits. Another attempt for faster biomarker detection was the development of Point-Of-Care (POC) devices, which are simple, fast, and inexpensive to use without the need for sample transport to a laboratory (McDonnell et al. 2009).

However, these advantages come at the cost of lower sensitivity and the need for several biomarkers testing to obtain the certainty required for a treatment.

Silicon nanowires for cardiac biomarker detection

Nanotechnology can optimize the detection of cardiac biomarkers, and even aid in the discovery of new ones. In this line, probably one of the most promising platforms is silicon nanowire (SiNW). SiNWs act as field effect transistors, able to control the size and consequently the conductivity of a channel by using an electric field (Zhang 2012). They can be surface functionalized with antibodies by covalently or electrostatic interactions. When a protein binds to the antibody, the change in charge density triggers a change in the surface electric field of the SiNW, this allows the quantification of the analyte concentration. SiNWs have been engineered for multiple detection in serum samples of cTnT, creatine kinase isoform MM, and creatine kinase isoform MB. These nanoplatforms were not only applied as a POC biomarker detection device, but also demonstrated significantly greater detection ranges (fg/mL) compared to conventional methods (pg/mL). SiNW applications also extend to the areas of pH fluctuations detection, determination of Ca^{2+} ion concentration as well as traces of important chemical and biological molecules (Cui et al. 2001). Accurate measurements of low quantities of biomarkers can help in the early detection of an irregularity or disease. Furthermore, creation of POC nanodevices by combining micro-electric-mechanical systems and NPs has drastically improved the sensitivity of biomarkers present in acute myocardial infarction (Wang et al. 2009).

A pioneering perspective of nanoplatforms (apart from their *ex vivo* applications) is exploring their *in vivo* biomarker detection capabilities. Nanosensors implanted into the myocardium and coronary artery offer real-time detection of several cations (e.g., H^+, Na^+, K^+, Ca^{2+}) while simultaneously assessing the role of H^+ and K^+ ion activity in myocardial infarction (Vogt et al. 2004).

Nanofibers in Cardiovascular Medicine

Nanofibers as vascular grafts

Despite the increasing uptake of percutaneous angioplasty for the treatment of CV diseases, open surgical repair of arteries remain a cornerstone in the treatment options. Synthetic Vascular Grafts (VGs) are routinely used in peripheral vascular surgery and there is ongoing research to create synthetic VGs, but only few have been successfully employed in clinical practice. One example is the use of expanded polytetrafluoroethylene tubes (ePTFE) which still accounts as one of the favored materials for revascularization procedures (Twine and McLain 2010). Although these VGs were applied to larger diameter arteries, the problem still persists with the smaller diameter ones. Apart from the diameter, there are several hemodynamic differences in small arteries like lower blood flow velocity and consequently lower sheer stress. Use of synthetic grafts may lead to thrombosis, leaving only the option of autologous ones to be applied in small diameter artery revascularization (Twine and McLain 2010). Ideally the small-sized grafts should be able to mimic the biological and mechanical properties of the artery to be replaced.

Nanotechnology can be of great aid in the field of nanofiber VG creation. By using novel nanomaterials available, nanofibers can be engineered in a way to overcome the challenges presented when synthesizing small synthetic VGs. Furthermore, their already enhanced properties can be enriched with new ones, like drug delivery, thus providing a new generation of nanofiber VGs.

Electrospinning

This is the most effective method for creating such grafts. Although this technique has been known for almost a century, interest in it has resurfaced mostly due to recent advances in materials science and the fast growing need for new biomaterials. Electrospinning is a very simple method requiring only a polymer solution in a syringe pump, a high voltage generator, an electrode to charge the polymer solution, and a surface oppositely charged to collect the fibers. When the voltage applied to the droplet is sufficient, surface tension is counteracted by electrostatic repulsion, resulting in droplet stretching. At a critical point (also known as Taylor cone), a stream of liquid erupts from the surface. As the jet travels through the air, the fluid steam is elongated to form solid fibers which then accumulate on the collector (Greiner and Wendorff 2007) (Fig. 11.3).

More advanced electrospinning techniques allow for the creation of highly aligned fibers as well as double layered ones (core/shell). Better aligned nanofibers possess greater mechanical strength and were recently found to enhance cell migration towards the nanofiber orientation (He et al. 2006). Such attributes are much needed in VGs.

Materials used for vascular graft construction

Poly(ε-caprolactone) (PCL). PCL is a synthetic biocompatible and biodegradable aliphatic polyester with excellent mechanical properties and low degradation rate. Thus, it is the most widely used material for the construction of nanofiber VGs. It is also hydrophobic which can enhance its drug delivery capabilities. PCL-based VGs, when applied to a rat model and evaluated during 24 weeks, demonstrated greater healing and mechanical characteristics as well as rapid endothelialization, than their ePTFE counterparts (Pektok et al. 2008).

Collagen. Collagen is a protein encountered in abundance in the artery extracellular matrix, giving them the required mechanical strength and durability. There are several types of collagen with specific attributes,

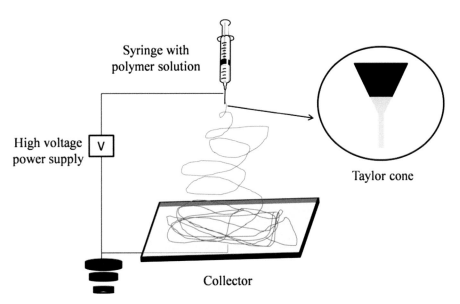

Figure 11.3. Overview of the electrospinning process. A viscous polymer solution is ejected at a controlled rate, charged by an electrode (10 to 30 kV). As the solutions travels through the air, solvent evaporation occurs and nanofibers are formed. These nanofibers finally deposit on the collector.

depending on their role and location in the extracellular matrix. Notably, collagen types I, III, and IV are mostly encountered in the three artery layers (the intima, the media, and the adventitia), making them ideal candidate materials for the construction of nanofibers. Collagen has been successfully electrospinned using appropriate solvents and can create highly biocompatible VGs (Sell et al. 2009).

Other Polymers. Several different combinations of polymeric materials have been employed to create nanofiber VGs. For instance, synthetic polymers such as polyurethanes, PLA, and poly(glycolide), and natural ones like fibrin and gelatin. Mix of natural and synthetic polymers can optimize their characteristics even more and solve some immunogenicity and biocompatibility issues that may arise when utilized as VGs.

Nanofibers with drug delivery activity as vascular grafts

VGs based on nanofibers can be further enhanced with drug delivery technologies. Drugs can either be physically incorporated into the polymer or covalently attached to it. In the first case, both polymer and the drug must be stable in the solvent used in electrospinning. This can be a limiting factor as these solvents are in most cases harsh and can damage fragile biomolecules and drugs. Covalent bonding of the therapeutic agent to the nanofiber after the electrospinning process can solve the aforementioned problem.

PCL-based nanofibers and loaded with the anticoagulant heparin were assessed for their therapeutic effect and heparin release rate (Luong-Van et al. 2006). It was demonstrated that the nanofibers achieved local release of heparin for longer periods, with almost half of the drug released in 14 days. Furthermore, the nanofibers did not cause inflammatory responses and inhibited smooth muscle cell proliferation *in vitro*.

Another example is the synthesis of PLGA-based nanofibers loaded with tacrolimus, widely used as an immunosuppressive agent (Mutsuga et al. 2009). These nanofibers with diameters ranging from 100 to 800 nm, demonstrated an initial burst drug release within the first day, followed up by a period of four weeks, proving to be an invaluable nanotool for the prevention of anastomotic strictures, which are the leading cause for prosthetic, arterial, and venous graft failure (Kapadia et al. 2008).

Nanotoxicity

The unique nature of nanomaterials makes them invaluable tools for nanomedicine applications. However, some of their intriguing properties account for their limitations as well. Given the fact that NP attributes are completely different than those of their larger counterparts, it is hard to predict their potential toxicity. Hence, it is imperative that new materials intended for nanomedicine purposes are thoroughly assessed individually and as a combination for any toxicological effects. All the parameters affecting NP synthesis (i.e., shape, size, chemical modification, solubility, functional groups) play a key role in their nanotoxicity effects. The small size of NPs confers an increased surface-to-volume ratio which attributes for their enhanced chemical and biological activity. This may result in undesired ROS production and consequently cause irreversible damage to important biomolecules such as DNA, RNA, proteins, and enzymes. Furthermore, several NPs are able to cross the blood-brain barrier and other membranes, gaining entrance into blood circulation and access into cells and organs. This may prove a challenge as NP local administration can potentially cause damage to seemingly irrelevant target areas. Biocompatibility and biodegradation issues need also to be addressed as they can further enhance their toxicological profile (Stern and McNeil 2008).

Another nanotoxicity issue, which also greatly hinders the performance of nanosystems, is their recognition and interaction with elements of the immune system. The immune systems are a complex and highly sophisticated defense mechanism tasked with protecting the host against pathogens, infections, or even the host's cancer cells. NP-immune system interactions may cause severe side effects. They can potentially result in immunostimulation which in return may lead to inflammatory responses or even "disorient" the immune system causing autoimmune diseases. On the other hand, they may weaken the immune system causing immunosuppression, crippling the host's ability to protect itself from pathogens resulting in infections or even cancer (Fig. 11.4).

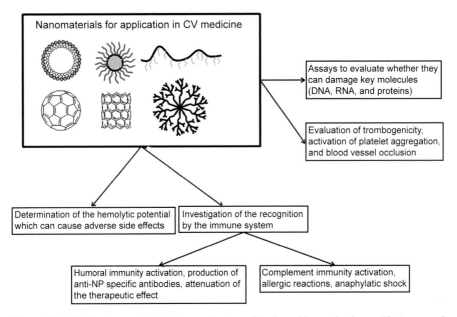

Figure 11.4. Critical nanotoxicity issues that need to be addressed when utilizing novel nanomaterials in CV diseases.

Humoral and complement activation

NPs may activate the humoral and complement immunities. The term humoral immunity refers to the immunity mediated by the secretion of antibodies produced by B cells. NPs may cause antibody secretion, which bind to the particle surface, effectively removing them from blood before they can reach their target and achieve their desired effect. There are reports of antibodies secreted against fullerene-protein conjugates. Furthermore, despite PEGylation as the most effective method increasing NP biocompatibility, there are reports of PEG antibodies when PEGylated liposomes have been administered (Ishida et al. 2007).

Complement immunity is a complex network of proteins that aids the humoral immune system, via activation of several biochemical cascades, aiming to kill a target cell by destroying its plasma membrane. When an allergen enters in the blood, it triggers an immune response causing allergic reactions, inflammation, or even an anaphylactic shock. NPs can act as allergens and the aforementioned side effects may occur as a result of their administration. Their allergenic potential is greatly influenced by their surface properties, e.g., surface charge, coating material used, functional groups present, etc. Biocompatibility is a critical feature in this case, as it can diminish such effects.

Hemolysis

An aspect of NP toxicity that needs to be addressed is their potential hemolytic ability. When NPs enter the blood, they can interact with erythrocytes. Inadequately constructed nanosystems have the potential to cause hemolysis and consequently anemia. Studies have stressed the role of NP surface electrical charge as a key factor for determining their hemolytic ability. For instance, fullerenes with a positive surface charge have demonstrated increased hemolytic potential compared to their negatively charged counterparts. In addition, PAMAM and PLL dendrimers exhibit increased hemolytic potential due to their positively charged primary amine groups (Bosi et al. 2004).

Thrombogenicity

The potential of NP to induce thrombogenicity is another important consideration. One of the main reasons for creating nanosystems is to assure longer plasma half-lives to ensure a prolonged and successful delivery of therapeutic and/or imaging agents. However, this might prove challenging as the longer a NP remains in circulation the greater the probability of interaction with coagulating molecules. Such interactions may result in platelet aggregation and thrombus formation. Studies have demonstrated that particle size has a definitive effect on the platelet activation pathway. Platelets are activated by the platelet glycoprotein integrin receptor IIb/IIIa (Radomski et al. 2005). For instance, microparticles do so via protein kinase C, while NPs trigger such activation in a protein kinase C independent manner. It has also been claimed that carbon-based particles induce platelet aggregation without thromboxane A2 and adenosine diphosphate (ADP) release as a prerequisite.

Conclusions

Over the last few years the interdisciplinary field of nanomedicine has witnessed a tremendous boost, due to rapid advances of its related fields (medicine, biology, chemistry, materials science, etc.) and the successful first results from clinical applications. CV disease will remain the foremost health care burden globally and remain a focus of medicinal research. Nanotechnology has been progressively introduced in the field of CV disease research and promising results are reported in the application of nanomedicine as a treatment strategy against CV diseases. Despite the encouraging progress, every nanomaterial utilized must be thoroughly assessed to avoid the potential nanotoxicity. It is likely that nanomedicine will eventually equip medical practitioners with a new array of tools in the management of CV diseases.

Abbreviations

ADP	:	adenosine diphosphate
AFM	:	atomic force microscopy
Apo	:	apolipoprotein
Au	:	gold
BNP	:	B type-natriuretic peptide or brain natriuretic peptide
CRP	:	C-reactive protein
CT	:	computed tomography
cTnI	:	cardiac troponin I
cTnT	:	cardiac troponin T
^{64}Cu	:	copper-64
CV	:	cardiovascular
Cy5.5	:	cyanine 5.5
DDS	:	drug delivery system
DNA	:	deoxyribonucleic acid
*ds*RNA	:	double stranded ribonucleic acid
ePTFE	:	expanded polytetrafluoroethylene
^{18}F	:	fluorine-18
FT	:	fluorescence tomography
Gd^{3+}	:	gadolinium
HDL	:	high density lipoprotein
ICAM-1	:	intracellular adhesion molecule-1
Ig	:	immunoglobulin
IL	:	interleukin
IMA	:	ischaemia modified albumin
^{111}In	:	indium-111
IO	:	iron oxide
LDL	:	low density lipoprotein
MMP	:	matrix metalloproteinase
MRI	:	magnetic resonance imaging
M_W	:	molecular weight
NF	:	neointimal formation
NOX2	:	nicotinamide adenine dinucleotide phosphate oxidase isoform 2
NP	:	nanoparticle
NT-proBNP	:	*N*-terminal prohormone brain natriuretic peptide
$^{1}O_2$	:	singlet oxygen
oxLDL	:	oxidized low density lipoprotein
PAI-1	:	plasminogen activator inhibitor type 1
PAMAM	:	polyamidoamine
PECAM-1	:	platelet endothelial cell adhesion molecule-1
PEG	:	poly(ethylene glycol)

PEI	:	polyethyleneimine
PET	:	positron emission tomography
PLA	:	poly(D,L-lactide)
PCL	:	poly(ε-caprolactone)
PLGA	:	poly(D,L-lactide-*co*-glycolide)
PlGF	:	placental growth factor
PLL	:	poly(L-lysine)
POC	:	point-of-care
PVP	:	poly(*N*-vinylpyrrolidone)
QD	:	quantum dot
RNA	:	ribonucleic acid
ROS	:	reactive oxygen species
sCD40L	:	soluble CD40 ligand
SiNW	:	silicon nanowire
*si*RNA	:	small interfering ribonucleic acid
SPECT	:	single photon emission computed tomography
TCP	:	5-(4-carboxyphenyl)-10,15,20-triphenyl-2,3-dihydroxychlorin
USPIO	:	ultrasmall superparamagnetic iron oxide
VCAM-1	:	vascular cell adhesion molecule-1
VG	:	vascular graft
VSMC	:	vascular smooth muscle cell
vWF	:	von Willebrand factor

References

Akagi, D. and M. Oba, H. Koyama, N. Nishiyama, S. Fukushima, T. Miyata, H. Nagawa and K. Kataoka. 2007. Biocompatible micellar nanovectors achieve efficient gene transfer to vascular lesions without cytotoxicity and thrombus formation. Gene Ther. 14: 1029–1038.

Antoniades, C. and C. Psarros, D. Tousoulis, C. Bakogiannis, C. Shirodaria and C. Stefanadis. 2010. Nanoparticles: a promising therapeutic approach in atherosclerosis. Curr. Drug Deliv. 7: 303–311.

Bai, S. and F. Ahsan. 2009. Synthesis and evaluation of pegylated dendrimeric nanocarrier for pulmonary delivery of low molecular weight heparin. Pharm. Res. 26: 539–548.

Bosi, S. and L. Feruglio, T. Da Ros, G. Spalluto, B. Gregoretti, M. Terdoslavich, G. Decorti, S. Passamonti, S. Moro and M. Prato. 2004. Hemolytic effects of water-soluble fullerene derivatives. J. Med. Chem. 47: 6711–6715.

Chnari, E. and H.B. Lari, L. Tian, K.E. Uhrich and P.V. Moghe. 2005. Nanoscale anionic macromolecules for selective retention of low-density lipoproteins. Biomaterials. 26: 3749–3758.

Chono, S. and Y. Tauchi, Y. Deguchi and K. Morimoto. 2005. Efficient drug delivery to atherosclerotic lesions and the antiatherosclerotic effect by dexamethasone incorporated into liposomes in atherogenic mice. J. Drug Target. 13: 267–276.

Christofidou-Solomidou, M. and A. Scherpereel, R. Wiewrodt, K. Ng, T. Sweitzer, E. Arguiri, V. Shuvaev, C.C. Solomides, S.M. Albelda and V.R. Muzykantov. 2003. PECAM-directed delivery of catalase to endothelium protects against pulmonary vascular oxidative stress. Am. J. Physiol. Lung Cell Mol. Physiol. 285: L283–L292.

Cormode, D.P. and E. Roessl, A. Thran, T. Skajaa, R.E. Gordon, J.P. Schlomka, V. Fuster, E.A. Fisher, W.J. Mulder, R. Proksa and Z.A. Fayad. 2010. Atherosclerotic plaque composition: analysis with multicolor CT and targeted gold nanoparticles. Radiology. 256: 774–782.

Cui, Y. and Q. Wei, H. Park and C.M. Lieber. 2001. Nanowire nanosensors for highly sensitive and selective detection of biological and chemical species. Science. 293: 1289–1292.

Douma, K. and R.T. Megens and M.A. van Zandvoort. 2011. Optical molecular imaging of atherosclerosis using nanoparticles: shedding new light on the darkness. Wiley Interdiscip. Rev. Nanomed. Nanobiotechnol. 3: 376–388.

Goldberg, M. and R. Langer and X. Jia. 2007. Nanostructured materials for applications in drug delivery and tissue engineering. J. Biomater. Sci. Polym. Ed. 18: 241–268.

Greiner, A. and J.H. Wendorff. 2007. Electrospinning: a fascinating method for the preparation of ultrathin fibers. Angew. Chem. Int. Ed. Engl. 46: 5670–5703.

He, W. and T. Yong, Z.W. Ma, R. Inai, W.E. Teo and S. Ramakrishna. 2006. Biodegradable polymer nanofiber mesh to maintain functions of endothelial cells. Tissue Eng. 12: 2457–2466.

Hsu, H.C. and Y.Y. Chiang, W.J. Chen and Y.T. Lee. 2000. Water-soluble hexasulfobutyl [60] fullerene inhibits plasma lipid peroxidation by direct association with lipoproteins. J. Cardiovasc. Pharmacol. 36: 423–427.

Ishida, T. and X. Wang, T. Shimizu, K. Nawata and H. Kiwada. 2007. PEGylated liposomes elicit an anti-PEG IgM response in a T cell-independent manner. J. Control. Release. 122: 349–355.

Jayagopal, A. and Y.R. Su, J.L. Blakemore, M.F. Linton, S. Fazio and F.R. Haselton. 2009. Quantum dot mediated imaging of atherosclerosis. Nanotechnology. 20: 165102.

Joner, M. and K. Morimoto, H. Kasukawa, K. Steigerwald, S. Merl, G. Nakazawa, M.C. John, A.V. Finn, E. Acampado, F.D. Kolodgie, H.K. Gold and R. Virmani. 2008. Site-specific targeting of nanoparticle prednisolone reduces in-stent restenosis in a rabbit model of established atheroma. Arterioscler. Thromb. Vasc. Biol. 28: 1960–1966.

Kapadia, M.R. and D.A. Popowich and M.R. Kibbe. 2008. Modified prosthetic vascular conduits. Circulation. 117: 1873–1882.

Kim, D. and D. Lee, Y.L. Jang, S.Y. Chae, D. Choi, J.H. Jeong and S.H. Kim. 2012. Facial amphipathic deoxycholic acid-modified polyethyleneimine for efficient MMP-2 siRNA delivery in vascular smooth muscle cells. Eur. J. Pharm. Biopharm. 81: 14–23.

Lee, S. and E.J. Cha, K. Park, S.Y. Lee, J.K. Hong, I.C. Sun, S.Y. Kim, K. Choi, I.C. Kwon, K. Kim and C.H. Ahn. 2008. A near-infrared-fluorescence-quenched gold-nanoparticle imaging probe for *in vivo* drug screening and protease activity determination. Angew. Chem. Int. Ed. Engl. 47: 2804–2807.

Lee, R. and K.M. Channon and C. Antoniades. 2012. Therapeutic strategies targeting endothelial function in humans: clinical implications. Curr. Vasc. Pharmacol. 10: 77–93.

Lewis, D.R. and K. Kamisoglu, A.W. York and P.V. Moghe. 2011. Polymer-based therapeutics: nanoassemblies and nanoparticles for management of atherosclerosis. Wiley Interdiscip. Rev. Nanomed. Nanobiotechnol. 3: 400–420.

Li, J.M. and P.E. Newburger, M.J. Gounis, P. Dargon, X. Zhang and L.M. Messina. 2010. Local arterial nanoparticle delivery of siRNA for NOX2 knockdown to prevent restenosis in an atherosclerotic rat model. Gene Ther. 17: 1279–1287.

Libby, P. and P.M. Ridker and G.K. Hansson. 2009. Inflammation in atherosclerosis: from pathophysiology to practice. J. Am. Coll. Cardiol. 54: 2129–2138.

Lu, Y. and Q. Gong, F. Lu, J. Liang, L. Ji, Q. Nie and X. Zhang. 2011. Preparation of sulfonated porous carbon nanotubes/activated carbon composite beads and their adsorption of low density lipoprotein. J. Mater. Sci. Mater. Med. 22: 1855–1862.

Luong-Van, E. and L. Grondahl, K.N. Chua, K.W. Leong, V. Nurcombe and S.M. Cool. 2006. Controlled release of heparin from poly(epsilon-caprolactone) electrospun fibers. Biomaterials. 27: 2042–2050.

Maximov, V.D. and V.V. Reukov, J.N. Barry, C. Cochrane and A.A. Vertegel. 2010. Protein-nanoparticle conjugates as potential therapeutic agents for the treatment of hyperlipidemia. Nanotechnology. 21: 265103.

McCarthy, J.R. and F.A. Jaffer and R. Weissleder. 2006. A macrophage-targeted theranostic nanoparticle for biomedical applications. Small. 2: 983–987.

McDonnell, B. and S. Hearty, P. Leonard and R. O'Kennedy. 2009. Cardiac biomarkers and the case for point-of-care testing. Clin. Biochem. 42: 549–561.
Mutsuga, M. and Y. Narita, A. Yamawaki, M. Satake, H. Kaneko, Y. Suematsu, A. Usui and Y. Ueda. 2009. A new strategy for prevention of anastomotic stricture using tacrolimus-eluting biodegradable nanofiber. J. Thorac. Cardiovasc. Surg. 137: 703–709.
Naghavi, M. and P. Libby, E. Falk, S.W. Casscells, S. Litovsky, J. Rumberger, J.J. Badimon, C. Stefanadis, P. Moreno, G. Pasterkamp, Z. Fayad, P.H. Stone, S. Waxman, P. Raggi, M. Madjid, A. Zarrabi, A. Burke, C. Yuan, P.J. Fitzgerald, D.S. Siscovick, C.L. de Korte, M. Aikawa, K.E. Airaksinen, G. Assmann, C.R. Becker, J.H. Chesebro, A. Farb, Z.S. Galis, C. Jackson, I.K. Jang, W. Koenig, R.A. Lodder, K. March, J. Demirovic, M. Navab, S.G. Priori, M.D. Rekhter, R. Bahr, S.M. Grundy, R. Mehran, A. Colombo, E. Boerwinkle, C. Ballantyne, W. Insull, Jr., R.S. Schwartz, R. Vogel, P.W. Serruys, G.K. Hansson, D.P. Faxon, S. Kaul, H. Drexler, P. Greenland, J.E. Muller, R. Virmani, P.M. Ridker, D.P. Zipes, P.K. Shah and J.T. Willerson. 2003. From vulnerable plaque to vulnerable patient: a call for new definitions and risk assessment strategies: part II. Circulation. 108: 1772–1778.
Parot, P. and Y.F. Dufrene, P. Hinterdorfer, C. Le Grimellec, D. Navajas, J.L. Pellequer and S. Scheuring. 2007. Past, present and future of atomic force microscopy in life sciences and medicine. J. Mol. Recognit. 20: 418–431.
Pektok, E. and B. Nottelet, J.C. Tille, R. Gurny, A. Kalangos, M. Moeller and B.H. Walpoth. 2008. Degradation and healing characteristics of small-diameter poly(epsilon-caprolactone) vascular grafts in the rat systemic arterial circulation. Circulation. 118: 2563–2570.
Psarros, C. and R. Lee, M. Margaritis and C. Antoniades. 2012. Nanomedicine for the prevention, treatment and imaging of atherosclerosis. Maturitas. 73: 52–60.
Radomski, A. and P. Jurasz, D. Alonso-Escolano, M. Drews, M. Morandi, T. Malinski and M.W. Radomski. 2005. Nanoparticle-induced platelet aggregation and vascular thrombosis. Br. J. Pharmacol. 146: 882–893.
Sanz, J. and Z.A. Fayad. 2008. Imaging of atherosclerotic cardiovascular disease. Nature. 451: 953–957.
Sato, H. 2002. Enzymatic procedure for site-specific pegylation of proteins. Adv. Drug Deliv. Rev. 54: 487–504.
Sell, S.A. and M.J. McClure, K. Garg, P.S. Wolfe and G.L. Bowlin. 2009. Electrospinning of collagen/biopolymers for regenerative medicine and cardiovascular tissue engineering. Adv. Drug Deliv. Rev. 61: 1007–1019.
Stern, S.T. and S.E. McNeil. 2008. Nanotechnology safety concerns revisited. Toxicol. Sci. 101: 4–21.
Stocker, R. and J.F. Keaney, Jr. 2004. Role of oxidative modifications in atherosclerosis. Physiol. Rev. 84: 1381–1478.
Strijkers, G.J. and E. Kluza, G.A. Van Tilborg, D.W. van der Schaft, A.W. Griffioen, W.J. Mulder and K. Nicolay. 2010. Paramagnetic and fluorescent liposomes for target-specific imaging and therapy of tumor angiogenesis. Angiogenesis. 13: 161–173.
Te Boekhorst, B.C. and G.A. van Tilborg, G.J. Strijkers and K. Nicolay 2012. Molecular MRI of inflammation in atherosclerosis. Curr. Cardiovasc. Imaging Rep. 5: 60–68.
Tu, C. and T.S. Ng, H.K. Sohi, H.A. Palko, A. House, R.E. Jacobs and A.Y. Louie. 2011. Receptor-targeted iron oxide nanoparticles for molecular MR imaging of inflamed atherosclerotic plaques. Biomaterials. 32: 7209–7216.
Twine, C.P. and A.D. McLain. 2010. Graft type for femoro-popliteal bypass surgery. Cochrane Database Syst. Rev. (5) CD001487.
Vasan, R.S. 2006. Biomarkers of cardiovascular disease: molecular basis and practical considerations. Circulation. 113: 2335–2362.
Vogt, S. and D. Troitzsch, S. Spath and R. Moosdorf. 2004. Efficacy of ion-selective probes in early epicardial *in vivo* detection of myocardial ischemia. Physiol. Meas. 25: N21–N26.
Walker, V.G. and Z. Li, T. Hulderman, D. Schwegler-Berry, M.L. Kashon and P.P. Simeonova. 2009. Potential *in vitro* effects of carbon nanotubes on human aortic endothelial cells. Toxicol. Appl. Pharmacol. 236: 319–328.
Wang, J. and B. Hong, J. Kai, J. Han, Z. Zou, C.H. Ahn and K.A. Kang. 2009. Mini sensing chip for point-of-care acute myocardial infarction diagnosis utilizing micro-electro-mechanical system and nano-technology. Adv. Exp. Med. Biol. 645: 101–107.

Wickline, S.A. and A.M. Neubauer, P.M. Winter, S.D. Caruthers and G.M. Lanza. 2007. Molecular imaging and therapy of atherosclerosis with targeted nanoparticles. J. Magn. Reson. Imaging. 25: 667–680.

Winter, P.M. and A.M. Neubauer, S.D. Caruthers, T.D. Harris, J.D. Robertson, T.A. Williams, A.H. Schmieder, G. Hu, J.S. Allen, E.K. Lacy, H. Zhang, S.A. Wickline and G.M. Lanza. 2006. Endothelial alpha(v)beta3 integrin-targeted fumagillin nanoparticles inhibit angiogenesis in atherosclerosis. Arterioscler. Thromb. Vasc. Biol. 26: 2103–2109.

Xiao, L. and H. Aoshima, Y. Saitoh and N. Miwa. 2011. Highly hydroxylated fullerene localizes at the cytoskeleton and inhibits oxidative stress in adipocytes and a subcutaneous adipose-tissue equivalent. Free Radic. Biol. Med. 51: 1376–1389.

Zhang, G.J. Cardiac biomarker and nanowire sensor arrays. pp. 121–140. *In*: R.J. Hunter and V.R. Preedy [eds.]. 2012. Nanomedicine and the Cardiovascular System. Science Publishers, Enfield, NH, USA.

CHAPTER 12

Nano(Neuro)Medicinal Interventions for Neurodegenerative Disorders
A Meta-Analysis of Concurrent Challenges and Strategic Solutions

Pradeep Kumar,[1,a] *Girish Modi,*[2] *Yahya E. Choonara*[1,b] and *Viness Pillay*[1,*]

ABSTRACT

The chapter highlights the recent nanomedicinal strategies and phenomena involved in the design of nanoarchitectures employed in neuropharmaceutical applications attempting to intervene the therapeutic process of imaging, preventing, modifying, and treating neurodegenerative disorders. An insight into the potential challenge of nanomedicine for combined theranostic strategies is provided here. A meta-analysis account of the recent investigations done for the translation from preclinical to concrete clinical applications is discussed in detail. A tabulated account of studies using nanomaterials for imaging in the central nervous system, transport of nanoparticles to the brain, neurotoxicity of nanoparticles, and drug-loaded nanoparticles tested for the

[1] Wits Advanced Drug Delivery Platform Research Unit, Department of Pharmacy and Pharmacology, School of Therapeutic Sciences, Faculty of Health Sciences, University of the Witwatersrand, 7 York Road, Parktown, 2193, Johannesburg, South Africa.
[a] Email: pradeep.kumar@wits.ac.za
[b] Email: yahya.choonara@wits.ac.za
[2] Department of Neurosciences, Division of Neurology, Faculty of Health Sciences, University of the Witwatersrand, 7 York Road, Parktown 2193, Johannesburg, South Africa.
Email: gmodicns@mweb.co.za
[*] Corresponding author: viness.pillay@wits.ac.za

treatment of Alzheimer's disease are also presented. Therefore, the chapter encompasses a combinatorial therapeutic approach derived from the science of drug delivery, cell tracking, nanoparticle synthesis, along with insights from fundamental aspects of neurodegeneration.

Introduction

Nano(*neuro*)medicine, application of nanotechnology to medicine in clinical neurosciences, is presented in terms of its impact on the diagnosis and treatment of neurodegenerative diseases, i.e., Alzheimer's Disease (AD), Parkinson's Disease (PD), multiple sclerosis, Human Immunodeficiency Virus (HIV)-associated Central Nervous System (CNS) diseases, CNS neoplasms, and other CNS disorders (Fig. 12.1) (Kanwar et al. 2012).

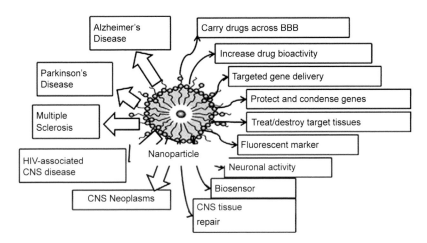

Figure 12.1. Multifunctional nanosystem labeled with functional molecules to target neurodegenerative and neurological disorders. It can be functionalized with suitable biomarkers, antibodies, genes, and drugs. BBB: blood-brain barrier. Reprinted with permission from Kanwar et al. (2012). Copyright Elsevier Science BV (2012).

Nanomedicinal conjugates such as tetanus toxin C for delivery of the tetanus toxin fragment via retrograde transport (Townsend et al. 2007), lactoferrin in poly(ethylene glycol) (PEG)-poly(D,L-lactide) (PLA) via uptake through lactoferrin receptor (Hu et al. 2009), trans-activating transcriptor for ritonavir bypassing the efflux transport (Rao et al. 2008), OX26 monoclonal antibody to transferrin for loperamide via receptor-mediated endocytosis (Ulbrich et al. 2009), vascular endothelial growth factor for Evans blue dye via enhanced permeability (Ay et al. 2008), apolipoproteins (Apos) for loperamide via Low Density Lipoprotein (LDL) receptor-related protein-mediated endocytosis (Michaelis et al. 2006), endothelins via endothelin receptor-mediated endocytosis (Narushima et al. 2003), pertussis toxin via enhanced permeability (Lu et al. 2008), and angiopep-2 for paclitaxel via LDL receptor-related protein-mediated endocytosis (Xin et al. 2011), are some typical examples of enhanced drug delivery into the brain (Kanwar et al. 2012). These nanomedicinal conjugates can be incorporated or fabricated in the form of various nanostructures (generally nanoparticles, NPs), e.g., nanocapsules, nanospheres, nanogels, Carbon Nanotubes (CNTs), nanofibers, nanomicelles, and nanoliposomes (NLPs) (Table 12.1), wherein the nanomedicinal systems employed consisted of clioquinol-loaded poly(butylcyanoacrylate) NPs for Cu^{2+}/Zn^{2+} chelator to solubilize amyloid beta ($A\beta$) plaques, thioflavin T (ThT)-loaded poly(butylcyanoacrylate) nanocapsules for the detection of $A\beta$ peptide in senile plaques, and D-penicillamine-loaded 1,2-dioleoyl-*sn*-glycero-3-phosphoethanolamine-N-(4-(*p*-maleimidophenyl) butyramide) phosphatidylethanolamine (PE), or pyridyldithio-propionyl phosphoethanolamine NPs for iron-chelating thereby limiting toxicity (Kanwar et al. 2012).

Table 12.1. Polymeric nanoparticulate systems against neurological diseases. Reprinted with permission from Kanwar et al. (2012). Copyright Elsevier Science BV (2012).

Polymeric nanostructure	Targeted against	Drug delivered	Significance
Nanocapsule, nanosphere	Neuroinflammation	Indomethacin	Neuroprotective
	$A\beta$ in AD	ThT	Diagnostic
	$A\beta$ in AD	Clioquinol	Inhibition of $A\beta$ aggregation
	$A\beta$ in AD	D-penicillamine	Dissolution of $A\beta$
Nanogel	Brain delivery	Oligonucleotides	Oligonucleotide delivery
	$A\beta$ in AD	Cholesterol (Chol)-bearing pullulan	Inhibition of $A\beta$ aggregation
CNT, nanofiber	Nerve growth	Human nerve growth factor (hNgf)	Neuronal outgrowth
	Dopamine release in PD	Biosensor	Therapeutic
	AD	Acetylcholine	Therapeutic
Nanomicelle	$A\beta$ in AD	Phospholipids	Neuroprotective against $A\beta$ aggregation
NLP	$A\beta$ aggregate in AD	Curcumin (Cur)	Diagnostic and therapeutic

Potential Role of Nanotechnologies in Neurodegenerative Diseases

Early diagnosis

1. Monitor the rate of cell loss in substantia nigra and other nuclei, and alert the immune system and the compensatory mechanism systems (neurogenesis included) when the rate exceeds the normal expected decline.
2. Monitor the state of defense and compensatory mechanisms.
3. Create biosensors to monitor neurotransmitter levels in precise locations within the brain (dopamine and others) which can be reduced long before the appearance of motor and non-motor symptoms.
4. Improve image technologies (fluorophores and Quantum Dots, QDs) which may also facilitate surgical approaches.

Study of pathogenetic mechanisms

Increase our knowledge about the mechanisms of cell death, thereby opening the doors to new drug targets.

Treatment [Reproduced with permission from Linazasoro et al. (2008). Copyright Elsevier Science BV (2008)]

1. Direct drugs to their target in a very specific way: targeted drug delivery systems. Drugs can act on signaling pathways required for neurotransmission (symptomatic effect) or on signaling pathways involved in neurodegeneration (neuroprotection and neurorescue), e.g., NPs (silica, vesicles, dendrimers, etc.), drug encapsulation strategies, multifunctional nanotherapeutics, ablation of areas with NPs.
2. Create biosensors to monitor neurotransmitter levels in precise locations within the brain (dopamine and others). Intracellular manipulations and interventions: repair deoxyribonucleic acid (DNA) and other damages, cleaning of deposits of aggregated abnormal proteins.
3. Introduce genes and proteins required for normal functioning in a highly controlled way (durable and controlled expression of the gene), avoiding the needs of viral vectors and complex control systems or of infusion pumps.
4. Create bridges from substantia nigra to striatum and other basal ganglia nuclei, and favor their development by blocking the expression of antireparative signals (no-go, etc.). Creating of the media to push the development of functional dopaminergic neurons from stem cells.

Mechanisms of nanoenabled drug delivery across the blood-brain barrier
[Reproduced with permission from Modi et al. (2009). Copyright Elsevier Science BV (2009)]

1. Increased NP retention in the brain blood capillaries combined with an adsorption to capillary walls could create a concentration gradient that would enhance the transport of NPs across the endothelial cell layer for drug delivery.
2. A surfactant effect characterized by solubilization of endothelial cell membrane lipids would lead to membrane fluidization and enhanced drug permeability.
3. NPs could lead to an opening of the tight junctions between endothelial cells, thus allowing the drug to permeate with the NPs in a bound or free form.
4. NPs may be endocytosed by endothelial cells, followed by drug release within these cells of the brain.
5. Drug-loaded NPs could be transcytosed through the endothelial cell layer.
6. Tween® 80 used as a coating agent could inhibit the P-glycoprotein efflux system.

Leading Research Reports

Nanoparticle-based receptor targeting

Roy et al. (2012) reported a "NP-based receptor targeting" wherein hNgf-EE ($_{85}$TFVKALTMDGKQAAWR$_{100}$, a short peptide mimetic of hNgf-beta) was conjugated to the surface of polymersomes formulated by self-assembling of PEG-b-poly(ε-caprolactone) (PCL) copolymer in an aqueous environment (Fig. 12.2). The research was based on the hypothesis that stimulation of the tyrosine kinase receptor B (TrkB) receptor by neurotrophic growth factors can be used as a possible therapeutic target for the treatment of neurodegenerative disorders. Additionally, Brain-Derived Neurotrophic Factor (BDNF) is known for reducing cell loss in animal models of PD, Huntington's disease, and stroke. In line with these results, the authors previously reported that hNgf-EE conjugation to the surface of polymersomes may increase NP uptake into TrkB positive spiral ganglion cells. However, it was postulated that the short *in vivo* half-life of BDNF and the difficulty of delivering neurotrophins to the targeted tissues are the major limitations to an effective BDNF-based treatment. The hNgf-EE conjugated polymersomes were investigated for their capability of activating the TrkB receptor *in vitro* in the SHSY-G7 cell line (Fig. 12.3). Confocal profiling demonstrated that TrkB receptors were phosphorylated when targeted by hNgf-EE-conjugated polymersomes as no TrkB phosphorylation was detected in cells incubated with non-functionalized polymersomes. Furthermore, the uptake of non-functionalized polymersomes

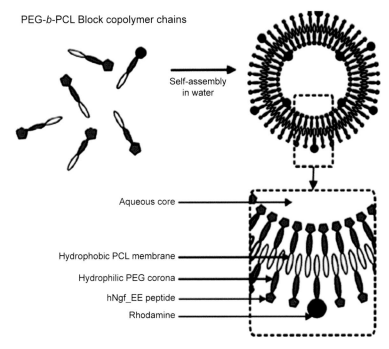

PEG-*b*-PCL Block copolymer chains

Self-assembly in water

Aqueous core

Hydrophobic PCL membrane

Hydrophilic PEG corona

hNgf_EE peptide

Rhodamine

Figure 12.2. PEG-*b*-PCL copolymers self-assemble in an aqueous environment to form polymersomes. The PCL units form the hydrophobic membrane, while the PEG units form the hydrophilic corona and line the interior cavity of the polymersome. The PEG-*b*-PCL polymer can be functionalized with a short peptide sequence (hNgf-EE) or a fluorophore (rhodamine B) before formation. Reprinted with permission from Roy et al. (2012). Copyright Elsevier Science BV (2012).

was low compared with hNgf-EE-conjugated polymersomes. Therefore, it was concluded that: (i) the functionalized polymersomes entered the cell by non-specific endocytosis; (ii) the binding mode of the peptide could be responsible for the activation of the TrkB, thus inducing survival signaling in the cell; (iii) the hNgf-EE peptide is capable of interacting and activating the TrkB receptor although conjugated to the surface of a polymersome; (iv) the polymersomes offer an attractive support for the delivery of hNgf-EE as a treatment for neurodegenerative diseases; and, (v) the advantage of using polymersomes as a support is that they would increase the *in vivo* half-life of the peptide.

Neuroprotective potential of rasagiline-loaded poly(D,L-lactide-*co*-glycolide) microspheres

Fernández et al. (2011) reported the efficacy of rasagiline mesylate (RM)-loaded poly(D,L-lactide-*co*-glycolide) (PLGA) microspheres against a rotenone-induced PD. The report was based on three research aspects: (i) RM was loaded to the microspheres to counteract the core pathological feature of PD (the

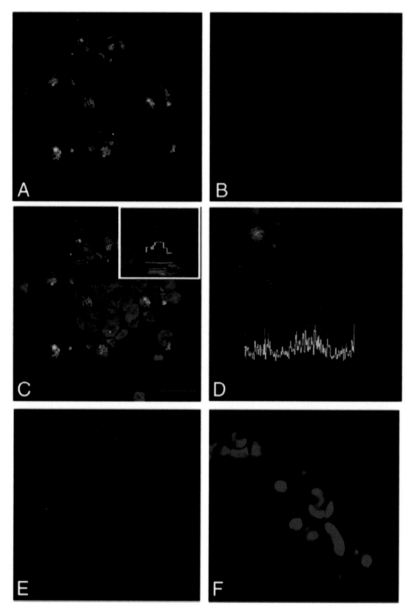

Figure 12.3. Confocal images of TrkB activation in SHSY-G7 cells by hNgf-EE-conjugated polymersomes. (A) Uptake of hNgf-EE and rhodamine B-labeled polymersomes (green). (B) Phospho-TrkB (red). (C) Merged image of A and B, nuclei stained with 4′,6-diamidino-2-phenylindole (DAPI) (blue). Inset shows a confocal profiling demonstrating the co-localization of the red and green signals. (D) Confocal profiling within a highly magnified cell where TrkB is phosphorylated by the hNgf-EE-conjugated polymersomes. (E) Cells incubated with non-functionalized polymersomes: no TrkB phosphorylation and low polymersome uptake (green). (F) Merged image of E with the nuclei stained with DAPI (blue). Reprinted with permission from Roy et al. (2012). Copyright Elsevier Science BV (2012).

accelerated loss of dopaminergic neurons in the substantia nigra, associated with abnormal protein aggregation, and leading to disorders in movements); (ii) rotenone-induced rat model of PD was employed to test the drug delivery system as compared to other models, e.g., 1-methyl-4-phenylpyridinium ion, 6-hydroxydopamine, and paraquat (systemic administration of rotenone to animals leads to the formation of Lewy bodies in the substantia nigra and loss of dopaminergic neurons which are in turn very close to PD pathogenesis, and therefore can act as a therapeutic approach representing different clinical stages of PD); and, (iii) pathophysiological changes following PD (e.g., greater cerebral blood flow and glucose consumption in the thalamus/capsula interna/lentiform intersection, the pons, cerebellum, and motor cortex/white matter) were monitored by Positron Emission Tomography (PET): fluorodeoxyglucose (^{18}F-FDG), considered to be a marker of cerebral glucose consumption, was used as the radiotracer for the determination of the neuronal viability.

The *in vitro* RM release from PLGA microspheres occurred at a constant rate of ≈ 60 g/day during ≈ 14 days. Catalepsy, akinesia, and swim tests in animals with intraperitoneal injection of rotenone (2 mg/Kg/day) demonstrated a reversal in descent latency after receiving RM (dose equivalent to 1 mg/Kg/day of RM intraperitoneally injected every 15 days). Specifically, RM-loaded microspheres reverted the degeneration of the substantia nigra dopaminergic neurons in rotenone treated animals, as confirmed by cresyl violet staining (Nissl staining) of brain sections. Additionally, results confirmed that high doses of microspheres reported a better *in vivo* efficacy than free RM (in solution), and significantly counteracted the substantia nigra cell loss following injection of rotenone in rats (Fig. 12.4, Table 12.2).

Functionalized self-targeting cerium oxide nanoparticles to counteract brain pathologies

The valence structure of cerium can undergo significant alterations depending on the surrounding chemical environment, thereby providing unique antioxidant properties to the surface of cerium oxide or ceria (CeO_2) NPs (Korsvik et al. 2007). Cimini et al. (2012) developed antibody-conjugated PEGylated CeO_2 NPs for the selective targeting of Aβ aggregates and modulation of neuronal survival pathways, based on previous findings wherein they demonstrated the superoxide dismutase (SOD) and catalase mimetic activity of CeO_2 NPs and proved their potential as redox active and biocompatible materials. Briefly, PEGylated CeO_2 NPs were conjugated with anti-Aβ antibody to assure a selective delivery to the Aβ plaques and a simultaneous increase in neuronal survival as well as BDNF signaling. Results demonstrated that the NPs may be a potential candidate for anti-neurodegenerative therapy. In fact, the NPs were proposed to counteract oxidative stress induced brain pathologies, to

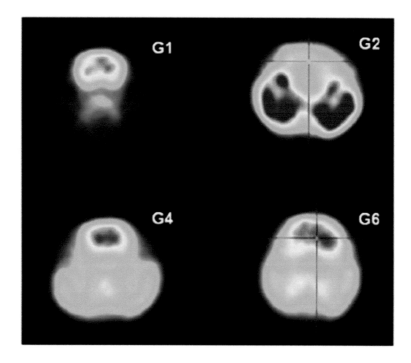

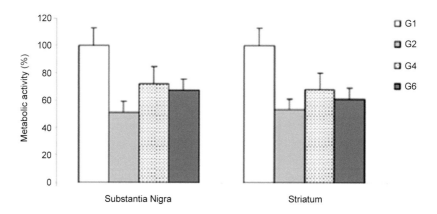

Figure 12.4. Above: representative PET/computed tomography (CT) ^{18}F-FDG neuroimages from animal groups [G1: control group. G2: rotenone treated control group. G4: rotenone treated animals also receiving RM-loaded PLGA microspheres (amount of microspheres equivalent to 15 mg/Kg of RM injected every 15 days). G6: rotenone treated animals also receiving RM in saline, 1 mg/Kg/day during 45 days]. Below: metabolic activity (%) of ^{18}F-FDG in substantia nigra and striatum of brains corresponding to the animal groups G1, G2, G4, and G6. Values are the mean ± standard error of the mean ($n = 4$). Reprinted with permission from Fernández et al. (2011). Copyright Elsevier Science BV (2011).

Table 12.2. Pathophysiological changes in the animal groups administered with different doses of rotenone and RM. Reprinted with permission from Fernández et al. (2011). Copyright Elsevier Science BV (2011).

Group	Dose	Pathophysiological changes
G1	Vehicle (sunflower oil, or saline)	Heterogeneous distribution of radioactivity with greater activity detected in deep lying brain structures which probably represent substantia nigra, globus pallidus, and/or thalamic nuclei
G2	Rotenone (2 mg/Kg/d)	^{18}F-FDG intensity of bilateral frontal cortex was reduced (reduction of glucose metabolism), but increased in the bilateral parietal cortex (increased glucose metabolism). Quantification of the metabolic activities in substantia nigra and striatum revealed significant decreases compares to the basal metabolic activity indicative of neuronal hypometabolism and/or loss of cellular tissue
G4	Rotenone + RM-loaded PLGA microspheres (15 mg/Kg RM)	A heterogeneous distribution of radioactivity which was increased in the frontal cortex and reduced in the parietal cortex as compared to G2. With respect to the substantia nigra, the increase in cerebral metabolism was more pronounced in G4 ($\approx 40\%$) than in G6 ($\approx 25\%$) ($p < 0.05$), thereby confirming the better efficacy achieved by RM given in microspheres than in solution
G6	Rotenone + RM in saline (1 mg/Kg/d)	Quantification of ^{18}F-FDG accumulation in substantia nigra and striatum demonstrated a greater metabolic activity in G4 and G6 when compared to G2, and a slightly greater activity in the parietal cortex of G6 compared to G4

ameliorate symptoms, and to counteract the disease progression by improving neuronal viability and neurite atrophy. Major findings of the study were (Fig. 12.5):

1. Functionalization of the PEGylated CeO$_2$ NPs: the NPs were functionalized with an amine group, and the anti-Aβ antibody was attached to this amine group by a two-step process: (i) alignment of the antibody in the proper orientation; and, (ii) covalent bond formation by the 1-ethyl-3-(3-dimethylaminopropyl)carbodiimide)/sulfo-N-hydroxysulfosuccinimide coupling reaction.
2. PEG coating decreased the non-specific interaction of CeO$_2$ NPs with Aβ: the interaction force of negatively charged Aβ is higher with amine-functionalized (positively charged) NPs. Minimal/no interaction was observed with PEGylated CeO$_2$ NPs (negative surface electrical charge).
3. NP targeting toward Aβ aggregates: conjugation of the anti-Aβ antibody to the NPs allowed the NPs to specifically recognize the aggregates with minimum or no interaction with nearby neuronal cells, and thus no effect on cell viability.
4. Protected by the neurons against Aβ-mediated cytotoxicity: NP-based treatment showed no significant differences with respect to the control,

whereas Aβ treatment induced a significant increase in apoptotic cell death. In addition, DAPI nuclear staining proved nuclear fragmentation in control and treated cells, whereas Aβ treatments lead to an increase in apoptotic nuclei and to an increase of nucleosome concentration. The NPs restored the control condition, thus indicating that they can play a protective effect against the Aβ cytotoxicity.

5. Preserved by the neuronal morphology: phase-contrast microscopy demonstrated that control cells showed neuronal clustering and neuronal aggregation, Aβ treatment induced an evident neurite loss, while the NPs protected the cells from neurite atrophy even in the presence of Aβ aggregates.

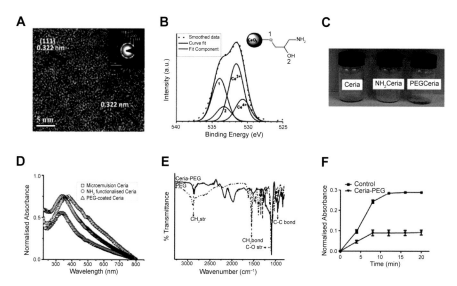

Figure 12.5. Characterization of CeO₂ NPs: (A) High resolution transmission electron microscopy image of the NPs showing controlled particle size distribution (3 to 5 nm). Bar length: 5 nm. The large d-spacing plane (111), focused at 300 kV, is indicated in the micrograph. Smaller d-spacing planes (220, 311) are not marked for clarity. Inset: selected-area electron diffraction pattern of NPs captured at low magnification, confirming the crystalline nature and fluorite structure of the NPs by calculation of each diffraction ring diameter. (B) Amine functionalization of CeO₂ NPs confirmed by X-ray photoelectron spectroscopy. Two O (1s) peaks corresponding to two different valence states of CeO₂ (Ce³⁺: 531.5 eV, and Ce⁴⁺: 530.6 eV) confirm the functionalization. Peak 1 is the O–C bond that connects epichlorohydrin to the CeO₂ (534.00 eV) and peak 2 is the epoxy group of epichlorohydrin (533.35 eV). (C) Change in the color of CeO₂ NPs (yellow) after amine functionalization (light yellow) and PEG conjugation (dark brown). (D) Ultraviolet-visible absorbance spectra of CeO₂ (□), NH₂-functionalized CeO₂ (○), and PEGylated CeO₂ (Δ) NPs, showing the shift in the absorbance maximum after amine functionalization (38.45 nm) and PEG conjugation (33.41 nm). (E) Fourier transform infrared spectra of PEGylated CeO₂ NPs confirming the PEGylation. (F) SOD mimetic activity of PEGylated CeO₂ NPs as compared to control, showing that the surface of PEGylated CeO₂ NPs is still active and scavenge the radical efficiently. a.u.: arbitrary units. Reprinted with permission from Cimini et al. (2012). Copyright Elsevier Science BV (2012).

6. Activation of signal transduction pathways involved in neuronal survival and plasticity: a reduction of pro-BDNF levels in Aβ-treated cells following NP-based treatment was observed, and significantly increased TrkB and extracellular signal-regulated kinase 5 (ERK5) levels: an activation of the neuronal survival pathway BDNF/TrkB/ERK5.

Nanozymes for improved delivery to the central nervous system

Synthetic SOD/catalase mimetics, EUK-189 and EUK-207, can provide neuroprotection under acute ischemic conditions by elimination of free radicals, but key improvements have not yet been achieved because of: (i) restricted transport across the BBB; (ii) rapid elimination from circulation; and, (iii) inactivation by proteases present in the body. Numerous attempts have been tried to overcome these limitations, e.g., incorporation into PEGylated polymeric NPs, but the encapsulation of enzymes into NPs may result in the inactivation and unsatisfactory loading, and decreased permeability of SOD1 across the brain microvessels.

To beat the challenges, electrostatic coupling of antioxidant enzymes, SOD1 and catalase, with cationic block copolymers, polyethyleneimine (PEI)-PEG or poly(L-lysine)-PEG has been recently reported by Klyachko et al. (2012). These nanostructures can be further stabilized by covalently cross-linking with different cross-linking strategies such as glutaraldehyde, bis-(sulfosuccinimidyl) suberate sodium salt, and 1-ethyl-3-(3-dimethylaminopropyl)carbodiimide hydrochloride with *N*-hydroxysulfosuccinimide. Active enzymes loaded to cross-linked NPs, termed "nanozymes", basically consists of a core of enzyme-polyelectrolyte complex/conjugate surrounded by a PEG shell (Fig. 12.6). The nanostructure provides protection to the encapsulated enzymes (SOD1 + catalase), as they are capable of reactive oxidative species decomposition without the need for release from the NPs (Klyachko et al. 2012). The increased

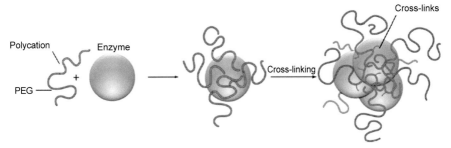

Figure 12.6. Schematic representation of polyion complexes. Complexes spontaneously form in aqueous solution as a result of electrostatic coupling of the enzyme and cationic block copolymer. Although only one protein globule is schematically represented, the polyion complex may contain several protein globules. Cross-linker was added to preformed complexes that resulted in covalent stabilization. Reprinted with permission from Klyachko et al. (2012). Copyright Elsevier Science BV (2012).

stability of the antioxidant enzyme complexes in both blood and brain, and the increased accumulation in CNS tissue was demonstrated. Future studies are encouraged to evaluate the potential of these nanoplatforms for antioxidant enzyme deliver to the CNS to attenuate the oxidative stress in neurodegenerative diseases.

Poly(D,L-lactide-*co*-glycolide) nanoparticles capable of estradiol delivery to the brain upon oral administration

Mittal et al. (2011) designed an estradiol delivery system based on surfactant-coated NPs for post-menopausal estrogen replacement therapy in order to reduce the risk or delay of the onset of AD in women. Clinically, the study was based on the fact that women are twice more likely than men to suffer from AD and that the deprivation of endogenous estrogen after menopause is implicated as a risk factor in the pathogenesis of AD in post-menopausal women. Pharmaceutically, the study challenged the estradiol delivery via the oral route, as a large dose is currently required to achieve therapeutic levels of estradiol (that increases the peripheral drug burden, and thus potentiates the risk of peripheral adverse effects, most notably breast cancer). Therefore, it was hypothesized that the surfactant-coated NPs may successfully transport drugs across the BBB by endocytosis.

Concretely, the research team developed Tween® 80-coated PLGA NPs for estradiol delivery to the brain upon oral administration. The NPs were formulated by single emulsion, and Tween® 80 coating was possible by incubating the re-constituted NPs at different concentrations of the surfactant. It was reported that Tween® 80 coating resulted in adsorption of Apo E and/or B from blood onto the NP surface, and the resulting coated NPs can mimic natural LDL particles, thus interacting with the LDL receptor family located in the brain capillary endothelial cells (endocytotic uptake).

Briefly, the significance of the surface coating of the NPs with Tween® 80 was tested in an ovariectomized rat model of AD mimicking the postmenopausal conditions wherein orally administered Tween® 80-coated NPs resulted in significantly higher brain estradiol levels after 24 hours ($\approx$ 1.97 ng/g tissue) as compared to uncoated NPs ($\approx$ 1.1 ng/g tissue) at a dose of 0.2 mg/rat. Interestingly, the brain estradiol levels were similar to those obtained after administration of a suspension via the 100% bioavailable intramuscular route. The nanosystem further prevented the expression of Aβ(42) immunoreactivity in the hippocampus region of brain. In conclusion, the orally delivered NPs were as effective as an intramuscular drug injection in preventing/reducing the pathological development of AD with the added benefits of patient compliance and reduced peripheral drug burden.

Curcumin-associated and lipid ligand-functionalized nanoliposomes

Cur, a naturally occurring phytochemical, is known to possess antioxidant and anti-inflammatory activities along with a favorable toxicity profile, with the potential to protect the brain from lipid peroxidation. Cur exhibits both neuroprotective and neurotherapeutic properties as it can inhibit Aβ(1-42) oligomer formation and cell toxicity at micromolar concentrations *in vitro*, and also binds to senile plaques, thus reducing Aβ levels *in vivo*. Aβ is also known to interact with certain membrane lipids (e.g., ionic lipids and gangliosides), being the aggregation process that is affected. Such binding was advantageously used by Taylor et al. (2011) in the development of NLPs incorporating (in their lipid membrane) or decorated (on their surface) with Cur or lipid ligands [phosphatidic acid (PA), cardiolipin (CL), or monosialoganglioside GM1]. Cur-loaded liposomes were prepared by adding Cur in the lipid phase during liposome preparation. Cur surface-decorated liposomes were prepared either by using a Cur-lipid conjugate to form lipid-S-Cur liposomes, or by attaching a Cur derivative on preformed liposomes by click chemistry (click-Cur liposomes). Lipid ligands were also incorporated into NLPs during their formation.

The NLPs were evaluated for their ability to influence Aβ(1-42) peptide aggregation *in vitro* using an assay based on the fluorescent dye ThT (which can bind to fibrillar forms of Aβ) and a highly sensitive sandwich immunoassay capable of detecting small oligomeric forms of Aβ. It was demonstrated that NLPs containing PA and CL have the ability to target the aggregated forms of Aβ(1-42) with high binding affinity (Gobbi et al. 2010). The NLPs loaded with Cur, or the Cur derivative, successfully inhibited the formation of fibrillar and/or oligomeric Aβ *in vitro*, thus proving the neuroprotective effect with click-Cur type being most effective (Figs. 12.7 and 12.8). This selective effectiveness of the click-Cur liposomes was attributed to the fact that Cur-derivative molecules protrude from the liposome surface rather than entering the liposome bilayer, and hence they are more amenable to the interaction with Aβ species. Click-Cur liposomes showed concentration-dependent inhibition of Aβ(1-42) fibril formation in the ThT assay. The NLPs with lipid ligands required a very high ratio of liposome to peptide for Aβ fibril inhibition. In conclusion, it was demonstrated that Cur-based liposomes and more specifically the click-Cur liposomes represent a very promising approach in AD therapy (Taylor et al. 2011).

Surface-functionalized nanoparticles and the Aβ fibrillogenesis

According to the molecular aspects of neurodegeneration associated with AD, controlling the nucleation/elongation-growth processes of monomeric Aβ peptides into insoluble oligomers, protofibrils, and fibrils could be a potential target for the therapeutic interventions for advanced nanomaterials and

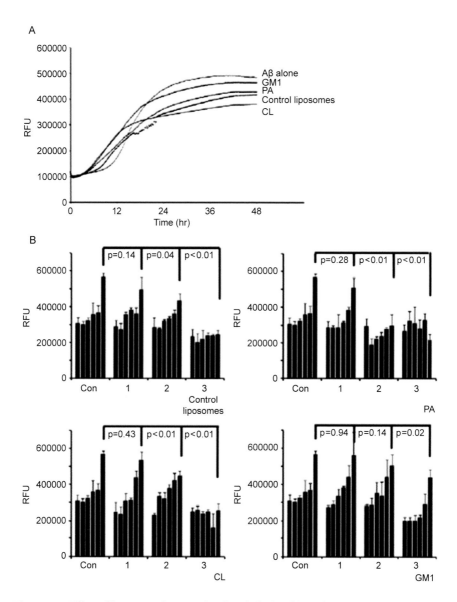

Figure 12.7. Effect of liposomes functionalized with the lipid ligands on Aβ(1-42) aggregation. (A) ThT assay data for liposomes containing the lipid ligands PA, CL, or monosialoganglioside GM1, plus control liposomes, all at 1 mM, and 25 μM Aβ alone (48 hours time course). (B) Immunoassay data for these liposomes. For each type of liposome, three 48-hour time courses are presented (data for 0, 2, 4, 8, 24, and 48 hours), plus a control time course with 12.5 μM Aβ(1-42) alone (Con), showing the effect of increasing liposome concentration, where *1*: 25 μM, *2*: 125 μM, and *3*: 500 μM liposomes. Also shown are the *p* values from paired t-tests for the 48-hour time-point data, comparing values for the control and liposome containing reactions. RFU: relative fluorescence units. Reprinted with permission from Taylor et al. (2011). Copyright Elsevier Science BV (2011).

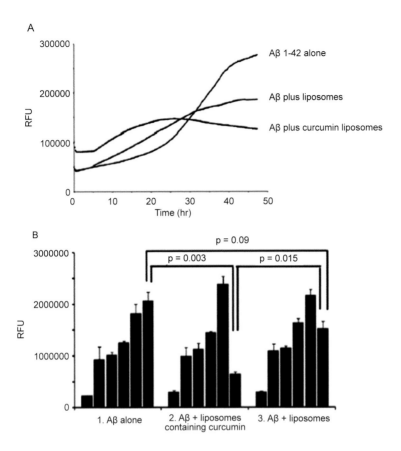

Figure 12.8. Effect of Cur-liposomes on Aβ(1-42) aggregation. (A) ThT assay of Aβ fibril formation in the presence and absence of 40 µM liposomes (total phospholipids). (B) Immunoassay data for Aβ oligomers in the presence and absence of 20 µM liposomes (total phospholipids). Three time courses are shown with samples taken at 0, 2, 4, 8, 24, and 48 hours. Also shown are the p values from paired t-tests, comparing data from 48-hour time points as indicated by the lines. Reprinted with permission from Taylor et al. (2011). Copyright Elsevier Science BV (2011).

nanostructures. However, there is a considerable debate over the promotion/ inhibition aspect of these nanostructures towards the self-assembling mechanism of Aβ peptides, particularly the fibrillogenesis, as discussed by Chan et al. (2012).

Wu et al. (2008) reported that $\approx$ 20 nm-sized titanium dioxide (TiO$_2$) NPs could promote the growth of Aβ, shortening the nucleation process. Cabaleiro-Lago et al. (2008) demonstrated that co-polymeric N-isopropylacrylamide (NiPAM)/N-tert-butylacrylamide (BAM) NPs ($\approx$ 40 nm in size) with different hydrophobic characters inhibited the growth of Aβ fibrils, adsorbing the monomers onto the particle surface. Cabaleiro-Lago et al. (2010) further reported that cationic amino-modified polystyrene NPs (mean diameter

$\approx$ 60 to 180 nm) induced both acceleration and retardation effects on Aβ fibrillation, based on the concentration and coverage of the peptide monomers on the particle surfaces. Yoo et al. (2011) have shown that functionalized QDs non-specifically interacted with the Aβ monomers, interrupting the nucleation process and inhibiting the growth of Aβ fibrils. Majzik et al. (2010) described the covalent interaction between gold (Au) NPs and cysteine-modified Aβ peptides, thus formation of the polypeptide chain structure was hindered. Finally, Xiao et al. (2010) illustrated that N-acetyl-L-cysteine (NAC)-capped QDs (hydrodynamic diameter $\approx$ 3 nm) could effectively quench both nucleation and elongation process of the Aβ fibrillogenesis at any time point in the seed-mediated growth of Aβ(1-40), blocking active sites of the seed fibrils or monomers. Therefore, precautionary measures should be applied on the rationality of the dose, size, shape, surface area, composition, and functionalities to be employed for therapeutics and diagnostics purposes.

Based on the earlier cited reports and their own previous findings, Chan et al. (2012) hypothesized that the nanomaterials not only regulate the nucleation but also the elongation phase of Aβ fibrillogenesis. Additionally, the inhibitory effect is concentration dependent, and a remarkable inhibition towards peptide can be observed in a dose dependent manner. In this line, they explored the effect of inorganic NPs on regulating the elongation of Aβ(1-40) fibrils under physiological conditions. Au NPs (diameter $\approx$ 15 nm) were synthesized and capped with the thiolated ligands NAC and 3-mercaptopropionic acid (MPA) via the hydrothermal method and the modified Frens method, respectively. The NPs were co-incubated with monomeric Aβ(1-40) peptides for seed-mediated growth such that the elongation phase in the amyloidogenesis was dominant. The effect of particle size, surface electrical charge, functionality, and composition toward Aβ fibrillogenesis was investigated (Fig. 12.9).

Single nanoparticulate platform for cancer and Alzheimer's disease

Le Droumaguet et al. (2012) developed a versatile and efficient functionalization strategy for polymeric NPs with a potential therapeutic application in the fields of cancer and AD. PEGylated, biodegradable poly(alkylcyanoacrylate) nanocarriers were designed as a versatile nanoparticulate platform. Briefly, the NPs exhibiting stealth, fluorescent, and targeting abilities were synthesized as shown below (Fig. 12.10):

1. CuAAC was used to covalently attach the ligand of interest: heterobifunctional azidoPEG was first derivatized with the selected ligand by CuAAC using copper sulfate/sodium ascorbate as the catalytic system and turned into its cyanoacetate derivative (ligand-PEG cyanoacetate) under DCC-assisted chemistry.
2. Copolymerization of different monomer species to introduce the desired features (fluorescence, targeting moiety, hydrophobic/hydrophilic

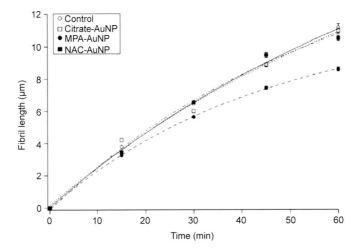

Figure 12.9. Fibrillation kinetics of Aβ(1-40) monitored by measuring the fibril length (µm) at different time points (minutes) by total internal reflection fluorescence microscopy (TIRFM) under the addition of functionalized Au NPs at 10^{-8} M: control (no NPs), Citrate-capped Au NPs, MPA-capped Au NPs, and NAC-capped Au NPs. The fibrillation kinetics follows the pseudo first order kinetics. Reprinted with permission from Chan et al. (2012). Copyright Elsevier Science BV (2012).

character): functionalized building block was terpolymerized with varying amounts of methoxyPEG cyanoacetate and hexadecylcyanoacrylate by tandem Knoevenagel condensation/Michael addition to obtain the corresponding ligand containing poly(methoxyPEG cyanoacetate-*co*-ligand-PEG cyanoacetate-*co*-hexadecylcyanoacrylate) amphiphilic copolymer.

3. Self-assembly in aqueous solution of the resulting amphiphilic copolymers: concomitant self-assembly in aqueous solution with a rhodamine B-tagged poly(hexadecylcyanoacrylate-*co*-rhodamine B cyanoacetate-*co*-methoxyPEG cyanoacetate) copolymer produced the desired colloidal nanocarrier.

The resulting functionalized polymeric NPs exhibited the requisite characteristics for drug delivery purposes, i.e., a biodegradable core made of poly(alkylcyanoacrylate), a hydrophilic PEG shell leading to colloidal stabilization, fluorescent properties provided by the covalent linkage of a rhodamine B-based dye to the polymer backbone, and surface functionalization with biologically active ligands that enabled specific targeting. The construction method is very versatile and was illustrated by the coupling of a small library of ligands (e.g., biotin, Cur derivatives, and antibodies), resulting in high affinity toward: (i) M109 murine lung carcinoma, and MCF7 human breast cancer cell lines, even in a coculture environment with healthy cells; and, (ii) the Aβ(1-42), believed to be the most representative and toxic species in AD, both under

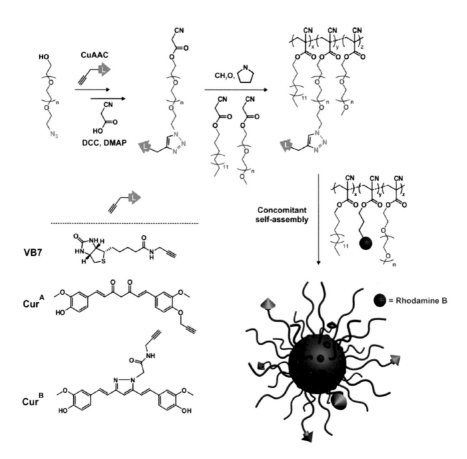

Figure 12.10. Synthetic pathway to prepare fluorescent, PEGylated, and biodegradable poly(alkylcyanoacrylate) NPs functionalized with biotin VB7 or Cur derivatives (Cur^A and Cur^B). CuAAC: copper-catalyzed azide-alkyne cycloaddition; DCC: N,N'-dicyclohexylcarbodiimide; DMAP: 4-(N,N-dimethylamino)pyridine. Reprinted with permission from Le Droumaguet et al. (2012). Copyright American Chemical Society (2012).

its monomeric and fibrillar forms (Fig. 12.11). In the case of AD, the ligand-functionalized NPs exhibited higher affinity toward Aβ(1-42) species compared to other colloidal systems, and led to significant aggregation inhibition and toxicity rescue of Aβ(1-42) at low molar ratios (Le Droumaguet et al. 2012).

Lipid-based nanoparticles with high binding affinity for Aβ(1-42) peptide

The neurotoxic Aβ, formed in anomalous amounts in AD, is released as monomer and then undergoes aggregation forming oligomers, fibrils, and plaques in diseased brains. On this basis, Gobbi et al. (2010) developed a nanosystem capable of targeting all of the forms of Aβ: NLPs (mean size ≈ 145 nm) and solid lipid nanoparticles (SLNs, mean size ≈ 75 nm) functionalized

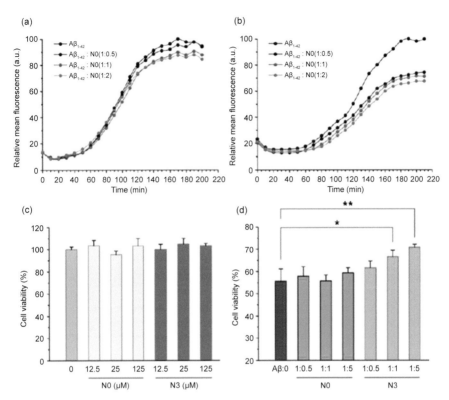

Figure 12.11. (a and b) Effects of NPs on the aggregation of Aβ(1-42) using the ThT binding assay. Aggregation kinetics of 25 μM Aβ(1-42) alone or coincubated with increasing molar ratios (1:0.5; 1:1, and 1:2) of non-functionalized (N0) (a) or Cur^B-functionalized (N3) (b) NPs. Data (relative mean fluorescence, a.u., vs. time, minutes) are shown as mean (n = 3) from a representative experiment of three independent experiments. (c and d) Effects of NPs on Aβ(1-42) toxicity using the 3-(4,5-dimethylthiazol-2-yl)-2,5-diphenyltetrazolium bromide (MTT) viability assay. Differentiated SK-N-SH cells were treated during 48 hours in the absence or in the presence of different concentrations of NPs N0 or N3 (12.5, 25, or 125 μM) to assess the toxicity of the NPs (c). Differentiated SK-N-SH cells were treated during 48 hours in the absence or presence of Aβ(1-42) (25 μM), preaggregated in phosphate buffered saline during 24 hours at 25°C, alone or in combination with three different molar ratios (1:0.5, 1:1, and 1:5) of N0 or N3 NPs (d), to address the interference of the NPs with Aβ toxicity. Cell viability (%) was measured using the MTT assay and it is depicted as a percentage of the untreated cells (control). Reprinted with permission from Le Droumaguet et al. (2012). Copyright American Chemical Society (2012).

with anionic phospholipids (PA and CL) to target Aβ(1-42) with high affinity. In detail, the NLPs were composed of a matrix of sphingomyelin (Sm) from bovine brain and Chol (Sm:Chol, 1:1 molar ratio) mixed with one of the following lipids: monosialogangliosides (GM1, GM2, and GM3), disialogangliosides (GD1a, GD1b, and GD3), trisialoganglioside (GT1b) from bovine brain gangliosides, 1-palmitoyl-oleoyl-phosphatidylcholine (1-palmitoyl-oleoyl-PC), PE, dimyristoylPA, diphosphatidylglycerol (diPG), or CL. SLNs were prepared by following the oil-in-water (o/w) warm microemulsion method using stearic acid as internal phase, phospholipon 90G (purified soy lecithin with PC) as surfactant, sodium taurocholate as cosurfactant, and ultrapure water as external phase.

NP targeting was identified using immunostaining studies: PA/CL-functionalized, but not plain, NPs interacted with Aβ(1-42) aggregates as indicated by ultracentrifugation experiments as the binding reaction occurred in solution. The targeting was further confirmed by Surface Plasmon Resonance (SPR) experiments as the NPs flowed onto immobilized Aβ(1-42) (Fig. 12.12). The SPR experimental session showed that negligible binding was detected when flowing liposomes composed of Sm/Chol alone, and even after embedding 20% PE, 20% PC, or 5% PG, no binding was observed. However, some binding was observed with liposomes containing 5% monosialoganglioside GM1. Interestingly, a very marked concentration-dependent binding response, specific for the surface coated with Aβ(1-42)

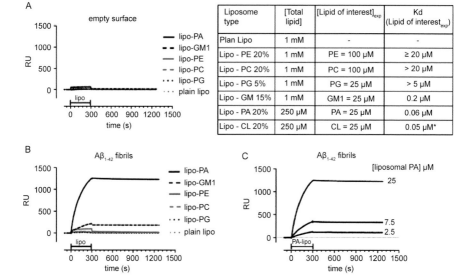

Figure 12.12. SPR studies comparing the binding properties of liposomes of different composition for Aβ(1-42) fibrils: raw sensorgrams, i.e., the SPR signal in resonance units (RU) vs. time(s). Plain liposomes (plain lipo, Sm:Chol, 1:1) containing or not the lipid of interest (PE, PC, PG, monosialoganglioside GM1, PA) were injected and flowed simultaneously over an empty sensor surface (used as reference) (A), or (B) over a sensor surface previously coated with Aβ(1-42) fibrils. They flowed for 5 minutes (as indicated by the bars) at a flow rate of 30 mL/minute. The proportion of lipid of interest and the lipid concentrations utilized (μM) are indicated in the inserted table which further summarized experimental conditions and the K_d values. PA-exposing liposomes (lipo-PA) showed the highest binding. (C) shows the specific binding of three different concentrations of lipo-PA (corresponding to 2.5, 7.5, and 25 μM exposed PA) to Aβ(1-42) fibrils obtained after subtraction of the binding of lipo-PA to the empty surface (non-specific binding). Lipo: liposome. Reprinted with permission from Gobbi et al. (2010). Copyright Elsevier Science BV (2010).

fibrils, was observed when flowing Sm/Chol liposomes embedding 20% PA. PA conferred a high affinity for Aβ(1-42) and fibrillar preparations of the peptide to the NLPs and SLNs, confirming the multivalent nature of the interaction.

Promotion of Aβ fibrillation by titanium dioxide nanoparticles

On the hypothesis that NPs in the brain may interact with Aβ and influence Aβ aggregation, Wu et al. (2008) investigated the relationship between NPs and AD. Briefly, the researchers tested the influence of TiO_2 NPs on the Aβ assembly and reported that TiO_2 NPs promoted Aβ assembly into amyloid fibrils by accelerating the nucleation process [Aβ(42) fibrillation by ThT assay], even at a very low concentration (Fig. 12.13). The promoting effect of NPs on Aβ fibrillation was proposed to be a result of a local high Aβ monomer concentration owing to the adsorption on NP surface. It was described that TiO_2 NPs adsorbed Aβ(42) monomers on their surface, while silica (SiO_2), ZrO_2, zirconia (ZrO_2), fullerene C60, and fullerene C70 NPs slightly adsorbed Aβ(42) monomers on their surface.

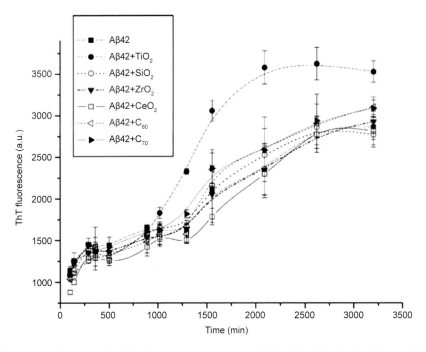

Figure 12.13. Kinetics of Aβ fibrillation in the presence of TiO_2, SiO_2, ZrO_2, CeO_2, fullerene C60, and fullerene C70 NPs. ThT fluorescence (a.u.) was plotted as a function of time (minutes) for 20 μM Aβ(42) at 37°C in phosphate buffered saline (pH 7.4) without or with NPs (0.01 mg/mL). Reprinted with permission from Wu et al. (2008). Copyright Elsevier Science BV (2008).

Therefore, although all the studies analyzed above have postulated the promising use of nanoparticulate-based strategies as promising therapeutic interventions against neurodegenerative disorders and conditions, the possible toxicity of these nanosystems cannot be ruled out.

Conclusion

Nanotechnological strategies provide a unique way to overcome the various brain delivery related challenges, e.g., the low permeability through the BBB which can be overcome by a wise surface functionalization of the nanoplatforms with suitable ligands. In fact, a synergistic therapeutic approach can be designed by incorporating the bioactives into nanostructures with directional cues and targeting abilities for controlled and site specific release of neuroregenerative and neuroprotective chemical entities. Most importantly, the design of NPs capable of releasing the drugs and biofactors at a predetermined and controlled rate is essential for the success of these neurointerventional approaches (Table 12.3). Unfortunately, these (nano)strategies suffer at the moment from various drawbacks (Fig. 12.14).

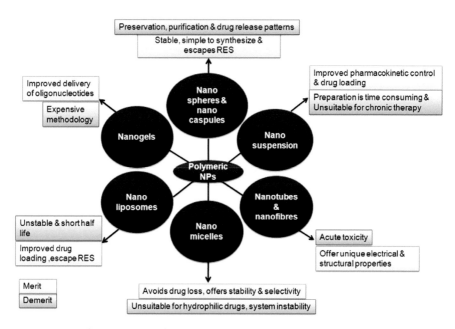

Figure 12.14. Polymeric NPs and their merits and demerits. RES: reticuloendothelial system. Reprinted with permission from Kanwar et al. (2012). Copyright Elsevier Science BV (2012).

Table 12.3. Bioactive-loaded nanoplatforms against neurological disorders. POPC: 1-palmitoyl-2-oleoyl-*sn*-glycero-3-phosphocholine; POPG: 1-palmitoyl-2-oleoyl-*sn*-glycero-3-phospho-*rac*-1-glycerol.

Nanoneuro-Architecture	Outstanding features and findings	Reference
Binary cross-linked alginate scaffold. Embedding with stable dopamine-loaded cellulose acetate phthalate NPs	Intracranial nanoenabled scaffold device for the site specific delivery of dopamine that minimize the peripheral side effects of conventional PD therapy. Dopamine release maintained favorable cerebrospinal fluid (10 µg/mL) vs. systemic concentrations (1 to 2 µg/mL) over 30 days following implantation in the parenchyma of frontal lobe of Sprague-Dawley rats	Pillay et al. 2009
NLPs surface engineered with chelating ligands, i.e., copper acetate, ethylene diamine tetraacetic acid (EDTA), histidine, and zinc acetate	*In vitro* and *ex vivo* results demonstrated the effectiveness of chelating ligand-bound NLPs for prevention of copper-Aβ(1-42) or zinc-Aβ(1-42) aggregate build up associated with neurotoxicity in PC12 neuronal cells, as well as promotion of intracellular uptake in the presence of copper or zinc ions	Mufamadi et al. 2012
Self-assembling peptide P11-2 (CH$_3$CO-Gln-Gln-Arg-Phe-Gln-Trp-Gln-Phe-Glu-Gln-Gln-NH$_2$) nanostructures	The peptide mimics Aβ(1-40) in terms of toxicity, and can produce intermediate oligomers showing higher toxicity against cells than the monomeric or higher aggregating counterparts. P11-2 binds to both zwitterionic (POPC) and negatively charged (POPC:POPG) liposomes, acquires a partial β-sheet conformation, and is protected against deuterium exchange in the presence of lipids	Salay et al. 2009
Carboxylic-functionalized polystyrene NPs conjugated with the iron chelator 2-methyl-*N*-(2'-aminoethyl)-3-hydroxyl-4-pyridinone (MAEHP)	Chelating agents selectively bind to, and remove and/or redox silence transition metals as an effective therapy for AD. MAEHP-conjugated NPs can protect human cortical neurons from Aβ-associated oxidative toxicity	Liu et al. 2009
Neurotensin-polyplex (Trojan horse) nanosystem	The nanosystem can enter dopaminergic neurons through neurotensin receptor internalization to deliver a genetic cargo	Martinez-Fong et al. 2012

Table 12.3. contd....

Table 12.3. contd.

Nanoneuro-Architecture	Outstanding features and findings	Reference
Single-walled CNTs	They were successfully used to deliver acetylcholine into the brain for treatment of experimentally induced AD. By precisely controlling the doses, the single-walled CNTs preferentially enter lysosomes (the target organelles) and not mitochondria (the target organelles for cytotoxicity)	Yang et al. 2010
Meloxicam-loaded PCL	Meloxicam can protect against learning and memory impairments, loss neuronal, and oxidative stress in a mouse model of AD induced by Aβ peptide	Ianiski et al. 2012
Vitamin E-functionalized PLGA NPs	With the increase of vitamin E ratio, more effective *in vitro* therapeutic effects were observed. The highest cell viability was achieved because NP degradation may release the D-α-tocopheryl PEG 1000 succinate components that have synergistic activity	Jalali et al. 2011
Pullulan-modified cholesteryl nanogels	Both neutral and positively charged nanogels interact with Aβ(1-42) monomers and oligomers. Neutral nanogel is non-toxic, but positively charged derivatives are toxic, particularly in primary cortical cultures. Binding of both monomeric and oligomeric Aβ(1-42) to the nanogel significantly reduces Aβ(1-42) toxicity in both the primary cortical and microglial cells	Boridy et al. 2009
Nitroxide radical-containing NPs coupled with piperine	The NPs significantly reduced the levels of reactive oxygen species and reactive oxygen species products, enhanced catalase and glutathione peroxidase activity, and augmented the antioxidant effect on an *in vitro* AD model. The NPs reduced the generation of reactive oxygen species and prevent apoptosis via scavenging enzyme action pathways	Chonpathompikunlert et al. 2011

Current nanotechnology and drug delivery approaches discussed in the chapter demonstrate that a combinatorial design can provide the desired characteristics required for CNS imaging, transport of bioactives to the CNS, and treatment of neurological disorders (Tables 12.4 and 12.5). The readers are encouraged to read various enlightening approaches in the form of drug loaded-NPs tested for the treatment of AD (Table 12.6).

Table 12.4. Neurodegenerative disorders and pharmaceutical nanoformulations. Reprinted with permission from Nowacek et al. (2009). Copyright Future Medicine Ltd. (2009).

Neurodegenerative disorder	Nanoformulation
AD	Aberrant homeostasis of transition metals has long been linked with Aβ aggregate formation, a potential cause of AD. Different methods are being explored for sequestering excess metal ions, e.g., chelator-NP complexes, as well as ways to supplement metal, such as PEI metal-transporting NPs
	Aβ aggregation is a multistep process involving many oligomeric intermediates. Preventing the process of Aβ fibrilization at any point may provide benefits. NPs such as polyamidoamine dendrimers, fullerene C60, and PEGylated phospholipid nanomicelles attempt to inhibit this process by depleting either the number of available monomers or critical nuclei
	The removal of fully formed Aβ aggregates from the blood and brain can reduce neural damage in AD. Metal NPs that bind Aβ fibrils are being used to selectively ablate, by the application of electromagnetic energy, or remove, by magnetization, Aβ aggregates
	Advancements in drug delivery are being made with the development of huperzine-packaged PLGA NPs, and in diagnosis with the engineering of Au NPs complexed with fragments of Aβ antibody or protein for imaging
PD	C60 fullerenes for treatment of PD and other neurodegenerative disorders are being explored. NPs such as C60-ascorbic acid and polyhydroxylated C60 show potential antioxidant and radical scavenging properties. However, concern has been raised about the toxicity of C60 fullerenes and much more must be learned about these NPs before they can be used clinically
	Cell-mediated delivery of catalase-containing NPs to the brain has been developed. This method offers great promise for delivering drugs specifically to areas of the brain that need them, not just for PD but for all neurodegenerative disorders
	Chronic neuroinflammation has been implicated in causing dopaminergic cell death. VP025, a PG-based phospholipid NP, has been described to cause an anti-inflammatory response by interacting with antigen presenting cells and decreasing cytokine production. Recent studies using animal models of PD have suggested that this NP could improve clinical outcomes in PD
	Delivery of functional proteins to degenerating neurons is being developed. Poly(butylcyanoacrylate) NPs may be used to deliver multiple proteins to hippocampal cells in culture
	Bromocriptine-loaded SLNs are being developed to improve the pharmacokinetics over free drug

Table 12.5. Nanomaterials for therapeutic interventions in the CNS. ATPase: adenosinetriphosphatase; IO: iron oxide; *m*RNA: messenger ribonucleic acid; TAT peptide: transactivator of transcription (GRKKRRQRRRPQ) peptide. Reprinted with permission from Hu and Gao (2010) and Nunes et al. (2012). Copyright Elsevier Science BV (2010 and 2012).

Nanomaterials for imaging in the CNS				
	Nanomaterial	**Model**	**Route of administration**	**Aim and main conclusions**
NPs	IO (Ferumoxtran®, Ferumoxytol®)	Patients with malignant brain tumors	Intravenous	Comparison between the MRI signal of ultrasmall superparamagnetic IO and gadolinium (Gd^{3+}) in patients with malignant brain tumors. Signal enhancement
	IO (Ferumoxtran®)	Patients with ischemic lesions	Intravenous	Investigation of the cellular imaging of human ischemic stroke (Phase II). Intravascular retention and lack of extravasation allowed better contrast between the vessel and adjacent tissue
	IO (Endorem®)	Rats with a cortical or spinal cord injury	Intracerebral and intravenous	Investigation of IO NPs as an adjuvant for MRI to study the fate of transplanted cell *in vivo*. Useful method for evaluating the migration and fate of stem cells in CNS
	Dextran-coated superparamagnetic IO	Mice with bilateral carotid artery occlusion	Intraperitoneal	Investigation of additional biomarkers of angiogenesis-associated pericytes. Gene transcript-targeted MRI non-invasively revealed neural progenitor cells during vascularization
	IO	Rats with glial brain tumor	Intravenous	Investigation of brain tumor vessels in glioblastoma. Single domain antibody IOs targeted MRI contrast agent and selectively binds to abnormal vessels

IO		Patients with spinal cord injury	Lumbar puncture technique	IO NPs for MRI to study the fate of transplanted cells. Cells labeled with magnetic NPs migrated into the injured site with chronic spinal cord injury
	Magnetite-dextran	Rats with glial brain tumor	Intra-carotid injection after disruption of BBB	Investigation of magnetic NPs as MRI agents for the diagnosis and treatment of brain tumors. Nanodispersed magnetite-dextran preparations penetrated into brain tumor and peritumoral tissue
QDs	QDs (TAT peptide-conjugated)	Rats	Intravenous	Investigation of the delivery of QDs for imaging the brain tissue. TAT peptide was necessary to overcome the BBB
	QDs coated with serum	Wild-type mice brain	Intravenous	Investigation of the *in vivo* microangiography of deep brain capillaries and blood vessels after injection with QDs. Deep *in vivo* microangiography provided a new approach for visualization microangiopathies, typical from AD
	QDs into a core of PEG-PLA NPs [wheat germ agglutinin (WGA)-conjugated]	BALB/c nude mice	Intranasal	Study of the biodistribution. Targeted QDs showed brain delivery by intranasal administration
	AminoPEG QDs	Rats with gliosarcoma	Intravenous	Identification of neoplastic tissue within normal brain during biopsy and tumor resection. QDs were visualized within the experimental brain tumor, outlining the tumor and potentially augmenting brain tumor biopsy and resection

Table 12.5. contd....

Table 12.5. contd.

Nanomaterials for imaging in the CNS				
	Nanomaterial	Model	Route of administration	Aim and main conclusions
Dendrimers	PEGylated G-5 dendrimer conjugated to 1,4,7,10-tetraazacyclododecane-1,4,7,10-tetraacetic acid (DOTA) (Gd^{3+}) [labeled with cyanine 5.5 (Cy5.5), rodhamine B, and angiopet-2]	Mice with glioblastoma	Intravenous	Investigation of imaging brain tumor by dendrimer-based optical paramagnetic nanoprobe. Tumor margins were successfully delineated holding potential for preoperative brain tumor localization and image-guided tumor resection during surgery
Nanowires	Array of platinum nanowires	–	Intravenous	Electrical recording of the activity of small groups of neurons by an array of platinum nanowires. Nanowires were guided to the brain through the circulatory system reaching specific targets
CNTs	Electrodes coated with multi-walled CNTs	Rats and monkeys	Intracranial insertion	Development of CNT-based electrodes to record neuronal electrical events. Multi-walled CNT-coated electrodes improved the recording of neuronal electrical events
Transport of NPs to the brain				
Non-degradable NPs	QDs coated by hydroxyl group-modified SiO_2 networks ($\approx$ 20 nm-sized)	Mice	Intravenous	QDs were found to rarely distribute in the brain
	SiO_2-overcoated magnetic NPs (size $\approx$ 50 nm)	Mice	Intraperitoneal	NPs were detected in the brain
	TiO_2 NPs (diameter $\approx$ 25, $\approx$ 80, and $\approx$ 155 nm)	Mice	Gastrointestinal	The mice had a slight brain lesion associated with exposure to TiO_2 NPs

	Maghemite NPs (size ≈ 300 nm)	Mice	Intranasal	A deep brain penetration of the NPs and its potential to disrupt the cellular morphology in the hippocampus were observed
	Fluorescent magnetic NPs (≈ 50 nm-sized)	Mice	Inhalation	NPs were found to distribute in the brain
	Manganese oxide NPs (size ≈ 30 nm)	Rats	Inhalation	NPs were detected in olfactory bulbs and in deep brain structures (cortex and cerebellum)
	^{13}C NPs (≈ 35 nm-sized)	Rats	Inhalation	A significant and persistent increase of ^{13}C NPs in the olfactory bulbs was reported
Degradable polymeric NPs	PEGylated poly(hexadecylcyanoacrylate) NPs (size ≈ 100 to 200 nm)	Mice and rats	Intravenous	NPs penetrated into the brain to a large extent
	Dalargin absorbed on Tween® 80-coated poly(butylcyanoacrylate) NPs (size ≈ 230 nm)	Mice	Intravenous	NPs deliver dalargin across the BBB
	Dalargin adsorbed on Tween® 80-coated poly(butylcyanoacrylate) NPs (size ≈ 200 to 300 nm)	Mice	Intravenous and oral	Tween® 80-stabilized and dalargin-loaded NPs can to induce a central analgesic effect
	Doxorubicin bound to Tween®-coated NPs (≈ 270 nm-sized)	Rats	Intravenous	Doxorubicin bound to NPs crossed the intact BBB, thus reaching therapeutic concentrations in the brain
	Lectin-conjugated PEGylated PLA NPs (size ≈ 75 nm)	Rats	Intranasal	Two-fold increase in the brain uptake of WGA-conjugated NPs
	Delivery of nimodipine by methoxyPEGylated PLA NPs (diameter ≈ 75 nm)	Rats	Intranasal	Significant enhancement of nimodipine in the cerebrospinal fluid and olfactory bulb was reported

Table 12.5. contd....

Table 12.5. contd.

	Nanomaterial	Model	Route of administration	Aim and main conclusions
Neurotoxicity of NPs				
NPs	Copper, silver, or aluminium (size ≈ 50 to 60 nm)	Rats and mice	Intravenous, intraperitoneal, intracerebral	NPs induced brain dysfunction in normal animals and aggravated the brain pathology caused by whole-body hyperthermia
	TiO_2 (≈ 5 nm-sized)	Mice	Injected into the abdominal cavity	The accumulation of TiO_2 NPs in the mice brain occurred and caused the oxidative stress and injury of the brain
	Manganese oxide (size ≈ 30 nm)	Rats	Inhalation	Manganese oxide NPs resulted in the increase of macrophage inflammatory protein-2, glial fibrillary acidic protein, and neuronal cell adhesion molecule mRNA level in the brain
	Silver (diameter ≈ 25 nm)	Mice	Intraperitoneal	Mice oxidative stress and antioxidant defense genes were significantly and differentially expressed in the caudate, frontal cortex and hippocampus, suggesting silver NPs have the potential to cause neurotoxicity
	Maghemite (size ≈ 300 nm)	Mice	Intranasal	The neuron fatty degeneration occurred in the hippocampus, implying an adverse impact of inhalation of maghemite NPs on CNS
	Ultrafine carbon black (size ≈ 15 nm or ≈ 95 nm)	Mice	Intranasal	Up-regulation of proinflammatory cytokines mRNA in brain olfactory bulb, not in the hippocampus

Fullerene C60 (diameter ≈ 30 to 100 nm)	Fish	–	Significant lipid peroxidation was found in brain. Glutathione was also marginally depleted in gills of fish
TiO_2 (size ≈ 20 nm)	Fish	–	The NPs increased the zinc levels, decreased the copper levels, and inhibited Na^+K^+-ATPase activity in the brain
Neutral emulsifying wax NPs (≈ 100 nm-sized)	Rats	Brain perfusion	Neutral NPs and low concentrations of anionic NPs induced no effect on BBB integrity, whereas high concentrations of anionic NPs and cationic NPs disrupted the BBB. Brain uptake rates of anionic NPs at lower concentrations were superior to neutral or cationic formulations at equal concentrations

Table 12.6. Drug-loaded NPs tested for the treatment of AD. Reprinted with permission from Sahni et al. (2011). Copyright Elsevier Science BV (2011).

Category	Drug	NP	Preparation method	Model	Route of administration	Advantages/Applications	Particle size (nm)
Metal chelators	Copper chelator, D-penicillamine	–	Conjugation of drug and NP	–	–	Deliver D-penicillamine to the brain to prevent $A\beta$(1-42) accumulation	≈ 120
	Iron chelator: MAEHP	Polystyrene	NPs activated by N-cyclohexyl-N'-(2-morpholinoethyl) carbodiimide methyl-p toluensulfonate and then reacted with MAEHP	–	–	NP-chelator conjugates can inhibit $A\beta$ fibril formation, and cross the BBB and protect human brain cells from $A\beta$-related toxicity	≈ 240
	Quinoline derivatives, clioquinol	Poly(butylcyanoacrylate)	Polymerization	AD transgenic mice	Intravenous	Drug-loaded NPs exhibited specificity for $A\beta$ plaques both *in vitro* and *in vivo*. Capable of aiding in the early diagnosis of AD	≈ 50
Cholinesterase inhibitors	Tacrine	Tween® 80-coated poly(butylcyanoacrylate)	–	Rats	Intravenous	Enhanced concentration of the drug in the brain	≈ 35
		Chitosan	Spontaneous emulsification	Rats	Intravenous	Increased bioavailability of the drug in the brain	≈ 40
	Rivastigmine	Poly(butylcyanoacrylate)	Emulsion polymerization	Rats	Intravenous	≈ 4-fold increase in brain concentration of the drug	≈ 40
$A\beta$ targeted drugs	ThT and thioflavin S	Polystyrene/poly(butylcyanoacrylate) (core/shell)	Emulsion polymerization	Mice	Intracerebro-ventricular	Tools to trace and clear $A\beta$ in the brain	≈ 90 to 100

Polyphenol epigallocatechin gallate	Nanolipidic	Cosolubilization	Rats	Oral	Prevent brain Aβ plaque formation	≈ 30 to 80
Coenzyme Q10	Trimethylated chitosan-conjugated PLGA	Nanoprecipitation	Mice	Intravenous	NPs greatly improved memory impairment, restoring it to a normal level	≈ 95 to 150
Apo E binding	Cur	Poly(butylcyanoacrylate)	Anionic polymerization	–	–	Attachment of Apo E3 to the NPs increased the uptake of Cur into cells as compared to controls	≈ 180 to 200
	–	Albumin	Desolvation	Mice	Intravenous	Enhanced brain uptake of NPs by cerebral endothelium (endocytosis + transcytosis)	≈ 250
Au NPs	–	–	Functionalization with the Cys-PEP peptide (H-Cys-Leu-Pro-Phe-Phe-Asp-NH$_2$) which was obtained following a solid phase peptide synthesis (Fmoc)	–	–	The NPs dissolve toxic Aβ deposits by the combined use of weak microwave fields and Au NPs without any bulk heating	–
Magnetite NPs	–	–	Nucleation followed by controlled growth of IO layers onto IO/ gelatin-rhodamine B isothiocyanate nuclei	–	–	Biomarkers for detecting the location and the removal of other Aβ plaques derived from different amyloidogenic proteins	≈ 15

Table 12.6. contd....

Table 12.6. contd.

Category	Drug	NP	Preparation method	Model	Route of administration	Advantages/ Applications	Particle size (nm)
Hormones	Estradiol	Chitosan	Ionic gelation of chitosan with tripolyphosphate anions	Rats	Intranasal	NPs significantly increased the transport of estradiol into the CNS	From < 100 to > 500 nm, depending on the type of chitosan
	Melatonin	Eudragit® S100	Interfacial deposition of preformed polymer	Mice	Intraperitoneal	Melatonin-loaded Tween® 80-coated nanocapsules significantly reduced lipid peroxidation levels, and increased the total antioxidant reactivity in the hippocampus	≈ 200 to 240
		Eudragit® S100	Nanoprecipitation	–	–	NPs increased the antioxidant effect of melatonin against lipid peroxidation	≈ 125 to 255
Proteins and peptides	Vasoactive intestinal neuroprotective peptide	PEGylated PLA modified with WGA	Emulsion/solvent evaporation	Mice	Intranasal	Improved brain delivery of estradiol using WGA NPs	≈ 90 to 120
	Aβ	Chitosan	Mechanical stirring emulsification and chemical cross-linking	Mice	Systemic	Nanovaccine. Potential carrier for Aβ	≈ 15

Abbreviations

AD	:	Alzheimer's disease
Apo	:	apolipoprotein
ATPase	:	adenosinetriphosphatase
Au	:	gold
a.u.	:	arbitrary units
$A\beta$	:	amyloid beta
BAM	:	N-tert-butylacrylamide
BBB	:	blood-brain barrier
BDNF	:	brain-derived neurotrophic factor
Chol	:	cholesterol
CeO_2	:	ceria or cerium oxide
CL	:	cardiolipin
CNS	:	central nervous system
CNT	:	carbon nanotube
CT	:	computed tomography
CuAAC	:	copper-catalyzed azide-alkyne cycloaddition
Cur	:	curcumin
Cy5.5	:	cyanine 5.5
DAPI	:	4',6-diamidino-2-phenylindole
DCC	:	N,N'-dicyclohexylcarbodiimide
DMAP	:	4-(N,N-dimethylamino)pyridine
DNA	:	deoxyribonucleic acid
DOTA	:	1,4,7,10-tetraazacyclododecane-1,4,7,10-tetraacetic acid
EDTA	:	ethylene diamine tetraacetic acid
ERK5	:	extracellular signal-regulated kinase 5
^{18}F-FDG	:	fluorodeoxyglucose
Gd^{3+}	:	gadolinium
HIV	:	human immunodeficiency virus
hNgf-beta	:	human nerve growth factor beta
^{125}I	:	iodine-125
IO	:	iron oxide
LDL	:	low density lipoprotein
MAEHP	:	2-methyl-N-(2'-aminoethyl)-3-hydroxyl-4-pyridinone
MPA	:	3-mercaptopropionic acid
*m*RNA	:	messenger ribonucleic acid
MTT	:	3-(4,5-dimethylthiazol-2-yl)-2,5-diphenyltetrazolium bromide
NAC	:	N-acetyl-L-cysteine
NiPAM	:	N-isopropylacrylamide
NLP	:	nanoliposome
NP	:	nanoparticle

o/w	:	oil-in-water
PA	:	phosphatidic acid
PC	:	phosphatidylcholine
PCL	:	poly(ε-caprolactone)
PD	:	Parkinson's disease
PE	:	phosphatidylethanolamine
PEG	:	poly(ethylene glycol)
PEI	:	polyethyleneimine
PET	:	positron emission tomography
PG	:	phosphatidylglycerol
PLA	:	poly(D,L-lactide)
PLGA	:	poly(D,L-lactide-*co*-glycolide)
POPC	:	1-palmitoyl-2-oleoyl-*sn*-glycero-3-phosphocholine
POPG	:	1-palmitoyl-2-oleoyl-*sn*-glycero-3-phospho-*rac*-1-glycerol
QD	:	quantum dot
RES	:	reticuloendothelial system
RFU	:	relative fluorescence units
RM	:	rasagiline mesylate
RU	:	resonance units
SiO_2	:	silicon dioxide or silica
SLN	:	solid lipid nanoparticle
Sm	:	sphingomyelin
SOD	:	superoxide dismutase
SPR	:	surface plasmon resonance
TAT peptide	:	transactivator of transcription (GRKKRRQRRRPQ) peptide
ThT	:	thioflavin T
TiO_2	:	titanium dioxide
TIRFM	:	total internal reflection fluorescence microscopy
TrkB	:	tyrosine kinase receptor B
WGA	:	wheat germ agglutinin
ZrO_2	:	zirconium dioxide or zirconia

References

Ay, I. and J.W. Francis and R.H. Brown, Jr. 2008. VEGF increases blood-brain barrier permeability to Evans blue dye and tetanus toxin fragment C but not adeno-associated virus in ALS mice. Brain Res. 1234: 198–205.

Boridy, S. and H. Takahashi, K. Akiyoshi and D. Maysinger. 2009. The binding of pullulan modified cholesteryl nanogels to Aβ oligomers and their suppression of cytotoxicity. Biomaterials. 30: 5583–5591.

Cabaleiro-Lago, C. and F. Quinlan-Pluck, I. Lynch, S. Lindman, A.M. Minogue, E. Thulin, D.M. Walsh, K.A. Dawson and S. Linse. 2008. Inhibition of amyloid beta protein fibrillation by polymeric nanoparticles. J. Am. Chem. Soc. 130: 15437–15443.

Cabaleiro-Lago, C. and F. Quinlan-Pluck, I. Lynch, K.A. Dawson and S. Linse. 2010. Dual effect of amino modified polystyrene nanoparticles on amyloid beta protein fibrillation. ACS Chem. Neurosci. 1: 279–287.

Chan, H.M. and L. Xiao, K.M. Yeung, S.L. Ho, D. Zhao, W.H. Chan and H.W. Li. 2012. Effect of surface-functionalized nanoparticles on the elongation phase of beta-amyloid (1-40) fibrillogenesis. Biomaterials. 33: 4443–4450.

Chonpathompikunlert, P. and T. Yoshitomi, J. Han, H. Isoda and Y. Nagasaki. 2011. The use of nitroxide radical-containing nanoparticles coupled with piperine to protect neuroblastoma SH-SY5Y cells from Ab-induced oxidative stress. Biomaterials. 32: 8605–8612.

Cimini, A. and B. D'Angelo, S. Das, R. Gentile, E. Benedetti, V. Singh, A.M. Monaco, S. Santucci and S. Seal. 2012. Antibody-conjugated PEGylated cerium oxide nanoparticles for specific targeting of Ab aggregates modulate neuronal survival pathways. Acta Biomater. 8: 2056–2067.

Fernández, M. and S. Negro, K. Slowing, A. Fernández-Carballido and E. Barcia. 2011. An effective novel delivery strategy of rasagiline for Parkinson's disease. Int. J. Pharm. 419: 271–280.

Gobbi, M. and F. Re, M. Canovi, M. Beeg, M. Gregori, S. Sesana, S. Sonnino, D. Brogioli, C. Musicanti, P. Gasco, M. Salmona and M.E. Masserini. 2010. Lipid based nanoparticles with high binding affinity for amyloid-β1-42 peptide. Biomaterials. 31: 6519–6529.

Hu, K. and J. Li, Y. Shen, W. Lu, X. Gao, Q. Zhang and X. Jiang. 2009. Lactoferrin conjugated PEG-PLA nanoparticles with improved brain delivery: *in vitro* and *in vivo* evaluations. J. Control. Release. 134: 55–61.

Hu, Y.L. and J.Q. Gao. 2010. Potential neurotoxicity of nanoparticles. Int. J. Pharm. 394: 115–121.

Ianiski, F.R. and C.B. Alves, A.C.G. Souza, S. Pinton, S.S. Roman, C.R.B. Rhoden, M.P. Alves and C. Luchese. 2012. Protective effect of meloxicam-loaded nanocapsules against amyloid-β peptide-induced damage in mice. Behav. Brain Res. 230: 100–107.

Jalali, N. and F. Moztarzadeh, M. Mozafari, S. Asgari, M. Motevalian and S.N. Alhosseini. 2011. Surface modification of poly(lactide-co-glycolide) nanoparticles by d-α-tocopheryl polyethylene glycol 1000 succinate as potential carrier for the delivery of drugs to the brain. Colloids Surf. A Physicochem. Eng. Aspects. 392: 335–342.

Kanwar, J.R. and X. Sun, V. Punj, B. Sriramoju, R.R. Mohan, S.F. Zhou, A. Chauhan and R.K. Kanwar. 2012. Nanoparticles in the treatment and diagnosis of neurological disorders: untamed dragon with fire power to heal. Nanomedicine. 8: 399–414.

Klyachko, N.L. and D.S. Manickam, A.M. Brynskikh, S.V. Uglanova, S. Li, S.M. Higginbotham, T.K. Bronich, E.V. Batrakova and A.V. Kabanov. 2012. Cross-linked antioxidant nanozymes for improved delivery to CNS. Nanomedicine. 8: 119–129.

Korsvik, C. and S. Patil, S. Seal and W.T. Self. 2007. Superoxide dismutase mimetic properties exhibited by vacancy engineered ceria nanoparticles. Chem. Commun. (Camb.). 14: 1056–1058.

Le Droumaguet, L. and J. Nicolas, D. Brambilla, S. Mura, A. Maksimenko, L. De Kimpe, E. Salvati, C. Zona, C. Airoldi, M. Canovi, M. Gobbi, M. Noiray, B. La Ferla, F. Nicotra, W. Scheper, O. Flores, M. Masserini, K. Andrieux and P. Couvreur. 2012. Versatile and efficient targeting using a single nanoparticulate platform: application to cancer and Alzheimer's disease. ACS Nano. 6: 5866–5879.

Linazasoro, G. 2008. Potential applications of nanotechnologies to Parkinson's disease therapy. Parkinsonism Relat. Disord. 14: 383–392.

Liu, G. and P. Men, W. Kudo, G. Perry and M.A. Smith. 2009. Nanoparticle–chelator conjugates as inhibitors of amyloid-b aggregation and neurotoxicity: a novel therapeutic approach for Alzheimer disease. Neurosci. Lett. 455: 187–190.

Lu, C. and S. Pelech, H. Zhang, J. Bond, K. Spach, R. Noubade, E.P. Blankenhorn and C. Teuscher. 2008. Pertussis toxin induces angiogenesis in brain microvascular endothelial cells. Neurosci. Res. 86: 2624–2640.

Majzik, A. and L. Fulop, E. Csapo, F. Bogar, T. Martinek, B. Penke, G. Bíró and I. Dékány. 2010. Functionalization of gold nanoparticles with amino acid, beta-amyloid peptides and fragment. Colloids Surf. B Biointerfaces. 81: 235–241.

Martinez-Fong, D. and M.J. Bannon, L.E. Trudeau, J.A. Gonzalez-Barrios, M.L. Arango-Rodriguez, N.G. Hernandez-Chan, D. Reyes-Corona, J. Armendáriz-Borunda and I. Navarro-Quiroga. 2012. NTS-Polyplex: a potential nanocarrier for neurotrophic therapy of Parkinson's disease. Nanomedicine. 8: 1052–1069.

Michaelis, K. and M.M. Hoffmann, S. Dreis, E. Herbert, R.N. Alyautdin, M. Michaelis, J. Kreuter and K. Langer. 2006. Covalent linkage of apolipoprotein to albumin nanoparticles strongly enhances drug transport into the brain. J. Pharmacol. Exp. Ther. 317: 1246–1253.

Mittal, G. and H. Carswell, R. Brett, S. Currie and M.N.V. Ravi Kumar. 2011. Development and evaluation of polymer nanoparticles for oral delivery of estradiol to rat brain in a model of Alzheimer's pathology. J. Control. Release. 150: 220–228.

Modi, G. and V. Pillay, Y.E. Choonara, V.M.K. Ndesendo, L.C. du Toit and D. Naidoo. 2009. Nanotechnological applications for the treatment of neurodegenerative disorders. Prog. Neurobiol. 88: 272–285.

Mufamadi, M.S. and Y.E. Choonara, P. Kumar, G. Modi, D. Naidoo, V.M.K. Ndesendo, L.C. du Toit, S.E. Iyuke and V. Pillay. 2012. Surface-engineered nanoliposomes by chelating ligands for modulating the neurotoxicity associated with β-amyloid aggregates of Alzheimer's disease. Pharm Res. 29: 3075–3089.

Narushima, I. and T. Kita, K. Kubo, Y. Yonetani, C. Momochi, I. Yoshikawa, N. Ohno and T. Nakashima. 2003. Highly enhanced permeability of blood-brain barrier induced by repeated administration of endothelin-1 in dogs and rats. Pharmacol. Toxicol. 92: 21–26.

Nowacek, A. and L.M. Kosloski and H.E. Gendelman. 2009. Neurodegenerative disorders and nanoformulated drug development. Nanomedicine (Lond.). 4: 541–555.

Nunes, A. and K.T. Al-Jamal and K. Kostarelos. 2012. Therapeutics, imaging and toxicity of nanomaterials in the central nervous system. J. Control. Release. 161: 290–306.

Pillay, S. and V. Pillay, Y.E. Choonara, D. Naidoo, R.A. Khan, L.C. du Toit, V.M.K. Ndesendo, G. Modi, M.P. Danckwerts and S.E. Iyuke. 2009. Design, biometric simulation and optimization of a nano-enabled scaffold device for enhanced delivery of dopamine to the brain. Int. J. Pharm. 382: 277–290.

Rao, K.S. and M.K. Reddy, J.L. Horning and V. Labhasetwar. 2008. TAT-conjugated nanoparticles for the CNS delivery of anti-HIV drugs. Biomaterials. 29: 4429–4438.

Roy, S. and A.H. Johnston, S.T. Moin, J. Dudas, T.A. Newman, B. Hausott, A. Schrott-Fischer and R. Glueckert. 2012. Activation of TrkB receptors by NGFβ mimetic peptide conjugated polymersome nanoparticles. Nanomedicine. 8: 271–274.

Sahni, J.K. and S. Doggui, J. Ali, S. Baboota, L. Dao and C. Ramassamy. 2011. Neurotherapeutic applications of nanoparticles in Alzheimer's disease. J. Control. Release. 152: 208–231.

Salay, L.C. and W. Qi, B. Keshet, L.K. Tamm and E.J. Fernandez. 2009. Membrane interactions of a self-assembling model peptide that mimics the self-association, structure and toxicity of Aβ(1-40). Biochim. Biophys. Acta. 1788: 1714–1721.

Taylor, M. and S. Moore, S. Mourtas, A. Niarakis, F. Re, C. Zona, B. La Ferla, F. Nicotra, M. Masserini, S.G. Antimisiaris, M. Gregori and D. Allsop. 2011. Effect of curcumin-associated and lipid ligand-functionalized nanoliposomes on aggregation of the Alzheimer's Aβ peptide. Nanomedicine. 7: 541–550.

Townsend, S.A. and G.D. Evrony, F.X. Gu, M.P. Schulz, R.H. Brown and R. Langer. 2007. Tetanus toxin C fragment-conjugated nanoparticles for targeted delivery to neurons. Biomaterials. 28: 5176–5184.

Ulbrich, K. and T. Hekmatara, E. Herbert and J. Kreuter. 2009. Transferrin- and transferrin-receptor-antibody-modified nanoparticles enable drug delivery across the blood-brain barrier (BBB). Eur. J. Pharm. Biopharm. 71: 251–256.

Wu, W.H. and X. Sun, Y.P. Yu, J. Hu, L. Zhao, Q. Liu, Y.F. Zhao and Y.M. Li. 2008. TiO2 nanoparticles promote beta-amyloid fibrillation *in vitro*. Biochem. Biophys. Res. Commun. 373: 315–318.

Xiao, L.H. and D. Zhao, W.H. Chan, M.M.F. Choi and H.W. Li. 2010. Inhibition of beta 1-40 amyloid fibrillation with n-acetyl-l-cysteine capped quantum dots. Biomaterials. 31: 91–98.

Xin, H. and X. Jiang, J. Gu, X. Sha, L. Chen, K. Law, Y. Chen, X. Wang, Y. Jiang and X. Fang. 2011. Angiopep conjugated poly(ethylene glycol)-co-poly(e-caprolactone) nanoparticles as dual-targeting drug delivery system for brain glioma. Biomaterials. 32: 4293–4305.

Yang, Z. and Y. Zhang, Y. Yang, L. Sun, D. Han, H. Li and C. Wang. 2010. Pharmacological and toxicological target organelles and safe use of single-walled carbon nanotubes as drug carriers in treating Alzheimer disease. Nanomedicine. 6: 427–441.

Yoo, S.I. and M. Yang, J.R. Brender, V. Subramanian, K. Sun, N.E. Joo, S.H. Jeong, A. Ramamoorthy and N.A. Kotov. 2011. Inhibition of amyloid peptide fibrillation by inorganic nanoparticles: functional similarities with proteins. Angew. Chem. Int. Ed. Engl. 50: 5110–5115.

CHAPTER 13

Nanomedicines against Infectious Diseases

Leticia H. Higa,[a] *Ana Paula Perez,*[b] *Priscila Schilrreff,*[c] *Maria Jose Morilla*[d] and *Eder Lilia Romero**

ABSTRACT

An attractive alternative to the urgent need of developing new medicines against infectious diseases (not generating resistances, and resulting in less toxic and more effective than current therapies) is offered by the introduction of nanotechnology in the pharmaceutical and immunological fields. Thanks to this approach to the problem, therapeutic molecules loaded into nanoparticulate carriers can be satisfactorily delivered to intracellular compartments of selected tissues, enabling both their targeting and physicochemical protection independent of their chemical structure.

This chapter evaluates the use of nanoparticulate and microparticulate carriers in drug therapy and vaccine development against malaria, tuberculosis, leishmaniasis, and Chagas disease. The benefits from the incorporation of antimalarial drugs to particles administered intravenously will be discussed. The latest preclinical strategies demonstrating how the inhalation of antituberculosis drugs loaded into particulate platforms can result in a direct targeting of alveolar macrophages will also be analyzed, thus reducing the number of administrations and providing surfactant material to atelectatic lungs. In addition, the chapter will focus on the

Departamento de Ciencia y Tecnologia, Programa de Nanomedicina, Universidad Nacional de Quilmes, Roque Saenz Peña 352, Bernal B1876BXD, Buenos Aires, Argentina.
[a] Email: lhiga@unq.edu.ar
[b] Email: apperez@unq.edu.ar
[c] Email: pschilrreff@unq.edu.ar
[d] Email: jmorilla@unq.edu.ar
* Corresponding author: elromero@unq.edu.ar

satisfactory use of nanomedicines against visceral leishmaniasis, despite the cutaneous and mucocutaneous clinical forms needs improved delivery (micro/nano)strategies. It will be further explored how Chagas disease, with intracytoplasmic targets within non-phagocytic cells in tissues where inflammation is almost absent, remains as an unsurpassed challenge for conventional and nanomedical approaches. Finally, the contribution will emphasize how (micro/nano)particulate adjuvants can increase the immunogenicity and the delivery of the protein or genetic material to target cells, inducing type 1 T helper and type 2 T helper responses.

Introduction

Tuberculosis, malaria, leishmaniasis, and Chagas disease affect more than two billion people globally and cause substantial morbidity and mortality, particularly among the world's poorest people. Unfortunately, the morbidity and mortality of these diseases is increased in patients infected with Human Immunodeficiency Virus (HIV). Conventional therapeutic approaches habitually fail in the fight against infectious diseases. To beat the challenge, it is hypothesized that Drug Delivery Systems (DDSs) based on microparticles and nanoparticles (NPs) can be wisely engineered to assure an efficient therapy. Concretely, it is suggested that nanotechnology can help in modifying drug's pharmacokinetics, biodistribution, and intracellular traffic with the help of appropriate carriers. In the field of adjuvancy, by loading antigens within particulate carriers it can be possible to modify the route of administration, raising intense and controlled immune responses, because of the preference of antigen presenting cells of taking up particulate solids instead of soluble materials. This chapter will critically analyze the use of nanoparticulate and microparticulate carriers as drug/vaccine delivery systems against experimental models of tuberculosis, malaria, leishmaniasis, and Chagas disease.

Malaria

The elimination of malaria is now considered a realistic goal because of good surveillance and high intervention coverage between the years 2000 and 2007 which resulted in the reduction of malaria cases and deaths by $\geq 50\%$ in some countries of Africa. However, each year 300 to 500 million people suffer from acute malaria, and 0.5 to 2.5 million die of the disease of which 90% are in sub-Saharan Africa. Malaria is caused by four species of *Plasmodium* (*P. falciparum*, *P. vivax*, *P. malariae*, and *P. ovale*). *P. falciparum* infection (80% of malaria cases) causes severe malaria, where neurological symptoms occur and may result in death if treatment is not promptly instituted, especially in acute primary infections. *P. vivax* and *P. ovale* infections cause chronic malaria. The disease can relapse months or years after exposure, due to the presence of dormant liver stage parasites. Finally, *P. malariae* produces long-lasting infections and if untreated it can persist asymptomatically in the human host for years, even a lifetime.

Plasmodium parasites enter humans by the bites of female mosquito of *Anopheles* genus. The inoculated sporozoites migrate to the liver and invade the hepatocytes. Sporozoites generate new invasive forms of the parasites (merozoites) that are released to the bloodstream. There, merozoites enter erythrocytes where parasite undergoes a rapid phase of growth, forming the trophozoite stage, during which the parasite digests the majority of the hemoglobin and grows to fill > 50% of the volume of the host cell. At the end of the trophozoite stage the parasite divides several times (the schizont stage) before the host cell lyses ($\approx$ 48 hours after invasion) to release the newly formed merozoites that continue the cycle. Some merozoites turn into male and female gametocytes that also invade erythrocytes.

The erythrocytic stages (trophozoites, schizontes, and gametocytes) living inside parasitophorous vacuole and the exoerythrocytic stages (intrahepatocyte hypnozoites) present major structural and phenomenological barriers that antimalarial drugs have to overcome.

Conventional treatments

Therapy depends on *Plasmodium* specie, severity of infection, previous exposition to infection, clinic status of the patient, and area where the infection was acquired and its drug-resistance status. Most drugs are active against the parasite forms in blood, including chloroquine, primaquine atovaquone/proguanil, artemether/lumefantrine, mefloquine, quinine, quinidine, doxycycline/quinine, clindamycin/quinine, and artesunate. The main drawbacks of chemotherapy are the development of multiple drug resistances and the non-specific targeting to non-infected cells, resulting in high dose requirements and subsequent intolerable toxicity.

Preclinical drug delivery systems against malaria

Santos-Magalhães and Furtado Mosqueira (2010) thoroughly reviewed the latest preclinical developments against malaria. Most of the approaches were based on changing pharmacokinetics by drug loading into liposomes, nanocapsules, and lipid NPs, while a minority fraction of articles were found to be focused on targeting to infected erythrocytes or hepatocytes (Table 13.1). The main findings can be grouped according to the delivery strategy:

1. Increased half-life upon intravenous administration. Halofantrine-loaded poly(D,L-lactide) (PLA) nanocapsules surface functionalized with poly(ethylene glycol) (PEG, PEGylated) demonstrated higher area under the plasma drug concentration-time curve (AUC) and faster control of parasitemia in the absence of toxic effects (up to 100 mg/Kg) than free halofantrine, after a single dose (Mosqueira et al. 2004). Halofantrine

Table 13.1. DDSs against malaria. PC: phosphatidylcholine; DOPC: 1,2-dioleoyl-*sn*-glycero-3-phosphatidylcholine; DSPE-PEG(2000): 1,2-distearoyl-*sn*-glycero-3-phosphoethanolamine-*N*-[amino(polyethylene glycol)-2000]; MPB-PE: 1,2-dipalmitoyl-*sn*-glycero-3-phosphoethanolamine-*N*-[4-(*p*-maleimidophenyl) butyramide].

DDS	Drug	Route of administration, dose	Main results	References
Multilamellar liposomes (egg PC:cholesterol, 4:3 molar ratio)	*β*-arteether	Intraperitoneal to mice infected with *P. chabaudi*	Cleared the parasitaemia	Chimanuka et al. 2002
Liposomes (200 nm-sized; DOPC:cholesterol:MPB-PE, 77.5:20:2.5 molar ratio) grafted to antibodies against *P. falciparum* infected erythrocytes	Chloroquine	Intravenous	Cleared ≈ 26% of *Plasmodium*-infected red blood cells	Urban et al. 2011
Liposomes [size: 90–140 nm; surface electrical charge: –20 mV; soybean PC:cholesterol:DSPE-PEG(2000), 5.0:6:0.25 molar ratio]	Artemisinin and/ or curcumin	Intraperitoneal (12 d) to mice infected with *P. berghei* NK-65	Less variability in plasma concentrations than the free drugs	Isacchi et al. 2012
Medium chain triglycerides/PEGylated PLA (core/shell) nanocapsules	Halofantrine	Intravenous to mice infected with *P. berghei*	6-fold higher plasma AUC and activity than free drug (up to 70 hours)	Mosqueira et al. 2004
PCL nanocapsules	Halofantrine	Intravenous, 1 mg/Kg to mice infected with *P. berghei*	Reduced drug cardiotoxicity	Leite et al. 2007
PCL and Tween® 80 nanocapsules	Quinine	Intravenous to rats infected with *P. berghei*	Pharmacokinetic parameters of quinine in nanocapsules were similar to those of the free drug	Haas et al. 2009
CS-tripolyphosphate NPs (diameter: 150–300 nm; surface electrical charge: +30 mV)	Chloroquine	Intraperitoneal to Swiss mice, 250 mg/Kg for 15 d	Eliminate ≈ 98% of parasite and protect lymphocytes, serum and red blood cells against *P. berghei* infection	Satyajit et al. 2012

Table 13.1. contd....

Table 13.1. contd.

DDS	Drug	Route of administration, dose	Main results	References
SLNs [blend of solid lipid trimyristin (triglyceride of C14) with the liquid soybean oil]	Artemether	Intravenous to mice infected with *P. berghei*	Prolonged survival period in comparison to drug solution and to marketed formulation	Aditya et al. 2010a
NLCs [made of glyceryl dilaurate (solid lipid), Capmul® MCM (liquid lipid), Tween® 80, and Solutol® HS 15; size ≈ 60 nm]	Artemether	Intraperitoneal to mice infected with *P. berghei*	Increased survival time as compared to the commercial formulation	Joshi et al. 2008a
NLCs (trimyristin, tristerin, and glyceryl monostearate as solid lipids, and medium chain triglyceride as liquid)	Curcumin	Intraperitoneal, 3 doses	Increased the survival period of mice as compared to free drugs	Aditya et al. 2010b
Miglyol® nanoemulsions	Primaquine	Oral to mice infected with *P. berghei*	Increased ≈ 1.3-fold the AUC, and generated high drug levels in the liver	Singh and Vingkar 2008
Self-emulsifying DDS	Artemether	Oral	Antimalarial activity	Mandawgade et al. 2008
Self-emulsifying DDS (groundnut or sesame oil, Maisine™ 35-1, Tween® 80 or Cremophor® EL, and absolute ethanol)	Artemether	Oral, 24 mg/Kg for 4 d	Complete cure for more than 45 days in 100% of *P. berghei* infected mice	Memvanga and Préat 2012

loaded to poly(ε-caprolactone) (PCL) particles showed better results than PEGylated PLA nanocapsules (Leite et al. 2007). On the other hand, quinine-loaded PCL nanocapsules demonstrated increased efficacy compared to the free drug, with enhanced drug penetration into infected red blood cells (Haas et al. 2009). Finally, artemether-loaded Solid Lipid Nanoparticles (SLNs) significantly prolonged the survival period of animals without parasitemia due to the burst drug release followed by a sustained release of the drug. As a result of this drug release profile, the fast metabolism of artemether could be minimized reducing thereafter the production of high toxicity levels of dihydroartemisinin (Aditya et al. 2010a).

2. Sustained drug release. Artemether-loaded multilamellar liposomes produced $\approx 100\%$ cure of mice infected with a virulent rodent malaria parasite upon intraperitoneal administration (Chimanuka et al. 2002). Artemisinin in combination with curcumin, encapsulated in PEGylated liposomes showed an immediate antimalarial effect and cured all infected mice upon intraperitoneal administration (Isacchi et al. 2012). Liposomal encapsulation generates a modified drug release and a constant antimalarial effect during time. Nanostructured Lipid Carriers (NLCs) loaded with artemether (Joshi et al. 2008a) and curcuminoids (Aditya et al. 2010b) increased the survival time of mice upon intraperitoneal administration thanks to a sustained drug release from the NLC. On the other hand, chitosan (CS) NPs containing chloroquine, eliminate $\approx 98\%$ of parasite upon intraperitoneal administration by decreasing free radical generation, and lipid and protein damage, and increasing the antioxidant status (Satyajit et al. 2012).

3. Increased bioavailability upon oral administration. Primaquine-loaded Miglyol® nanoemulsions suppressed parasitemia ($\approx 93\%$) and extended survival at doses $\approx 25\%$ lower than free drug (Singh and Vingkar 2008). Artemether incorporation into self-emulsifying DDSs (Mandawgade et al. 2008) and solid microemulsions (Joshi et al. 2008b) produced an improvement in antimalarial activity after oral administration compared to the intramuscular administration of commercial formulation. Recently, it was demonstrated that the antimalarial efficacy of β-arteether loaded to self-emulsifying DDSs was comparable to that of an oily solution of β-arteether administered intramuscularly, and significantly higher than that given orally (Memvanga and Préat 2012).

4. Increased brain delivery. The transferrin receptor is highly polarized at the blood-brain barrier. It is localized only on the apical membrane of endothelial cells where it transports iron by receptor-mediated endocytosis from the luminal membrane of brain capillaries to the brain parenchyma. On these bases, transferrin-conjugated SLNs were investigated for their ability to deliver quinine dihydrochloride to the

brain, for the management of cerebral malaria (Gupta et al. 2007). Upon intravenous administration, conjugation of SLNs significantly enhanced brain uptake of quinine as compared with non-conjugated SLNs or drug solution. However, neither the presence of quinine in brain parenchima nor the antimalarial activity was determined.

5. Targeted delivery to erythrocytes. First works showed a single dose of chloroquine-loaded liposomes surface functionalized with F(ab')2 fragments of a mouse monoclonal antibody (raised against cell membranes isolated from *P. berghei*-infected mouse erythrocytes) can effectively control chloroquine-susceptible and resistant infections (Owais et al. 1995). These studies were discontinued, probably due to the structural complexity of the carrier construct that made it difficult to further scaling up. Recently, liposomes covalently functionalized with oriented specific half-antibodies against infected red blood cells with late form of *P. falciparum* showed high affinity to *Plasmodium*-infected red blood cells (Urbán et al. 2011). In preliminary assays, chloroquine (dose 2 nM, $\geq$ 10 times below its half maximal inhibitory concentration, IC_{50}) cleared $\approx$ 26% of *Plasmodium*-infected red blood cells when delivered by targeted immunoliposomes. Because chloroquine targets a metabolic pathway inside the food vacuole, these results provide additional confirmation of the delivery of immunoliposomal contents inside *Plasmodium*-infected red blood cells.

6. Targeted delivery to hepatocytes. Two different strategies could successfully target hepatocytes, however the antimalarial activity was not determined. The first one used a reconstituted artificial chylomicron emulsion made of commercially available lipids (Dierling and Cui 2005). Chylomicrons are recognized by the remnant receptor, uniquely localized on hepatocytes. Being endogenous, lipoproteins are biodegradable, do not trigger immune reactions, and are not recognized by the reticuloendothelial system. Primaquine loaded into a chylomicron emulsion showed an enhanced accumulation in the liver, as compared to free primaquine. The second strategy employed large unilamellar vesicles grafted to the sporozoite recognizing peptide that is partially responsible for *Plasmodium* binding to the heparan sulfate proteoglycans found in the liver (Longmuir et al. 2006). Fluorescence and electron microscopy studies demonstrated that these liposomes were accumulated both by non-parenchymal cells (endothelial and Kupffer cells) and hepatocytes, with the majority of the liposomal material associated with hepatocytes. Further works demonstrated that liver cell uptake was more than 600-fold higher than uptake by heart cells, and more than 200-fold higher than uptake by lung or kidney cells. Effective targeting *in vivo* to liver was successful after repeated (up to three) administrations at 14 day intervals (Haynes et al. 2008). Intracellular localization of drugs as well as its antimalarial activity remained to be determined.

Vaccine delivery systems against malaria

The practical implementation of vaccination programs to millions of receptors, involves high costs and compliance failures. Most of the conventional vaccines are administered by the parenteral route in multiple shoots. However, an ideal vaccine for massive administration in countries without economical resources should be inexpensive, safe, and capable of inducing lifetime immunity. It should also be stable under the environmental conditions to avoid the cold chain necessity, easy to administer (preferably by non-invasive routes), allowable during childhood and, if possible, by a single shot.

An optimal malaria vaccine should have the ability to elicit protective immunity blocking infection, prevent pathology, and block transmission of parasite. Current preclinical efforts are divided in three groups that target different stages of the parasite life cycle: (i) the pre-erythrocytic strategies generate sporozoites neutralizing antibodies to prevent them from invading the hepatocyte, and cell-mediated immune response to interfere with the intrahepatic multiplication cycle of the parasites and further development into tissue schizonts. A subunit vaccine directed against *P. falciparum* sporozoites employing the recombinant protein sporozoite RTS, S is currently being assessed in a large multicenter Phase III trial in Africa and is likely to become the first registered malaria vaccine (Cohen et al. 2010); (ii) the asexual blood stage (erythrocytic stage) generate antibodies that could inactivate merozoites and/or target malaria antigens (Ags) expressed on the erythrocyte surface through antibody-dependent cellular cytotoxicity, and/or cell mediated complement lysis and T-cell responses to inhibit the development of the parasite in red blood cells. These vaccines are intended to protect against severe malaria, by decreasing the exponential multiplication of merozoites therefore decreasing morbidity and mortality. Effective vaccination with a blood stage vaccine would also prevent parasite sequestration and its complications, e.g., cerebral malaria, anemia, renal failure, and all of the manifestations of severe malaria in pregnancy. These complications are likely due to the cytoadherence of the *P. falciparum* Erythrocyte Membrane Protein-1 (PfEMP-1, expressed on the surface of infected red cells) to CD36, or intercellular adhesion molecule-1 on microvascular endothelial cells, or chondroitin sulfate A or other glycosaminoglycans in placenta; and finally, (iii) sexual stage/transmission-blocking vaccines are altruistic vaccines not aimed to prevent illness or infection in vaccinated individual, but to prevent or decrease transmission of the parasite to new hosts (Tyagi et al. 2012). The complex life cycle of the parasite and antigenic diversity are two additional reasons why a malaria vaccine is still elusive.

1st generation malaria vaccines based on whole parasites [irradiated (Hoffman et al. 2010) or genetically modified] are of high cost, and possess manufacturing problems and logistic difficulties (e.g., cryopreservation and/ or extensive assessment of safety) that make them unaffordable in endemic countries (Pinder et al. 2010). 2nd generation vaccines use Ag subunits of the parasite which were naive fractions purified from parasites, or synthetic Ag made by deoxyribonucleic acid (DNA) recombinant technology. However, malaria vaccines directed against a single Ag are unable to mount a complete immune response. Because of this, there is an active search for vaccines based in Ag subunits from different stages of the parasite and of DNA vaccines. 3rd generation vaccines include genes coding for a protective Ag and cloned into a vector containing a eukaryotic promoter. However, most protein and peptide vaccines, and plasmid DNA exhibit only low immunological activity when administered alone. This is the reason why 2nd and 3rd generation vaccines depend on the development of microparticulate/nanoparticulate adjuvants capable of increasing the immunogenicity and the delivery of the protein or genetic material to target cells. In this sense, microparticles and NPs have the potential to be stable at room temperature, stored in liquid form, and have lower manufacturing costs than biological vaccines, thus broadening access in resource-poor areas (Hubbell et al. 2009, Griffiths et al. 2010). Moreover, endocytic uptake of particulate materials by immature Antigen Presenting Cells (APCs) is a key step for induction of type 1 T helper (Th1) and type 2 T helper (Th2) immune responses, probably by affecting initial Ag uptake, processing, and presentation (Kensil et al. 2004). Representative vaccine delivery systems against malaria are summarized in Table 13.2.

The first attempts to develop particulate vaccines against malaria employed oral poly(D,L-lactide-*co*-glycolide) (PLGA) microparticles loaded with SPf66 (a chimeric molecule of 45 aminoacids, that is a combination of pre-erythrocytic and blood stage merozoite vaccine) in an effort to simplify the immunization protocols (Carcaboso et al. 2003) (Table 13.2). The microparticles administered orally showed an immunoglobulin (Ig) G2a isotype compared to the absent levels of this isotype for intramuscularly immunized group. Microparticles administered intranasally improved and maintained higher antibody levels characterized as a combined IgG2a/IgG1 response (suggesting a Th1/Th2 response), compared to the conventional adjuvant and to the administration of the particles by the subcutaneous or oral routes (Carcaboso et al. 2004).

Another approach employed intravenously administered pH-sensitive liposomes for direct cytosolic delivery of the carboxyl-terminal 19 kDa fragment of *P. falciparum* merozoite surface protein-1 (PfMSP-1) as vaccine against the asexual blood stage (Vyas et al. 2007). The PfMSP-1 is one of the Ag more successfully used because antibodies to MSP-1 C-terminal portion can be found at all stages of invasion. pH-sensitive liposomes induced a combined serum IgG2a/IgG1 response, more intense and perdurable than that generated by the free Ag or within conventional liposomes. Gel core liposomes loaded with the CpG ODN and the Pfs25 protein (found on the surface of zygote and ookinet stage of parasite, a transmission blocking recombinant protein Ag with low immunogenicity needing repeated administration) were recently tested as a vaccine against the sexual blood stage (Tiwari et al. 2009). Synthetic ODNs, containing non-methylated CpG motifs, are extremely efficient inducers of Th1 response and generation of cytotoxic T lymphocyte,

Table 13.2. Vaccine delivery systems against malaria. ODN: oligodeoxynucleotide; PGA: poly(γ-glutamic acid). PEI: polyethyleneimine; PyMSP-1: *P. yoelii* merozoite surface protein-1.

Vaccine delivery system	Ag	Immunization protocol, animal model, dose	Route of administration	Challenge	References
PLGA 50:50 and 75:25 (1.4 µm-sized)	SPf66	Days 0, 1, and 2, and boost days 21, 22, and 23. BALB/c mice. 500 µg	Oral	–	Carcaboso et al. 2003
PLGA (1.5 µm-sized, 500 nm-sized)	SPf66	Days 0, 1, and 2. BALB/c mice. 10 µg	Intranasal	–	Carcaboso et al. 2004
Liposomes ($\approx$ 250 nm, 11 mV; PC:cholesteryl hemisuccinate:Tween® 80:oleyl alcohol, 50:50:2:80 molar ratio)	PfMSP-1	Day 0, and boost day 15. BALB/c mice. 25 µg	Intramuscular	–	Vyas et al. 2007
Gel core liposomes [1.1 µm-sized; surface electrical charge: –37 mV; PC:cholesterol 7:3 molar ratio, with a poly(acrylic acid) 0.3% w/v core that becomes a sol at pH < 4.5]	Pfs25	Once. Mice. 0.5 µg with or without 2 µg of CpG ODN	Intramuscular	–	Tiwari et al. 2009
Plasmid DNA/PEI/PGA NPs ($\approx$ 60 nm-sized; surface electrical charge: –14 mV)	Plasmid DNA encoding the carboxyl-terminal 19 kDa fragment of PyMSP-1	3 times at 3 weeks interval. C57BL/6 mice. 80 µg plasmid DNA	Intravenous	10^5 *P. yoelii*-infected erythrocytes	Shuaibu et al. 2011
		3 times at 3 weeks interval. C57BL/6 mice. 100 µg plasmid DNA	Intravenous, subcutaneous, intraperitoneal		Cherif et al. 2011

which have shown to induce protection against an extensive range of viral, bacterial, and some parasitic pathogens in animal models (Wilson et al. 2009). Gel core liposomes elicited maximum levels of interleukin (IL)-2 and interferon gamma (IFN-γ), and a combined IgG2a/IgG1 response, thus suggesting Th1 and Th2 activations. Nonetheless, the clinical efficacy of these formulations remains to be tested. Unlike pre-erythrocytic vaccine candidates, this could be due to the current lack of a human artificial challenge model (humanized model) for the blood stage vaccine candidates.

DNA and recombinant viral subunit vaccines codify for a protein or series of epitopes inserted into either a circular *Escherichia coli* derived purified plasmid DNA or the genome of a double-stranded DNA virus such as *Vaccinia*. After capture by APCs, the plasmid expression will lead to intracellular synthesis, processing, and presentation of Major Histocompatibility Complex (MHC) class I and class II T-cell epitopes by Human Leukocyte Antigen (HLA) molecules for strong CD8+ and CD4+ T-cell immunogenicities. In theory, DNA vaccination can elicit both humoral and cellular immune responses by designing sequences that integrate Ag and immunostimulatory sequences. Disappointingly, the levels of antibody induced and protection observed in immunized mice against *Plasmodium* are variable (from lower antibody response and no protection to higher antibody response and partial protection). In particular, in spite of the partial and full protective immunity reported following DNA vaccination against malaria and other parasitic diseases in laboratory models, similar results were not observed in higher animals (Shuaibu et al. 2011). This is mostly attributable to the amount of DNA delivered, the amount that gets transfected and subsequently the amount of target Ag expressed. Naked DNA is rapidly degraded *in vivo* by extracellular deoxyribonucleases and exhibits poor cellular uptake by myocytes, requiring larger dose administration often into regenerating muscles. Besides, although myocytes carry MHC class I molecules, they are not APCs due to insufficient co-stimulatory molecules. This low potency of naked malaria DNA vaccines has led to the exploration and development of enhanced delivery strategies aimed to protect the DNA structure against nucleases and achieve its efficient delivery into the cytosol. After being released into the cytosol, the DNA has to travel across the nuclear pores that only allow the passive diffusion of small molecules. Hence, unless the nuclear envelope is disorganized when the cell is under division, DNA transport across the nucleus remains as a major barrier for successful transfection. Another drawback associated to DNA vaccines is that the intravenous injection of cationic lipid-DNA complexes is often accompanied by a dose-dependent toxicity, apoptosis of endothelial cells, piloerection, production of reactive oxygen intermediates, lung toxicity, lethargy, liver damage and necrosis, and can induce death. However, anionic lipoplexes have demonstrated low toxicities and high transcription levels. For instance, anionic NPs (plasmid DNA/PEI/PGA NPs) were tested as vaccine against the asexual blood stage (Shuaibu et al. 2011). These NPs have proved to be taken up by cells via a PGA-specific receptor mediated pathway showing high transfection efficiency and low toxicity. The plasmid DNA/ PEI/PGA NPs generated a dose-dependent antibody response dominated by IgG1 and IgG2b and 33 to 60% of survival. The elevation of IL-12p40 and IFN-γ was marginal but IL-4 levels were significantly high, thus suggesting a predominant Th2 CD4+ T cell response. The same NPs at a higher dose and administered intravenously and intraperitoneally resulted in a 100% survival after a lethal *P. yoelii* challenge. However, when administered subcutaneously the survival fell to $\approx$ 50% (Cherif et al. 2011).

Tuberculosis

Mycobacterium tuberculosis (*Mtb*) is the main cause of tuberculosis (TB), a deadly infection, considered one of the main challenges in public health. Approximately two billion people ($\approx$ 30% of the global population) are currently infected. After HIV, TB is the second most deadly infectious disease, every year 9.2 million people develop the disease and the annual mortality rate is 1.7 million people. TB disease presents as pulmonary TB (80%), extrapulmonary TB (20%), or a combination of both. Acute TB meningitis or disseminated TB can sometimes result in death. Only 6 to 10% of HIV-negative patients develop the disease and, in most of cases, because of the reactivation of a preexisting infection. In contrast, 50 to 60% of HIV infected patients have chances to show reactivation during their lifetime.

Tubercle bacilli are spread out by infected patients coughing, sneezing, or speaking. Upon entering the respiratory system the majorities of *Mtb* are phagocytosed by alveolar macrophages and are destroyed. Bacilli that are not destroyed multiply and are released after macrophage lysis (7 to 21 days after infection), and infect other circulating macrophages. Extracellular bacilli attract macrophages from the bloodstream, and at the end of this stage, a huge number of macrophages and bacilli are concentrated at early pulmonary lesions. Within 2 to 10 weeks after infection, the immune system is usually able to halt the multiplication of the tubercle bacilli, preventing further spread and leading to the formation of a granuloma. At this point the person is infected with TB. TB results when the immune system is not able to halt the multiplication of tubercle bacilli. Three months after infection, these bacilli can spread through the lymphatic channels to regional lymph nodes, and then through the bloodstream to more distant tissues and organs from the apices of the lungs, kidneys, genitalia, and spongy bone to the brain.

Conventional treatments

Pharmacotherapy consisted of an initial intensive stage (two months) of a combination of isoniazid (INH), pyrazinamide (PYZ), and rifampicin (RIF) administered together with ethambutol (ETB). The second phase (four months) comprises exclusively RIF and INH. These four drugs together with the aminoglycoside streptomycin constitute the first-line therapy. Even though these drugs successfully act against TB, the complexity of the treatment, the adverse side effects, and the development of drug resistances are impediments to eradicate this infection. Misuse or mismanagement of first-line drugs results in the emergence of multidrug resistant TB, which takes even longer to treat with second-line drugs, which are more expensive and have higher toxicity. When second-line drugs are misused, extensive drug resistant TB develops. The prolonged pharmacotherapy and the pill burden can hamper patient lifestyle, and thus decrease compliance and adherence to administration schedules remain the main reasons for therapeutic failure, therefore contributing to the development of multidrug resistant strains.

Preclinical drug delivery systems against tuberculosis

DDSs against *Mtb* were by far the most varied, outnumbering those used against other bacterial infections. In first place, the performance of oral polymeric NPs, which are not absorbed but increased drug bioavailability was extensively explored. Their use led to a reduced number of administrations and increased accumulation of drug in tissues. On the other hand, intravenously administered NPs (being captured by fixed accessible or circulating macrophages) allowed a targeted delivery of drugs to infected macrophages. Once phagocitosed, drugs within NPs probably followed the same intracellular pathway and, unless being carried by pH-sensitive NPs, drugs were delivered inside phagosomes. Alveolar macrophages were refractary to the uptake of intravenously administered NPs, and so the disease burden was less diminished than in the liver and spleen. Only pulmonary administration allowed an effective targeting to alveolar macrophages, and therefore the frequency of administrations could be pronouncedly reduced as compared to the other methods. In a recent review by Sosnik et al. (2010), strategies based in the use of NPs for sustained or targeted delivery of antibiotics against TB are extensively discussed. In this chapter only works on preclinical studies in disease models will be included.

Oral and parenteral administration

First-line drugs were loaded into PLGA NPs and administered orally. For instance, RIF-, INH-, and PYZ-loaded PLGA NPs extent drug detection in plasma and tissues (Pandey et al. 2003a), and five oral doses reduced the bacterial count and lung histopathology of infected guinea pigs to the same extent than free drugs daily administered for six weeks (Johnson et al. 2005). Addition of ETB to this formulation eliminated the bacteria in the meninges of infected mice (Pandey and Khuller 2006).

A single dose of econazole (ECZ, an imidazole that potentially replace INH and RIF) and moxifloxacin (MOX, a 4th generation synthetic fluoroquinolone that may be used to shorten the duration of chemotherapy) loaded to PLGA

NPs extent therapeutic drug levels in plasma and tissues (Ahmad et al. 2008), while eight oral doses resulted equipotent to 56 doses of free MOX daily administered or 112 doses of free ECZ administered twice daily in infected mice. Addition of RIF to this combination resulted in total bacterial clearance from the organs of mice in eight weeks. Similarly, RIF, INH, PYZ, and ETB loaded to alginate NPs, extent duration of drugs in plasma and in tissues (Ahmad et al. 2006). On the other hand, eight oral doses of ECZ loaded to alginate NPs resulted equipotent to 112 doses of free ECZ administered twice daily in reducing bacterial burden by > 90% in the lungs and spleen of infected mice (Ahmad et al. 2007). A single oral dose of SLNs loaded with RIF, INH, and PYZ also extent drugs detection in plasma, and no tubercle bacilli were detected in the lungs and spleen of infected mice after five oral doses; whereas 46 daily doses of the free drugs administered orally were necessary to reach the same therapeutic effect (Pandey et al. 2005). An active targeting strategy did not lead to superior results as compared to non-targeted carriers. Plasma half-lives of RIF, INH, and PYZ loaded to PLGA NPs surface grafted with lectins (recognizable by glycosylated structures in the gut and the lung mucosa) were increased and total bacterial clearance was achieved in the lungs, liver, and spleen after three doses (Sharma et al. 2004).

The intravenous via has been barely explored. The intravenous administration of RIF-loaded gelatin NPs allowed reduction of 28 doses (RIF daily administered orally) to 10 doses (intravenously administered every three days) (Saraogi et al. 2010). INH-loaded mannosylated gelatin NPs significantly reduced bacterial counts in the lungs and spleen of infected mice, and also reduced the hepatotoxicity of the drug (Saraogi et al. 2011). Gelatin NPs offer a number of benefits compared with other delivery systems, e.g., biocompatibility, biodegradability, low antigenicity, low cost, and ease of use as parenteral formulation. PYZ-loaded liposomes administered intravenously showed high therapeutic efficacy (El-Ridy et al. 2007). Rigid liposomes loaded with rifabutin (a drug used for patients taking antiretroviral drugs that have unacceptable interactions with RIF) caused lower bacterial loads in the spleen, liver, and lungs, than in tissues of mice treated with free rifabutin (Gaspar et al. 2008a,b). Rifabutin-loaded liposomes could be a promising approach for the treatment of TB in HIV co-infected patients. Finally, sustained drug release formulations help guard against the development of drug resistances, as there is less chance for missed doses leading to suboptimal drug concentrations in the blood (Kisich et al. 2007). A single subcutaneous administration of RIF-, INH-, and PYZ-loaded PLGA NPs maintained plasma, lungs, and spleen drugs concentrations for more than one month, and completely eliminated bacterial in the different organs of infected mice (Pandey and Khuller 2004).

Pulmonary administration

There are two objectives for targeting alveolar macrophages using inhaled therapies: (i) deliver large amounts of antimycobacterial drugs to macrophage cytosol, even potentially sufficient to overcome drug resistances; and, (ii) activation of infected macrophages. Representative examples of DDSs against TB are collected in Table 13.3.

Between the years 2001 and 2009, the performance of RIF (alone or together with other antibiotics) was investigated loaded in microspheres and PLGA NPs administered by nebulization or instillation. For instance, RIF-loaded PLGA microspheres nebulizated directly to the lungs of infected guinea pigs decreased burden of bacteria in lungs in a dose-effect relationship (Suárez et al. 2001). Further assays demonstrated that a single nebulization of RIF-, INH-, and PYZ-loaded PLGA microspheres significantly prolonged the elimination half-life and mean residence time of drugs compared to free drugs administered orally, thus resulting in an enhanced relative bioavailability for encapsulated drugs ($\approx$ 13-, $\approx$ 33-, and $\approx$ 15-fold for RIF, INH, and PYZ, respectively) (Pandey et al. 2003b). Nebulization of PLGA microspheres to infected guinea pigs every day 10 resulted in no tubercle bacilli detected in the lung after five doses of treatment whereas 46 daily doses of orally administered drug were required to obtain an equivalent therapeutic benefit. Hence, these PLGA microspheres could be used for intermittent treatments. In another approach, RIF-loaded PLGA microspheres were superior to free RIF for killing intracellular bacilli and preventing granuloma formation in lobes (Yoshida et al. 2006).

The performance of alginate microparticles was also assayed. Concentration of RIF-, INH-, and PYZ-loaded alginate microparticles were detected in plasma faster than when loaded into PLGA microparticles, and were detectable up to two weeks. Nebulization of drugs-loaded alginate NPs was as effective in clearing the lungs and the spleen of *Mtb*-infected guinea pigs as 45 oral daily doses of the free drugs. Therefore, alginate microparticles could also be suitable for intermittent treatments (Ahmad et al. 2005).

Vaccine delivery systems against tuberculosis

The conventional anti-TB vaccine, an attenuated strain of *M. bovis* Bacillus Calmette-Guérin (BCG), has been widely used to prevent TB since 1921. However, the protective efficacy of BCG against adult pulmonary TB is questionable, even though it continues to be used in many countries to prevent meningitis and phthisis miliaris in children (Kaufmann and McMichael 2005). Furthermore, the World Health Organization no longer recommends BCG vaccination of children with HIV or HIV+ mothers due to safety concerns, leaving many infants without any protection against this disease (Kaufmann et al. 2010). Because of the emergence of multidrug resistant *Mtb* strains and HIV infection, as well as the lack of success of the TB vaccine, there have been ongoing efforts to develop more effective vaccines using different strategies, such as 2nd generation protein vaccines or 3rd generation DNA vaccines. The best hope for the control or elimination of TB is a safer and more effective vaccine that drive robust T-cell immunity against *Mtb*. Research has

Table 13.3. DDSs against TB. DPPC: dipalmitoylphosphatidylcholine; DPPG: dipalmitoylphosphatidylglycerol.

DDS	Drug	Route of administration	Dose, animal model	Main results	References
PLGA (190 to 290 nm in size)	RIF, INH, and PYZ	Oral	RIF 12 mg/Kg, INH 10 mg/Kg, and PYZ 25 mg/Kg, 5 doses every 10 days. Guinea pigs infected with aerosolized *Mtb*	Drugs detected 9 days in plasma. Therapeutic concentrations in tissues were maintained during 9 to 11 days	Pandey et al. 2003a, Johnson et al. 2005
PLGA (190 to 290 nm in size)	RIF, INH, PYZ, and ETB	Oral	RIF 10 mg/Kg, INH 25 mg/Kg, PYZ 150 mg/Kg, and ETB 100 mg/Kg, 5 doses every 10 days. Mice intravenously infected with *Mtb*	Therapeutic drug levels maintained during 5 to 8 days and 9 days in plasma and brain, respectively	Pandey and Khuller 2006
PLGA (220 nm-sized)	ECZ and MOX	Oral	MOX 8 mg/Kg and ECZ 3.3 mg/Kg, 8 doses administered weekly	Therapeutic drug levels in plasma were extended for 5 (ECZ) or 4 days (MOX); while in lungs, liver, and spleen they were up to 6 days. Free drugs were cleared in 12 to 24 hours	Ahmad et al. 2008
Alginate (235 nm-sized)	RIF, INH, PYZ, and ETB	Oral	–	Drugs levels detected up to 7 to 11 days in plasma, and until 15 days in tissues. Free drugs were cleared in 12 to 24 hours and were detected in spleen, liver, and lung for 1 day	Ahmad et al. 2006
Alginate (235 nm-sized)	ECZ	Oral	ECZ 3.3 mg/Kg, 8 doses. Mice intravenously infected with *Mtb*	Reduced bacterial burden by 90% in the lungs and spleen	Ahmad et al. 2007

Table 13.3. contd....

Table 13.3. contd.

DDS	Drug	Route of administration	Dose, animal model	Main results	References
PLGA (350 to 400 nm in size) surface grafted with lectins	RIF, INH, and PYZ	Oral, pulmonar	RIF 12 mg/Kg, INH 10 mg/Kg, and PYZ 25 mg/Kg, 3 doses (1 every 14 days). Guinea pigs intramuscularly infected with *Mtb*	Drug levels were extended from 4 to 9 days (uncoated NPs) to 6 to 14 days	Sharma et al. 2004
PLGA (186 to 290 nm in size)	RIF, INH, and PYZ	Subcutaneous	RIF 12 mg/Kg, INH 10 mg/Kg, and PYZ 25 mg/Kg. Mice intravenously infected with *Mtb*	Maintained plasma, lungs, and spleen drugs concentrations for more than 1 month, while free drugs were cleared in 12 to 24 hours	Pandey and Khuller 2004
Gelatin (265 nm-sized)	RIF	Intravenous	10 mg/Kg every 3 days for 4 weeks. BALB/c mice infected with aerosolized *Mtb*	2-fold reduction in *Mtb* colony forming units (CFUs) in the lungs and spleen	Saraogi et al. 2010
Mannosylated gelatin (260 to 380 nm in size)	INH	Intravenous	Mice infected with *Mtb*	Reduction in bacterial counts in the lungs and spleen	Saraogi et al. 2011
Poly(butylcyanoacrylate)	MOX	Intravenous	Mice infected with *Mtb*	Decrease *Mtb* counts in lungs of infected mice	Shipulo et al. 2008
PLGA (≈ 2.8 to 3.4 μm in size)	RIF	Nebulization	1 to 1.7 mg/Kg, Guinea pig infected with an aerosolized low dose of virulent H37Rv strain of *Mtb*	Decreased number of viable bacteria, and reduced inflammation and lung damage, compared to free RIF	Suárez et al. 2001
PLGA (≈ 1.9 μm-sized)	RIF, INH, and PYZ	Nebulization	RIF 12 mg/Kg, INH 10 mg/Kg, and PYZ 25 mg/Kg. Guinea pigs	Sustained therapeutic drug levels in plasma for 6 to 8 days, and in the lungs for 11 days	Pandey et al. 2003b

PLGA (≈ 3.5 μm-sized)	RIF	Intratraqueal	RIF 0.4 and 0.04 mg/Kg. Rats infected with *Mtb* (Kurono strain)	Kill intracellular bacilli	Yoshida et al. 2006
Alginate (≈ 1.1 μm-sized)	RIF, INH, and PYZ	Nebulization	1 dose biweekly, 3 doses over the course of 45 days. Guinea pigs infected with *Mtb*	INH, RIF, and PYZ were detectable up to 14, 10, and 14 days, respectively. Fast clearance of the free drugs after 12 to 24 hours	Ahmad et al. 2005
SLNs	RIF, INH, and PYZ	Oral	5 doses administered every 10 days	Drug detected during 8 days in therapeutic concentrations in the lungs, and during 10 days in liver and spleen. Free drugs were cleared after 1 to 2 days	Pandey et al. 2005
Liposomes (DPPC:cholesterol, 7:2 molar ratio)	PYZ	Intravenous	Twice weekly. Mice infected with *Mtb*	Reduction in bacterial counts in lungs. Severity of infection: empty liposomes > PYZ-loaded liposomes > free PYZ (6 days/week)	El-Ridy et al. 2007
Liposomes (DPPC and DPPG)	RFB	Intravenous	Mice model of disseminated TB	Higher concentration in liver, spleen, and lungs 24 hours after administration compared with free drug	Gaspar et al. 2008a,b

indicated that DNA vaccine is a very powerful and easy method for inducing a strong immune response in mice. However, clinical results of the DNA vaccine have been disappointing with regard to the magnitude of induced immune responses.

Between these preclinical developments aiming to generate a protective cellular response by plasmid DNA combined with micro/nanoparticulate materials (Table 13.4), based on plasmid DNA/PEI/magnetite electrostatic complexes was recently published (Yu et al. 2012). Plasmid DNA encoded a fusion protein of: (i) the Ag85A of *Mtb*; (ii) the 6-kDa early secretory antigen target (ESAT-6, one of the most immunodominant and highly specific target Ag containing multiple immunogenic T-cell epitopes to enhance cell-mediated responses); and, (iii) secreted IL-21, involved in Natural Killer (NK) and T-cell activation (immunostimulatory adjuvant for enhancing effector/memory lymphocyte responses). Although the plasmid DNA vaccine alone and BCG also elicited an effective immune response and protective efficacy against *Mtb* challenge, the efficacy was greater in mice vaccinated with plasmid DNA/ PEI/magnetite. This vaccine enhanced the *Mtb*-specific antibody levels and the number of IFN-γ spot secreting cells (SSCs) (IL-4 SSCs was much less). The cytotoxicities of the NK cells, splenocytes, and CD8+ splenocytes, as well as splenocyte proliferative responses to Ag85A were enhanced. This vaccine induced a marked inhibition of lung injury, CFU, and increased net weight in mice after the *Mtb* challenge.

One of the reasons for the low efficacy of DNA vaccines is that an important fraction of cells that are not under division are refractory to plasmid DNA transfection. These could be circumvented by the presence of specialized cargo proteins such as the NLSs, a short peptide sequence within proteins that allows its association with cargo proteins that will provide nuclear transport. It has been reported that cationic NLSs allow DNA condensation, thus increasing the internalization efficiency up to 4.5-fold, decreasing the percentage of lysosomal DNA by 2.1-fold, and increasing the efficiency of nuclear accumulation by three-fold (Rea et al. 2009). In this context, Rosada et al. (2012) tested the activity of preformed cationic liposomes electrostatically complexed with plasmid DNA and NLS, where the plasmid DNA expresses hsp65 from *M. leprae* that has demonstrated prophylactic and therapeutic effects in mice with TB by inducing CD4 and CD8 memory T cell cytotoxic activity, and IFN-γ needed for killing mycobacteria. Plasmid DNA immunotherapy alone suppressed Th2 cytokine levels (which oppose IFN-γ effects) and controlled the intensity of local inflammation. In this work, it was found that the administration of these liposomes intranasally induced the same immune response as naked plasmid DNA administered intramuscularly, but with a four-fold lower amount of plasmid DNA due to the presence of NLSs.

Vaccine delivery by inhalation has been suggested for eliciting mucosal and systemic immunity to airborne viruses, bacteria, potential biological weapons, and even to secondary infection in chronic occlusive pulmonary disease. Unfortunately, there is limited effort directed at developing inhaled

Table 13.4. Vaccine delivery systems against TB. DOPE: 1,2-dioleoyl-*sn*-glycero-3-phosphoethanolamine; DOTAP: 1,2-dioleoyl-3-trimethylammonium propane; hsp65: 65-kDa heat shock protein; NLS: nuclear localization signal.

Vaccine delivery system	Ag	Immunization protocol, animal model, dose	Route of administration	Challenge	References
Magnetite NPs coated with PGA complexed with PEI at 5:1 ratio (2:1, NP:plasmid DNA ratio)	Plasmid DNA encoding fusion protein of Ag85A-ESAT-6 and IL-21	3 times with 3 weeks intervals. 100 µg plasmid DNA	Intramuscular	Intravenous 10^4 CFU of virulent *Mtb* H37Rv strain	Yu et al. 2012
Liposomes ($\approx$ 250 nm-sized; surface electrical charge: 11 mV; egg PC:DOPE:DOTAP, 2:1:1 molar ratio)	DNA-hsp65 and cationic NLSs	30 days after TB induction 4 times at 10 day intervals. Mice. 100 µg plasmid DNA	Intranasal	Intratraqueal	Rosada et al. 2012
Pluronic®-stabilized poly(propylene sulfide) NPs ($\approx$ 30 nm-sized)	Ag85B	Days 0, 7, and 21. Mice. 5 µg of Ag85B and 15 µg of CpG ODN	Pulmonar, intradermal	*Mtb* aerosol challenge	Ballester et al. 2011

vaccines for TB. In contrast to the area of intranasal vaccination, only a few recent studies have focused on pulmonary immunization and the involvement of the pulmonary immune system in eliciting protective immune responses against inhaled pathogens (Bivas-Benita et al. 2005). This is a complex area where vaccine platforms must ensure that damage to the lung is limited during both vaccination and when memory cells respond to pathogenic infection.

Whereas most viral lung infections target lung parenchymal and epithelial cells, pathogenic TB bacilli establish infection in APCs of the lung: alveolar macrophages and, to a lesser extent, Dendritic Cells (DCs). Establishment of *Mtb* infection leads to an alternative activation of infected alveolar macrophages and suppression of DC functions, thus subverting innate bactericidal, immunological, and signaling mechanisms. Alveolar macrophages are equipped to detect pathogens with the aid of Pattern Recognition Receptors (PRRs) that recognize pathogen-associated molecular patterns. One family of PRRs found on alveolar macrophages, known as C-type Lectin Receptors (CLRs), recognize conserved carbohydrate structures, including mannose and galactose, found on the surface of many respiratory pathogens, e.g., *Yersinia pestis*, *Mtb*, *Streptococcus pneumonia*, and *Influenza* viruses. CLRs also function as phagocytic receptors, and include members of the mannose receptor family and dendritic cell-specific intercellular adhesion molecule-3-grabbing nonintegrin (DC-SIGN). Alveolar macrophages constitute > 80% of the total cells obtained by bronchoalveolar lavage of a healthy individual, and they constitutively migrate from the lung to the draining lymph nodes. It was recently reported that random copolymer polyanhydride NPs derivatized with D-mannose and galactose can increase the immunomodulatory activity on alveolar macrophages. Co-culture of these NPs with alveolar macrophages significantly increased cell surface expression of MHC class I and class II, CD86, CD40, and the CLRs CIRE (a 238 amino acid type II membrane protein of ≈ 33 kDa in size) over non-functionalized NPs. It was shown that D-mannose and galactose functionalization also enhanced the expression of the macrophage mannose receptor and the macrophage galactose lectin, respectively. These NPs also promoted an increase in the alveolar macrophage production of the pro-inflammatory cytokines IL-1β, IL-6, and Tumor Necrosis Factor alpha (TNF-α). These findings confirm that the targeted engagement of macrophage mannose receptor and other CLRs is a viable strategy for enhancing the intrinsic adjuvant properties of vaccine adjuvants and promoting robust pulmonary immunity after pulmonary administration (Chavez-Santoscoy et al. 2012).

On the other hand, TB vaccines are most commonly administered by the intradermal or subcutaneous routes, as it is the case for BCG. It was shown that intradermal injection of ≈ 30 nm-sized Pluronic®-stabilized poly(propylene sulfide) NPs, efficiently targeted half of the lymph node-residing DCs, whereas 100 nm-sized poly(propylene sulfide) NPs were only 10% as efficient. The surface chemistry of these poly(propylene sulfide) NPs activated the complement cascade, thus generating a danger signal *in situ* and potently activating DCs. Moreover, intramuscular administration of the

NPs conjugated to ovalbumin induces humoral and cellular immunity in a size- and complement-dependent manner (Reddy et al. 2007). The efficacy of these intradermal and pulmonary poly(propylene sulfide) NPs containing Ag85B conjugated via a reducible disulfide bond in combination with the CpG ODNs has been recently compared (Ballester et al. 2011). It was found that the pulmonary administration of this nanovaccine, independent of BCG pre-vaccination, can enhance type 17 T helper (Th17) responses and increases the polyfunctionality of Th1 responses in the spleen, the lung, and lung-draining lymph nodes, thus leading to improved protection against *Mtb* aerosol challenge, as compared to soluble Ag85B with CpG ODN and to the intradermally delivered formulations. *In vitro*, poly(propylene sulfide) NPs matured DCs (as revealed by coexpression of the maturation markers CD86 and MHC class II) in a concentration-dependent manner. This effect was significantly enhanced in the presence of CpG ODN. CpG-induced secretion of IL-6, essential for Th17 induction, was significantly enhanced when poly(propylene sulfide) NPs were present. IL-1β, indicative of inflammasome activation, was secreted only when DCs were co-stimulated by both CpG ODN and poly(propylene sulfide) NPs, not in the presence of one or the other alone. In contrast, poly(propylene sulfide) NPs did not significantly influence CpG-induced secretion of IL-12p70, required for the generation of IFN-γ-producing CD4+ T cells. In the absence of CpG ODN, poly(propylene sulfide) NPs did not stimulate any of these cytokines. *In vivo*, mucosal and systemic Th17 responses were observed especially in the lung, generating a substantial reduction of the lung bacterial burden.

Leishmaniasis

Leishmaniasis is caused by flagellated promastigotes of the *Leishmania* genus that is injected in the skin by sand flies. Depending on the *Leishmania* genus, different clinical manifestations are produced: ulcerative skin lesions (Cutaneous Leishmaniasis, CL), destructive mucosal inflammation (mucocutaneous leishmaniasis), multiple non-ulcerative nodules (diffuse CL), and disseminated visceral infection (visceral leishmaniasis, VL, kala-azar). VL is mortal if untreated; CL heals by reepithelization with scarring, but it is treated to avoid disfiguring lesions; mucocutaneous leishmaniasis can produce potentially life-threatening inflammatory disease and must be treated. About 1.5 million new cases of CL and 500,000 new cases of VL occur each year. However, the number of cases is increasing globally at an alarming rate, mainly due to sand fly vectors expansion caused by ecological chaos. There are also a growing number of cases of HIV/leishmaniasis co-infection. Leishmaniasis is an important opportunistic infection in HIV patients, which is potentially fatal, even when treated appropriately. HIV infection can also increase the risk of development of VL by 10- to 100-fold in endemic areas.

Once injected into the skin, the parasites invade the local phagocytic host cells, including neutrophils. Promastigotes inhibit phagosome-endosome fusion through unique lipophosphoglycan molecules on their surface and transform into amastigotes, and after that the inhibition is lifted. Amastigotes, that are metabolically most active at an acidic environment, depend on the harsh environment of the phagolysosome of resident macrophages where they survive and multiply. Then, dissemination occurs locally and distant macrophages are infected. In VL, liver, spleen, and bone marrow macrophages are colonized; while in CL and mucocutaneous leishmaniasis, skin macrophages and DCs including Langerhans cells are colonized. The amastigotes living inside the macrophage's phagolysosomes located in different anatomical areas present major structural and phenomenological barriers that antileishmanial drugs have to overcome.

Conventional treatments

Pentavalent antimonials (meglumine antimoniate and sodium stibogluconate) were introduced in 1945 and remain an effective treatment for some forms of leishmaniasis, but some disadvantages limit the usefulness of the drug. Diamidine pentamidine and amphotericin B (AmB) (Fungizone®, colloidal dispersion of AmB and deoxycholate) are used as second-line drugs when pentavalent antimonials have proved to be ineffective, although they are highly toxic. The choice of treatment also depends on the causative *Leishmania* species. The development of lipid-associated AmB formulations has reduced the toxicity and extended plasma half-life in comparison to the parent drug. High cost of AmB-loaded liposomes (AmBisome®) has limited its use.

Preclinical drug delivery systems against leishmaniasis

Visceral leishmaniasis

From the mid '70s, a series of articles addressed the use of antileishmanial drugs loaded into liposomes for selective delivery to the liver and spleen macrophages infected with VL. Pentavalent antimonials-loaded liposomal formulations have shown to be 700 times more active than the free drug (Alving et al. 1978, New et al. 1978), while multilamellar liposomes containing AmB were 170–750 and 60 times more active than pentavalent antimonials in *L. donovani* infected hamsters and monkeys, respectively (Berman et al. 1986). Once AmBisome® was marketed, it was rapidly confirmed that it can eliminate liver parasites to the same extent but faster than treatment with pentavalent antimonials (Gradoni et al. 1993). AmBisome® was effective in cases of pentavalent antimonial unresponsiveness in *L. infantum* and *L. donovani*, both in immunocompetent and in immunosuppressed patients, as well as being less toxic than other AmB lipid formulations, e.g., Amphocil® (mixed micelles of AmB and surfactant) (Minodier et al. 2003). A comparison of the efficacy of AmB formulations, including AmBisome®, in the treatment of leishmaniasis has been previously reviewed (Barratt and Legrand 2005, Bern et al. 2006). A significant regional variation in response to AmBisome® is reflected in the total dose required for 100% cure: it is low in India (6 mg/Kg for *L. donovani*), higher in Kenya (14 mg/Kg for *L. donovani*), and the highest in Brazil (> 20 mg/Kg for *L. chagasi*) (Meyerhoff 1999). In India, Fungisome™, an AmB-loaded liposomal formulation, was developed and commercialized from May 2003 (Kshirsagar et al. 2005).

Besides, several other drugs like inosine analogs, atovaquone, harmine, and miltefosine improved their performance compared with free drugs when loaded into liposomes (being intravenously administered against experimental VL) (Romero and Morilla 2008). Also furazolidone and buparvaquone improved their performance compared with free drugs when loaded into liposomes (being intraperitoneally administered) (Tempone et al. 2010, Reimão et al. 2012).

On the other hand, cationic liposomes [egg PC:stearylamine (SA)] can display leishmanicidal activities (Dey et al. 2000, Afrin et al. 2001), and entrapment of pentavalent antimonials enhanced their potentiality in chronic VL mice models (Pal et al. 2004). Recently, it was demonstrated that only one intravenous administration of these liposomes containing pentavalent antimonials suppressed liver ($\approx$ 95%), spleen ($\approx$ 97%), and bone marrow ($\approx$ 85%) parasitic load in BALB/c mice infected with pentavalent antimonials-resistant *L. donovani* strains, which were comparable to AmB deoxycholate therapy (2 mg/Kg). There was a 10^5-fold fall in viable parasites with < 100 viable parasites observed in the organs after therapy, which was a clear indication of a nearly complete healing (Roychoudhury et al. 2011). Interestingly, in comparison to AmB, mice treated with these liposomes were more resistant to re-infection, and treated mice showed enhanced T cell proliferation, persistent IgG1 levels, increased IgG2a, and upregulated IL-12, IFN-γ, and TNF-α production in leishmania-pulsed splenocytes.

Other strategies based on the use of grafted liposomes to increase targeting to Kupffer cells have demonstrated improved activity over free drugs on experimental VL, thanks to an increased macrophage uptake. Meanwhile, niosomes, emulsions, and polymeric microparticles/NPs augmented the efficacy of carried drugs upon parenteral administration to different diseased animal models (Romero and Morilla 2008).

Polymer-drug conjugates are taken into cells by endocytosis and then trafficked through endosomes to lysosomes. Quinolone was linked to a biocompatible hydrophilic lysosomotropic polymer [*N*-(2-hydroxypropyl) methacrylamide, HPMA] bearing a 5% mole mannose targeting moiety. The mannose-grafted polymers were designed to mimic the invasion process of *Leishmania* that is dependent on the interaction between the mannose-containing lipopolysaccharides on the parasite cell surface and the macrophage mannose receptors. These conjugates showed high *in vivo* antileishmanial activity upon intravenous administration (Nan et al. 2004). Later, AmB was attached to poly(HPMA) through a degradable glycine-phenylalanine-leucine-glycine linker (Nicoletti et al. 2009). The copolymers developed a potent *in vivo* activity with 50% inhibition of parasite burden at 1 mg/Kg upon intravenous administration. Recently, the poly(HPMA)-AmB conjugate was functionalized with alendronic acid (Nicoletti et al. 2010). However, no advantage of the combinatorial conjugates was observed as compared to single poly(HPMA)-AmB conjugates.

First attempts of using less invasive treatments administered orally employed nanosuspensions made of AmB in an aqueous solution of Tween® 80, Pluronic® F-68, and sodium cholate, but they only reduced the liver parasite by up to 29% on experimental VL (Kayser et al. 2003). Recently, formulations composed of the lipid Peceol®, the surfactant Gelucire® 44/14, and the cosurfactant vitamin E-D-α-tocopheryl poly(ethylene glycol) 1000 succinate (TPGS) were developed to enhance the absorption and efficacy of AmB. These formulations could be considered as self-emulsifying DDSs, being able to form instant submicron-sized emulsions on mixing with simulated gastrointestinal fluids (Wasan et al. 2009a). The dispersed AmB solubilized within the emulsion after mixing with gastrointestinal fluids, resulted in improved oral absorption. Additionally, prolongation of gastrointestinal transit time and increase of intestinal wall permeability could be involved in enhancing oral absorption of AmB. It was determined that treatment with a single intravenous dose of AmBisome® (2 mg/Kg) administered one week after infection completely eradicated liver parasites, while miltefosine given orally in five daily doses (3 mg/Kg) resulted in ≈ 48% of inhibition of liver parasites (Wasan et al. 2010). However, oral AmB formulations at 10 mg/Kg twice daily for five days resulted in 99.5% inhibition of parasitemia (Wasan et al. 2009b). Moreover, nephrotoxicity associated with AmB from the lipid-based formulations administered orally was significantly lower than those of AmBisome® and Fungizone® (Leon et al. 2011, Sivak et al. 2011).

Cutaneous leishmaniasis

The success of treatment at early stages of CL depends on how physically accessible are the infected macrophages in the *stratum spinosum* to the DDS. Circulating NPs can become close to the *stratum spinosum* only from local extravasation. The higher IC_{50} values (25 mg/Kg) for CL than for VL (0.3 mg/Kg) of intravenously administered AmBisome® reflect the difficulty for particulate materials to target infected cells (Yardley and Croft 2000). Although clinical applications of intravenously administered AmBisome® against CL have been reported, up to date there are no available data on an optimum dose regimen (Wortmann et al. 2010). Successful short term treatments (five days at 3 mg/Kg and a reinforcement dose on day 10) in adults have been reported (Solomon et al. 2007). Other authors recommend total doses of 40 mg/Kg (Brown et al. 2005). However, the need for intravenous administration together with its high cost may limit the use of AmBisome®. AmB-loaded to apolipoprotein-stabilized phospholipids bilayer disk complexes, completely cleared parasites with no lesions remaining on experimental CL upon intraperitoneal administration (Nelson et al. 2006). It was proposed that the small size (8 to 20 nm) of these nanodisks was responsible for their identification by class A scavenger receptors on macrophages. In the search for a less invasive route of administration, oral administration of meglumine antimoniate-β-cyclodextrin complexes led to smaller skin lesions on experimental CL (Demicheli et al. 2004, Frézard et al. 2008).

Equally less invasive are the topical treatments. For example, topically applied dispersions of Amphocil® in 5% ethanol have been successfully assayed in patients infected with *L. major* in Israel (Vardy et al. 2001, Zvulunov et al. 2003). An ointment of 15% paromomycin, associated to the permeation enhancer methylbenzethonium chloride (12%) (marketed in Israel as Leshcutan®) has resulted relatively effective against *L. major*, *L. tropica*, *L. mexicana*, and *L. panamensis* (El-On et al. 1986, 1992), but local side effects were frequently observed due to the permeation enhancer (Arana et al. 2001, Armijos et al. 2004). A cream formulation containing paromomycin and gentamicin induced high cure rates (94 vs. 71% placebo) in treating patients infected with *L. major* with only mild local irritation (Ben Salah et al. 2009). However, no significant differences in cure rates were reported in a clinical trial in comparison with a placebo (Soto et al. 2002).

The effect of paromomycin sulfate-loaded liposomes administered topically was evaluated in mice infected with *L. major* (Jaafari et al. 2009). Mice which received $\approx$ 500 nm-sized liposomes twice a day for four weeks showed a significant reduction of the lesion size and eight weeks later were completely cured. Currently, this formulation is in clinical trial. Recently, topical application of transfersomes containing paromomycin (soybean PC:sodium cholate:with or without ethanol; 20:2:5 % w/w ratio; 200 nm-sized) twice a day for four weeks caused significant reductions in the lesion sizes and lower parasite burden in the spleen in mice infected with *L. major* compared to a paromomycin cream (Bavarsad et al. 2012). Using a similar approach, it was demonstrated that 300 to 500 nm-sized liposomes containing paromomycin enhanced *in vitro* drug permeation across stripped skin and improved the *in vivo* antileishmanial activity in mice infected with *L. major* (Carneiro et al. 2010). Finally, topical administration was also addressed by our research group (Montanari et al. 2010). Briefly, the antipromastigote ($\approx$ 20%) and antiamastigote ($\approx$ 20%) activities of the hydrophobic zinc phthalocyanine against *L. braziliensis* after 15 min of sunlight irradiation (15 J/cm^2) was enhanced up to 100 and 80%, respectively, when loaded into ultradeformable liposomes. Interestingly, it was reported that these liposomes also showed non-photodynamic leishmanicidal activity without producing host cells toxicity. When loaded into the ultradeformable liposomes, phthalocyanine was capable of penetrating homogeneously in the *stratum corneum*, accumulating a seven-fold higher amount and eight-fold deeper than conventional liposomes. Preliminary *in vivo* results further demonstrated that topical administration of zinc phtalocyanine loaded into ultradeformable liposomes for five days to BALB/c mice infected with *L. braziliensis* (and after 15 minutes sunlight irradiation) produced a significant reduction of the lesion size.

Vaccine delivery systems against leishmaniasis

Current control strategies of leishmaniasis are either ineffective or hard to maintain in many foci, available drugs are expensive, need multiple injections, accompanied with side effects, and are not always effective. Therefore, a mass vaccination of the entire population of an endemic area would be the most cost-effective tool to diminish *Leishmania* burden. The feasibility of developing a vaccine against CL has been sustained by the fact that long lasting protection was observed upon recovery from CL or by leishmanization (LZ). LZ consists of inducing the infection by injecting live virulent parasites in an aesthetically acceptable site of the body in healthy individuals. LZ has been used for centuries in various Asian countries to protect against further infection. Due to various reasons (e.g., development of uncontrolled lesion), LZ practice was stopped except in Uzbekistan (Noazin et al. 2009).

1st generation *Leishmania* vaccines consisting of whole killed parasites with or without adjuvants have reached phase III trials but failed to show enough efficacies. A vaccine comprising a single dose of whole-cell autoclave-killed *L. major* was mixed with BCG and compared with BCG alone against leishmaniasis in Bam (Iran). However, this vaccine was shown to have low efficacy ($\approx 55\%$) (Mutiso et al. 2010). On the other hand, the subunit vaccine has not reached clinical trials. Previous studies confirm that the use of adjuvants increases the efficacy of purified Ag by up to $\approx 80\%$. Recombinant 2nd generation vaccines and 3rd generation DNA vaccines achieved mean parasite load reductions of ≈ 70 and 60%, respectively, in laboratory animal models, but their success in field trials has not yet been reported (Palatnik-de-Sousa 2008). There is an open avenue for improved particulate adjuvants bearing recombinant Ag, that from the pharmaceutical point of view can be massively produced in a safer and accurate way, and better controlled with Good Manufacturing Practice rules, than mass production of killed or dangerously modified microorganisms. For example, active substances assay (for dose adjustment) is possible for recombinant Ag and macromolecules by new chemical/biotechnological instrumentation, while for weak or dead microbes, the assay is complicated and imprecise (Danesh-Bahreini et al. 2011).

In all forms of leishmaniasis, a cure is achieved through a cellular immune response involving IL-12 produced by macrophages, DCs, B-lymphocytes, and other accessory cells. IL-12 stimulates proliferation and production of IFN-γ, to promote the oxidative burst that eliminates the parasites through a nitric oxide-mediated mechanism in host macrophages (Tripathi et al. 2007). BCG is the only available adjuvant to induce Th1 response with enough safety profile in humans, but in experimental *Leishmania* vaccines it was shown to be problematic. Thus, it seems again that one of the major drawbacks in the development of an effective vaccine against leishmaniasis is the lack of an appropriate adjuvant (Noazin et al. 2008, 2009). So far, no *Leishmania* vaccine candidate has been able to induce the required potent, effective, and safe cell mediated immune response that can confer effective immunity against the parasite.

The performance of SLNs, PLGA, and alginate nanospheres, CS NPs, liposomes, and metallo-lipid NPs tested in preclinical assays between the years 1987 and 2011 has been thoroughly described before (Doroud and Rafati 2012). Representative examples of vaccine delivery systems against leishmaniasis can be seen in Table 13.5. Here the main approaches aimed to improve the protective immune response by loading Ags within particulate materials targeting APC to obtain a Th1 response are outlined. For instance, immunization with neutral liposomes loaded with rgp63 (the first recombinant Ag used as a vaccine against leishmaniasis, also known as leishmaniolysin, a membrane protease present in the promastigotes of all species that showed limited immunogenic properties in clinical trials) induced a significantly smaller footpad swelling, lower splenic parasite burden, higher IgG2a/IgG1 ratio and IFN-γ production, and the lower IL-4 level upon challenge with *L. major,* compared with negatively or positively surface charged liposomes (Badiee et al. 2009). However, Bhowmick et al. (2010) demonstrated that cationic SA-based multilamellar liposomes loaded with the *L. donovani* promastigote membrane Ag induced almost complete protection, as well as highly significant delayed type hypersensitivity (DTH, index of cell-mediated immunity). Ag-loaded liposomes demonstrated durable cell-mediated immunity, and mice challenged 10 weeks after vaccination could also strongly resist the experimental challenge. Ravindran et al. (2010) also demonstrated that the intraperitoneal administration of SA-based liposomes loaded with the Soluble *Leishmania* Antigen (SLA) provided significant protection against murine VL compared with BCG and monophosphoryl lipid-trehalose dicorynomycolate (MPL-TDM) as adjuvants. Liposomal formulations reduced parasite loads by ≈ 93 and $\approx 98\%$ in the liver and spleen, respectively. Higher levels of IgG2a than IgG1 were detected in serum, and highest DTH responses as well as IFN-γ levels, together with lowest IL-4 were detected in animals immunized with liposomes.

Cationic SLNs (containing the synthetic quaternary ammonium DOTAP, an active stimulator of DCs resulting in extracellular-signal-regulated kinase activation and β-chemokine induction) loaded with plasmid DNA (encoding CpG ODN) and *L. major* cysteine proteinase types I, II, and III showed high protection levels with specific Th1 response (Doroud et al. 2011a). It was demonstrated that mice vaccinated with these SLNs increased the specific Th1 response, leading to parasite inhibition (Doroud et al. 2011b). Interestingly, PLGA nanospheres loaded with autoclaved *L. major* induced strong protection against a challenge with a small increase in footpad thickness. Surprisingly, a reverse effect on protective immune responses were seen in the presence

Table 13.5. Vaccine delivery systems against *Leishmania* species. DDAB: dimethyldioctadecylammonium bromide; KMP-11: 11-kDa kinetoplastid membrane protein; SOD: superoxide dismutase.

Vaccine delivery system	Ag	Immunization protocol, animal model, dose	Route of administration	Challenge	References
Liposomes (1.2 μm-sized; DPPC:cholesterol, 2:1 molar ratio; DPPC:cholesterol:DDAB and DPPC:cholesterol:dicetyl phosphate, 2:1:1 molar ratio)	rgp63	3 times at 3 week intervals. BALB/c mice. 2 μg rgp63	Subcutaneous	Subcutaneous into the footpad with 1.5×10^6 *L. Major*, 3 wk after the last booster	Badiee et al. 2009
Multilamellar liposomes (surface electrical charge ≈ 45 mV; distearoyl PC:cholesterol:SA, 7:2:2 molar ratio)	SLA *L. donovani*	3 doses at 2 week intervals BALB/c mice. 20 μg	Intraperitoneal	Intravenous 2×10^7 promastigotes, 10 d after last booster	Bhowmick et al. 2010
Liposomes (200 to 500 nm-sized; surface electrical charge ≈ 60 mV; DOTAP:cholesterol, 1:1 molar ratio, with CpG ODN)	SLA *L. major*	3 times at 2 week intervals. BALB/c mice. 25 μg SLA, 10 μg CpG ODN	Subcutaneous	Subcutaneous in the left footpad, 10^6 promastigotes, 2 week after the last booster	Shargha et al. 2012
Liposome (surface electrical charge ≈ 60 mV; DOTAP:cholesterol with protamine CpG ODN)	Live *L. major* parasites	10^6 parasites. BALB/c mice	Subcutaneous	–	Alavizadeh et al. 2012
CS NPs (≈ 275 nm-sized)	SOD B1	3 doses at 3 week intervals. BALB/c mice	Subcutaneous	–	Danesh et al. 2011
PLGA NPs with DOTAP (300 to 450 nm in size; surface electrical charge ≈ 25 mV)	KMP-11 and plasmid DNA encoding KMP-11	Days 0, 14, and 28. BALB/c mice. 100 μg plasmid DNA or prime with 30 μg plasmid DNA NPs; and day 21, 10 μg KMP-11 NPs with 25 μg CpG ODN	Intramuscular, intradermal	Intradermal *L. braziliensis* with sand fly saliva	Santos et al. 2012

Liposomes (≈ 300 nm-sized; egg PC:cholesterol:SA, 7:2:2 molar ratio)	SLA *L. donovani*	3 doses at 2 week intervals. 20 µg SLA	Intraperitoneal	Intravenous 2 × 10^7 promastigotes, 10 days after last booster	Ravindran et al. 2010
Liposomes (≈ 330 nm-sized; surface electrical charge ≈ 40 mV; egg PC:cholesterol:SA, 7:2:2 molar ratio mixed with MPL-TDM)	SLA *L. donovani*	Days 0 and 22. 15 µg SLA	Subcutaneous, intraperitoneal	Intravenous 2 × 10^7 promastigotes, 10 days or 12 weeks after last booster	Ravindran et al. 2012
Alginate microspheres and CpG ODN (≈ 1.8 µm-sized)	Autoclaved *L. major*	3 times at 3 week intervals. BALB/c mice. 180 µg parasites	Subcutaneous	Subcutaneous into the footpad, promastigotes 3 weeks after last booster	Tafaghodi et al. 2011
Cationic SLNs (≈ 240 nm-sized; surface electrical charge ≈ 25 mV; DOTAP 0.4% w/v, and cetyl palmitate:cholesterol:Tween® 80, 3.2:1 molar ratio)	Plasmid DNA encoding cysteine proteinases	Days 0 and 21. 50 µg plasmid DNA	Right-hind footpad	3 weeks after booster	Doroud et al. 2011a,b

of Quillaja saponins as immunomodulators (Tafaghodi et al. 2010). Alginate microspheres loaded with CpG ODN and autoclaved *L. major* induced the lowest lesion development with significantly high IgG2a/IgG1 ratio and IFN-γ (Tafaghodi et al. 2011).

The most recent approaches include DOTAP-based cationic liposomes loaded with the nuclease-sensitive phosphodiester CpG ODN and SLA, tested in BALB/c mice (Shargh et al. 2012). In this investigation, it was found that free nuclease-sensitive phosphodiester CpG ODN induced a lower protection rate than the free nuclease-resistant phosphorothioate CpG ODN, a more costly and toxic derivative. However, it was determined that protection of nuclease-resistant phosphorothioate CpG ODN loaded into liposomes (in terms of smaller footpad swelling and parasite loads, higher IFN-γ and variable IL-4 levels, together with an increase of a two-fold in the IgG2a/IgG1 ratio) was indistinguishable from the generated by nuclease-sensitive phosphodiester CpG ODN loaded to liposomes. These results suggested that nuclease-sensitive phosphodiester CpG ODN-loaded liposomes might be used instead of nuclease-resistant phosphorothioate CpG ODN-loaded liposomes. Immunization with nuclease-sensitive phosphodiester CpG ODN-loaded liposomes raised an early IL-4 response in spleen cells that decreased significantly at nine weeks post-infection. The authors claimed that the early IL-4 production does not hinder the Th1 response, thus being crucial for the priming of long-term CD8+ T cell memory responses.

The same cationic liposomes but complexed with the cationic polymer protamine (condensing CpG ODN) were recently employed to induce a milder *Leishmania* lesion and enhance immunogenicity of LZ (Alavizadeh et al. 2012). The liposomal formulation was originally designed for gene therapy and consists of a virus-like structure (100 to 150 nm in size) with the condensed DNA located inside the lipid membranes. The administration of these NPs was previously observed to induce rapid production of several Th1 cytokines, mainly TNF-α, IL-12, and IFN-γ (Cui et al. 2005). It was further found that mice receiving these NPs and parasites developed a significantly smaller lesion and showed minimum number of *L. major* in spleen and lymph nodes, accompanied by a Th1 response with a preponderance of IgG2a isotype which is concurrent with the production of IFN-γ in the spleen of the mice. Taken together, the results suggested that immune modulation using NPs might be a practical approach to improve the safety of LZ.

DOTAP-based PLGA NPs loaded with a plasmid DNA encoding for KMP-11 were used to immunize mice challenged with *L. braziliensis* (Santos et al. 2012). Vaccination was accomplished by a heterologous prime-boost regimen (a strategy proved effective in models of VL and CL), consisting of priming with these NPs followed by a boost with PLGA NPs loaded with the recombinant KMP-11 protein in the presence of CpG ODN. KMP-11 is a promising vaccine candidate against leishmaniasis because it is a strong inducer of IFN-γ production by cells from cured patients and it is highly conserved among the trypanosomatids. It was previously observed that vaccination with plasmid

DNA encoding for KMP-11 was able to confer protection against LV (*L. donovani*) and against CL (*L. major*), when used in combination with IL-12. In this work, it was found that the immunization with naked plasmid DNA encoding for KMP-11 elicited a mixed Th1/Th2 response. However, immunization with plasmid loaded into the NPs in the presence of CpG ODN, induced a significant increase in TNF-α upon restimulation *in vitro*. The increased levels of IL-2, IFN-γ, TNF-α were ascribed to the presence of DOTAP, while CpG motifs (able to trigger plasmacytoid DCs) contributed to the increased TNF-α production. The presence of IgG1 and IgG2a antibodies suggested the participation of both IL-4 and IFN-γ in antibody isotype switching, even though levels of these cytokines were not significantly increased in mice immunized with the NPs. Following immunization, the mice were challenged with live parasites in the presence of sand fly saliva, mimicking the context of natural infection with *Leishmania* species. It was also hypothesized the immunomodulatory role of saliva from *L. intermedia*. Salivary molecules at the time of parasite challenge can modulate the microenvironment, favoring lesion development. If well neither immunization strategy prevented lesion development upon challenge, a significant reduction in parasite load as well as an increased IFN-γ expression was detected at the infection site. Moreover the greater parasite killing at the challenge site was observed in the group immunized with the NP, ascribed to the upregulation of IFN-γ and TNF-α, combined with downregulation of IL-10. In mice immunized with plasmid DNA alone, upregulation of IFN-γ expression was accompanied by a strong elevation of IL-10 expression. Despite resolution of dermal lesions and parasite clearance from the infection site, the draining lymph nodes were not cleared by any treatment. This parasite persistence in CL has been due to the presence of regulatory T cells that could counteract the presence of effector cells.

The main problem with recombinant Ags (i.e., lack of stability and loss of potency during handling and transportation that could lead to severe problems with future scale up production) could be overcome by the increased stability of a nanoparticulate formulation. In this context, CS NPs prepared by ionotropic gelation with tripolyphosphate, and containing recombinant *Leishmania* SOD B1, were used to get a sustained release of the Ag, aiming to develop a single dose vaccine (Danesh-Bahreini et al. 2011). SOD B1 has a similar structure in many protozoans, and it could be used as a potential vaccine for diverse protozoan infections, including malaria, trypanosomiasis, trichomoniasis, and toxoplasmosis. The structure of protozoan SOD B1 is different from that of human SOD, so there would be no risk of an autoimmune response. In the investigation, it was found that both single dose and triple dose vaccinations of mice with SOD B1-loaded CS NPs showed identical results, being more effective in inducing cell-mediated immunity than control and other groups which received the soluble form of SOD B1.

Finally, SA-based liposomes loaded with SLA plus MPL-TDM (administered subcutaneously) were evaluated in terms of immune response and short/long term protections induced (Ravindran et al. 2012). Meanwhile,

SLA entrapped in liposomes alone, and SLA plus MPL-TDM elicited partial protection, while the SLA-loaded liposomes plus MPL-TDM induced high levels of short term ($\approx$ 90%) and long term ($\approx$ 85%) protection in the liver and spleen ($\approx$ 87 and $\approx$ 83%, respectively), which was similar to that induced by intraperitoneal immunization (Ravindran et al. 2010). Highest and significant levels of DTH were exhibited by mice immunized with the SLA-loaded liposomes injected subcutaneously, intraperitoneally, or in combination with MPL-TDM injected subcutaneously. Protection conferred by this formulation was sustained up to 12 weeks, and infection was controlled for at least four months. An analysis of cellular immune responses demonstrated the induction of IFN-γ and IgG2a antibody production not only 10 d or 12 weeks post-vaccination but also four months after the challenge infection, and a downregulation of IL-4 production after infection. Moreover, long term immunity elicited by this formulation was associated with IFN-γ production also by CD8+ T cells. Taken together, these results suggest that this could be a good vaccine formulation for the induction of durable protection against *L. donovani* through a human administrable route.

Chagas Disease

The causative agent of Chagas disease is the flagellate protozoan *Trypanosoma cruzi* which is transmitted to humans by hematophagous *Reduviidae* bugs. *T. cruzi* infect 10 to 12 million people in endemic areas of Latin America with 15,000 deaths each day. After the generally asymptomatic acute phase (characterized by detectable parasitemia of trypomastigotes) that lasts from a few weeks to several months, the infection is well controlled by the host immune response. Nevertheless, without specific treatment during the acute phase, the infection progresses to a long chronic asymptomatic period, probably lasting for years. It is estimated that in 1/3 of those infected develop clinical symptoms of different degrees of severity, which include cardiomyopathy, heart failure, and digestive tract anomalies (e.g., megacolon and megaoesophagous), appearing in what it is known as symptomatic chronic Chagas disease. The irreversible structural damage to the heart, the oesophagus, and the colon, with severe disorders of nerve conduction in these organs are caused by the intracellular amastigotes.

After entering a mammal through skin wound or mucosal membrane, trypomastigote forms of *T. cruzi* invade many different cell types. In the cytoplasm, they are transformed in amastigotes that multiply by means of binary fission producing cell lysis, and releasing new trypomastigotes into the bloodstream that can invade any nucleated cell to begin a new reproductive cycle. *T. cruzi* parasites are not only taken up by phagocytic cells via classic phagocytosis, but can also actively invade cells by induced phagocytosis. Because of the short and asymptomatic acute phase, cytoplasmatic amastigotes present the major structural and phenomenological barriers that antichagasic drugs have to overcome.

Conventional treatments

Benznidazole and nifurtimox were introduced for clinical use in the late 1960s and early 1970s. They have significant activity in the acute (up to $\approx$ 80% of cures) and early chronic phases (up to $\approx$ 60% cures) but are not active in the chronic phase.

Preclinical drug delivery systems against Chagas disease

The state-of-the-art in the development of nanotechnological strategies against Chagas disease (Romero and Morilla 2010, Morilla and Romero 2015) has been recently reviewed. The activities of 4 AmB formulations (Fungizone®, AmBisome®, Amphocil®, and Abelcet®) were compared *in vitro* and *in vivo* on an acute murine model infected with the Y and the Tulahuen strains (Yardley and Croft 1999). On *T. cruzi* Y strain infected BALB/c mice, the administration of six doses of Fungizone® (0.5 mg/Kg, maximum tolerated dose) or AmBisome® (12.5 mg/Kg) enabled almost 100% mice to survive until the end of the experiment (60 days post-infection, dpi). The effect of AmBisome® was not curative since trypomastigotes were observed in the blood of treated mice for three weeks post-treatment. Untreated control animals died 18 dpi. On *T. cruzi* Tulahuen strain infected mice, the lowest dose of AmBisome® (6.25 mg/Kg) produced survival of all animals until 60 dpi, meanwhile untreated controls survived until 13 dpi. Used as a single dose (25 mg/Kg), AmBisome® induced the survival of 100% mice, whereas Abelcet® and Amphocil® and five oral doses of benznidazole (45 mg/Kg) only induced the survival of three of the five mice at the end of 60 days. In general terms, *in vivo* AmBisome® was more effective and less toxic than other lipid AmB formulations, despite of a delayed elimination of blood parasites when compared to benznidazole (three weeks vs. one week). A crucial difference between the use of AmBisome® against leishmaniasis (a parasite that colonizes the phagolysosomal system in cells of the reticuloendothelial system) and against Chagas disease is that in the latter, even if properly biodistributed, the intracellular pathway followed by AmB could not be appropriate. It is possible that once inside the target cell, the hydrophobic nature of the AmB impaired its diffusion from the endolisosomal/phagolisosomal confinement.

Recently, the effect of AmBisome® intraperitoneally administered during the acute parasitemic phase, the chronic phase, or both phases of infection were studied on BALB/c mice infected with *T. cruzi* Tulahuen strain (Cencig et al. 2011). Administration of AmBisome® (25 mg/Kg, six injections given on alternate days starting on dpi 10) to acutely infected mice significantly reduced the acute phase mean parasitemias by five times, though blood parasites remained detectable at dpi 21 in all mice. AmBisome® treatment reduced parasite loads as compared to untreated mice in spleen and adipose tissue. On dpi 74, blood parasite DNA levels were similar to untreated mice, but in contrast all other tissues exhibited a significant reduction in parasite

DNA amounts compared with untreated animals. An earlier administration (starting on dpi 1) was able to improve the treatment efficiency of AmBisome®. All treated mice survived and displayed reduced parasitemias compared to the untreated group. Administration of AmBisome® to chronically infected mice, showed blood parasite DNA amounts roughly similar to those of untreated animals, whereas they displayed a significant reduction of parasite DNA loads in all tested tissues when compared to untreated mice. Mice treated in acute and chronic phase also presented similar blood parasite DNA amounts than untreated. However, this second round of AmBisome® allowed a significant reduction of parasite DNA loads in all tested tissues when compared to untreated mice. However, whatever the treatment schedule, cyclophosphamide injections boosted infection to parasite amounts comparable to those observed in acutely infected and untreated mice. Taken together, these results indicate that AmBisome® prevents mice from fatal issue in the acute phase of infection, contributes to drastically reduce parasite loads in the heart, liver, spleen, skeletal muscle, and adipose tissues in acute as well as in chronic infection, but fails to completely cure animals from *T. cruzi* infection.

To minimize opsonization (reticuloendothelial system uptake, thus acting as a long circulating drug depot), different azoles (itraconazole, ketokonazole, and the 4th generation bistriazole D0870) were loaded to PEGylated PLA nanospheres. Nanospheres were daily intravenously administered for 30 days to Swiss albino mice infected with a nitroimidazoles/nitrofurans susceptible strain and a partially resistant strain (Molina et al. 2001). D0870-loaded nanospheres (drug equivalent dose: 3 mg/Kg) produced similar percentages of cure (≈ 90%) than free D0870 (30 oral doses, 5 mg/Kg, cure ≈ 80%) on the susceptible strain. In the case of the resistant strain, D0870-loaded nanospheres were more effective (cure ≈ 60%) than itraconazole-loaded and ketokonazole-loaded nanospheres (cure: 0%) and 30 daily oral doses of benznidazole (100 mg/Kg) (cure ≈ 45%). However, 20 oral doses of free D0870 (5 mg/Kg) in the same animal model produced 100% cure.

Aiming to increase the efficacy of benznidazole by modifying its pharmacokinetics and biodistribution, a benznidazole-loaded multilamellar liposomal formulation (hydrogenated soybean PC:cholesterol:DPPG, 2:2:1 molar ratio) was developed. When intravenously administered in rats (drug equivalent dose: 0.2 mg/Kg), a three-fold higher benznidazole accumulation in the liver was found than that achieved with the same dose of the free drug. However, benznidazole-loaded liposomes (intravenous administration, 0.4 mg/Kg, and twice a week from 5 to 22 dpi) did not decrease parasitemia levels in mice infected with the *T. cruzi* RA strain. These results indicated that the relationship between the increased liver delivery and the therapeutic effect of benznidazole-loaded liposomes was not that simple. The hydrophobic benznidazole remained associated to the liposomal bilayer that kept trapped within the endolysosomal pathway, instead of being released to the cell cytoplasm (Morilla et al. 2004). To beat the challenge, pH-sensitive liposomes were engineered (Morilla et al. 2005). In the investigation, it was reported that the acid media trigger a phase transition in pH-sensitive liposomes from bilayer (at neutral or alcaline media) to inverted hexagonal phase II (at pH values < 6). The hexagonal phase II is responsible for the fusion of liposomes with the endolysosomal bilayer. As a result, the aqueous content of pH-sensitive liposomes is released to the cell cytoplasm. The hydrophobic nature of benznidazole made it unsuitable for its delivery by pH-sensitive liposomes. Hence, pH-sensitive liposomes (DOPE:cholesteryl hemisuccinate, 6:4 molar ratio, ≈ 400 nm-sized) containing the hydrophilic etanidazole were formulated. This nanoformulation ensured a fast and massive delivery of etanidazole into the cytosol of murine J774 macrophages. Intravenous administration of etanidazole-loaded pH-sensitive liposomes (drug equivalent dose: 0.56 mg/Kg, starting 5 dpi, three days a week over three weeks) resulted in a significant decrease in parasitemia (day 12, 19, 21, and 23) of BALB/c mice infected with *T. cruzi* RA strain. Administration of a 180-fold higher dose of free etanidazole failed to reduce the number trypomastigotes in blood.

Vaccine delivery systems against Chagas disease

There is only one work where *T. cruzi* trypomastigote and amastigote membrane proteins were loaded into liposomes (DPPC:DPPS:cholesterol, 5:1:4 weight ratio), and BALB/c mice were intraperitoneally immunized (Migliacio et al. 2008). Despite the fact that immunized mice generated antibodies and activated the macrophages, the immunized mice were not protected against *T. cruzi* Y strain intraperitoneal challenge. Although inoculation of BALB/c mice with the liposomal formulation delayed the death of the animals, later in the infection their mortality was equivalent to controls.

More recently, immune response and efficacy of archaeosomes (liposomes made from lipids extracted from the Archaea *Halorubrum tebenquichense*) loaded with soluble *T. cruzi* Ags upon subcutaneous administration (day 0, 14, and 21) on C3H/HeN mice was investigated (Higa et al. 2013). It was found that mice rapidly developed higher levels of circulating antibodies than those measured in the sera from animals receiving the Ag alone with a dominant IgG2a isotype. In addition, mice displayed reduced parasitemia during early infection and were protected against an otherwise lethal challenge with the virulent Tulahuen strain of the parasite (100% of survival of animals immunized with archaeosomes at 30 dpi vs. 100% mortality of control groups at 25 dpi).

Conclusions

The current pace of evolution of therapeutic and prophylactic nanomedical strategies against neglected diseases is undoubtedly slow. DDSs acting as drug depots against malaria have been administered by the intraperitoneal route (of non-realistic use in humans). On the other hand, the significantly increased bioavailability of artemisin and derivatives (conventionally administered by the intramuscular route) achieved by oral self-emulsifying DDSs could lead to the appearance of new resistances. The two major challenges remaining are targeting to infected erythrocytes by cost effective scaled up nanomaterials, together with demonstrating the therapeutic efficacy of liver targeting. In adjuvancy, only two preclinical investigations demonstrated the protective efficacy of plasmid DNA/PEI/PGA NPs administered by the intravenous and intraperitoneal routes, while that achieved by the subcutaneous route resulted poor. The use of plasmid DNA is still controversial because of the toxicity of its ionic complexes and the absence of succeeding results in animals other than rodents.

The oral administration of drug-loaded polymeric NPs against TB allowed reducing the number of administrations and increased drug tissue accumulation, but alveolar macrophages were not targeted by this route of administration. Only when alveolar macrophages were targeted by pulmonary administration, a pronounced reduction in frequency of administrations was possible as compared to other routes of administration. Good protection levels were achieved by plasmid DNA-loaded liposomal and Pluronic®-stabilized poly(propylene sulfide) nanovaccines administered by intranasal and pulmonary routes in mice. Their performance in animals other than rodents and the security profile of the pulmonary administration remain to be demonstrated.

In spite of its unsurpassed efficacy against VL, AmBisome® is unaffordable for underdeveloped countries. Other less invasive routes of administration for nanomedicines, such as oral, seem to be promising, economical, and of high stability. Despite an important number of drug-loaded liposomes against Old World CL administered topically entered clinical trials, a clinical cure is still waiting to be achive. Preclinical approaches of vaccination using plasmid DNA-loaded SLNs against CL recently showed satisfactory results. Finally, Chagas disease remains the most neglected of the parasitosis, with scarce preclinical approaches testing the efficacy of nanomedicines against acute phase murine models.

Overall, no preclinical approaches using drug nanocarriers against these neglected diseases (except the clinical forms of the Old World leishmaniasis) have entered clinical trials yet. Preclinical vaccination strategies against leishmaniasis are showing encouraging results as well. In this scenario the scarce interest of using nanomedicines against neglected diseases could be due to affordability issues together with lack of technical knowledge and absence of key strategic health plans by the governments of the endemic countries.

Abbreviations

Ag	:	antigen
AmB	:	amphotericin B
APC	:	antigen presenting cell

AUC	:	area under the plasma drug concentration-time curve
BCG	:	bacillus Calmette-Guérin
CFU	:	colony forming unit
CL	:	cutaneous leishmaniasis
CLR	:	C-type lectin receptor
CS	:	chitosan
DC	:	dendritic cell
DC-SIGN	:	dendritic cell-specific intercellular adhesion molecule-3-grabbing nonintegrin
DDAB	:	dimethyldioctadecylammonium bromide
DDS	:	drug delivery system
DNA	:	deoxyribonucleic acid
DOPC	:	1,2-dioleoyl-*sn*-glycero-3-phosphatidylcholine
DOPE	:	1,2-dioleoyl-sn-glycero-3-phosphoethanolamine
DOTAP	:	1,2-dioleoyl-3-trimethylammonium propane
dpi	:	days post-infection
DPPC	:	dipalmitoylphosphatidylcholine
DPPG	:	dipalmitoylphosphatidylglycerol
DSPE-PEG(2000)	:	1,2-distearoyl-*sn*-glycero-3-phosphoethanolamine-*N*-[amino(polyethylene glycol)-2000]
DTH	:	delayed type hypersensitivity
ECZ	:	econazole
ESAT-6	:	6-kDa early secretory antigen target
ETB	:	ethambutol
HIV	:	human immunodeficiency virus
HLA	:	human leukocyte antigen
HPMA	:	*N*-(2-hydroxypropyl)methacrylamide
hsp65	:	65-kDa heat shock protein
IL	:	interleukin
IFN-γ	:	interferon gamma
Ig	:	immunoglobulin
INH	:	isoniazid
IC$_{50}$	:	half maximal inhibitory concentration
KMP-11	:	11-kDa kinetoplastid membrane protein
LZ	:	leishmanization
MHC	:	major histocompatibility complex
MOX	:	moxifloxacin
MPB-PE	:	1,2-dipalmitoyl-*sn*-glycero-3-phosphoethanolamine-*N*-[4-(*p*-maleimidophenyl) butyramide]
MPL-TDM	:	monophosphoryl lipid-trehalose dicorynomycolate
Mtb	:	*Mycobacterium tuberculosis*

NK	:	natural killer
NLC	:	nanostructured lipid carrier
NLS	:	nuclear localization signal
NP	:	nanoparticle
ODN	:	oligodeoxynucleotide
PC	:	phosphatidylcholine
PCL	:	poly(ε-caprolactone)
PEG	:	poly(ethylene glycol)
PEI	:	polyethyleneimine
PfEMP-1	:	*P. falciparum* erythrocyte membrane protein-1
PfMSP-1	:	*P. falciparum* merozoite surface protein-1
PGA	:	poly(γ-glutamic acid)
PLA	:	poly(D,L-lactide)
PLGA	:	poly(D,L-lactide-*co*-glycolide)
PRR	:	pattern recognition receptor
PyMSP-1	:	*P. yoelii* merozoite surface protein-1
PYZ	:	pyrazinamide
RIF	:	rifampicin
SA	:	stearylamine
SLA	:	soluble *Leishmania* antigen
SLN	:	solid lipid nanoparticle
SOD	:	superoxide dismutase
TB	:	tuberculosis
Th1	:	type 1 T helper
Th2	:	type 2 T helper
Th17	:	type 17 T helper
TNF-α	:	tumor necrosis factor alpha
TPGS	:	D-α-tocopheryl poly(ethylene glycol) 1000 succinate
VL	:	visceral leishmaniasis

References

Aditya, N.P. and S. Patankar, B. Madhusudhan, R.S. Murthy and E.B. Souto. 2010a. Arthemeter-loaded lipid nanoparticles produced by modified thin RSR -film hydration: pharmacokinetics, toxicological and *in vivo* anti-malarial activity. Eur. J. Pharm. Sci. 40: 448–455.

Aditya, P.N. and W. Tiyaboonchai, S. Patankar, B. Madhusudhan and E.B. Souto. 2010b. Curcuminoids loaded in lipid nanoparticles: novel approach towards malaria treatment. Colloids Surf. B Biointerfaces. 81: 263–273.

Afrin, F. and T. Dey, K. Anam and N. Ali. 2001. Leishmanicidal activity of stearylamine bearing liposomes *in vitro*. J. Parasitol. 87: 188–193.

Ahmad, Z. and S. Sharma and G.K. Khuller. 2005. Inhalable alginate nanoparticles as antitubercular drug carriers against experimental tuberculosis. Int. J. Antimicrob. Agents. 26: 298–303.

Ahmad, Z. and R. Pandey, S. Sharma and G.K. Khuller. 2006. Pharmacokinetic and pharmacodynamic behavior of antitubercular drugs encapsulated in alginate nanoparticles at two doses. Int. J. Antimicrob. Agents. 27: 409–416.

Ahmad, Z. and S. Sharma and G.K. Khuller. 2007. Chemotherapeutic evaluation of alginate nanoparticle encapsulated azole antifungal and antitubercular drugs against murine tuberculosis. Nanomedicine. 3: 239–243.

Ahmad, Z. and R. Pandey, S. Sharma and G.K. Khuller. 2008. Novel chemotherapy for tuberculosis: chemotherapeutic potential of econazole- and moxifloxacin-loaded PLG nanoparticles. Int. J. Antimicrob. Agents. 31: 142–146.

Alavizadeh, H. and A. Badiee, A. Khamesipour, S.A. Jalali, H. Firouzmand, A. Abbasi and M.R. Jaafari. 2012. The role of liposome–protamine–DNA nanoparticles containing CpG oligodeoxynucleotides in the course of infection induced by *Leishmania major* in BALB/c mice. Exp. Parasitol. 132: 313–319.

Alving, C.R. and E.A. Steck, W.L. Chapman, V.B. Waits, L.D. Hendricks, G.M. Swartz, Jr. and W.L. Hanson. 1978. Therapy of leishmaniasis: superior efficacies of liposome-encapsulated drugs. Proc. Natl. Acad. Sci. U.S.A. 75: 2959–2963.

Arana, B.A. and C.E. Mendoza, N.R. Rizzo and A. Kroeger. 2001. Randomized, controlled, double-blind trial of topical treatment of cutaneous leishmaniasis with paromomycin plus methylbenzethonium chloride ointment in Guatemala. Am. J. Trop. Med. Hyg. 65: 466–470.

Armijos, R.X. and M.M. Weigel, M. Calvopina, M. Mancheno and R. Rodriguez. 2004. Comparison of the effectiveness of two topical paromomycin treatments versus meglumine antimoniate for New World cutaneous leishmaniasis. Acta Trop. 91: 153–160.

Badiee, A. and M.R. Jaafari, A. Khamesipour, A. Samiei, D. Soroush, M.T. Kheiri, F. Barkhordari, W.R. McMaster and F. Mahboudi. 2009. The role of liposome charge on immune response generated in BALB/c mice immunized with recombinant major surface glycoprotein of Leishmania (rgp63). Exp. Parasitol. 121: 362–369.

Ballester, M. and C. Nembrini, A. Dhar Neeraj de Titta, C. de Piano, M. Pasquiera, E. Simeonia, A.J. van der Vlies, J.D. McKinney, J.A. Hubbell and M.A. Swartz. 2011. Nanoparticle conjugation and pulmonary delivery enhance the protective efficacy of Ag85B and CpG against tuberculosis. Vaccine. 29: 6959–6966.

Barratt, B. and P. Legrand. 2005. Comparison of the efficacy and pharmacology of formulations of amphotericin B used in treatment of leishmaniasis. Curr. Opin. Infect. Dis. 18: 527–530.

Bavarsad, N. and B.S.F. Bazzaz, A. Khamesipour and M.R. Jaafari. 2012. Colloidal, *in vitro* and *in vivo* anti-leishmanial properties of transfersomes containing paromomycin sulfate in susceptible BALB/c mice. Acta Trop. 124: 33–41.

Ben Salah, A. and P.A. Buffet, G. Morizot, N. Ben Massoud, A. Zâatour, N. Ben Alaya, N.B. Haj Hamida, Z. El Ahmadi, M.T. Downs, P.L. Smith, K. Dellagi and M. Grögl. 2009. WR279 a third generation aminoglycoside ointment for the treatment of *Leishmania major* cutaneous leishmaniasis: a phase 2, randomized, double blind, placebo controlled study. PLoS Negl. Trop. Dis. 3: e432.

Berman, J.D. and W.L. Hanson, W.L. Chapman, C.R. Alving and G. Lopez-Berestein. 1986. Antileishmanial activity of liposome-encapsulated amphotericin B in hamsters and monkeys. Antimicrob. Agents Chemother. 30: 847–851.

Bern, C. and J. Adler-Moore, J. Berenguer, M. Boelaert, M. den Boer, R.N. Davidson, C. Figueras, L. Gradoni, D.A. Kafetzis, K. Ritmeijer, E. Rosenthal, C. Royce, R. Russo, S. Sundar and J. Alvar. 2006. Liposomal amphotericin B for the treatment of visceral leishmaniasis. Clin. Infect. Dis. 43: 917–924.

Bhowmick, S. and T. Mazumdar, R. Sinhá and N. Ali. 2010. Comparison of liposome based antigen delivery systems for protection against *Leishmania donovani*. J. Control. Release. 141: 199–207.

Bivas-Benita, M. and T.H.M. Ottenhoff, H.E. Junginger and G. Borchard. 2005. Pulmonary DNA vaccination: concepts, possibilities and perspectives. J. Control. Release. 107: 1–29.

Brown, M. and M. Noursadeghi, J. Boyle and R.N. Davidson. 2005. Successful liposomal amphotericin B treatment of *Leishmania braziliensis* cutaneous leishmaniasis. Br. J. Dermatol. 153: 203–205.

Carcaboso, A.M. and R.M. Hernández, M. Igartua, A.R. Gascón, J.E. Rosas, M.E. Patarroyo and J.L. Pedraz. 2003. Immune response after oral administration of the encapsulated malaria synthetic peptide SPf66. Int. J. Pharm. 260: 273–282.

Carcaboso, A.M. and R.M. Hernández, M. Igartua, J.E. Rosas, M.E. Patarroyo and J.L. Pedraz. 2004. Potent, long lasting systemic antibody levels and mixed Th1/Th2 immune response after nasal immunization with malaria antigen loaded PLGA microparticles. Vaccine. 22: 1423–1432.

Carneiro, G. and D.C. Santos, M.C. Oliveira, A.P. Fernandes, L.S. Ferreira, G.A. Ramaldes, E.A. Nunan and L.A. Ferreira. 2010. Topical delivery and *in vivo* antileishmanial activity of paromomycin loaded liposomes for treatment of cutaneous leishmaniasis. J. Liposome Res. 20: 16–23.

Cencig, S. and N. Coltel, C. Truyens and Y. Carlier. 2011. Parasitic loads in tissues of mice infected with *Trypanosoma cruzi* and treated with AmBisome. PLoS Negl. Trop. Dis. 5: e1216.

Chavez-Santoscoy, A.V. and R. Roychoudhury, N.L.B. Pohl, M.J. Wannemuehler, B. Narasimhan and A.E. Ramer-Tait. 2012. Tailoring the immune response by targeting C-type lectin receptors on alveolar macrophages using "pathogen-like" amphiphilic polyanhydride nanoparticles. Biomaterials. 33: 4762–4772.

Cherif, M.S. and M.N. Shuaibu, T. Kurosaki, G.K. Helegbe, M. Kikuchi, T. Yanagi, T. Tsuboi, H. Sasaki, and K. Hirayama. 2011. Immunogenicity of novel nanoparticle-coated MSP-1 C-terminus malaria DNA vaccine using different routes of administration. Vaccine. 29: 9038–9050.

Chimanuka, B. and M. Gabriëls, M.R. Detaevernier and J.A. Plaizier-Vercammen. 2002. Preparation of betaartemether liposomes, their HPLC-UV evaluation and relevance for clearing recrudescent parasitaemia in Plasmodium chabaudi malaria-infected mice. J. Pharm. Biomed. Anal. 28: 13–22.

Cohen, J. and V. Nussenzweig, R. Nussenzweig, J. Vekemans and A. Leach. 2010. From the circumsporozoite protein to the RTS, S/AS candidate vaccine. Hum. Vaccin. 6: 90–96.

Danesh-Bahreini, M.A. and J. Shokri, A. Samiei, E. Kamali-Sarvestani, M. Barzegar-Jalali and S. Mohammadi-Samani. 2011. Nanovaccine for leishmaniasis: preparation of chitosan nanoparticles containing Leishmania superoxide dismutase and evaluation of its immunogenicity in BALB/c mice. Int. J. Nanomedicine. 6: 835–842.

Demicheli, C. and R. Ochoa, J.B.B. Da Silva, C.A. Falcão, B. Rossi-Bergmann, A.L. de Melo, R.D. Sinisterra and F. Frézard. 2004. Oral delivery of meglumine antimoniate-cyclodextrin complex for treatment of leishmaniasis. Antimicrob. Agents Chemother. 48: 100–103.

Dey, T. and K. Anam, F. Afrin and N. Ali. 2000. Antileishmanial activities of stearylamine bearing liposomes. Antimicrob. Agents Chemother. 44: 1739–1742.

Dierling, A.M. and Z. Cui. 2005. Targeting primaquine into liver using chylomicron emulsions for potential vivax malaria therapy. Int. J. Pharm. 303: 143–152.

Doroud, D. and F. Zahedifard, A. Vatanara, A.R. Najafabadi, Y. Taslimi, R. Vahabpour, F. Torkashvand, B. Vaziri and S. Rafati. 2011a. Delivery of a cocktail DNA vaccine encoding cysteine proteinases type I, II and III with solid lipid nanoparticles potentiate protective immunity against *Leishmania major* infection. J. Control. Release. 153: 154–162.

Doroud, D. and F. Zahedifard, A. Vatanara, Y. Taslimi, R. Vahabpour, F. Torkashvand, B. Vaziri, A. Rouholamini Najafabadi and S. Rafati. 2011b. C-terminal domain deletion enhances the protective activity of cpa/cpb loaded solid lipid nanoparticles against *Leishmania major* in BALB/c mice. PLoS Negl. Trop. Dis. 5: e1236.

Doroud, D. and S. Rafati. 2012. Leishmaniasis: focus on the design of nanoparticulate vaccine delivery systems. Expert. Rev. Vaccines. 11: 69–86.

El-On, J. and R. Livshin, Z. Even-Paz, D. Hamburge and L. Weinrauch. 1986. Topical treatment of cutaneous leishmaniasis. J. Invest. Dermatol. 87: 284–288.

El-On, J. and S. Halevy, M.H. Grunwald and L. Weinrauch. 1992. Topical treatment of Old World cutaneous leishmaniasis caused by *Leishmania major*: a double-blind control study. J. Am. Acad. Dermatol. 27: 227–231.

El-Ridy, M.S. and D.M. Mostafa, A. Shehab, E.A. Nasr and S.A. El- Alim. 2007. Biological evaluation of pyrazinamide liposomes for treatment of Mycobacterium tuberculosis. Int. J. Pharm. 330: 82–88.

Frézard, F. and P.S. Martins, A.P. Bahia, L. Le Moyec, A.L. de Melo, A.M. Pimenta, M. Salerno, J.B. da Silva and C. Demicheli. 2008. Enhanced oral delivery of antimony from meglumine antimoniate/beta-cyclodextrin nanoassemblies. Int. J. Pharm. 347: 102–108.

Gaspar, M.M. and A. Cruz, A.G. Fraga, A.G. Castro, M.E.M. Cruz and J. Pedrosa. 2008a. Developments on drug delivery systems for the treatment of mycobacterial infections. Curr. Trop. Med. Chem. 8: 579–591.

Gaspar, M.M. and A. Cruz, A.F. Penha, J. Reymao, A.C. Sousa, C.V. Eleuterio, S.A. Domingues, A.G. Fraga, A. Longatto Filho, M.E.M. Cruz and J. Pedrosa. 2008b. Rifabutin encapsulated in liposomes exhibits increased therapeutic activity in a model of disseminated tuberculosis. Int. J. Antimicrob. Agents. 31: 37–45.

Gradoni, L. and R.N. Davidson, S. Orsini, P. Betto and M. Giambenedetti. 1993. Activity of liposomal amphotericin B (AmBisome) against Leishmania infantum and tissue distribution in mice. J. Drug Target. 1: 311–316.

Griffiths, G. and B. Nyström, S.B. Sable and G.K. Khuller. 2010. Nanobead-based interventions for the treatment and prevention of tuberculosis. Nat. Rev. Microbiol. 8: 827–834.

Gupta, Y. and A. Jain and S.K. Jain. 2007. Transferrin-conjugated solid lipid nanoparticles for enhanced delivery of quinine dihydrochloride to the brain. J. Pharm. Pharmacol. 59: 935–940.

Haas, S.E. and C.C. Bettoni, L.K. de Oliveira, S.S. Guterres and T. Dalla Costa. 2009. Nanoencapsulation increases quinine antimalarial efficacy against *Plasmodium berghei in vivo*. Int. J. Antimicrob. Agents. 34: 156–161.

Haynes, S.M. and K.J. Longmuir, R.T. Robertson, J.L. Baratta and A.J. Waring. 2008. Liposomal polyethyleneglycol and polyethyleneglycol-peptide combinations for active targeting to liver *in vivo*. Drug Deliv. 15: 207–217.

Higa, L.H. and R.S. Corral, M.J. Morilla, E.L. Romero and P.B. Petray. 2013. Archaeosomes display immunoadjuvant potential for a vaccine against Chagas disease. Hum. Vaccin. Immunother. 9: 409–412.

Hoffman, S.L. and P.F. Billingsley, E. James, A. Richman, M. Loyevsky, T. Li, S. Chakravarty, A. Gunasekera, R. Chattopadhyay, M. Li, R. Stafford, A. Ahumada, J.E. Epstein, M. Sedegah, S. Reyes, T.L. Richie, K.E. Lyke, R. Edelman, M.B. Laurens, C.V. Plowe and B.K. Sim. 2010. Development of a metabolically active, non-replicating sporozoite vaccine to prevent *Plasmodium falciparum* malaria. Hum. Vaccin. 6: 97–106.

Hubbell, J.A. and S.N. Thomas and M.A. Swartz. 2009. Materials engineering for immunomodulation. Nature. 462: 449–460.

Isacchi, B. and M.C. Bergonzi, M. Grazioso, C. Righeschi, A. Pietretti, C. Severini and A.R. Bilia. 2012. Artemisinin and artemisinin plus curcumin liposomal formulations: enhanced antimalarial efficacy against *Plasmodium berghei*-infected mice. Eur. J. Pharm. Biopharm. 80: 528–534.

Jaafari, M.R. and N. Bavarsad, B.S.F. Bazzaz, A. Samiei, D. Soroush, S. Ghorbani, M.M.L. Heravi and A. Khamesipour. 2009. Effect of topical liposomes containing paromomycin sulfate in the course of *Leishmania major* infection in susceptible BALB/c mice. Antimicrob. Agents Chemother. 53: 2259–2265.

Johnson, C.M. and R. Pandey, S. Sharma, G.K. Khuller, R.J. Basaraba, I.M. Orme and A.J. Lenaerts. 2005. Oral therapy using nanoparticle-encapsulated antituberculosis drugs in guinea pigs infected with Mycobacterium tuberculosis. Antimicrob. Agents Chemother. 49: 4335–4338.

Joshi, M. and S. Pathak, S. Sharma and V. Patravale. 2008a. Design and *in vivo* pharmacodynamic evaluation of nanostructured lipid carriers for parenteral delivery of artemether: Nanoject. Int. J. Pharm. 364: 119–126.

Joshi, M. and S. Pathak, S. Sharma and V. Patravale. 2008b. Solid microemulsion preconcentrate (NanOsorb) of artemether for effective treatment of malaria. Int. J. Pharm. 362: 172–178.

Kaufmann, S.H. and A.J. McMichael. 2005. Annulling a dangerous liaison: vaccination strategies against AIDS and tuberculosis. Nat. Med. 11: S33–S44.

Kaufmann, S.H. and G. Hussey and P.H. Lambert. 2010. New vaccines for tuberculosis. Lancet. 375: 2110–2119.

Kayser, O. and C. Olbrich, V. Yardley, A.F. Kiderlen and S.L. Croft. 2003. Formulation of amphotericin B as nanosuspension for oral administration. Int. J. Pharm. 254: 73–75.

Kensil, C.R. and A.X. Mo and A. Truneh. 2004. Current vaccine adjuvants: an overview of a diverse class. Front. Biosci. 9: 2972–2988.

Kirby, A.C. and M.C. Coles and P.M. Kaye. 2009. Alveolar macrophages transport pathogens to lung draining lymph nodes. J. Immunol. 183: 1983–1989.

Kisich, K.O. and S. Gelperina, M.P. Higgins, S. Wilson, E. Shipulo, E. Oganesyan and L. Heifets. 2007. Encapsulation of moxifloxacin within poly(butyl cyanoacrylate) nanoparticles enhances efficacy against intracellular Mycobacterium tuberculosis. Int. J. Pharm. 345: 154–162.

Kshirsagar, N.A. and S.K. Pandya, B.G. Kirodian and S.S. Sanath. 2005. Liposomal drug delivery systems from laboratory to clinic. J. Postgrad. Med. 51: 5–15.

Leite, E.A. and A. Grabe-Guimarães, H.N. Guimarães, G.L.L. Machado-Coelho, G. Barratt and V.C.F. Mosqueira. 2007. Cardiotoxicity reduction induced by halofantrine entrapped in nanocapsule devices. Life Sci. 80: 1327–1334.

Lenaerts, A.J. and V. Gruppo, K.S. Marietta, C.M. Johnson, D.K. Driscoll, N.M. Tompkins, J.D. Rose, R.C. Reynolds and I.M. Orme. 2005. Preclinical testing of the nitroimidazopyran PA-824 for activity against Mycobacterium tuberculosis in a series of *in vitro* and *in vivo* models. Antimicrob. Agents Chemother. 49: 2294–2301.

Leon, C.G. and J. Lee, K. Bartlett, P. Gershkovich, E.K. Wasan, J. Zhao, J.G. Clement and K.M. Wasan. 2011. *In vitro* cytotoxicity of two novel oral formulations of Amphotericin B (iCo-009 and iCo-010) against Candida albicans, human monocytic and kidney cell lines. Lipids Health Dis. 10: 144.

Longmuir, K.J. and R.T. Robertson, S.M. Haynes, J.L. Baratta and A.J. Waring. 2006. Effective targeting of liposomes to liver and hepatocytes *in vivo* by incorporation of a Plasmodium amino acid sequence. Pharm. Res. 23: 759–769.

Mandawgade, S.D. and S. Sharma, S. Pathak and V.B. Patravale. 2008. Development of SMEDDS using natural lipophile: application to beta-Artemether delivery. Int. J. Pharm. 362: 179–183.

Memvanga, P.B. and V. Préat. 2012. Formulation design and *in vivo* antimalarial evaluation of lipid-based drug delivery systems for oral delivery of b-arteether. Eur. J. Pharm. Biopharm. 82: 112–119.

Meyerhoff, A. 1999. U.S. Food and Drug Administration approval AmBisome (liposomal amphotericin B) for treatment of viseral leishamiasis. Clin. Infect. Dis. 28: 42–48.

Migliaccio, V. and F.R. Santos, P. Ciancaglini and F.J. Ramalho-Pinto. 2008. Use of proteoliposome as a vaccine against Trypanosoma cruzi in mice. Chem. Phys. Lipids. 152: 86–94.

Minodier, P. and K. Retornaz, A. Horelt and J.M. Garnier. 2003. Liposomal amphotericin B in the treatment of visceral leishmaniasis in immunocompetent patients. Fundam. Clin. Pharmacol. 17: 183–188.

Molina, J. and J.A. Urbina, R. Gref, Z. Brener and M.J.J. Rodrigues. 2001. Cure of experimental Chagas disease by the bis-triazole D0870 incorporated into stealth polyethyleneglycol-polylactide nanospheres. J. Antimicrob. Chemother. 47: 101–104.

Montanari, J. and C. Maidana, M.I. Esteva, C. Salomon, M.J. Morilla and E.L. Romero. 2010. Sunlight triggered photodynamic ultradeformable liposomes against Leishmania braziliensis are also leishmanicidal in the dark. J. Control. Release. 147: 368–376.

Morilla, M.J. and J.A. Montanari, M.J. Prieto, M.O. Lopez, P.B. Petray and E.L. Romero. 2004. Intravenous liposomal benznidazole as trypanocidal agent: increasing drug delivery to liver is not enough. Int. J. Pharm. 278: 311–318.

Morilla, M.J. and J. Montanari, F. Frank, E. Malchiodi, R. Corral, P. Petray and E.L. Romero. 2005. Etanidazole in pH-sensitive liposomes: design, characterization and *in vitro/in vivo* anti-Trypanosoma cruzi activity. J. Control. Release. 103: 599–607.

Morilla, M.J. and E.L. Romero. 2015. Nanomedicines against Chagas disease: an update on therapeutics, prophylaxis and diagnosis. Nanomedicine (Lond). 10: 465–481.

Mosqueira, V.C.F. and P.M. Loiseau, C. Bories, P. Legrand, J.P. Devissaguet and G. Barratt. 2004. Efficacy and pharmacokinetics of intravenous nanocapsule formulations of halofantrine in Plasmodium berghei-infected mice. Antimicrob. Agents Chemother. 48: 1222–1228.

Mutiso, J.M. and J.C. Macharia and M.M. Gicheru. 2010. A review of adjuvants for vaccine candidates. J. Biomed. Res. 24: 16–25.

Nan, A. and S.L. Croft, V. Yardley and H. Ghandehari. 2004. Targetable water-soluble polymer–drug conjugates for the treatment of visceral leishmaniasis. J. Control. Release. 94: 115–127.

Nelson, K.G. and J.V. Bishop, R.O. Ryan and R. Titus. 2006. Nanodisk-associated amphotericin B clears leishmanis major cutaneous infection in susceptible Balb/c mice. Antimicrob. Agents Chemother. 50: 1238–1244.

New, R.R.C. and M.L. Chance, S.C. Thomas and W. Peters. 1978. Antileishmanial activity of antimonials entrapped in liposomes. Nature. 272: 55–56.

Nicoletti, S. and K. Seifert and I.H. Gilbert. 2009. N-(2-hydroxypropyl)methacrylamide-amphotericin B (HPMA-AmB) copolymer conjugates as antileishmanial agents. Int. J. Antimicrob. Agents. 33: 441–448.

Nicoletti, S. and K. Seifert and I.H. Gilbert. 2010. Water-soluble polymer–drug conjugates for combination chemotherapy against visceral leishmaniasis. Bioorg. Med. Chem. 18: 2559–2565.

Noazin, S. and F. Modabber, A. Khamesipour, P.G. Smith, L.H. Moulton, K. Nasseri, I. Sharifi, E.A. Khalil, I.D. Bernal, C.M. Antunes, M.P. Kieny and M. Tanner. 2008. First generation leishmaniasis vaccines: a review of field efficacy trials. Vaccine. 26: 6759–6767.

Noazin, S. and A. Khamesipour, L.H. Moulton, M. Tanner, K. Nasseri, F. Modabber, I. Sharifi, E.A. Khalil, I.D. Bernal, C.M. Antunes and P.G. Smith. 2009. Efficacy of killed whole-parasite vaccines in the prevention of leishmaniasis: a meta-analysis. Vaccine. 27: 4747–4753.

Owais, M. and G.C. Varshney, A. Choudhury, S. Chandra and C.M. Gupta. 1995. Chloroquine encapsulated in malaria-infected erythrocyte-specific antibody-bearing liposomes effectively controls chloroquine- resistant Plasmodium berghei infections in mice. Antimicrob. Agents Chemother. 39:180–184.

Pal, S. and R. Ravindran and N. Ali. 2004. Combination therapy using sodium antimony gluconate in stearylamine-bearing liposomes against established and chronic *Leishmania donovani* infection in BALB/c Mice. Antimicrob. Agents Chemother. 48: 3591–3593.

Palatnik-de-Sousa, C.B. 2008. Vaccines for leishmaniasis in the fore coming 25 years. Vaccine. 26: 1709–1724.

Pandey, R. and A. Zahoor, S. Sharma and G.K. Khuller. 2003a. Nanoparticle encapsulated antitubercular drugs as a potential oral drug delivery system against murine tuberculosis. Tuberculosis. 83: 373–378.

Pandey, R. and A. Sharma, A. Zahoor, S. Sharma, G.K. Khuller and B. Prasad. 2003b. Poly(DL-lactide-co-glycolide) nanoparticle-based inhalable sustained drug delivery system for experimental tuberculosis. J. Antimicrob. Chemother. 52: 981–986.

Pandey, R. and G.K. Khuller. 2004. Subcutaneous nanoparticle-based antitubercular chemotherapy in an experimental model. J. Antimicrob. Chemother. 54: 266–268.

Pandey, R. and S. Sharma and G.K. Khuller. 2005. Oral solid lipid nanoparticle based antitubercular chemotherapy. Tuberculosis. 85: 415–420.

Pandey, R. and G.K. Khuller. 2006. Oral nanoparticle-based antituberculosis drug delivery to the brain in an experimental model. J. Antimicrob. Chemother. 57: 1146–1152.

Pinder, M. and V.S. Moorthy, B.D. Akanmori, B. Genton and G.V. Brown. 2010. MALVAC 2009: progress and challenges in development of whole organism malaria vaccines for endemic countries, 3-4 June 2009 Dakar, Senegal. Vaccine. 28: 4695–4702.

Ravindran, R. and S. Bhowmick, A. Das and N. Ali. 2010. Comparison of BCG, MPL and cationic liposome adjuvant systems in leishmanial antigen vaccine formulations against murine visceral leishmaniasis. BMC Microbiol. 10: 181.

Ravindran, R. and M. Maji and N. Ali. 2012. Vaccination with liposomal Leishmanial antigens adjuvanted with Monophosphoryl Lipid-Trehalose Dicorynomycolate (MPL-TDM) confers long-term protection against Visceral Leishmaniasis through a human administrable route. Mol. Pharm. 9: 59–70.

Rea, J.C. and R.F. Gibly, A.E. Barron and L.D. Shea. 2009. Self-assembling peptide-lipoplexes for substrate-mediated gene delivery. Acta Biomater. 5: 903–912.

Reddy, S.T. and A.J. van der Vlies, E. Simeoni, V. Angeli, G.J. Randolph, C.P. O'Neil, L.K. Lee, M.A. Swartz and J.A. Hubbell. 2007. Exploiting lymphatic transport and complement activation in nanoparticle vaccines. Nat. Biotechnol. 25: 1159–1164.

Reimão, J.Q. and F.A. Colombo, V.L. Pereira-Chioccola and A.G. Tempone. 2012. Effectiveness of liposomal buparvaquone in an experimental hamster model of Leishmania (L.) infantum chagasi. Exp. Parasitol. 130: 195–199.

Romero, E.L. and M.J. Morilla. 2008. Drug delivery systems against leishmaniasis? Still an open question. Expert. Opin. Drug Deliv. 5: 805–823.

Romero, E.L. and M.J. Morilla. 2010. Nanotechnological approaches against Chagas disease. Adv. Drug Deliv. Rev. 62: 576–588.

Rosada, R.S. and C.L. Silva, M.H. Santana, C.R. Nakaie and L.G. de la Torre. 2012. Effectiveness, against tuberculosis, of pseudo-ternary complexes: peptide-DNA-cationic liposome. J. Colloid Interface Sci. 373: 102–109.

Roychoudhury, J. and R. Sinhá and N. Ali. 2011. Therapy with sodium stibogluconate in stearylamine-bearing liposomes confers cure against SSG-resistant Leishmania donovani in BALB/c mice. PLoS One. 6: e17376.

Santos, D.M. and M.W. Carneiro, T.R. de Moura, K. Fukutani, J. Clarencio, M. Soto, S. Espuelas, C. Brodskyn, A. Barral, M. Barral-Netto and C.I. de Oliveira. 2012. Towards development of novel immunization strategies against leishmaniasis using PLGA nanoparticles loaded with kinetoplastid membrane protein-11. Int. J. Nanomedicine. 7: 2115–2127.

Santos-Magalhães, N.S. and V.C. Furtado Mosqueira. 2010. Nanotechnology applied to the treatment of malaria. Adv. Drug Deliv. Rev. 62: 560–575.

Saraogi, G.K. and P. Gupta, U.D. Gupta, N.K. Jain and G.P. Agrawal. 2010. Gelatin nanocarriers as potential vectors for effective management of Tuberculosis. Int. J. Pharm. 385: 143–149.

Saraogi, G.K. and B. Sharma, B. Joshi, P. Gupta, U.D. Gupta, N.K. Jain and G.P. Agrawal. 2011. Mannosylated gelatin nanoparticles bearing isoniazid for effective management of tuberculosis. J. Drug Target. 19: 219–227.

Satyajit, T. and D. Sabyasachi, P.C. Subhankari, K.S. Sumanta, P. Panchanan and R. Somenath. 2012. Synthesis, characterization of chitosan–tripolyphosphate conjugated chloroquine nanoparticle and its *in vivo* anti-malarial efficacy against rodent parasite: a dose and duration dependent approach. Int. J. Pharm. 434: 292–305.

Shargh, V.H. and M.R. Jaafari, A. Khamesipour, I. Jaafari, S.A. Jalali, A. Abbasi and A. Badiee. 2012. Liposomal SLA co-incorporated with PO CpG ODNs or PS CpG ODNs induce the same protection against the murine model of leishmaniasis. Vaccine. 30: 3957–3964.

Sharma, A. and S. Sharma and G.K. Khuller. 2004. Lectin functionalised poly(lactide-co-glycolide) nanoparticles as oral/aerosolized antitubercular drug carriers for treatment of tuberculosis. J. Antimicrob. Chemother. 54: 761–766.

Shuaibu, M.N. and M.S. Cherif, T. Kurosaki, G.K. Helegbe, M. Kikuchi, T. Yanagi, H. Sasaki and K. Hirayama. 2011. Effect of nanoparticle coating on the immunogenicity of plasmid DNA vaccine encoding P. yoelii MSP-1 C-terminal M.N. Vaccine. 29: 3239–3247.

Singh, K.K. and S.K. Vingkar. 2008. Formulation, antimalarial activity and biodistribution of oral lipid nanoemulsion of primaquine. Int. J. Pharm. 347: 136–143.

Sivak, O. and P. Gershkovich, M. Lin, E.K. Wasan, J. Zhao, D. Owen, J.G. Clement and K.M. Wasan. 2011. Tropically stable novel oral lipid formulation of amphotericin B (iCo-010): biodistribution and toxicity in a mouse model. Lipids Health Dis. 10: 135.

Solomon, M. and S. Baum, A. Barzilai, A. Scope, H. Trau and E. Schwartz. 2007. Liposomal amphotericin B in comparison to sodium stibogluconate for cutaneous infection due to Leishmania braziliensis. J. Am. Acad. Dermatol. 56: 612–616.

Sosnik, A. and A.M. Carcaboso, R.J. Glisoni, M.A. Moretton and D.A. Chiappetta. 2010. New old challenges in tuberculosis: potentially effective nanotechnologies in drug delivery. Adv. Drug Deliv. Rev. 62: 547–559.

Soto, J.M. and J.T. Toledo, P. Gutierrez, M. Arboleda, R.S. Nicholls, J.R. Padilla, J.D. Berman, C.K. English and M. Grogl. 2002. Treatment of cutaneous leishmaniasis with a topical antileishmanial drug (WR279396): phase 2 pilot study. Am. J. Trop. Med. Hyg. 66: 147–151.

Suárez, S. and P. O'Hara, M. Kazantseva, C.E. Newcomer, R. Hopfer, D.N. McMurray and A.J. Hickey. 2001. Respirable PLGA microspheres containing rifampicin for the treatment of tuberculosis: screening in an infectious disease model. Pharm. Res. 18: 1315–1319.

Tafaghodi, M. and M. Eskandari, M. Kharazizadeh, A. Khamesipour and M.R. Jaafari. 2010. Immunization against leishmaniasis by PLGA nanospheres loaded with an experimental autoclaved *Leishmania major* (ALM) and Quillaja saponins. Trop. Biomed. 27: 639–650.

Tafaghodi, M. and M. Eskandari, A. Khamesipour and M.R. Jaafari. 2011. Alginate microspheres encapsulated with autoclaved Leishmania major (ALM) and CpG-ODN induced partial protection and enhanced immune response against murine model of leishmaniasis. Exp. Parasitol. 129: 107–114.

Tempone, A.G. and R.A. Mortara, H.F. de Andrade, Jr. and J.Q. Reimão. 2010. Therapeutic evaluation of free and liposome-loaded furazolidone in experimental visceral leishmaniasis. Int. J. Antimicrob. Agents. 36: 159–163.

Tiwari, S. and A.K. Goyal, N. Mishra, K. Khatri, B. Vaidya, A. Mehta, Y. Wu and S.P. Vyas. 2009. Development and characterization of novel carrier gel core liposomes based transmission blocking malaria vaccine. J. Control. Release. 140: 157–165.

Tripathi, P. and V. Singh and S. Naik. 2007. Immune response to Leishmania: paradox rather than paradigm. Immunol. Med. Microbiol. 51: 229–242.

Tyagi, R.K. and N.K. Garg and T. Sahu. 2012. Vaccination strategies against Malaria: novel carrier(s) more than a tour de force. J. Control. Release. 162: 242–254.

Urbán, P. and J. Estelrich, A. Cortés and X. Fernàndez-Busquets. 2011. A nanovector with complete discrimination for targeted delivery to Plasmodium falciparum-infected versus non-infected red blood cells *in vitro*. J. Control. Release. 151: 202–211.

Vardy, D. and Y. Barenholz, N. Naftoliev, S. Klaus, L. Gilead and S. Frankenburg. 2001. Efficacious topical treatment for human cutaneous leishmaniasis with ethanolic lipid amphotericin B. Trans. R. Soc. Trop. Med. Hyg. 95: 184–186.

Vyas, S.P. and R.S. Jadon, A.K. Goyal, N. Mishra, P.N. Gupta, K. Khatri and R. Tyagi. 2007. pH sensitive liposomes enhances immunogenicity of 19 kDa carboxyl-terminal fragment of Plasmodium falciparum, Int. J. Pharm. Sci. Nanotech. 1: 78–86.

Wasan, E.K. and K. Bartlett, P. Gershkovich, O. Sivak, B. Banno, Z. Wong, J. Gagnon, B. Gates, C.G. Leon and K.M. Wasan. 2009a. Development and characterization of oral lipid-based amphotericin B formulations with enhanced drug solubility, stability and antifungal activity in rats infected with Aspergillus fumigatus or Candida albicans. Int. J. Pharm. 372: 76–84.

Wasan, K.M. and E.K. Wasan, P. Gershkovich, X. Zhu, R.R. Tidwell, K.A. Werbovetz, J.G. Clement and S.J. Thornton. 2009b. Highly effective oral Amphotericin B formulation against murine visceral leishmaniasis. J. Infect. Dis. 200: 357–360.

Wasan, E.K. and P. Gershkovich, J. Zhao, X. Zhu, K. Werbovetz, R.R. Tidwell, J.G. Clement, S.J. Thornton and K.M. Wasan. 2010. A novel tropically stable oral Amphotericin B formulation (iCo-010) exhibits efficacy against visceral Leishmaniasis in a murine model. PLoS Negl. Trop. Dis. 4: e913.

Wilson, K.D. and S.D. de Jong and Y.K. Tam. 2009. Lipid-based delivery of CpG oligonucleotides enhances immunotherapeutic efficacy. Adv. Drug Deliv. Rev. 61: 233–242.

Wortmann, G. and M. Zapor, R. Ressner, S. Fraser, J. Hartzell, J. Pierson, A. Weintrob and A. Magill. 2010. Liposomal amphotericin B for treatment of cutaneous leishmaniasis. Am. J. Trop. Med. Hyg. 83: 1028–1033.

Yardley, V. and S.L. Croft. 1999. *In vitro* and *in vivo* activity of amphotericin B-lipid formulations against experimental *Trypanosoma cruzi* infections. Am. J. Trop. Med. Hyg. 61: 193–197.

Yardley, V. and S.L. Croft. 2000. A comparison of the activities of three amphotericin B lipid formulations against experimental visceral and cutaneous leishmaniasis. Int. J. Antimicrob. Agents. 13: 243–248.

Yoshida, A. and M. Matumoto, H. Hshizume, Y. Oba, T. Tomishige, H. Inagawa, C. Kohchi, M. Hino, F. Ito, K. Tomoda, T. Nakajima, K. Makino, H. Terada, H. Hori and G. Soma. 2006. Selective delivery of rifampicin incorporated into poly(DL-lactic-co-glycolic) acid microspheres after phagocytotic uptake by alveolar macrophages, and the killing effect against intracellular Mycobacterium bovis Calmettee Guérin. Microbes Infect. 8: 2484–2491.

Yu, F. and J. Wang, J. Dou, H. Yang, X. He, W. Xu, Y. Zhang, K. Hu and N. Gu. 2012. Nanoparticle-based adjuvant for enhanced protective efficacy of DNA vaccine Ag85A-ESAT-6-IL-21 against Mycobacterium tuberculosis infection. Nanomedicine. 8: 1337–1344.

CHAPTER 14

Nanomedicines against Chronic Inflammatory Diseases

Mazen M. El-Hammadi[1,2,a] and *José L. Arias*[1,3,4,*]

ABSTRACT

Chronic inflammatory diseases are serious health conditions that can have a negative socioeconomic impact. Chronic inflammation normally requires extended periods of therapy which aims to ameliorate symptoms. Frequent and long-term dosing often causes serious adverse effects due to unselective drug availability. In view of this, there is an urgent need to develop new formulation approaches that can selectively deliver the active ingredient to the inflammation site thereby protecting healthy tissues. Nanoparticle-based drug delivery systems could represent a promising therapeutic strategy in the management of chronic inflammatory diseases. Due to their unique physical chemistry, nanocarriers can augment the efficacy and safety by protecting drugs against environmental degradation, increasing drug solubility, enhancing drug absorption, and sustaining drug release. More importantly, the enhanced permeability promotes selective accumulation of nanomedicines in the inflamed tissues. In addition, certain cell receptors are overexpressed during inflammatory response, which can be exploited for active drug targeting using nanocarriers. As a result, higher local drug concentrations are achieved, less amount of drug is required, and less frequent adverse effects are

[1] Department of Pharmacy and Pharmaceutical Technology, Faculty of Pharmacy, University of Granada, Campus Universitario de Cartuja s/n, 18071 Granada, Spain.
[a] Email: mazenhammadi@yahoo.co.uk
[2] Department of Pharmaceutics and Pharmaceutical Technology, Faculty of Pharmacy, Damascus University, Damascus, Syria.
[3] Institute of Biopathology and Regenerative Medicine (IBIMER), University of Granada, 18100 Granada, Spain.
[4] Biosanitary Institute of Granada (ibs.GRANADA), Andalusian Health Service (SAS) – University of Granada, 18012 Granada, Spain.
* Corresponding author: jlarias@ugr.es

encountered. The chapter presents potential applications of nanoparticulate drug delivery systems towards treatment of chronic inflammatory diseases. The focus is placed on nanotherapy advancements in four common chronic inflammatory diseases, i.e., arthritis, inflammatory bowel disease, chronic airway inflammation, and uveitis. Current challenges, particulate engineering innovations, and drug targeting opportunities in nanomedicines for these diseases are also discussed in detail.

Introduction

Inflammation is a protective response of the organism to harmful stimuli, such as pathogens, damaged cells, or irritants, as an attempt to remove the injurious stimuli and to heal tissue damage. Inflammation can be classified as either acute or chronic. Acute inflammation characterized by pain, redness, warmth, and swelling (tumor) is typically triggered by external stimuli. It is a short inflammatory response (only for hours to days) which recovers completely after treatment with anti-inflammatory agents and other therapies of the causing stimuli (e.g., antimicrobials for bacterial infection). On the other hand, chronic inflammation is a prolonged disorder that can take place without an external stimulus. It is often associated with a more serious condition, and an extended period of therapy is normally needed.

Traditionally, the objective of chronic inflammation therapy is to ameliorate the symptoms using Non-Steroidal Anti-Inflammatory Drugs (NSAIDs) and corticosteroids. However, these drugs alone do not possess the ability to target inflammation sites and, consequently, greater drug doses are normally required to produce efficient therapeutic response (Ulbrich and Lamprecht 2010). As a result, elevated drug concentrations may unspecifically accumulate in normal tissues leading to undesirable adverse reactions. Unfortunately, prolonged use of these therapeutics, which is the case in chronic inflammatory conditions, has been linked with high incidence rates of serious side effects such as cardiovascular disorders (myocardial infarction, stroke, hypertension), renal disorders (reduction in renal blood flow and glomerular filtration rate), hepatic disorders, bleeding, ulcers, skin bruising, weight gain, cataract, abdominal pain, bone thinning, bone marrow depression, diabetes, pain, and possible infection at injection location.

Nanoparticle (NP)-based Drug Delivery Systems (DDSs) are promising tools for chronic inflammation therapy. In general, these systems provide several substantial advantages including drug protection against environmental degradation, improved drug solubility, enhanced absorption, and sustained drug release. More importantly, nanomedicines can specifically accumulate at inflamed tissues due to an increased permeability at these tissues. Furthermore, certain cell receptors are overexpressed during inflammatory response, which can be exploited for active drug targeting using nanovehicles.

Herein we review recent achievements in NP-based DDSs for Chronic Inflammatory Diseases (CIDs). The chapter focuses on nanotherapy advancements in four common CIDs including arthritis (e.g., rheumatoid arthritis, RA, and osteoarthritis, OA), Inflammatory Bowel Diseases (IBDs) (e.g., Crohn's disease, CD, and Ulcerative Colitis, UC), Chronic Lung Inflammatory Diseases (CLIDs) (e.g., asthma and Chronic Obstructive Pulmonary Disease, COPD), and uveitis. Current challenges, particulate engineering innovations, and drug targeting opportunities in nanomedicines for CIDs are also discussed in detail.

Challenges against Nanotherapy in Chronic Inflammatory Diseases

Although remarkable progress has been achieved, several challenges still hinder the use of nanosystems in clinical treatment of CIDs. These challenges can be categorized as nanosystem-related and *in vivo* challenges.

Nanosystem-related challenges

Key functions of a nanovehicle are to retain the drug material and protect it from *in vitro* and *in vivo* degradation, enhance drug pharmacokinetics (minimize absorption variations, increase biological half-life, enhance localization at site of action, etc.), produce controlled drug release exclusively into the non-healthy site, and reduce the frequency and severity of drug side effects. While supplying the nanosystem with the above listed functions can be quite challenging, physical and chemical stability of the drug and the carrier, scaling-up, immunogenicity, and toxicity are also considered major challenges for the commercialization and clinical application of NP-based DDSs.

In vivo challenges

Challenges that a nanosystem can face in the living organism can be subdivided into extracellular and cellular. Extracellular challenges include route of administration, stability in biological media, biological half-life, and localization at the site of action. Upon *in vivo* administration, a nanosystem will be introduced to biological media with a variety of composition and pH conditions, such as gastrointestinal fluids, pulmonary mucus, blood, endosomal fluids, etc. These media can compromise drug/carrier stability and promote formation of aggregations as a consequence of random steric, electrostatic, or hydrophobic interactions with constituents of these fluids, e.g., proteins. When administered systemically, nanosystems with undesirable properties, such as large diameter, high net surface charge, and hydrophobic surface, will be subject to recognition and consequent capture by the reticuloendothelial system. It is mainly for this reason that local administration of anti-inflammatory nanosystems may be favorable and lead to more pronounced efficiency as observed in intra-articular injection in arthritis, oral and colonic administration in IBD, pulmonary delivery in lung inflammatory conditions, and topical application in uveitis.

Cellular challenges include NP-cell interaction, cellular uptake, and endosomal escape and intracellular trafficking. For internalization to take place it is necessary that the nanosystem is first interacted with the cell membrane surface. NP-cell interactions are mainly dictated by surface characteristics of the nanosystem including positive surface charge for electrostatic interaction with the negatively charged cell membrane and ligand functionalization for specific binding to membrane receptors. Interacted NPs are usually taken up by endocytosis, with the involvement of other mechanisms such as macropinocytosis (He et al. 2013). Following internalization, NPs and their therapeutic loads may undergo acidic and lysosomal enzyme degradation which can be avoided by endosomal escape.

Addressing nanosystem-related and *in vivo* challenges against NP delivery to inflammatory diseases requires sophisticated engineering of the DDS thanks to the development of numerous nanocarriers and to recent advances in surface functionalization techniques.

Nanosystem Engineering against Chronic Inflammatory Diseases

A distinctive aspect of nanosystems is their engineering flexibility which enables their fabrication with a broad spectrum of shape, size, and surface characteristics using a wide variety of polymer-based and/or lipid-based materials, and preparation techniques (Fig. 14.1). This versatility in NP design allows the control of pharmacokinetics properties including absorption, biodistribution, and elimination of the encapsulated drug, leading to improved drug efficiency and specificity.

Ideally, it is highly advantageous to obtain a nanosystem which exhibits a spherical shape, a small particle size (preferably < 200 nm), a relatively good hydrophilic character, and neutral surface electrical charge. Optimized properties ascertain that the nanosystem is physically and chemically stable in biological media, can overcome recognition by the reticuloendothelial system, and, subsequently, has longer biological half-life and less immunogenicity and toxicity effects.

Formulating materials

Selection of a nanocarrier forming material is usually performed based on a number of criteria including nanosystem stability, drug loading capacity, biodegradability and biocompatibility, and low/no toxicity or immunogenicity of the material and its degradation products. Materials utilized for the formulation of nanosystems against CIDs are classified into polymer and lipid materials.

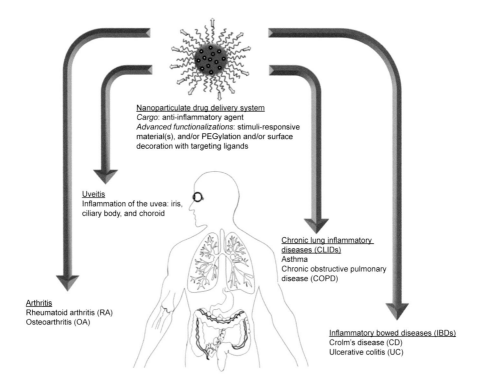

Figure 14.1. Drug-loaded nanocarrier and CIDs.

Polymers

Polymers are promising materials for the formulation of NP-based DDSs. They are very versatile, and characteristics of polymer NPs can be rather easily optimized based on the particular application thus allowing optimized drug vehiculization capabilities (maximum drug loading capacity and sustained drug release). A variety of methods can be employed to fabricate polymeric NPs: coacervation, interfacial polymer disposition, dialysis, solvent evaporation, salting-out, and emulsification techniques, to cite some illustrative examples. When selecting a suitable method of preparation several factors are considered, such as, particle size, particle size distribution, and area of application.

Although recent advances in polymer science have enabled the synthesis of numerous novel polymers, many of these exhibit high toxicity or require comprehensive toxicity studies to evaluate their suitability for biomedical applications. Among polymers suggested for the formulation of NP-based DDSs against CIDs, chitosan (CS), poly(D,L-lactide-*co*-glycolide) (PLGA), and poly(ε-caprolactone) (PCL) are the most extensively examined. The common properties of these polymers are biodegradability, biocompatibility, and low toxicity.

Lipids

Lipid-based nanocarriers are self-assembled macromolecular structures formed by spontaneous association of varieties of structural lipids in aqueous solution. Among various lipid-based nanosystems, liposomes, niosomes, and Solid Lipid Nanoparticles (SLNs) have been examined for CIDs therapy.

The classical and the most studied model of lipid-based nanovehicles are liposomes which consist of phospholipid bilayer(s) surrounding an aqueous cavity with a typical diameter of ≈ 100 nm. The general preparation method involves dissolving lipids in an organic solvent followed by solvent evaporation. The formed dry lipid film is then dispersed into an aqueous phase and liposomes are obtained by sonication, extrusion, or thin lipid film hydration. A major advantage of liposomes is that polar and apolar drugs can be entrapped either in the internal aqueous compartment or in the lipid bilayer(s), respectively.

Niosomes have been developed from self-assembly of non-ionic amphiphilic bilayer into a liposome-like vesicular system. They provide several advantages over liposomes, including larger stability, lower cost, and relative higher storage stability.

More recently, SLNs have been designed to minimize toxicity and increase stability of lipid-based nanosystems. SLNs are lipid crystal matrices which remain in solid form at physiological temperature. They are fabricated by melting and dispersing of lipids into nanodroplets often by solvent emulsification-evaporation or diffusion, high-using pressure homogenization, or microemulsification. These methods avoid the use of organic solvents and are easy for scaling-up.

Targeting strategies to chronic inflammatory diseases

Numerous changes are observed in inflamed tissues, compared with normal ones, including changes in angiogenesis, pH, temperature, and expression of receptors. A profound understanding of the microenvironment changes in inflammation can be exploited to improve selectivity and increase localization of NP-based DDSs at the inflammation site. Thus, drug nanocarriers with targeting ability have been developed by smart engineering of their characteristics including shape, size, composition, and surface functionalization. Here we will discuss strategies for developing nanostructures facilitating passive and/or active drug targeting.

Passive drug targeting

Passive targeting refers to strategies that exploit the inherent properties of the nanoparticulate system as well as the diseased tissue, without the attachment of a targeting ligand.

One strategy is to target macrophages, which play a critical role in the initiation and maintenance of inflammation (Ye et al. 2008, Howard et al. 2009, Lo et al. 2010, Ulbrich and Lamprecht 2010). When administered systemically, nanoparticulate systems with a hydrophobic surface and large diameter, more than 200 nm, are subject to adsorption of proteins, such as immunoglobulin G and fibrinogen, a process known as opsonization. As a result, opsonized nanosystems are rapidly taken up by macrophages, located in the liver (termed Küpffer cells) and the spleen. Thus, macrophage targeting can be particularly useful for targeting inflammation in these organs. It is noteworthy that efficient anti-inflammatory therapy of other tissues, such as the synovial in arthritis, may require local administration or other targeting strategies. This also applies to an inflamed intestine where oral and colonic administration of a nanosystem improves targeting of inflamed intestine and uptake by presenting macrophages (Lamprecht et al. 2001, Jubeh et al. 2004, Niebel et al. 2012, Valerii et al. 2013).

Inflamed tissues show significantly enhanced capillary permeability to macromolecules, which is beneficial for successful passive targeting of nanosystems to these tissues (Higaki et al. 2005). This enhanced accumulation can be further boosted by making particle surface more hydrophilic and neutral. This surface modification reduces opsonization in the circulation and leads to a remarkable increase in circulating half-life of the nanoparticulate system. Several hydrophilic polymers, such as poly(ethylene glycol) (PEG), poloxamers, poloxamines, or polysaccharides, can be physically or chemically attached onto the surface of the particle to form a protective hydrophilic neutral surface shell (Schroeder et al. 2008, Matsuo et al. 2009, Sakai et al. 2011, Prabhu et al. 2012). The resulting enhancement in NP accumulation in inflamed tissues is also accompanied by improved targeting of macrophages in these tissues. For instance, Ishihara et al. (2010) were able to show that PEGylated poly(D,L-lactide) (PLA) NPs first accumulated in the inflammatory lesion owing to the enhanced permeability and retention effect. As NPs lost their PEG segment at this stage, they were internalized by inflammatory macrophages, and finally the encapsulated drug was released in macrophages during polymer hydrolysis.

Active drug targeting

The term "active targeting" is used to describe drug delivery to a specific site based on molecular recognition, i.e., ligand-receptor interactions. For this purpose, a nanosystem can be surface functionalized with a targeting ligand that is able to bind to unique targeted molecules in the inflamed tissues. Active targeting ensures more specific activity of the drug at the pathology site and much less non-specific distribution to normal tissues. Based on their interactions with receptors overexpressed in inflamed tissues, a variety of biomolecules are useful for targeting of inflammation (Ulbrich and Lamprecht 2010, Clares et al. 2012). Examples include cell-adhesion molecules (P-selectin,

E-selectin, L-selectin), arginine-glycine-aspartic acid (RGD) peptides and integrins, folate moieties, and monoclonal antibodies (mAbs).

Several studies examined active targeting of arthritis using surface functionalized nanosystems. To study the effect of dextran sulfate as a ligand for targeting macrophage, Kim et al. (2013) synthesized an amphiphilic block copolymer using dextran sulfate as a hydrophilic block and PCL as a hydrophobic block. On systemic administration into Collagen-Induced Arthritis (CIA) mice, the self-assembled NPs showed selective accumulation into the inflamed synovia. This inflammatory joint-targeting behavior resulted primarily from binding to the macrophage scavenger receptors (scavenger receptor class A) that were overexpressed in the synovia of CIA mice. Similarly, intravenously administered sialyl-Lewis X (sLex)-conjugated liposomes were able to target activated endothelial cells in mice arthritic joints and were detected within the phagosomes of synovial macrophages (Maehara et al. 2014). Zhou et al. (2012) employed $\alpha_v\beta_3$ integrin antagonist for targeting angiogenic endothelium overexpressing $\alpha_v\beta_3$ integrin in inflammatory arthritis. The perfluorooctylbromide-based NPs loaded with a lipase-labile prodrug of fumagillin, a mycotoxin produced by *Aspergillus fumagatus* with antiangiogenic effect, were surface decorated with $\alpha_v\beta_3$ integrin antagonist conjugated to PEG_{2000}-phosphatidylethanolamine. Biodistribution studies demonstrated that $\alpha_v\beta_3$-functionalized NPs accumulated mainly in the small blood vessel wall in the arthritic paw of a KRN serum-mediated inflammatory arthritis mouse model. In addition, the targeted nanosystem efficiently suppressed the clinical disease indices as compared with control NPs. In another study, the expression of the folate receptor in synovial mononuclear cells and CD14+ cells in patients with RA was also exploited for targeting joint inflammation. Interleukin (IL)-1 receptor antagonist gene-loaded folate-CS NPs showed low cytotoxicity and protective bone effects in arthritic rats. Moreover, the nanotherapy was accompanied with an increased IL-1 receptor antagonist protein synthesis and decreased expression levels of IL-1β and prostaglandin E2 (Fernandes et al. 2008).

The inflamed intestine was also the target of several ligand-functionalized drug nanocarriers after local or systemic administration. In an example, Coco and co-workers (2013) demonstrated that active targeting using mannose (for targeting immune cells) or a specific peptide (for targeting inflamed colon) grafted NPs improves accumulation of the loaded drug in the site of action (Coco et al. 2013). Peer et al. (2008) used a mAb against $\beta7$ integrins to provide CyD1-small interfering ribonucleic acid (*si*RNA)-loaded liposomes with inflamed intestine targeting function. Following intravenous administration of the silencing system in mice with dextran sodium sulfate-induced colitis, colitis was successfully reversed by suppressing leukocyte proliferation and T-helper cell type 1 cytokine expression. In another study, a galactosylated NP was produced using CS-cysteine conjugate and encapsulated with a *si*RNA to suppress Tumor Necrosis Factor-alpha (TNF-α) production in macrophages. Owing to galactose receptor-mediated endocytosis, the promoted uptake by activated macrophages resulted in enhanced localization in the inflamed colon after oral administration of the targeted gene system (Zhang et al. 2013).

Although eye targeting by systematic administration is difficult due to the blood-retinal barrier, Hashida et al. (2008) reported specific targeting of inflamed eyes using sLex-conjugated liposomes loaded with dexamethasone (DEX). The intravenously injected liposomes accumulated in the inflamed lesions due to interaction with E-selectin and P-selectin on the activated endothelial cells. Finally, the interaction between Hyaluronic Acid (HA) and the CD44 receptor was also useful in targeting CD44-positive retinal pigment epithelium cells using intravitreal injected HA-modified NPs (Gan et al. 2013).

Alternatively, the conceptualization of stimuli-responsive drug nanovehicles is based on drug release at a suitable rate in response to stimuli. Thus, materials that reverse their physical properties (e.g., disruption/ aggregation, swelling/de-swelling) in response to a specific external stimulus can be used to formulate stimuli-responsive nanosystems. Environmentally-sensitive anti-inflammation nanosystems have the ability to release their therapeutic cargo exclusively into the inflamed tissues (acid-, thermosensitive-, light-, ultrasound-, or enzyme-triggered drug release) or to enhance accumulation at the inflamed site (e.g., magnetically responsive NPs).

Light-triggered nanosystems contain photosensitive bonds which release their encapsulated drug by exposure to various exciting light waves. For example, light-sensitive liposomes can be prepared from photofragmentation components. This concept was tested by Banerjee and Chen (2009) who prepared a DEX-NP conjugate using a photosensitive linker. Upon exposure to near-infrared radiation, the linker was cleaved triggering DEX release from the ultra-small nanoassemblies ($\approx$ 13 nm in size) (Banerjee and Chen 2009).

Enzyme-responsive nanosystems can be formulated to retain the loaded drug while circulating in the body and to deliver it at the target site due to cleavage by specifically overregulated enzymes at this site. This can be achieved by synthesizing an enzyme-cleaved drug-nanocarrier conjugate. An example is the PEGylated (PEG surface functionalized) ibuprofen-polyamidoamine dendrimer conjugate which was synthesized to trigger drug release when specifically cleaved by esterase (Kurtoglu et al. 2010). In addition, several enzyme-triggered liposomal systems have been developed with susceptibility to endogenous enzymes, e.g., secretory phospholipase A2, elastase, sphingomyelinase, phospholipase C, alkaline phosphatase, or transglutaminase.

A pH-sensitive nanosystem is designed to deliver its cargo at a particular pH environment, while the integrity of the system is maintained at other pH values. For this purpose, nanovehicles that are stable at physiological pH (pH 7.4) but degrade and release the loaded drug under acidic conditions, such as NPs formulated using poly(N-vinylpyrrolidone-co-dimethylmaleic anhydride) and poly(β-benzyl-L-aspartate)-b-poly(N-vinylpyrrolidone) diblock copolymer, have been developed (Wang et al. 2009a). Similar results can be achieved using NPs formulated using drug-polymer conjugates with a pH-sensitive linker. For example, Hornig et al. (2009) prepared self-assembled NPs using ibuprofen- and naproxen-dextran conjugates. Drug release from these NPs was pH-dependent and influenced by the degree of substitution.

Conversely, drug delivery to inflamed colon requires a nanovehicle that retains the encapsulated drug in the acidic stomach pH, however as the nanosystem travels to the colonic neutral environment drug release is triggered. Several mechanisms can be employed to trigger drug release at colonic pH. One mechanism is pH-dependant dissolution, e.g., NPs formulated using Eudragit® S100 are insoluble in acidic pH but dissolve at pH > 7 (Coco et al. 2013). Another mechanism is electrostatic repulsion, as observed in mesoporous silica NPs in which silanol groups are deprotonated in pH 7.4 forcing a loaded anionic drug, e.g., sulfasalazine, to be released (Lee et al. 2008).

Thermosensitive nanosystems can be prepared using temperature-sensitive polymers which show a remarkable change in their hydration degree below and above their Low Critical Solution Temperature (LCST). For example, NPs based on the thermosensitive polymer poly(N-isopropylacrylamide), which has a LCST between 31°C and 33°C, loaded with the cell-penetrating anti-inflammatory KAFAK peptide can selectively and effectively suppress proinflammatory cytokines TNF-α and IL-6 within inflamed bovine knee cartilage explants (Bartlett et al. 2013).

Using a magnetic gradient, a nanosystem with a magnetic core (generally an iron oxide: magnetite, or maghemite) is forced to accumulate and remain at a target site until complete drug release is achieved. For this purpose, Arias et al. (2009) developed diclofenac sodium-loaded magnetic nanocomposites consisting of magnetic cores (iron) embedded within an ethylcellulose matrix with high drug loading efficiency and prolonged drug release. It was speculated that this system can be useful for efficient delivery of the NSAID to inflammation sites.

Nanosystems which combine several targeting and stimuli-responsive drug delivery strategies have emerged as tools for efficient anti-inflammation therapy. In this line, Lee et al. (2013) produced PEGylated PLGA NPs loaded with methotrexate (MTX). The NP was designed to contain a gold half-shell, for photothermally controlled drug release, which was surface decorated with RGD peptide, a targeting moiety for inflammation. When administered systemically to CIA mice and upon exposure to near-infrared irradiation, the NP with multi-targeting strategies exhibited superior therapeutic efficacy at a much smaller drug dose, as compared with a free MTX solution.

A number of multi-targeting strategies gene delivery nanosystems with anti-inflammation effects have been recently engineered. For example, He et al. (2013) developed mannose-modified trimethyl CS-cysteine conjugate-based NPs for oral administration of TNF-α siRNA. At the complexation level, the positive charge of the trimethyl and thiol groups in the NPs provides efficient condensation of siRNA. When the NPs with multi-targeting strategies are administered orally, the trimethyl groups allows electrostatic interactions with negatively charged components in epithelial mucosa, while the cysteine residues can form disulfide bonding with mucin glycoproteins in the mucosa, which improves intestinal mucoadhesion of CS to promote permeation. In addition, the mannose moieties enhance the intestinal permeation by enabling active targeting of NPs toward M cells that express mannose receptors. Consequently, the NPs effectively suppressed macrophageal TNF-α production in mice with acute hepatic injury. Likewise, a mannosylated bioreducible cationic polymer was used to prepare NPs loaded with TNF-α *si*RNA, with the assistance of sodium tripolyphosphate, for IBD therapy. The reducible polymer was synthesized by conjugation of cystamine bisacrylamide and branched polyethyleneimine (PEI), and further coupled with mannose. The resulting non-toxic NPs with multi-targeting strategies demonstrated enhanced cellular uptake by macrophages, due to receptor-mediated endocytosis, and reduction-triggered release of *si*RNA to the cytoplasm (Xiao et al. 2013).

Advances in Nanomedicines against Chronic Inflammatory Diseases

Arthritis

Arthritis is a serious health problem that involves inflammation of one or more joints. It is the most common cause of disability in the United Stated of America. Chronic arthritis is characterized by a progressive joint degeneration and severe pain. Among a range of inflammatory disorders, the two most common forms of chronic arthritis are RA, a systemic autoimmune form of inflammation, and OA, also known as degenerative joint disease, the most frequent cause of pain, loss of function, and disability in adults. The pathophysiologic cause of arthritis is still unclear. Nonetheless, it is well-established that chronic inflammation and immune response as well as trauma, infection, and age all contribute to the development of the degenerative joint disease.

A complete recovery from arthritis is still far from realization. Current strategies for treating arthritis focus on improving quality of life by minimizing pain and local inflammation and decelerating the progressive joint damage. Medicinal groups used in arthritis management include NSAIDs, corticosteroids, and disease-modifying antirheumatic drugs (DMARDs) such as MTX, actarit, and anti-TNF-α mAbs such as infliximab and adalimumab.

Because of the chronic nature of the disease, efficient drug therapy of arthritis necessitates the development of a selective DDS to boost therapeutic effects and reduce side effects. For this purpose, anti-arthritic NP-based systems can be useful tools for arthritis management (Table 14.1) (Arias et al. 2009, Arias 2010, Ulbrich and Lamprecht 2010).

Several NSAID-loaded NPs have been recently developed and examined. For instance, Arias et al. (2010) proposed PCL-based NPs for prolonged release of diclofenac sodium. The NSAID-loaded NPs, produced following an interfacial polymer disposition method, exhibited a diameter of ≈ 200 nm, drug

Table 14.1. NP-based DDSs for arthritis.

NP-based carrier	Drug	Size (nm)	Route of administration	Targeting/Stimuli-responsive strategy	Reference
PCL	Diclofenac sodium	≈ 200	No *in vivo* studies	–	Arias et al. 2010
Dextran sulfate-PCL	–	≈ 200	Intravenous	Ligand-receptor targeting of macrophages: dextran	Kim et al. 2013
PLGA	Betamethasone sodium phosphate	≈ 100–200	Intravenous	–	Higaki et al. 2005
	Glucosamine	≈ 75	No *in vivo* studies	–	Marimuthu et al. 2013
Gold-PLGA	MTX	≈ 100–115	Intravenous	PEGylation, photothermally-triggered drug release (gold half-shell), thermosensitive drug release, ligand-receptor targeting (RGD peptide)	Lee et al. 2013
CS	IL-1 receptor antagonist gene or IL-10	Not indicated	Intra-articular	–	Zhang et al. 2006
	Anti-TNF-α DsiRNA	≈ 350–450	Intraperitoneal	–	Howard et al. 2009
	IL-1 receptor antagonist gene	≈ 110	Intravenous	–	Fernandes et al. 2008
Perfluorooctylbromide	Fumagillin prodrug	≈ 230–260	Intravenous	PEGylation, ligand-receptor targeting of angiogenic endothelium (α$_v$β$_3$-integrin antagonist)	Zhou et al. 2012
poly(N-isopropylacrylamide)	KAFAK peptide	≈ 100–400	No *in vivo* studies	Thermosensitive drug release	Bartlett et al. 2013
Iron/ethylcellulose (core/shell)	Diclofenac sodium	≈ 430	No *in vivo* studies	Magnetic responsiveness	Arias et al. 2009

Table 14.1. contd....

Table 14.1. contd.

NP-based carrier	Drug	Size (nm)	Route of administration	Targeting/Stimuli-responsive strategy	Reference
Liposome	MTX	≈ 210–260	Intravenous	PEGylation	Prabhu et al. 2012
	Diclofenac sodium	Not indicated	Intra-articular	–	Turker et al. 2008
sLex-conjugated liposome	–	Not indicated	Intravenous	Ligand-receptor targeting of endothelial cells: sLex	Maehara et al. 2014
Ethosome	Tetrandrine	≈ 80	No *in vivo* studies	–	Fan et al. 2013
SLN	Actarit	≈ 240	Intravenous	Passive targeting of macrophages in the spleen	Ye et al. 2008
	Celecoxib	Not indicated	Intra-articular	–	Thakkar et al. 2007
	TwHF	≈ 100	Intra-articular	–	Xue et al. 2012

entrapment efficiency ≈ 45%, and drug loading ≈ 20%. More importantly, the NPs produced burst effect in the first two hours (≈ 40% drug release), which was followed by a sustained drug release profile over the subsequent 94 hours. In another report, an intra-articular injected liposome-based nanosystem was shown to significantly improve the anti-inflammatory effect of diclofenac sodium in RA (Turker et al. 2008).

Celecoxib was also investigated as a candidate drug for NP-based anti-arthritic therapy. The selective cyclooxygenase 2 inhibitor NSAID has been incorporated into SLNs (Thakkar et al. 2007), niosomes (Kaur et al. 2007), and liposomes (Dong et al. 2013). Enhanced sustained drug release properties and greater intra-articular retention was reported when these nanosystems were administered as injectable gel (Kaur et al. 2007, Dong et al. 2013). For example, after a single intra-articular injection in a rabbit knee OA model, celecoxib-loaded liposomes (embedded in a HA gel) were more effective than free drug in pain control and cartilage protection (Dong et al. 2013).

Among corticosteroids, betamethasone sodium phosphate was loaded into PLGA NPs, with diameter ≈ 100–200 nm. When administered intravenously to rats with adjuvant arthritis and to mice with anti-type II collagen antibody induced arthritis, betamethasone-loaded NPs reduced paw inflammation over seven days. This improved anti-arthritic effect provided evidence for selective inflammation targeting and sustained drug release by the nanomedicine (Higaki et al. 2005).

DMARDs represented by MTX and actarit have also been under focus of nanotechnology-based arthritis therapy. When administered intravenously to the rabbit and mouse models, actarit-loaded into SLNs resulted in prolonged mean retention time (from ≈ 1 to ≈ 14 hours), greater bioavailability, enhanced localization in the spleen from ≈ 6–16%, and reduced renal distribution (and, thus, decreased nephrotoxicity) compared to actarit solution (Ye et al. 2008). In addition, Prabhu et al. (2012) explored the effect of PEGylated liposomes on MTX efficacy. While prolonged drug release profile was observed *in vitro*, the stealth lipid vesicles significantly reduced edema volume after intravenous injection to rats with induced RA. The *in vivo* anti-rheumatoid effects were higher than that produced by MTX-loaded conventional liposomes coated with CS.

As a chronic disease, arthritis can be a good candidate for gene therapy. In this context, two studies reported the use of CS-based NPs as gene nanotherapy of arthritis. In one study, IL-1 receptor antagonist gene-loaded CS NPs were injected into the knee joint cavities of OA rabbits. The gene nanosystems produced measurable levels of IL-1 receptor antagonist leading to reduced severity of histological cartilage lesions (Zhang et al. 2006). In the second study, anti-TNF-*α* Dicer-substrate *si*RNA (D*si*RNA)-loaded CS NPs were tested for their ability to delay the onset of arthritis in CIA mice. *si*RNA-CS NPs injected intraperitoneally resulted in efficient TNF-*α*-induced inflammatory response down-regulation and joint swelling prevention. Only minimal cartilage destruction and inflammatory cell infiltration was observed in joints of treated animals (Howard et al. 2009).

Due to low patient compliance associated with parenteral route and in search for a more convenient administration method, the potential of transdermal route for anti-arthritic nanomedicines delivery has been examined (Fan et al. 2013, Marimuthu et al. 2013). For example, self-assembled PLGA-conjugated glucosamine NPs enhanced *ex vivo* drug transdermal permeation through human skin (Marimuthu et al. 2013). In addition, the oral administration of SLNs loaded with *Tripterygium wilfordii Hook F* (TwHF), a traditional Chinese herb with anti-inflammatory and immunosuppressive effects, has also been investigated. When administered to rats with adjuvant-induced arthritis, drug-loaded SLNs demonstrated greater anti-inflammatory effects as compared to free drug (Xue et al. 2012).

Preclinical studies of arthritis nanotherapy have shown encouraging results. Various therapeutic strategies and routes of administration using anti-arthritic nanomedicines have shown promise. However, the introduction of these systems to the clinic is awaiting feasibility studies, and clinical efficacy and safety data.

Inflammatory bowel diseases

IBDs are relapsing and remitting chronic inflammatory disorders of the gastrointestinal tract. IBDs are characterized by the development of intestinal inflammation which results from the transmural infiltration of neutrophils, macrophages, lymphocytes, and mast cells, eventually leading to mucosal disruption and ulceration. These disorders have relatively high incidence rates in western countries ranging from 0.1 to 0.15% of population. The two major forms of IBDs are CD and UC.

CD and UC share several similar symptoms including diarrhea, rectal bleeding, anemia, nausea, weight loss, abdominal spasms, fever, and fatigue. However, they show several differences in their pathogenesis and the typical clinical manifestations. In CD, the inflammation is transmural, extending through the bowel wall to the serosal layer, and may occur anywhere along the digestive tract from the mouth to the anus. Whereas in UC, the innermost mucosa is completely inflamed and the colon and rectum are typically the only sites that are affected. Based on the inflamed region of the gastrointestinal tract, drug delivery strategies in the treatment of CD and UC can be challenging and quite different. To achieve efficient drug administration it is preferred to use the rectal route in UC and the oral route in CD.

The common therapeutic agents of IBD include aminosalicylates, especially 5-aminosalicylic acid (5-ASA), corticosteroids, and immunosuppressive. Several drug delivery strategies to target inflamed tissues in IBDs, such as sustained drug release devices, pH-sensitive formulations, and prodrugs, have been developed. However, these approaches are not completely efficient and have many drawbacks including ineffective control of drug release, therapeutic variation owing to IBD symptoms (such as diarrhea, modified colonic environment), and difficulties to target inflamed areas (Moulari et al. 2013). Furthermore, the enhanced permeability in the intact non-inflamed tissues of the upper intestinal tract in patients with IBD may lead to serious adverse effects (Teahon et al. 1996, Bruewer et al. 2003).

NP-based DDSs offer a new strategy for targeting IBD due to the ability to selectively accumulate in the intestinal inflamed regions (Table 14.2). This effect of oral nanomedicines is a consequence of several pathophysiological modifications associated with intestinal inflammation, e.g., disruption of the intestinal barrier, increased mucus production, and enhanced uptake initiated by immune-related cells, including macrophages and dendritic cells, presenting in high levels at the inflamed tissues (Lamprecht et al. 2001). In addition, unlike conventional dosage forms such as tablets and capsules, NP-based drug delivery is not influenced by diarrhea, the most frequent symptom of IBD.

Many experimental animal models have been used to study human IBD. One of the most studied models is the mouse with dextran sodium sulfate-induced acute and chronic UC. This animal model is characterized by remarkable body weight loss, rectal bleeding, colon length reduction, and intestinal epithelium destruction.

The potential of NP-based DDSs for enhanced IBD therapy was first explored by Lamprecht et al. (2001). This research group examined the influence of particle size on accumulation using polystyrene beads. Following oral application in rats with induced UC, fluorescent polystyrene particles with diameters of 0.1, 1, or 10 μm resulted in size-dependent deposition. Smaller NPs (≈ 100 nm in diameter) accumulated considerably more in the inflamed than in non-inflamed regions of the intestinal mucosa. This effect was reduced with 1 μm-sized particles, and there was very little effect by the 10 μm-sized particles. Unfortunately, these encouraging findings in small animal models were not in agreement with clinical findings in human patients. A recent study in human IBD patients demonstrated practically no accumulation of NPs (mean size ≈ 250 nm) in the inflamed mucosa, whereas deposition of microparticles (3 μm-sized) in ulcerous lesions was clearly observed, after rectal administration. Using chamber studies revealed that microparticles adhered to the ulcerated tissue were not absorbed across the epithelial barrier. On the other hand, enhanced translocation of NPs was observed, possibly leading to undesirable systemic absorption. This data may provide an explanation for the enhanced disposition of larger particles in inflamed mucosa (Schmidt et al. 2013). Similar findings were obtained with PLGA NPs (300 nm in size) and microparticles (3 μm-sized) (Lautenschlager et al. 2013).

These studies importantly indicate that the use of NPs alone may not meet expected outcomes of IBD therapy in human patients. One strategy to improve the therapeutic efficiency is to incorporate drug-loaded NPs into a carrier with an ability to adhere to inflamed tissues providing a sustained release of the incorporated particles. For this purpose, a polysaccharide hydrogel

Table 14.2. NP-based DDSs for IBDs.

NP-based carrier	Drug	Size (nm)	Route of administration	Targeting/Stimuli-responsive strategy	Reference
PLA	Lysine-proline-valine (KPV)	≈ 400	Oral	NP incorporation into a pH sensitive alginate-CS hydrogel	Laroui et al. 2010
	Prohibitin 1	≈ 450	Oral	–	Theiss et al. 2011
	TNF-α siRNA	≈ 380	Oral	–	Laroui et al. 2011
	CD98 siRNA	≈ 480	Oral	–	Laroui et al. 2014
PLGA/Eudragit® P-4135F	Tacrolimus	≈ 450	Oral	pH-sensitive drug release	Meissner et al. 2006
PLGA	Tacrolimus	≈ 100	Oral/rectal	–	Lamprecht et al. 2005
PCL	5-ASA	≈ 200–350	Oral	Sustained drug release: drug-polymer conjugate	Pertuit et al. 2007
Silica	5-ASA	≈ 140	Oral	Sustained drug release: drug-silica	Moulari et al. 2008
Mesoporous silica	Sulfasalazine	≈ 100	No *in vivo* studies	pH-responsive drug release	Lee et al. 2008
Eudragit® RL	Clodronate	≈ 120	Rectal	–	Niebel et al. 2012
Ethylcellulose	Betamethasone	≈ 200	Rectal	–	Wachsmann et al. 2013
Polystyrene-*b*-poly(methylacrylate) micelle	Prednisone	≈ 25	No *in vivo* studies	–	Valerii et al. 2013
Mannose-PEG-poly(cystamine bisacrylamide-*b*-branched PEI)	TNF-α siRNA	≈ 200–275	No *in vivo* studies	Ligand-receptor targeting: mannose, reduction-triggered drug release, PEGylation	Xiao et al. 2013

Galactosylated trimethyl CS-cysteine	*siRNA* of mitogen-activated protein kinase kinase kinase 4 (Map4k4)	≈ 150	Oral	Ligand-receptor targeting: galactose	Zhang et al. 2013
Eudragit® S100/trimethyl CS/a mix of PLGA, PEG-PLGA and PEG-PCL	–	≈ 200–600	No *in vivo* studies	pH-responsiveness (Eudragit® S100), PEGylation, ligand-receptor targeting (mannose or specific peptides)	Coco et al. 2013
Liposome	CyD1 *siRNA*	≈ 100	Intravenous	Ligand-receptor targeting: mAb against β7 integrins	Peer et al. 2008
	Nov038	≈ 150	Intravenous	–	Arranz et al. 2013
Nanostructured lipid carrier	Budesonide	≈ 200	Oral	–	Beloqui et al. 2013

system based on alginate and CS (1:1 molar ratio), which collapses at colonic pH (pH 5–6), have been suggested (Laroui et al. 2010, Theiss et al. 2011). The concept is based on the formation of *in situ* NPs encapsulating hydrogel in the animal stomach. To achieve this, an alginate-CS solution containing NPs is administered first, followed by a chelation solution containing calcium chloride and sodium sulfate. This approach was tested using anti-inflammatory agent (peptide KPV/protein prohibitin 1)-loaded PLA NPs in mice with dextran sodium sulfate-induced colitis (Laroui et al. 2010, Theiss et al. 2011). Oral administration of the NPs-hydrogel formulations significantly increased drug levels in inflammatory region and reduced inflammation severity. Moreover, the effective KPV dose in the NP formulation (≈ 25 ng/d) was 12,000 times lower than free drug solution (200 µg/d) (Laroui et al. 2010).

Effects of surface electrical charge, another important NP characteristic, on IBD therapy have also been under investigation. When applied intrarectally to colitis-induced rats, anionic liposomes showed improved adherence to inflamed colonic mucosa, which was twice more than neutral or cationic liposomes. In contrast, cationic liposomes adhered significantly to healthy colonic mucosa and their adherence was three times greater than neutral or anionic liposomes. The overexpression of the positively charged protein transferrin in ulcerated colonic tissues may explain the enhanced adherence of negatively charged liposomes to these tissues (Jubeh et al. 2004). On the other hand, positively charged Eudragit® RL-based NPs (diameter ≈ 120 nm, zeta potential ≈ 50 mV) were also demonstrated to improve anti-inflammatory efficiency by promoting macrophage uptake upon rectal administration in mice models of colitis (Niebel et al. 2012). While these studies show significant influence of particle surface charge on interaction of locally administered NPs with inflamed regions, oral administration may show less pronounced effect. Possible unspecific interaction with healthy mucous throughout the intestinal tube may impede NP transport to the inflamed sites.

The choice of surfactant in NP formulation is of significant importance with regard to targeting efficiency in IBD. Wachsmann et al. (2013) studied the effects of surface properties on the accumulation selectivity and intensity of non-degradable ethylcellulose nanospheres after rectal administration in a murine colitis model. The NPs (≈ 200 nm in size) were obtained by the emulsification solvent evaporation technique using a number of charged and non-charged surfactants (polysorbate 20, sodium dodecyl sulphate, sodium cholate, cetyltrimethylammonium bromide, polyvinyl alcohol). NPs prepared with polysorbate 20 as surfactant showed the highest selectivity and resulted in a ≈ 35-fold higher particle content in the inflamed regions of the colon compared to healthy animals, and led to ≈ 4.5-fold higher particle content in the inflamed regions as compared to particles formulated with sodium dodecyl sulphate. These observations were translated into a considerably higher therapeutic efficiency when NPs were loaded with betamethasone. Polysorbate 20 NPs were more effective in reducing myeloperoxidase activity levels in inflamed tissues as compared to cetyltrimethylammonium bromide or sodium dodecyl sulphate NPs.

Interestingly, variations in IBD targeting efficiency among different animal species have also been reported. When administered orally to colitis-induced mice, PLGA and Eudragit® P-4135F NPs encapsulating tacrolimus, an immune-suppressant agent with nephrotoxic effects, demonstrated an increased effect in mitigating the inflammation in comparison with drug solution (Meissner et al. 2006). However, oral administration of tacrolimus PLGA NPs to colitis-induced rats did not enhance the therapeutic efficiency. Nonetheless, rectal application of these NPs improved selective drug accumulation into the inflamed regions in the rat model (Lamprecht et al. 2005). Several factors can be suggested for these different observations between mice and rats. The longer intestinal tract in rats, as compared to mice, means that orally administered nanosystems will have to travel a longer passage to reach the inflamed regions. As a consequence, the efficiency of these systems may be weakened by a number of causes such as degradation by digestive enzymes and uptake by Peyer's patches. Another factor to be considered is the particle diameter difference in these two reports. While NPs administered to rats had a diameter of ≈ 100 nm, those administered to mice were ≈ 450 nm in diameter.

To further improve therapeutic efficiency and selectivity of IBD, several new nanocarriers have been developed and investigated. NPs obtained using drug-polymer conjugates of 5-ASA covalently bound to PCL (Pertuit et al. 2007) or silica (Moulari et al. 2008) produced selective accumulation in the inflamed tissues. In addition, polymeric micelles prepared by self-assembly of polystyrene-poly(methylacrylate) block copolymer significantly improved the efficacy of anti-inflammatory and anticancer compounds to colonocytes and colon mucosa (Valerii et al. 2013). Moreover, nanostructured lipid carriers loaded with budesonide and fabricated by high-pressure homogenization significantly increased the efficacy of the corticosteroid in a murine model of colitis (Beloqui et al. 2013).

IBD gene therapy using *si*RNA strategy has been under assessment. TNF-*α si*RNA was complexed with PEI and then loaded into PLA NPs. Upon oral administration to lipopolysaccharide-treated mice, NPs encapsulated into a hydrogel system, comprised of alginate and CS (as described above), were efficiently taken up by inflamed macrophages resulting in specific reduction of TNF-*α* expression/secretion in colonic tissues (Laroui et al. 2011). A similar PLA-based NPs and alginate-CS hydrogel combined system was used to deliver a *si*RNA of CD98, a cell-surface amino acid with important roles in controlling homeostatic and innate immune responses in the gut, via the oral route to the mouse model of colitis. As a result, CD98 expression in colonic tissues was decreased leading to reduced colitis (Laroui et al. 2014). The successful application of TNF-*α si*RNA for IBD therapy was also reported using multi-targeting strategies NPs prepared from a mannosylated bioreducible cationic polymer (Xiao et al. 2013). Zhang et al. (2013) developed galactosylated trimethyl CS-cysteine NPs containing a *si*RNA of Map4k4, a key upstream mediator of TNF-α action. The NPs, produced by ionic gelation of galactosylated trimethyl CS-cysteine with tripolyphosphate or HA and delivered orally to mice with colitis, showed efficient localization of *si*RNA in the colon, thereby inhibiting TNF-α production. Active targeting of *si*RNA to inflamed intestines by intravenous injection into mice was also reported. This approach was achieved using liposomes surface decorated with a mAbs against β7 integrins, which are highly expressed in gut mononuclear leukocytes, and encapsulated with a *si*RNA of CyD1, a pivotal cell cycle-regulatory molecule that is up-regulated at inflammation regions in IBD (Peer et al. 2008).

A variety of stimuli-responsive strategies have been introduced for enhanced efficiency of IBD therapy. For example, Lee et al. (2008) suggested a pH-sensitive system based on mesoporous silica NPs for controllable release of anionic drugs in the intestines. At pH similar to that of the stomach (pH 2–5), the positively charged mesoporous silica NPs were able to load and retain sulfasalazine, an anionic anti-inflammatory prodrug used for IBD. However, at intestinal pH (pH 7.4) the deprotonated silanol groups produced a partial negative charge triggering a sustained release of the loaded negative drug, due to electrostatic repulsion. The same concept was adapted by Arranz et al. (2013) who developed an amphoteric liposomal system which is cationic at low pH values, to facilitate efficient drug loading, but becomes anionic at physiological conditions, to enhance uptake by macrophages and dendritic cells in inflamed intestinal regions.

The wide range of colon-specific delivery strategies available provides flexibility for NP formulation. Coco et al. (2013) compared several NP-based targeting strategies of IBD using Eudragit® S100, for pH-responsiveness (dissolves when pH > 7), trimethyl CS, for mucoadhesion, a mix of PLGA, PEG-PLGA, and PEG-PCL, for sustained drug delivery, or NPs surface functionalized with mannose (for targeting immune cells) or specific peptides (for targeting the inflamed colon), for ligand-receptor targeting. The study revealed that mannose-grafted NPs produced the greatest particle accumulation in the inflamed colon.

The remarkable success of oral nanotherapy in IBD small animal models still lack ability for translation into clinical use. Despite failing to cure human IBD, there is evidence of efficiency when nanosystems are applied on human samples. For example, butyrate and DEX-loaded SLNs were shown to effectively reduce cytokine production in human peripheral blood mononuclear cells (Serpe et al. 2010). These findings indicate the necessity to optimize nanosystems to be suitable for human oral drug delivery in IBD. Barriers posed by human gastrointestinal tract and species variation concerning intestinal surface area, lumen conditions, and mucosal physiology are issues to be addressed.

Chronic lung inflammatory diseases

CLIDs are serious global public health problems characterized by chronic airway inflammation and various degrees of airflow limitation and tissue remodeling. CLIDs are a group of diseases among which asthma and COPD are the most common. The two pulmonary disorders have clearly distinct characteristics. Asthma develops in childhood, is associated with allergies and eosinophils, and its inflammation involves all airways apart from the lung parenchyma. In contrast, COPD occurs in adults, is generally caused by tobacco smoke, involves neutrophils, affects the peripheral airways (bronchioles) and lung parenchyma, and is characterized by progressive decline in lung function (Barnes et al. 2003, Kim and Rhee 2010).

Inflammation plays an important role in the progress of lung inflammatory diseases. It contributes to mucous hypersecretion and bronchial epithelium damage. Furthermore, together with the associated immune response and mucous hypersecretion, inflammation poses a major obstacle against efficient drug delivery in lung inflammatory conditions. For these reasons, inflammation's therapy is essential for CLIDs management.

Thus far, no curative therapy is available for these conditions. For therapeutic control of CLIDs bronchodilators, anti-inflammatory agents, and glucocorticoids are usually used. Attempts to improve the efficiency of these medicinal groups using nanotechnology have been under intensive research. In general, drug nanonization has been proposed for enhanced steric stability and facilitated dissolution of inhaled drugs, as observed with budesonide (El-Gendy et al. 2009). Similarly, although the mechanism is unknown, silver NPs (mean diameter $\approx$ 6 nm) demonstrated an ability to reduce lung inflammation and hyper responsiveness in a murine model of asthma (Park et al. 2010). In addition, the application of NP-based DDSs to address delivery challenges and produce controlled drug delivery in CLIDs has been investigated (Table 14.3).

A variety of NP forming polymers has been assessed via different routes of administration, including oral, pulmonary, and nasal routes. Due to its mucoadhesive properties and ability to enhance drug absorption by opening tight junctions between epithelial cells (Fernández-Urrusuno et al. 1999), CS formulated as NPs and loaded with a range of therapeutic agents, including small drug molecules, macromolecules, and DNA, has been the subject of intensive research for lung inflammation treatment. CS conjugated with thiol groups, for improved mucoadhesive and permeation properties, was used to produce NPs loaded with theophylline, a bronchodilator that possesses anti-inflammatory properties. When applied intranasally to mice with allergic asthma, CS NPs significantly increased the anti-inflammatory activity of the encapsulated drug, thus leading to decreased eosinophils in bronchoalveolar lavage fluid, inhibited mucus hypersecretion, reduced bronchial damage,

Table 14.3. NP-based DDSs for CLIDs.

NP-based carrier	Drug	Size (nm)	Route of administration	Targeting/Stimuli-responsive strategy	Reference
Thiolated CS	Theophylline	≈ 220	Intranasal	–	Lee et al. 2006
HA-CS	Heparin	≈ 200	No *in vivo* studies	–	Oyarzun-Ampuero et al. 2009
CS-cyclodextrin	Heparin	≈ 200–700	No *in vivo* studies	–	Oyarzun-Ampuero et al. 2012
CS	Interferon-gamma plasmid deoxyribonucleic acid (DNA)	Not indicated	Intranasal	–	Kumar et al. 2003
	Vessel dilator plasmid DNA	Not indicated	Intranasal	–	Wang et al. 2009
PLGA	Alpha 1-antitrypsin	≈ 100–1000	No *in vivo* studies	–	Pirooznia et al. 2012
	Pyridone 6	Not indicated	Intraperitoneal	–	Matsunaga et al. 2011
PEG-PLA	Betamethasone disodium phosphate	≈ 100	Intravenous	PEGylation	Matsuo et al. 2009
PEG-dendritic block telodendrimer micelle	DEX	≈ 10–20	Intravenous	PEGylation	Kenyon et al. 2013
SLN	Curcumin	≈ 200	Intraperitoneal	–	Wang et al. 2012

and augmented apoptosis of lung cells (Lee et al. 2006). In other works, CS-based NPs loaded with unfractionated or low molecular weight heparin, a macromolecular anticoagulant with potent anti-allergic and anti-inflammatory effects, were produced by ionotropic gelation of the positively charged CS with the negatively charged drug, pentasodium tripolyphosphate, and HA (Oyarzun-Ampuero et al. 2009) or carboxymethyl-β-cyclodextrin (Oyarzun-Ampuero et al. 2012). *Ex vivo* experiments in rat mast cells demonstrated that only CS/carboxymethyl-β-cyclodextrin NPs, and at the highest drug dose used in the study, resulted in enhanced prevention of mast cell degranulation, as compared to free heparin. Nonetheless, considering their mucoadhesive property and ability to protect the loaded drug against enzymatic degradation, CS NPs may still possess potential for *in vivo* delivery of heparin. Intranasal gene delivery for the protection or treatment of mouse airway inflammation has been successfully reported using CS NPs loaded with two plasmid DNAs one encoded for interferon-gamma, a pleiotropic cytokine that promotes T-helper cell type 1 responses which down-regulates T-helper cell type 2-associated airway inflammation and hyper responsiveness (Kumar et al. 2003), and the second encoded for vessel dilator, an *N*-terminal natriuretic peptide of the pro-atrial natriuretic factor (Wang et al. 2009b).

PLGA-based NPs designed for systemic delivery of anti-inflammatory agents to the lungs have also been explored. Matsunaga et al. (2011) used an emulsion-solvent evaporation technique for the preparation of PLGA NPs loaded with pyridone 6, a pan-Janus kinase inhibitor with potential effects against allergic asthma. The preparation method enabled the encapsulation of a 10-fold greater drug amount than the maximum injectable dose. When injected intraperitoneally to ovalbumin-challenged mice by ovalbumin, pyridone 6 NPs effectively inhibited T-helper cell type 2 inflammation and consequently suppressed asthmatic responses. A PLGA-based nanocarrier for enhanced stability and sustained release of alpha 1-antitrypsin, a glycoprotein inhibitr of proteases with ability to protect the lung against cellular inflammatory enzymes, was also proposed (Pirooznia et al. 2012).

Beside efficient control of asthma by inhalation, steroids are also administered systemically as a treatment of intractable asthma and asthmatic exacerbation. For this purpose, PEGylated PLA NPs loaded with betamethasone were produced and injected intravenously to ovalbumin-exposed mice. Enhanced drug accumulation at airway inflammation sites and significant anti-inflammatory activity was developed by the stealth NPs (Matsuo et al. 2009). PEG-dendritic block telodendrimer, composed of PEG, cholic acid, and lysine, with self-assembling ability, was used to prepare DEX-loaded NPs. *In vivo* experiments in ovalbumin-exposed mice demonstrated that intravenously administered NPs targeted lungs and reduced allergic lung inflammation and airways hyper responsiveness to a greater degree in comparison to equivalent doses of free DEX (Kenyon et al. 2013). Following intraperitoneal injection to rats with ovalbumin-induced asthma, SLNs prepared using a combination of stearic acid and lecithin and loaded with curcumin, a natural polyphenol compound with anti-inflammatory properties, were shown to increase drug accumulation in lungs and considerably diminish airway inflammation (Wang et al. 2012).

Potential side effects induced by pulmonary delivery of nanosystems should be given particular attention. Several serious health consequences, such as oxidative inflammatory reactions and pulmonary diseases, have been linked to nanosystem inhalation. Moreover, due to their improved absorption, NPs can reach the systemic circulation leading to undesired systemic adverse reactions (Madl and Pinkerton 2009). Nevertheless, research in this field indicates that NP-based local and systemic therapy may present an immense promise for CLIDs treatment.

Uveitis

Uveitis is the inflammation of the tissues forming the "uvea", the middle layer of the eye between the retina and the sclera. The exact cause of uveitis is often unknown, although it is linked to infections, autoimmune disorders, and injuries. Uveitis can be serious, causing permanent vision loss or even blindness. Therefore, urgent diagnosis and treatment are crucial to control the inflammation and prevent complications.

Due to its complex structure, an eye exhibits high resistance to foreign substances including drugs and, as a consequence, topical ocular drug delivery suffers from several restrictions. Because of tearing and blinking defensive mechanisms, a large proportion of topically instilled drug is eliminated quickly to the nose via the nasolacrimal drainage. Besides, reaching intraocular tissues requires drug permeation through a large distance of corneal tight junctions. For these reasons, no more than 5% of the administered dose reaches intraocular target tissues. Conventionally, this problem is addressed by increasing drug concentration. However, this approach may lead to greater incidence of systemic side effects associated with increased drug absorption from the nose. Other routes of drug administration used for ophthalmic treatment also show disadvantages. Intraocular injection causes some serious complications, e.g., accelerated cataract formation, hemorrhage, retinal detachment, endophthalmitis, and increased intraocular pressure (Parke 2003). While, owing to the blood-ocular barriers, systemic drug delivery is inefficient and results in low intraocular drug concentrations.

Generally, ophthalmic delivery of nano-sized drugs improves their absorption and efficiency (Kassem et al. 2007). In uveitis therapy (Table 14.4), NP-based DDSs provide several important benefits including enhanced absorption of particularly poorly soluble drugs by topical administration, improved accumulation by systemic administration, reduced dosing frequency when intraocular injection is used, as well as general advantages of nanosystems such as drug protection and sustained drug release. Moreover, the miniature particle size and composition of topically applied nanosystems ensure low irritation, low toxicity, biocompatibility, and mucoadhesiveness.

Table 14.4. NP-based DDSs for ocular inflammation.

NP-based carrier	Drug	Size (nm)	Route of administration	Targeting/Stimuli-responsive strategy	Reference
Eudragit® RS100	Piroxicam	≈ 230–250	Ocular (topical)	–	Adibkia et al. 2007
PLGA	Triamcinolone acetonide	≈ 200–800	Ocular (topical)	–	Sabzevari et al. 2013
HA-modified core-shell lipo-CS	–	≈ 320	Intravitreal	HA for targeting CD44 receptors in the retinal pigment epithelium	Gan et al. 2013
PEG-*b*-PLA	Betamethasone disodium phosphate	≈ 120	Intravenous	PEGylation	Sakai et al. 2011
Liposome	Prednisolone acetate	≈ 70	Ocular (topical)	–	Elbialy et al. 2013
	Vasoactive intestinal peptide	≈ 300–600	Intravitreal	PEGylation	Lajavardi et al. 2007, Camelo et al. 2009
sLex-conjugated liposome	DEX	≈ 50–300	Intravenous	sLex to target E-selectin and P-selectin on activated endothelial cells	Hashida et al. 2008

For *in vivo* studies using NP-based DDSs, experimental animals with endotoxin-induced uveitis (by lipopolysaccharide) are often used. The evaluation of the anti-inflammatory efficiency is performed by clinical examinations, normally using Hogan's classification method, and local inflammation intensity assessments, by measuring leukocytes infiltration and other inflammatory mediators in the aqueous humor.

Topical delivery of ophthalmic anti-inflammatory agents using various polymer-based and lipid-based nanosystems has been examined. When applied in rabbits with endotoxin-induced uveitis, piroxicam-loaded Eudragit® RS100 NPs produced greater inhibition of inflammation as compared to the pure drug microsuspension. The positive charge of Eudragit® RS100 contributes to its ability to encapsulate negatively charged drugs and to enhance cellular uptake by electrical interaction with cellular membranes (Adibkia et al. 2007). Similarly, following topical administration to endotoxin-induced uveitis rabbits, PLGA-based NPs containing triamcinolone acetonide demonstrated higher anti-inflammatory activity than triamcinolone acetonide microsuspension and prednisolone acetate microsuspension, and comparable effects to triamcinolone acetonide subconjunctive injection (Sabzevari et al. 2013). In an attempt to study the effects of charge and particle size on drug delivery efficiency using various formulations of prednisolone acetate-loaded liposomes, Elbialy et al. (2013) demonstrated that positive unilamellar liposomes (mean size ≈ 70 nm) increased ability for drug delivery across the cornea, as compared to neutral multilamellar liposomes and positive multilamellar liposomes (≈ 5 μm in diameter).

Formulation of intraocular drug injections using nanovehicles is an attractive approach because it offers reduced dosing frequency. Following intravitreal injection to rats with uveitis (Lajavardi et al. 2007) or with experimental autoimmune uveoretinitis (Camelo et al. 2009), vasoactive intestinal peptide, an immunosuppressive factor, loaded in sterically stabilized PEGylated liposomes effectively reduced clinical and pathological ocular inflammation signs. When incorporated into HA gel, vasoactive intestinal peptide-loaded liposomes showed increased anti-inflammatory efficacy and prolonged drug action (Lajavardi et al. 2007). Gan et al. (2013) designed HA-modified core-shell lipo-CS NPs for drug targeting of the retinal pigment epithelium. Following intravitreal injection to experimental autoimmune uveoretinitis rats, HA-modified core-shell lipo-CS NPs specifically targeted retinal pigment epithelium, as compared to CS NPs, which were limited to the vitreous cavity, and lipo NPs, which only reached the inner layers of the retina. The mechanism of retinal pigment epithelium targeting is based on the interaction between the HA moiety from the HA-modified core-shell lipo-CS NPs and the CD44 receptor.

In addition to drug delivery using topical and intraocular injection, systemic administration using surface engineered NPs have been tested. Following a single intravenous injection to rats with experimental autoimmune uveoretinitis, PEGylated PLA NPs loaded with betamethasone phosphate significantly increased drug localization in the inflamed retina up to seven days after injection (Sakai et al. 2011). Likewise, the intravenous injection of DEX-loaded sLex-conjugated liposomes to mice with experimental autoimmune uveoretinitis resulted in doubled DEX concentration in the inflamed eyes, in comparison to free drug solution. This effect was due to sLex-conjugated liposomes targeting of E-selectin and P-selectin on the activated endothelial cells (Hashida et al. 2008).

Efficient, specific, and prolonged therapy of ocular inflammation using nanomedicines has been achieved in experimental animals. However, the eye is a very sensitive organ and therefore any likelihood to generate immune response development or loss of vision must be ruled out prior to human use of these systems.

Conclusion

NP-based DDSs have shown great potential for CIDs therapy. Major attractions in nanomedicine are its specific accumulation in target inflamed tissues and enhanced uptake by inflammation cells, which lead to greater efficacy in drug delivery, reduced adverse effects, and will ultimately increase patient compliance. Another important advantage of nanocarriers is formulation flexibility. Using a variety of formulating materials, engineering approaches, and surface functionalization strategies the generation of multi-targeting strategies nanosystems with ability to specifically target inflammatory sites and to provide controlled release at these sites have been made possible. A major challenge for nanotherapy of CIDs is the specificity of each disease in this group, which should be considered during nanomedicine formulation and administration route selection. Furthermore, there is a general concern associated with nanocarrier use because of possible toxicity. For this purpose, comprehensive toxicity studies prior to intensive clinical experiments are essential. Moreover, due to differences observed between humans and experimental animals, studies in human patients are essential to direct future research efforts in CIDs nanotherapy. Finally, industrial scale-up is another challenge due to the inherent complexity of these systems.

Abbreviations

5-ASA	:	5-aminosalicylic acid
CD	:	Crohn's disease
CIA	:	collagen-induced arthritis
CID	:	chronic inflammatory disease
CLID	:	chronic lung inflammatory disease
COPD	:	chronic obstructive pulmonary disease
CS	:	chitosan
DDS	:	drug delivery system

DEX	:	dexamethasone
DMARD	:	disease-modifying antirheumatic drug
DNA	:	deoxyribonucleic acid
D*si*RNA	:	Dicer-substrate small interfering ribonucleic acid
HA	:	hyaluronic acid
IBD	:	inflammatory bowel disease
IL	:	interleukin
KPV	:	lysine-proline-valine
LCST	:	low critical solution temperature
mAb	:	monoclonal antibody
Map4k4	:	mitogen-activated protein kinase kinase kinase kinase 4
MTX	:	methotrexate
NP	:	nanoparticle
NSAID	:	non-steroidal anti-inflammatory drug
OA	:	osteoarthritis
PEI	:	polyethyleneimine
PEG	:	poly(ethylene glycol)
PLA	:	poly(D,L-lactide)
PCL	:	poly(ε-caprolactone)
PLGA	:	poly(D,L-lactide-*co*-glycolide)
RA	:	rheumatoid arthritis
RGD	:	arginine-glycine-aspartic acid
*si*RNA	:	small interfering ribonucleic acid
SLN	:	solid lipid nanoparticle
sLex	:	sialyl-Lewis X
TNF-α	:	tumor necrosis factor-alpha
TwHF	:	*Tripterygium wilfordii Hook F*
UC	:	ulcerative colitis

References

Adibkia, K. and M.R. Siahi Shadbad, A. Nokhodchi, A. Javadzedeh, M. Barzegar-jalali, J. Barar, G. Mohammadi and Y. Omidi. 2007. Piroxicam nanoparticles for ocular delivery: physicochemical characterization and implementation in endotoxin-induced uveitis. J. Drug Target. 15: 407–416.

Arias, J.L. and M. López-Viota, J. López-Viota and A.V. Delgado. 2009. Development of iron/ethylcellulose (core/shell) nanoparticles loaded with diclofenac sodium for arthritis treatment. Int. J. Pharm. 382: 270–276.

Arias, J.L. and M. López-Viota, E. Sáez-Fernández and M.A. Ruiz. 2010. Formulation and physicochemical characterization of poly(epsilon-caprolactone) nanoparticles loaded with ftorafur and diclofenac sodium. Colloids Surf. B Biointerfaces. 75: 204–208.

Arias, J.L. 2010. Drug Targeting by Magnetically Responsive Colloids. Nova Science Publishers, Inc., New York, USA.

Arranz, A. and C. Reinsch, K.A. Papadakis, A. Dieckmann, U. Rauchhaus, A. Androulidaki, V. Zacharioudaki, A.N. Margioris, C. Tsatsanis and S. Panzner. 2013. Treatment of experimental murine colitis with cd40 antisense oligonucleotides delivered in amphoteric liposomes. J. Control. Release. 165: 163–172.

Banerjee, S.S. and D.H. Chen. 2009. A multifunctional magnetic nanocarrier bearing fluorescent dye for targeted drug delivery by enhanced two-photon triggered release. Nanotechnology. 20: 185103.

Barnes, P.J. and S. Shapiro and R.A. Pauwels. 2003. Chronic obstructive pulmonary disease: molecular and cellular mechanisms. Eur. Respir. J. 22: 672–688.

Bartlett, R.L. 2nd and S. Sharma and A. Panitch. 2013. Cell-penetrating peptides released from thermosensitive nanoparticles suppress pro-inflammatory cytokine response by specifically targeting inflamed cartilage explants. Nanomedicine. 9: 419–427.

Beloqui, A. and R. Coco, M. Alhouayek, M.A. Solinis, A. Rodríguez-Gascón, G.G. Muccioli and V. Preat. 2013. Budesonide-loaded nanostructured lipid carriers reduce inflammation in murine dss-induced colitis. Int. J. Pharm. 454: 775–783.

Bruewer, M. and A. Luegering, T. Kucharzik, C.A. Parkos, J.L. Madara, A.M. Hopkins and A. Nusrat. 2003. Proinflammatory cytokines disrupt epithelial barrier function by apoptosis-independent mechanisms. J. Immunol. 171: 6164–6172.

Camelo, S. and L. Lajavardi, A. Bochot, B. Goldenberg, M.C. Naud, N. Brunel, B. Lescure, C. Klein, E. Fattal, F. Behar-Cohen and Y. de Kozak. 2009. Protective effect of intravitreal injection of vasoactive intestinal peptide-loaded liposomes on experimental autoimmune uveoretinitis. J. Ocul. Pharmacol. Ther. 25: 9–21.

Clares, B. and M.A. Ruiz, V. Gallardo and J.L. Arias. 2012. Drug delivery to inflammation based on nanoparticles surface decorated with biomolecules. Curr. Med. Chem. 19: 3203–3211.

Coco, R. and L. Plapied, V. Pourcelle, C. Jerome, D.J. Brayden, Y.J. Schneider and V. Preat. 2013. Drug delivery to inflamed colon by nanoparticles: comparison of different strategies. Int. J. Pharm. 440: 3–12.

Dong, J. and D. Jiang, Z. Wang, G. Wu, L. Miao and L. Huang. 2013. Intra-articular delivery of liposomal celecoxib-hyaluronate combination for the treatment of osteoarthritis in rabbit model. Int. J. Pharm. 441: 285–290.

El-Gendy, N. and E.M. Gorman, E.J. Munson and C. Berkland. 2009. Budesonide nanoparticle agglomerates as dry powder aerosols with rapid dissolution. J. Pharm. Sci. 98: 2731–2746.

Elbialy, N.S. and B.M. Abdol-Azim, M.W. Shafaa, L.H. El Shazly, A.H. El Shazly and W. Khalil. 2013. Enhancement of the ocular therapeutic effect of prednisolone acetate by liposomal entrapment. J. Biomed. Nanotechnol. 9: 2105–2116.

Fan, C. and X. Li, Y. Zhou, Y. Zhao, S. Ma, W. Li, Y. Liu and G. Li. 2013. Enhanced topical delivery of tetrandrine by ethosomes for treatment of arthritis. Biomed. Res. Int. 2013: 161943.

Fernandes, J.C. and H. Wang, C. Jreyssaty, M. Benderdour, P. Lavigne, X. Qiu, F.M. Winnik, X. Zhang, K. Dai and Q. Shi. 2008. Bone-protective effects of nonviral gene therapy with folate-chitosan DNA nanoparticle containing interleukin-1 receptor antagonist gene in rats with adjuvant-induced arthritis. Mol. Ther. 16: 1243–1251.

Fernandez-Urrusuno, R. and D. Romani, P. Calvo, J.L. Vila-Jato and M.J. Alonso. 1999. Development of a freeze-dried formulation of insulin-loaded chitosan nanoparticles intended for nasal administration. S.T.P. Pharm. Sci. 9: 429–436.

Gan, L. and J. Wang, Y. Zhao, D. Chen, C. Zhu, J. Liu and Y. Gan. 2013. Hyaluronan-modified core-shell liponanoparticles targeting cd44-positive retinal pigment epithelium cells via intravitreal injection. Biomaterials. 34: 5978–5987.

Hashida, N. and N. Ohguro, N. Yamazaki, Y. Arakawa, E. Oiki, H. Mashimo, N. Kurokawa and Y. Tano. 2008. High-efficacy site-directed drug delivery system using sialyl-Lewis X conjugated liposome. Exp. Eye Res. 86: 138–149.

He, C. and L. Yin, C. Tang and C. Yin. 2013. Multifunctional polymeric nanoparticles for oral delivery of TNF-α siRNA to macrophages. Biomaterials. 34: 2843–2854.

Higaki, M. and T. Ishihara, N. Izumo, M. Takatsu and Y. Mizushima. 2005. Treatment of experimental arthritis with poly(D, L-lactic/glycolic acid) nanoparticles encapsulating betamethasone sodium phosphate. Ann. Rheum. Dis. 64: 1132–1136.

Hornig, S. and H. Bunjes and T. Heinze. 2009. Preparation and characterization of nanoparticles based on dextran-drug conjugates. J. Colloid Interface Sci. 338: 56–62.

Howard, K.A. and S.R. Paludan, M.A. Behlke, F. Besenbacher, B. Deleuran and J. Kjems. 2009. Chitosan/siRNA nanoparticle-mediated TNF-alpha knockdown in peritoneal macrophages for anti-inflammatory treatment in a murine arthritis model. Mol. Ther. 17: 162–168.

Ishihara, T. and M. Takahashi, M. Higaki, Y. Mizushima and T. Mizushima. 2010. Preparation and characterization of a nanoparticulate formulation composed of PEG-PLA and PLA as anti-inflammatory agents. Int. J. Pharm. 385: 170–175.

Jubeh, T.T. and Y. Barenholz and A. rubinstein. 2004. Differential adhesion of normal and inflamed rat colonic mucosa by charged liposomes. Pharm. Res. 21: 447–453.

Kassem, M.A. and A.A. Abdel Rahman, M.M. Ghorab, M.B. Ahmed and R.M. Khalil. 2007. Nanosuspension as an ophthalmic delivery system for certain glucocorticoid drugs. Int. J. Pharm. 340: 126–133.

Kaur, K. and S. Jain, B. Sapra and A.K. Tiwary. 2007. Niosomal gel for site-specific sustained delivery of anti-arthritic drug: *in vitro-in vivo* evaluation. Curr. Drug Deliv. 4: 276–282.

Kenyon, N.J. and J.M. Bratt, J. Lee, J. Luo, L.M. Franzi, A.A. Zeki and K.S. Lam. 2013. Self-assembling nanoparticles containing dexamethasone as a novel therapy in allergic airways inflammation. PLoS One. 8: e77730.

Kim, S.R. and Y.K. Rhee. 2010. Overlap between asthma and COPD: where the two diseases converge. Allergy Asthma Immunol. Res. 2: 209–214.

Kim, S.H. and J.H. Kim, D.G. You, G. Saravanakumar, H.Y. Yoon, K.Y. Choi, T. Thambi, V.G. Deepagan, D.G. Jo and J.H. Park. 2013. Self-assembled dextran sulphate nanoparticles for targeting rheumatoid arthritis. Chem. Commun. (Camb.). 49: 10349–10351.

Kumar, M. and X. Kong, A.K. Behera, G.R. Hellermann, R.F. Lockey and S.S. Mohapatra. 2003. Chitosan IFN-gamma-pDNA nanoparticle (CIN) therapy for allergic asthma. Genet. Vaccines Ther. 1: 3.

Kurtoglu, Y.E. and M.K. Ishra, S. Kannan and R.M. Kannan. 2010. Drug release characteristics of PAMAM dendrimer-drug conjugates with different linkers. Int. J. Pharm. 384: 189–194.

Lajavardi, L. and A. Bochot, S. Camelo, B. Goldenberg, M.C. Naud, F. Behar-Cohen, E. Fattal and Y. de Kozak. 2007. Downregulation of endotoxin-induced uveitis by intravitreal injection of vasoactive intestinal peptide encapsulated in liposomes. Invest. Ophthalmol. Vis. Sci. 48: 3230–3238.

Lamprecht, A. and U. Schafer and C.M. Lehr. 2001. Size-dependent bioadhesion of micro- and nanoparticulate carriers to the inflamed colonic mucosa. Pharm. Res. 18: 788–793.

Lamprecht, A. and H. Yamamoto, H. Takeuchi and Y. Kawashima. 2005. Nanoparticles enhance therapeutic efficiency by selectively increased local drug dose in experimental colitis in rats. J. Pharmacol. Exp. Ther. 315: 196–202.

Laroui, H. and G. Dalmasso, H.T. Nguyen, Y. Yan, S.V. Sitaraman and D. Merlin. 2010. Drug-loaded nanoparticles targeted to the colon with polysaccharide hydrogel reduce colitis in a mouse model. Gastroenterology. 138: 843–853.e1–2.

Laroui, H. and A.L. Theiss, Y. Yan, G. Dalmasso, H.T. Nguyen, S.V. Sitaraman and D. Merlin. 2011. Functional TNFα gene silencing mediated by polyethyleneimine/TNFα siRNA nanocomplexes in inflamed colon. Biomaterials. 32: 1218–1228.

Laroui, H. and D. Geem, B. Xiao, E. Viennois, P. Rakhya, T. Denning and D. Merlin. 2014. Targeting intestinal inflammation with CD98 siRNA/PEI-loaded nanoparticles. Mol. Ther. 22: 69–80.

Lautenschlager, C. and C. Schmidt, C.M. Lehr, D. Fischer and A. Stallmach. 2013. PEG-functionalized microparticles selectively target inflamed mucosa in inflammatory bowel disease. Eur. J. Pharm. Biopharm. 85: 578–586.

Lee, D.W. and S.A. Shirley, R.F. Lockey and S.S. Mohapatra. 2006. Thiolated chitosan nanoparticles enhance anti-inflammatory effects of intranasally delivered theophylline. Respir. Res. 7: 112.

Lee, C.H. and L.W. Lo, C.Y. Mou and C.S. Yang. 2008. Synthesis and characterization of positive-charge functionalized mesoporous silica nanoparticles for oral drug delivery of an anti-inflammatory drug. Adv. Funct. Mater. 18: 3283–3292.

Lee, S.M. and H.J. Kim, Y.J. Ha, Y.N. Park, S.K. Lee, Y.B. Park and K.H. Yoo. 2013. Targeted chemo-photothermal treatments of rheumatoid arthritis using gold half-shell multifunctional nanoparticles. ACS Nano. 7: 50–57.

Lo, C.T. and P.R. Van Tassel and W.M. Saltzman. 2010. Poly(lactide-co-glycolide) nanoparticle assembly for highly efficient delivery of potent therapeutic agents from medical devices. Biomaterials. 31: 3631–3642.

Madl, A.K. and K.E. Pinkerton. 2009. Health effects of inhaled engineered and incidental nanoparticles. Crit. Rev. Toxicol. 39: 629–658.

Maehara, A. and K. Nishida, M. Furutani, E. Matsumoto, A. Ohtsuka, Y. Ninomiya and T. Oohashi. 2014. Light and electron microscopic detection of inflammation-targeting liposomes encapsulating high-density colloidal gold in arthritic mice. Inflamm. Res. 63: 139–147.

Marimuthu, M. and D. Bennet and S. Kim. 2013. Self-assembled nanoparticles of PLGA-conjugated glucosamine as a sustained transdermal drug delivery vehicle. Polym. J. 45: 202–209.

Matsunaga, Y. and H. Inoue, S. Fukuyama, H. Yoshida, A. Moriwaki, T. Matsumoto, K. Matsumoto, Y. Asai, M. Kubo, A. Yoshimura and Y. Nakanishi. 2011. Effects of a Janus kinase inhibitor, pyridone 6, on airway responses in a murine model of asthma. Biochem. Biophys. Res. Commun. 404: 261–267.

Matsuo, Y. and T. Ishihara, J. Ishizaki, K. Miyamoto, M. Higaki and N. Yamashita. 2009. Effect of betamethasone phosphate loaded polymeric nanoparticles on a murine asthma model. Cell Immunol. 260: 33–38.

Meissner, Y. and Y. Pellequer and A. Lamprecht. 2006. Nanoparticles in inflammatory bowel disease: particle targeting versus pH-sensitive delivery. Int. J. Pharm. 316: 138–143.

Moulari, B. and D. Pertuit, Y. Pellequer and A. Lamprecht. 2008. The targeting of surface modified silica nanoparticles to inflamed tissue in experimental colitis. Biomaterials. 29: 4554–4560.

Moulari, B. and A. Beduneau, Y. Pellequer and A. Lamprecht. 2013. Nanoparticle targeting to inflamed tissues of the gastrointestinal tract. Curr. Drug Deliv. 10: 9–17.

Niebel, W. and K. Walkenbach, A. Beduneau, Y. Pellequer and A. Lamprecht. 2012. Nanoparticle-based clodronate delivery mitigates murine experimental colitis. J. Control. Release. 160: 659–665.

Oyarzun-Ampuero, F.A. and J. Brea, M.I. Loza, D. Torres and M.J. Alonso. 2009. Chitosan-hyaluronic acid nanoparticles loaded with heparin for the treatment of asthma. Int. J. Pharm. 381: 122–129.

Oyarzun-Ampuero, F.A. and J. Brea, M.I. Loza, M.J. Alonso and D. Torres. 2012. A potential nanomedicine consisting of heparin-loaded polysaccharide nanocarriers for the treatment of asthma. Macromol. Biosci. 12: 176–183.

Park, H.S. and K.H. Kim, S. Jang, J.W. Park, H.R. Cha, J.E. Lee, J.O. Kim, S.Y. Kim, C.S. Lee, J.P. Kim and S.S. Jung. 2010. Attenuation of allergic airway inflammation and hyperresponsiveness in a murine model of asthma by silver nanoparticles. Int. J. Nanomedicine. 5: 505–515.

Parke, D.W. 2003. Intravitreal triamcinolone and endophthalmitis. Am. J. Ophthalmol. 136: 918–919.

Peer, D. and E.J. Park, Y. Morishita, C.V. Carman and M. Shimaoka. 2008. Systemic leukocyte-directed siRNA delivery revealing cyclin D1 as an anti-inflammatory target. Science. 319: 627–630.

Pertuit, D. and B. Moulari, T. Betz, A. Nadaradjane, D. Neumann, L. Ismaili, B. Refouvelet, Y. Pellequer and A. Lamprecht. 2007. 5-amino salicylic acid bound nanoparticles for the therapy of inflammatory bowel disease. J. Control. Release. 123: 211–218.

Pirooznia, N. and S. Hasannia, A.S. Lotfi and M. Ghanei. 2012. Encapsulation of alpha-1 antitrypsin in PLGA nanoparticles: *in vitro* characterization as an effective aerosol formulation in pulmonary diseases. J. Nanobiotechnology. 10: 20.

Prabhu, P. and R. Shetty, M. Koland, K. Vijayanarayana, K.K. Vijayalakshmi, M.H. Nairy and G.S. Nisha. 2012. Investigation of nano lipid vesicles of methotrexate for anti-rheumatoid activity. Int. J. Nanomedicine. 7: 177–186.

Sabzevari, A. and K. Adibkia, H. Hashemi, A. Hedayatfar, N. Mohsenzadeh, F. Atyabi, M.H. Ghahremani and R. Dinarvand. 2013. Polymeric triamcinolone acetonide nanoparticles as a new alternative in the treatment of uveitis: *in vitro* and *in vivo* studies. Eur. J. Pharm. Biopharm. 84: 63–71.

Sakai, T. and T. Ishihara, M. Higaki, G. Akiyama and H. Tsuneoka. 2011. Therapeutic effect of stealth-type polymeric nanoparticles with encapsulated betamethasone phosphate on experimental autoimmune uveoretinitis. Invest. Ophthalmol. Vis. Sci. 52: 1516–1521.

Schmidt, C. and C. Lautenschlaeger, E.M. Collnot, M. Schumann, C. Bojarski, J.D. Schulzke, C.M. Lehr and A. Stallmach. 2013. Nano- and microscaled particles for drug targeting to inflamed intestinal mucosa: a first *in vivo* study in human patients. J. Control. Release. 165: 139–145.

Schroeder, A. and A. Sigal, K. Turjeman and Y. Barenholz. 2008. Using PEGylated nano-liposomes to target tissue invaded by a foreign body. J. Drug Target. 16: 591–595.

Serpe, L. and R. Canaparo, M. Daperno, R. Sostegni, G. Martinasso, E. Muntoni, L. Ippolito, N. Vivenza, A. Pera, M. Eandi, M.R. Gasco and G.P. Zara. 2010. Solid lipid nanoparticles as anti-inflammatory drug delivery system in a human inflammatory bowel disease whole-blood model. Eur. J. Pharm. Sci. 39: 428–436.

Teahon, K. and S. Somasundaram, T. Smith, I. Menzies and I. Bjarnason. 1996. Assessing the site of increased intestinal permeability in coeliac and inflammatory bowel disease. Gut. 38: 864–869.

Thakkar, H. and R. Kumar Sharma and R.S. Murthy. 2007. Enhanced retention of celecoxib-loaded solid lipid nanoparticles after intra-articular administration. Drugs R. D. 8: 275–285.

Theiss, A.L. and H. Laroui, T.S. Obertone, I. Chowdhury, W.E. Thompson, D. Merlin and S.V. Sitaraman. 2011. Nanoparticle-based therapeutic delivery of prohibitin to the colonic epithelial cells ameliorates acute murine colitis. Inflamm. Bowel Dis. 17: 1163–1176.

Turker, S. and S. Erdogan, Y.A. Ozer, H. Bilgili and S. Deveci. 2008. Enhanced efficacy of diclofenac sodium-loaded lipogelosome formulation in intra-articular treatment of rheumatoid arthritis. J. Drug Target. 16: 51–57.

Ulbrich, W. and A. Lamprecht. 2010. Targeted drug-delivery approaches by nanoparticulate carriers in the therapy of inflammatory diseases. J. R. Soc. Interface. 7: S55–S66.

Valerii, M.C. and M. Benaglia, C. Caggiano, A. Papi, A. Strillacci, G. Lazzarini, M. Campieri, P. Gionchetti, F. Rizzello and E. Spisni. 2013. Drug delivery by polymeric micelles: an *in vitro* and *in vivo* study to deliver lipophilic substances to colonocytes and selectively target inflamed colon. Nanomedicine. 9: 675–685.

Wachsmann, P. and B. Moulari, A. Beduneau, Y. Pellequer and A. Lamprecht. 2013. Surfactant-dependence of nanoparticle treatment in murine experimental colitis. J. Control. Release. 172: 62–68.

Wang, L. and R. Zeng, C. Li and R. Qiao. 2009a. Self-assembled polypeptide-block-poly(vinylpyrrolidone) as prospective drug-delivery systems. Colloids Surf. B Biointerfaces. 74: 284–292.

Wang, X. and W. Xu, X. Kong, D. Chen, G. Hellermann, T.A. Ahlert, J.D. Giaimo, S.A. Cormier, X. Li, R.F. Lockey, S. Mohapatra and S.S. Mohapatra. 2009b. Modulation of lung inflammation by vessel dilator in a mouse model of allergic asthma. Respir. Res. 10: 66.

Wang, W. and R. Zhu, Q. Xie, A. Li, Y. Xiao, K. Li, H. Liu, D. Cui, Y. Chen and S. Wang. 2012. Enhanced bioavailability and efficiency of curcumin for the treatment of asthma by its formulation in solid lipid nanoparticles. Int. J. Nanomedicine. 7: 3667–3677.

Xiao, B. and H. Laroui, S. Ayyadurai, E. Viennois, M.A. Charania, Y. Zhang and D. Merlin. 2013. Mannosylated bioreducible nanoparticle-mediated macrophage-specific TNF-α RNA interference for IBD therapy. Biomaterials. 34: 7471–7482.

Xue, M. and Z.Z. Jiang, T. Wu, J. Li, L. Zhang, Y. Zhao, X.J. Li, L.Y. Zhang and S.Y. Yang. 2012. Anti-inflammatory effects and hepatotoxicity of tripterygium-loaded solid lipid nanoparticles on adjuvant-induced arthritis in rats. Phytomedicine. 19: 998–1006.

Ye, J. and Q. Wang, X. Zhou and N. Zhang. 2008. Injectable actarit-loaded solid lipid nanoparticles as passive targeting therapeutic agents for rheumatoid arthritis. Int. J. Pharm. 352: 273–279.

Zhang, X. and C. Yu, X. Shi, C. Zhang, T. Tang and K. Dai. 2006. Direct chitosan-mediated gene delivery to the rabbit knee joints *in vitro* and *in vivo*. Biochem. Biophys. Res. Commun. 341: 202–208.

Zhang, J. and C. Tang and C. Yin. 2013. Galactosylated trimethyl chitosan-cysteine nanoparticles loaded with Map4k4 siRNA for targeting activated macrophages. Biomaterials. 34: 3667–3677.

Zhou, H.F. and H. Yan, A. Senpan, S.A. Wickline, D. Pan, G.M. Lanza and C.T. Pham. 2012. Suppression of inflammation in a mouse model of rheumatoid arthritis using targeted lipase-labile fumagillin prodrug nanoparticles. Biomaterials. 33: 8632–8640.

CHAPTER 15

Nanomedicine Biopharmaceuticals for Metabolic Diseases

Filipa Antunes[1,a] and *Bruno Sarmento*[1,2,]*

ABSTRACT

Modern biotechnology applications in the world of pharmaceutical industries are focused on the production of biopharmaceutical drugs. Biopharmaceuticals are increasingly used in therapy to treat many metabolic and oncologic diseases, to which the advances in the field of pharmaceutical biotechnology have been fundamental for these achievements. Metabolic diseases are caused by inborn errors of metabolism corresponding to an enzyme defect that can lead to disruption of a metabolic pathway. Over the last few decades there were numerous advances on the treatment of these incapacitated diseases, especially using biopharmaceutical drugs, but there are still many new challenges to developing safe and effective biopharmaceuticals for the treatment of metabolic diseases. Nanoparticulate platforms have become very important elements in novel drug delivery systems, being usually associated with the formulation and delivery of biopharmaceutical drugs. Nanoparticles can be used to effectively deliver biopharmaceuticals to a target site and thus increase the therapeutic benefit, while minimizing side effects. This chapter intends to review the recent advances on nanomedicine biopharmaceuticals for the treatment of metabolic diseases like diabetes, phenylketonuria, osteoporosis, growth hormone deficiency, Niemann-Pick disease, and Fabry's disease.

---

[1] Instituto de Engenharia Biomédica (INEB), Universidade do Porto, Rua do Campo Alegre 823, 4150-180 Porto, Portugal.
[2] Instituto de Investigação e Inovação em Saúde, Universidade do Porto, Portugal.
* Corresponding author: bruno.sarmento@ineb.up.pt

Introduction

In recent years, biotechnologically derived drugs, including proteins, peptides, monoclonal antibodies, and antibody fragments, as well as antisense oligonucleotides and deoxyribonucleic acid (DNA) preparations for gene therapy, have been a major focus of research and development efforts in the pharmaceutical industry. The big pharmaceutical companies and biotechnology companies that have emerged in recent years concentrated on the production of biopharmaceuticals, as well as industry research and development. Biopharmaceuticals are complex drug molecules manufactured by biotechnological means, usually involving live organisms or their active components. Biopharmaceuticals are increasingly used in therapy to treat many metabolic and oncologic diseases, to which the advances in the field of pharmaceutical biotechnology were fundamental for these achievements (Tang et al. 2004). More than 150 biopharmaceuticals have now gained medical approval and several hundred are in the pipeline. Most are protein-based, although two nucleic acid-based products are now on the United States of America/European market. An increasing proportion of approvals are engineered in some way, and advances in alternative production systems and delivery methods will also likely impact upon the approvals profile over the remainder of this decade (Walsh 2005).

The main applications of modern biotechnology in the world of pharmaceutical industries are the production of biopharmaceuticals like therapeutic proteins (e.g., insulin, growth hormone, erythropoietin) or vaccine (recombinant vaccines against hepatitis), and genomic studies for the prevention and cure of various diseases (gene therapy and pharmacogenomics). These companies are mainly located in developed countries like the United States of America, European countries, and Japan, but, in many cases, the development of these products involves partnerships between large multinational laboratories, biotechnology companies, and universities and research institutions. Biopharmaceuticals have been gaining attention due to scientific breakthroughs and the large volume of investments because it is a promising market. Moreover, the pharmaceutical industry is based on technological innovation and intellectual property in the form of patents. These patents grant exclusive rights to the market and generate high financial gains (Butler 2005).

For the pharmaceutical biotechnology industries operating under increasing pressure to reduce production costs, the use of high performance tools has emerged as a facilitator needed in a limited time and resources environment. So the concept of "quality by design" is gaining industry acceptance as an approach to the development and commercialization of therapeutic biotechnology products, as in "quality by design", the process is designed and controlled to deliver quality attributes specified consistently (Bhambure et al. 2011).

Because the development of biotech drugs generally lies on a fundamental understanding of the related disease, their clinical development is frequently more successful than it is for drug products based on conventional small molecules (Tang et al. 2004).

Metabolic Diseases

Metabolic diseases are caused by inborn errors of metabolism and affect one in five thousand live births (Vangala and Tonelli 2007). Inborn errors of metabolism are disorders of genetic origin that generally correspond to an enzyme defect leading to disruption of a metabolic pathway. These disorders are also characterized by a failure of synthesis (anabolism) and degradation (catabolism), storage, or transport of molecules in the body (Erez et al. 2011).

Inborn errors of metabolism fall into a number of classifications. They include disorders of intermediary metabolism (protein, carbohydrate, or fatty acid oxidation disorders), mitochondrial disorders, peroxisomal disorders, and disorders of carbohydrate glycosylation, creatine, or neurotransmitters. Additional inherited disorders are linked to defects in cytochrome P_{450} enzymes catalyzing cholesterol, bile acid, steroid, and vitamin D_3 synthesis and metabolism (Vangala and Tonelli 2007). The clinical and laboratory manifestations of Inborn Metabolic Disorders (IMDs) can include acute metabolic encephalopathy, hyperammonemia, metabolic acidosis, hypoglycemia, jaundice and liver dysfunction, lipid and liposomal storage disorders, and altered morphological features (Vangala and Tonelli 2007).

The most common disorder of amino acid metabolism is phenylketonuria (PKU). PKU is also the best characterized and most researched inborn error of protein metabolism. The amino acid phenylalanine (Phe) is normally transaminated to tyrosine by the enzyme Phe hydroxylase (with the assistance of a pterin cofactor). IMDs, most notably the organic acidemias/acidurias urea cycle defects, and certain amino acid metabolism disorders, present with acute life-threatening symptoms of encephalopathy and measurable clinical pathology parameters. These symptoms are primarily the result of the toxic effects of accumulating metabolites on the central nervous system.

In neonates, IMDs involving urea cycle defects and many of the organic acidemias are the primary cause of hyperammonemia, whereas in the older infant, fatty acid oxidation defects may be considered. Among the inherited disorders, the largest group typically associated with overwhelming metabolic acidosis in infancy is the group of organic acidemias, including methylmalonic aciduria, propionic acidemia, glutaric acidemia type II, and isovaleric acidemia. On the other hand, defects in pyruvate metabolism or in the respiratory chain may lead to lactic acidosis, which is present in infancy as severe metabolic acidosis but with normal urine organic acids.

Hypoglycemia and its associated symptoms are commonly seen in disorders of carbohydrate metabolism or fatty acid oxidation, although protein intolerance can also cause hypoglycemia. Among the best-known IMDs associated with hypoglycemia are the hepatic glycogen storage disorders. The hypoglycemia in these disorders is related to the inability of the liver to release glucose from glycogen, and it is most profound during periods of fasting. Hypoglycemia, hepatomegaly, and lactic acidosis are prominent features of these disorders.

Liver dysfunction has also been frequently found in several IMDs in infancy. For most of the IMDs associated with jaundice, the elevated serum bilirubin is of the direct reacting type. The best known metabolic disease associated with jaundice is galactosemia, in which deficiency of the enzyme galactose-1-phosphate uridyl transferase results in accumulation of galactose-1-phosphate and other metabolites such as galactitol that are thought to have a direct toxic effect on the liver and other organs (Vangala and Tonelli 2007). Another disorder that may be associated with neonatal jaundice is 1-antitrypsin deficiency. A determination of serum 1-antitrypsin is part of the initial evaluation of children with this syndrome. Hereditary tyrosinemia is also the cause of liver disease in early infancy (Vangala and Tonelli 2007).

Lipid storage disorders are due to an inherited deficiency of a lysosomal hydrolase that leads to lysosomal accumulation of the enzyme's specific sphingolipid substrate (Parkinson-Lawrence et al. 2010). Disorders include GM 1 gangliosidosis, GM 2 gangliosidosis, Gaucher's disease, Niemann-Pick disease (NPD), Fabry's disease, fucosidosis, Schindler's disease, metachromatic leukodystrophy, Krabbe's disease, multiple sulfatase deficiency, Farber disease, and Wolman's disease. Many of these diseases are not typically present in early infancy.

The above-mentioned metabolic diseases are considered later for the application of nanomedicine biopharmaceuticals.

Biopharmaceuticals in Therapy

Biopharmaceuticals as therapeutic drugs

A classic definition of biologics used in both academia and industry is "medical products, therapeutics, prophylactics, or *in vivo* diagnostics, whose active ingredient is biological in nature and is produced by biotechnology". This class of therapeutics generates in excess of €30 billion in sales annually, with several individual product commanding multi-billion annual revenues (Walsh 2005). Biological therapeutic agents are much larger than chemically synthesized compounds folding after translation into an elaborate three-dimensional structure. This molecular structure determines their function (Covic and Kuhlmann 2007). Biopharmaceuticals are increasingly used in therapy to treat many metabolic and oncologic diseases, for which the advances in the field of pharmaceutical biotechnology were fundamental for these achievements.

The delivery of therapeutic proteins still prevents them reaching their maximum pharmacodynamic potential, owing to their physicochemical properties, and poor stability, permeability, and biodistribution. Although the parenteral route is still the primary route of protein administration, research continues on non-parenteral delivery routes. However, the high Molecular weight (M_w) of proteins, combined with their hydrophilic and electrically charged natures, renders transport through membranes very difficult (Sarmento 2010). New technologies are applied for constructing innovative formulations and delivering biopharmaceuticals. The focus is more and more on targeted drug delivery, namely nanotechnological-based systems, as described later. In the pharmaceutical industry, there is potential to provide new formulations and routes of drug delivery. Simultaneously, the rapid advances in molecular biology and genetics contribute to an in depth understanding of mechanisms involved in disease development, and generate possibilities for novel indications for biopharmaceuticals.

The research on biopharmaceuticals is either in development or undergoing clinical trials for treatment of a number of serious diseases. Nevertheless, formulating biopharmaceuticals with the optimal therapeutic efficacy, and the possibility of large scale production of the required formulation as well as optimal storage stability is highly challenging. The exclusive structural characteristics of both amino acid-based as well as nucleic acid-based biopharmaceuticals make the formulation development more interesting than for more conventional drugs. The backbone and folding structure of the drug must be retained during processing and storage for the drug to exert its effect on its target. In addition, upon administration to the patient, the formulation must protect the drug under degradative conditions, such as the gastrointestinal (GI) tract, in order to ensure an efficient delivery to the site of action. Ideally, the formulation should ensure targeted delivery to the site of action and controlled release of the drug from the formulation at this site, thus enabling the easy administration and high efficacy of the formulated drug. The active biopharmaceutical usually requires an individualized delivery system for each drug due to its structure and complexity. Successful formulation of delivery systems for biopharmaceuticals depends on a systematic understanding of the molecular structure, stability, and biological activity of the biopharmaceutical drug, and the effect of processing it into a pharmaceutical dosage form. Developing advanced drug delivery systems thus requires interdisciplinary science, and a successful formulation of a biotechnology-based drug is very likely to be individual for each drug due to their structural complexity.

Advances in understanding the mechanism of metabolic diseases, such as diabetes and short stature, led to the discovery of polypeptide hormones. The early polypeptide hormone drugs were purified from organs, such as insulin from animal pancreas or growth hormone from cadaver pituitary. Although these products were breakthroughs in the treatment of these metabolic diseases, there were serious limitations with this type of production, including availability of organs and issues with transmission of infectious diseases. Advances in the synthesis of peptides in solution made it possible to produce peptides on the industrial scale. However, until the beginning of recombinant DNA technology, purification from natural or semi-synthetic sources, with the attendant limitations of scale and/or concerns about impurities and infectious agents, remained the only means of producing the large polypeptide therapeutics, such as insulin and human Growth Hormone (hGH).

Since the introduction of recombinant therapeutic proteins in the 1980s, a lot of products have been successfully commercialized, and new ones are currently in clinical trials. These products provide uniquely effective treatments for numerous human diseases and disorders. But the most promising protein-based drug will not be of benefit to patients unless it can be manufactured, shipped, stored, and delivered to the patient, while minimizing protein degradation. This is an overwhelming challenge because proteins can readily aggregate, even under solution conditions that greatly favor the native state. Also, proteins are susceptible to numerous pathways of chemical degradation. Adding to the challenge is the potential that even if a small fraction of the protein molecules in a dose is degraded, an immunogenic response may be triggered with the potential to cause adverse effects in patients. Also, each patient has its own characteristics and may react differently to the treatment. Furthermore, the therapeutic protein must be produced at a commercial scale using a complicated process that has been developed and documented to consistently result in a high-quality product. The appropriate analytical methods must be developed and validated to ensure that degradation products can be accurately and precisely quantified. Evidently, the successful development of a commercialized therapeutic protein product requires multidisciplinary efforts of experienced and skilled scientists, engineers, and managers, and tremendous expenditure of capital. It is very important for management to be cognizant of these challenges and to provide the appropriate resources to the development efforts for therapeutic proteins, as well as to establish reasonable timelines for this work, which is so vital to ensure product quality and protecting patients' safety.

As recombinant therapeutic proteins have been developed, there were no established academic or industrial foundations for these efforts, because recombinant proteins had never been used before to treat human diseases and disorders. Fortunately, during this time, many of the leaders in key disciplines have published papers and books describing the continually improving approaches to stabilize proteins, to analyze degradation products, and to develop successful formulations.

Challenges in the formulation of biopharmaceutical drugs

Over the last few decades there were numerous advances in the field. But there are still many new challenges to developing safe and effective therapeutic proteins. For example, monoclonal antibody products that have doses with relatively high protein concentrations (e.g., ≥ 100 mg/mL) can be difficult to manufacture, stabilize sufficiently, and analyze properly. Additionally, the use of prefilled syringes as product containers has recently led to new issues with protein stability that had to be resolved. In general, it is important to gain more fundamental insights into the effects of the various product containers and their component materials on protein stability.

During the years of development of therapeutic proteins, the types of degradation products that could be studied and the quality and resolution of analytical methods have vastly improved. These improvements allow for better understanding of causes and pathways for degradation. However, they also lead to more stringent criteria for the definition of a stable protein product. There are still many analytical challenges in this field. For example, Size Exclusion Chromatography (SEC) is the key method used to quantify levels of protein aggregates and monomers. But this method can provide misleading results because aggregates can dissociate or form during SEC and/or adsorb to the column resin. Thus, values obtained from SEC may not actually represent the true aggregate levels in the protein drug container, so there is a continued effort to investigate methods that can be used to corroborate results from SEC. Currently, the most promising approach is analytical ultracentrifugation (AUC), but this method has its own challenges in proper sample handling, data analysis, and appropriate training of personnel. The field must continue to improve SEC and AUC methods for aggregate quantification and to explore new methods (e.g., field flow fractionation).

Another challenge facing many companies is the need to develop consistent approaches for protein formulation studies, to characterize analytical methods, and to study protein stability during various processing steps. Rather, it is crucial to incorporate the scientific knowledge that has been gained across the industry in rational approaches that are developed and agreed on by educated and experienced personnel to ensure product quality and safety. As more companies develop global operations, such an approach may have the added benefits of promoting best practices between sites and individual researchers, minimizing unproductive conflicts, and speeding product development.

All biopharmaceuticals carry the potential risk of initiating an immunogenic response in the patient. The immunogenic potential of biopharmaceuticals is influenced by many factors, including the chemical structure of the molecule (e.g., variations in the amino acid sequence and glycosylation patterns), physical degradation (such as the formation of aggregates), and chemical decomposition (such as oxidation). Autoimmune condition (disease profile) or major histocompatibility class type of the patient are also known to play a role in the immunogenic response. Although the exact mechanism(s) remain unknown, the route of administration can also have an effect. Changing the route of administration does not eliminate the immunogenic response to a given protein and the risk of immunogenicity progressively increases from local, intravenous, intramuscular, to subcutaneous administration. In addition to the above factors, downstream processing (such as protein purification) as well as the formulation of a biopharmaceutical product can affect its immunogenic potential. For example, trace amounts of contaminants or impurities have been implicated in antibody development against insulin and growth hormone products. As new and improved techniques for protein purification are developed the problem of impurities may be reduced. Another important factor for consideration is the formulation of the protein product. Product formulation is critical to stabilize protein molecules to maintain the integrity of the protein structure (i.e., avoiding the formation of aggregates) and biological activity until delivery to the patient. Patient immunogenic response may be triggered by the administration of inadequately stabilized proteins that are aggregated or denatured. Some molecules, such as interferons, have a greater propensity to form aggregates under certain conditions, such as low pH or low denaturant concentrations. Interferon α protein aggregates have been found to be significantly more immunogenic than monomers *in vivo*. The use of specific assays to detect neutralizing antibodies is a key to monitoring product quality, along with close surveillance of efficacy in order to immediately detect increases in antibody production and drops in pharmacological effects (Covic and Kuhlmann 2007).

As has been the case throughout the history of working with recombinant therapeutic proteins, the field will take on current and future challenges, and will learn how to overcome them. Certainly, with future insights into disease pathologies and creation of new therapeutic protein categories, delivery approaches, and analytical methods, even more challenges will arise. With the strong foundation of excellence in therapeutic protein product development and rational approaches to delineate and solve problems, the field will successfully overcome these barriers, and new medicines will be made available for the benefit of patients.

The role of peptides and proteins in metabolic diseases

Peptide-based drugs represent a significant part of the new pharmaceuticals reaching the market every year. Most therapeutic proteins are used for life-threatening and seriously debilitating diseases such as diabetes, cancer, rheumatoid arthritis, or hepatitis. The high activity and specificity of proteins compared with the more conventional low M_W drugs often allows for a better treatment of these diseases.

Proteins may undergo a number of co- and post-translational modifications to "fine-tune" their activity. These include enzymatic cleavage (which can lead, i.e., to the activation of hormones), and attachment of lipids (for the localization of the protein to a cell membrane) or glycans (which can affect properties such as the serum half-life) (Covic and Kuhlmann 2007). Far less is known of the way in which protein and peptide drugs degrade in solution and of the factors influencing their stability. Consequently, the formulation of this increasingly important class of compounds presents more of a challenge. Protein pharmaceuticals can suffer both physical and chemical instability. Physical instability refers to changes in the higher-order structure (secondary and above) of the protein, whereas chemical instability can be thought of as any kind of modification of the protein via bond formation or cleavage, yielding a new chemical entity (Florence and Attwood 2006).

The most important feature of a therapeutic protein product is to demonstrate its safety and clinical efficacy, which comes from the combination of disease state, target biology, potency, safety margin, dosing, and selection of patient population, among other factors. All of these issues, in particular clinical efficacy, can differentiate one candidate from the next. To address these and related issues, therapeutic biologic programs desiring to generate competitive molecules need to take several factors into consideration, including: (i) molecules that provide the highest margin of efficacy, safety and lack of toxicity; (ii) route of administration (e.g., intravenous, subcutaneous), ease of administration, lack of reaction at the site of administration, and potential for self-administration; (iii) prolonged half-life and/or pharmacodynamic effect; (iv) tissue distribution and penetration; (v) stability, solubility, efficient folding, and general behavior of the molecule; and, (vi) the importance of the formulation process on the development of therapeutic proteins (Strohl and Knight 2009). In this context, therapeutic peptides and proteins may be potentially useful against numerous diseases and particularly against metabolic disorders.

The Value of Nanoparticles on the Delivery of Biopharmaceuticals

A broad spectrum of (biological, synthetic and semi-synthetic) materials assembled in a variety of conformational arrays has been designed to help in diagnostic and therapeutic interventions. These include carbon nanostructures, quantum dots, metal particles, liposomes, and formulations based on natural and/or synthetic polymers. The composition and architecture of these systems play an important role in their loading capacity, stability, biodegradability and overall biocompatibility, and various functional aspects (Sarmento 2010).

Nanoparticles (NPs) have become very important elements in novel drug delivery systems, being usually associated with the formulation and delivery of biopharmaceutical drugs. NPs are able to encapsulate biopharmaceutical molecules, thus providing protection against chemical and enzymatic degradation. In recent years, biodegradable polymeric NPs have attracted considerable attention in controlled drug release, in targeting particular organs/tissues, as DNA carriers in gene therapy, and in the delivery of proteins, peptides, hormones, antibodies, and genes (Wagner et al. 2006). NPs can be used to effectively deliver proteins to a target site, thus increasing the therapeutic benefit, while minimizing side effects (Soppimath et al. 2001). Furthermore, NPs are versatile in the method of formulation and materials to be used, can be designed to show sustained release properties, are of sub-cellular size, and can be biocompatible.

The use of NPs for the delivery of biopharmaceuticals has also been the focus in the field of long-term systemic delivery, intended to last for several days or weeks, depending on the degradability and erosion of the nanomatrix. To obtain desirable pharmacodynamic properties by altering the biopharmaceutic and pharmacokinetic characteristics of the molecule, nanoparticulate drug delivery systems show a promising approach (Sarmento 2010).

Nowadays, it is generally assumed that NPs can enhance the mucosal bioavailability of encapsulated therapeutic peptides and proteins, which might be pointed out as an advantage regarding the alternative routes of administration of biopharmaceutical drugs, rather than the classic parenteral route. Moreover, their size and their large specific surface area favor the absorption by cells of the whole particle compared to larger carriers like microparticles. It has been shown that nanoencapsulation of proteins protects them against the harsh environment of the mucosal fluids and increases their transmucosal diffusion. Nanoparticulate carriers can also be used for site-specific delivery of biopharmaceuticals, thus minimizing the toxicity associated to a non-specific biodistribution, improving patient compliance, and providing favorable clinical outcomes.

Particular interest has been focused on the oral administration of NPs containing proteins (Sarmento 2010). Peptides and proteins, unlike conventional small molecule drugs, are generally not therapeutically active upon oral administration. This lack of systemic bioavailability is mainly caused by two factors, high GI enzyme activity and the role of the GI mucosa as a barrier for absorption. There is substantial peptidase and protease activity in the GI tract, making it the most efficient body compartment for peptide and protein metabolism. Furthermore, the GI mucosa presents a major absorption barrier for water-soluble macromolecules like peptides and proteins. In addition, systemic availability of peptides is furthermore reduced by the activities of cytochrome P_{450} 3A and P-glycoprotein. Therefore, intravenous, subcutaneous, or intramuscular administration is frequently the preferred route of delivery for these drug products. During formulation, biopharmaceuticals must be assessed individually regarding their physicochemical and biological properties to develop the optimal delivery (Tang et al. 2004). One of the advantages of NPs, when administered orally, is that they can be absorbed transcellularly, although in small quantities, through the microfold cells of the Peyer's patches and also through enterocytes (Fröhlich and Roblegg 2012). NP size, electrical charge, and surface hydrophobic character are the main factors determining the NP uptake by Peyer's patches (Wells and Mercenier 2008). To improve NP uptake, surface modifications and enhanced mucoadhesive properties are usually explored with efficiency to promote the contact of proteins with the intestinal epithelium, thus increasing the concentration at the site of absorption. The NP surface can be easily modified by adsorption or chemical grafting of certain molecules such as poly(ethylene glycol) (PEG), poloxamers, and lectins. In the GI tract, cationic NPs are ideal to bind to the mucous layer, which is negatively charged, thus cationic polymers are selected as the preferred mucoadhesive coating (Sarmento 2010). Therapeutic proteins and peptides being explored for oral nanoparticulate delivery include insulin, calcitonin (CT), interferons, hGH, glucagons, gonadotropin-releasing hormones, enkephalins and, in general, vaccines, enzymes, hormone analogues, and enzyme inhibitors.

Nanomedicine biopharmaceuticals in metabolic diseases

Various nanotechnologies and other nanomaterials that are currently under investigation in medical research and diagnostics will soon find a practical application in medicine. Nanobiotechnologies are being used to create and study models of human disease, in the specific case, metabolic disorders. In the following sections, some metabolic diseases will be described and also treatments with biopharmaceuticals that are under investigation.

Diabetes

Diabetes mellitus is a metabolic disease and is a major cause of mortality and morbidity in epidemic proportions. Diabetes is a condition that occurs when the pancreas does not produce enough insulin or when the body cannot effectively use the insulin being produced. Insulin is a major anabolic hormone which regulates the carbohydrate and fat metabolism. Glucose uptake by organs such as liver, muscle, and fat tissues is possible by the action of insulin. In the absence of insulin, glucose uptake is affected thus leading to hyperglycemia, which, simultaneously with other related disturbances in the metabolic pathways cause serious damage to many of the physiological functions, especially the nerves and blood vessels. Primarily, there are two basic forms of diabetes, type 1 and type 2. In type 1 there is very little or no production of insulin, whereas in type 2, there will be insulin production but cells cannot use it effectively. A third type of diabetes, gestational diabetes mellitus, is developed during pregnancy but usually disappears after it. People with diabetes type 1 require daily injections of insulin to survive. A limited population of people with diabetes type 2 can manage their condition with lifestyle control alone, but for the majority of them oral drugs are often required (and less frequently insulin) to achieve a good metabolic control (Rekha and Sharma 2013).

The main opportunities offered by nanotechnology in diabetes are the miniaturization of the existing drug system and the improvement of the biocompatibility and bioavailability of drug carriers (Jain and Saraf 2009). Nanomedicine provides the delivery of anti-diabetic molecules which influences the disease origin rather than treating the symptoms. All of these molecules now can be delivered as new nanomedicines which require lower drug amounts, deliver selectively to the target organ or cell, and protect the drug molecules during their travel throughout the body. But so far, nanomedicine in the treatment of diabetes mellitus was used only to improve the existing administration forms of insulin, and try to improve the quality of life of patients by non-invasive administration and glucose monitoring (Rekha and Sharma 2013).

Diabetes is probably one of the metabolic disease with more studies on researching new insulin formulations (Sarmento et al. 2006, 2007a,b, Chaudhury and Das 2011), with special focus on developing oral formulations. However, insulin delivered by this route is not as effective as the one administered subcutaneously because of a poor absorption in the GI tract and its degradation by gastric acid or proteolytic enzymes, which are most important barriers limiting the insulin absorption. Encapsulation of insulin is a strategy that could protect it from digestive enzymes located in the GI tract, releasing it further down in the tract.

The oral or pulmonary delivery of insulin by polymeric NPs with focus on physiological changes, either related to the disease, or age-related metabolic variations, influence insulin bioavailability. The bioavailability of insulin being administered via routes other than the subcutaneous one is comparably low (up to 40%). Moreover factors like changed gut permeability as described for diabetes mellitus type 1 or other metabolic peculiarities such as insulin resistance in case of diabetes mellitus type 2 also play a role in affecting the development of novel nanoparticulate drug preparations, and it can be responsible for unsuccessful translation of promising *in vivo* results into human therapy. Future insulin-loaded NP development against diabetes must consider not only requirements imposed by the drug but also metabolic changes inflicted by the disease or by the age (Krol et al. 2012).

A recently published review on oral delivery of therapeutic protein/ peptides against diabetes focused on the advances reported during the past decade in the field of the oral administration of insulin and other peptidic incretin hormones such as Glucagon-Like Peptide-1 (GLP-1), and exendin-4 (Jain and Saraf 2009). From the very recent reports on oral delivery systems it is obvious that more focus is on polymeric nanoparticulate systems. Biocompatible non-toxic nanoplatforms being absorbed into the systemic circulation and cleared from the body will be the most appropriate means to improve the bioavailability of therapeutic proteins. Multifunctional NPs which can specifically protect the loaded insulin from enzymatic degradation, overcome the mucin barriers, enhance the insulin absorption by pathways such as transcellular or paracellular, and prolong the GI retention, holds the basis for improved insulin bioavailability. In addition, another approach which can be investigated is the use of nanoconjugates/nanocomplexes of the proteins/ peptides (i.e., insulin, GLP-1, and exendin-4) (Park et al. 2011, Rekha and Sharma 2013). By taking advantage of these multifunctional nanoplatforms for oral delivery, it is expected to define the definitive oral insulin formulation; however, safety remains a concern for any NP-based system.

Some studies have described the potential application of NPs containing insulin for the oral control of diabetes. As an example, nanosystems consisting of an enteric capsule and poly(D,L-lactide-*co*-glycolide) (PLGA) NPs for the oral delivery of insulin have been developed (Wu et al. 2012). The enteric capsule was coated with pH-sensitive hydroxypropyl methylcellulose phthalate, which could selectively release insulin from the NPs in the intestinal tract, instead of the stomach. Alginate (ALG) NPs have been applied to deliver insulin orally (Sarmento et al. 2007b). When administered orally to diabetic rats, basal serum glucose levels were lowered by more than 40%, thus sustaining a hypoglycemia over 18 hours. Insulin was also encapsulated within chitosan (CS) NPs through an ionotropic gelation technique. Following intratracheal administration to rats, quantitative analyses of the hypoglycemic effect and lung distribution studies demonstrated that this system is able to deliver CS NPs deep into the lungs and, thus, transport insulin in its bioactive form to the systemic circulation to induce a hypoglycemia. This effect was significantly pronounced and prolonged compared to the control formulations (Al-Qadi et al. 2012). In fact, progresses in the engineering of CS NPs for an efficient oral insulin delivery were recently reviewed (Mukhopadhyay et al. 2012). Several published reports state that certain modifications can protect insulin from the acidic environment and from the proteolytic deactivation in the stomach. NPs formulated with mild and straightforward methods are preferred. Moreover, maintaining the biocompatibility is the goal in all cases.

Finally, posttranscriptional gene silencing by ribonucleic acid interference (RNA*i*) represents a promising gene therapy approach to treat diabetes (Wang et al. 2010, Jean et al. 2012). However, direct delivery of RNA*i*-inducing entities such as synthetic small interfering ribonucleic acid (*si*RNA) or short hairpin ribonucleic acid (*sh*RNA) continues to be problematic owing to their rapid extracellular/intracellular degradation by nucleases, limited blood stability, poor cell uptake, and non-specific targeting (Katas and Alpar 2006). As a consequence, the translation of RNA*i* into the clinic is still pending the resolution of these issues.

Phenylketonuria

PKU is an inborn error of metabolism characterized by intolerance to the essential amino acid Phe in the diet, caused by a defect in the Phe hydroxylase, which is responsible for converting Phe to tyrosine, thus resulting in systemic Phe accumulation providing neurotoxic levels (and impaired cognitive development) (Sarkissian et al. 2011). Untreated, this disorder will result in severe intellectual disability. However, with proper management, the outcome is excellent. For many years, this disorder was managed exclusively with a Phe-restricted diet, but compliance with the diet is difficult. Therefore, the development of alternative treatments is desirable. Preclinical investigations of gene and cell therapies for PKU are ongoing (Bélanger-Quintana et al. 2011).

The Pahenu2/enu2 PKU mouse model to study oral enzyme substitution therapy with various chemically modified formulations of Phe ammonia lyase was developed. *In vivo* studies with the most therapeutically effective formulation (5 kDa PEGylated chemically modified Phe ammonia lyase) revealed that this conjugate, given orally, yielded statistically significant

(p = 0.0029) and therapeutically relevant reduction ($\approx$ 40%) in plasma Phe levels. Phe reduction occurred in a dose- and loading-dependent manner. A sustained clinically and statistically significant reduction of plasma Phe levels was observed with a treatment ranging from 0.3 to 9 IU, and with more frequent and smaller doses. Oral Phe ammonia lyase therapy could potentially serve as an adjunct therapy, perhaps with a dietary treatment, and will work independently of Phe hydroxylase, correcting such forms of hyperphenylalaninemias regardless of the Phe hydroxylase mutations carried by the patient. Phe ammonia lyase has the potential to correct the harmful metabolic phenotype in human patients and it might eliminate or reduce the need for dietary therapy in the treatment of PKU. Also, a chemically modified Phe ammonia lyase hydrogel protected NP formulation, a barium ALG microsphere formulation, an amorphous silica particle formulation, as well as a fusion protein formulation with protein transduction domains were investigated. Despite exhibiting varying levels of *in vitro* activities, *in vivo* activities for these formulations were unremarkable and did not produce statistically significant data (Sarkissian et al. 2011).

Osteoporosis

Osteoporosis is a metabolic bone disease characterized by a disorder of bone remodeling. Bone remodeling is the highly integrated process of resorption and successive formation of bone tissue that results in the maintenance of the skeletal mass with renewal of the mineralized matrix. The remodeling sites are known as basic multicellular units. The renewal of bone tissue occurs through cycles of activity. The first step includes the activation of quiescent osteoclasts and precursors that begin to excavate a cavity on a bony surface. Then, osteoblast precursors are activated and refill the excavation site.

Current treatments for osteoporosis can be divided into two categories: anti-resorptive modulators and anabolic therapies. Estrogen, estrogen receptor modulators, CT, and bisphosphonates (BPs) fall into the first category (Wang and Grainger 2012). Human clinical experience indicates that improved therapeutic strategies are needed in the context of osteoclastic bone resorption therapies. Researchers have attempted to quantify the importance of each component in the prevention or reversal of osteoporosis, but there still remains significant debate on the best means of preventing this disease. For these reasons, pharmaceutical agents have become the current last-resort treatment method. However, there are several risks that exist for the use of any pharmaceutical agents to stimulate new bone formation. First, these agents can cause non-specific bone formation in areas not selectively affected by the disease (Balasundaram et al. 2006).

In osteoporosis research there are several major barriers that exist for the use of any pharmaceutical agent to stimulate new bone formation. Because of these limitations, even the best strategies to sufficiently increase bone mass require at least one year to see any change; a time period not acceptable especially for the elderly. For these reasons, nanotechnology may be a reliable tool to explore in the development of novel drug-carrying systems that will specifically attach to the osteoporotic bone and distribute pharmaceutical agents locally to quickly increase bone mass.

Salmon CT is a single chain polypeptide hormone used in the long-term therapy of metabolic bone diseases characterized by excessive bone turnover, such as osteoporosis. Salmon CT therapy inhibits or slows osteoclast-mediated resorptive bone loss. However, the therapeutic utility of commercially available salmon CT to treat these conditions is severely restricted by the short plasma half-life of salmon CT (≈ 17 to ≈ 57 minutes) due to a rapid plasma clearance and enzymatic degradation via proteolysis in kidneys, liver, and blood. Recently, the therapeutic efficacy of a PEGylated salmon CT analog with improved bone targeting by BP conjugation was evaluated *in vivo*. Compared to the marketed unmodified salmon CT, the PEGylated salmon CT analog conjugated to BP showed a significantly improved efficacy in terms of preserving bone volume, bone mineral density, and trabecular micro-architecture in osteoporotic rats (Bhandari et al. 2012). This advanced formulation is expected to prolong the retention time of the protein in blood.

Metabolic skeletal disorders associated with impaired bone formation are a major clinical challenge. One approach to treat these defects is to silence bone formation inhibitory genes by *si*RNAs in osteogeniclineage cells that occupy the niche surrounding the bone formation surfaces. Dioleoyl trimethylammonium propane-based cationic liposomes surface functionalized with six repetitive sequences of aspartate-serine-serine for delivering *si*RNAs specifically to bone formation surfaces were developed. An osteogenic *si*RNA that targets casein kinase-2 interacting protein-1 was encapsulated to the liposomes. It was found that the *in vivo* systemic delivery of this *si*RNA in rats using this liposome-based system resulted in the selective enrichment of the *si*RNAs in osteogenic cells. A bioimaging analysis further showed that this approach markedly promoted bone formation, enhanced the bone micro-architecture, and increased the bone mass in both healthy and osteoporotic rats (Zhang et al. 2012).

The parathyroid hormone-related protein 1-34 (PTHrP1-34), another protein involved in bone homeostasis (promoting the proliferation of osteoblast and immature bone-like cells) was incorporated into *N*-(2-hydroxyl) propyl-3-trimethyl ammonium chitosan chloride (HTCC) NPs (100 to 180 nm in size). The encapsulation efficiency and loading capacity were related to the HTCC concentration and the initial concentration of PTHrP1-34. Maximum values reported were ≈ 78 and $\approx 14\%$, respectively. The *in vitro* release profile of PTHrP1-34 from the NPs was characterized by an initial burst release phase, followed by a slow release phase. The PTHrP1-34-loaded HTCC NPs were found to be appropriate for the treatment of osteoporosis because of their biphasic (slow) release properties (Zhao et al. 2010).

Growth hormone deficiency

Growth hormone deficiency is a condition in which the hGH is inadequately produced. Growth hormone, also known as somatotropin, is a polypeptide hormone that stimulates growth and cellular reproduction. At various stages of life, different symptoms and effects may be present. Children will experience stunted growth. Adults may have decreased lean body mass, poor bone density, and several physical and psychological problems. hGH deficiency can be either congenital or acquired in adult life (often due to a tumor). It is sometimes temporary, but it is most often permanent. hGH deficiency is treated by growth hormone replacement therapy.

Recombinant hGH (22 kDa) is currently administered by subcutaneous injection to children with a short stature due to growth hormone deficiency. The welfare of these patients would therefore greatly benefit from a non-invasive delivery method of hGH. The oral route would represent the most convenient alternative. However, the bioavailability of oral hGH is very low, given the enzymatic degradation in the GI tract.

In this context, there is a need for solutions less invasive than subcutaneous injection and there are several researchers studying other routes of administration and formulations for the delivery of hGH. A dry powder aerosol formed of hGH, lactose, and dipalmitoyl phosphatidylcholine was assessed for systemic delivery of the hormone in rats. The fate of the protein locally in the deep lung was examined post-delivery. A dry powder aerosol improved absorption of hGH in the lungs over a simple solution (Bosquillon et al. 2004).

The effectiveness of CS NPs in promoting the intranasal bioavailability of recombinant hGH has been evaluated (Cheng et al. 2005). In this study, hGH was formulated with CS to produce a powder blend and granules for intranasal administration. The *in vivo* pharmacokinetic performance of the formulations was evaluated in a group of six sheep in a randomized crossover study. A subcutaneous injection of hGH solution was administered as a control. The intranasal and subcutaneous doses of hGH were 0.3 and 0.03 mg/Kg, respectively. The intranasal formulations appeared to be well tolerated. It was concluded that CS-based intranasal powder formulations can provide a practical means for non-injectable delivery of hGH.

Although, the nasal route has many potential advantages over, for example, the oral route in terms of less demanding physiological barriers to peptide and protein transport across the mucosa, nasal absorption of such drugs is normally < 1%. Thus, the need for nasal absorption promoter systems to obtain an efficient nasal delivery of peptides and proteins is accepted. For instance, the absorption enhancing efficiency of CriticalSorb™ for hGH has been investigated *in vivo*. The absorption enhancing component of CriticalSorb™, Solutol® HS15, comprises polyglycol mono- and di-esters of 12-hydroxystearic acid, combined with free PEG. When administering hGH nasally in rats with increasing concentrations of Solutol® HS15, a bioavailability of 49% in the first 2 hours after administration were obtained. Furthermore, it was shown that the most effective ratio of Solutol® HS15 to hGH was 4:1 on a mg to mg basis. Histopathology studies in rats after five days of repeated nasal administration showed that Solutol® HS15 had no toxic effect on the nasal mucosa. These results were confirmed in a six month repeat nasal toxicity study in rats (Illum et al. 2012).

Recently, an effective and simple method was developed to prepare spherical and uniform-sized recombinant hGH-Zn^{2+}-dextran NPs. Recombinant hGH recovered from the NPs maintained its structural integrity and its bioactivity well, as demonstrated *in vitro*. The use of PEG and polysaccharide to mediate Zn^{2+}-induced precipitation has proved to be a promising method to prepare the protein-loaded NPs. It was demonstrated that drug loading was achieved without the aid of organic solvents or any other harmful treatment (Yuan et al. 2012).

Niemann-pick disease

NPD type B is a multiorgan system disorder caused by a genetic deficiency of acid sphingomyelinase (ASM), for which the lung is an important and challenging therapeutic target. New delivery vehicles for enzyme replacement therapy of the disease consisting of polystyrene and PLGA NPs targeted to the intercellular adhesion molecule 1 (ICAM-1), a protein expressed on endothelial cells throughout the vasculature up-regulated in NPD type B, were evaluated. Fluorescence microscopy of lung alveoli actin, tissue histology, and iodine-125 (^{125}I)-albumin blood-to-lung transport showed that anti-ICAM-loaded NPs can cause neither detectable lung injury, nor abnormal vascular permeability *in vivo*. Radioisotope tracing showed rapid disappearance from blood and enhanced accumulation of anti-ICAM/^{125}I-ASM-loaded NPs over the non-targeted (naked) enzyme in the kidney, heart, liver, spleen, and primarily the lungs, both in wild-type and ASM knockout mice (Fig. 15.1). These data demonstrated that ICAM-1-targeted NPs can enhance enzyme replacement therapy for NPD type B (Garnacho et al. 2008).

Fabry's disease

Fabry's disease, due to the deficiency of α-galactosidase (α-Gal), causes lysosomal accumulation of globotriaosylceramide in multiple tissues and prominently in the vascular endothelium. Although enzyme replacement therapy by injection of recombinant α-Gal improves the disease outcome, the effects on the vasculopathy associated with life-threatening cerebrovascular, cardiac, and renal complications are still limited. A strategy to enhance the delivery of α-Gal to organs and endothelial cells has been recently developed.

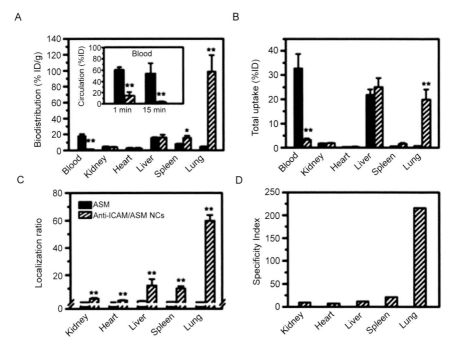

Figure 15.1. ASM delivery by anti-ICAM/ASM-loaded nanocarriers (NCs) in a NPD mouse model. Biodistribution of ^{125}I-labeled ASM 30 minutes after intravenous injection in anesthetized ASM knockout mice, calculated as percent of injected dose per gram (%ID/g) of tissue (A), %ID per organ (B), localization ratio (C), and specificity index (D). A comparison of naked ^{125}I-ASM (black bars) and 180 nm-sized anti-ICAM/^{125}I-ASM polystyrene particles (hatched bars) is shown. The inset in A shows NP clearance from blood (%ID). Data are mean ± standard error of mean ($n \geq 5$). Statistical differences between free enzyme and anti-ICAM-loaded NPs are depicted by asterisks: * ($p < 0.05$) and ** ($p < 0.01$) (Student's t test). Reproduced with permission from Garnacho et al. (2008). Copyright American Society for Pharmacology and Experimental Therapeutics (2008).

Concretely, α-Gal was targeted to ICAM-1 by loading this enzyme on NPs coated with anti-ICAM (anti-ICAM/α-Gal NPs). *In vitro* radioisotope tracing showed the efficient loading of α-Gal on the anti-ICAM NPs, stability of this formulation under storage and in model physiological fluids, and enzyme release in response to lysosome environmental conditions. In mice, the delivery of ^{125}I-α-Gal was markedly enhanced by the NPs coated with anti-ICAM in the brain, kidney, heart, liver, lung, and spleen, and transmission electron microscopy showed anti-ICAM/α-Gal NPs attached to and internalized into the vascular endothelium. Fluorescence microscopy proved targeting, endocytosis, and lysosomal transport of anti-ICAM/α-Gal NPs in macro- and micro-vascular endothelial cells, and a marked enhancement of globotriaosylceramide degradation (Fig. 15.2). Thus, ICAM-1 targeting strategy may help to improve the efficacy of therapeutic enzymes against Fabry's disease (Hsu et al. 2011).

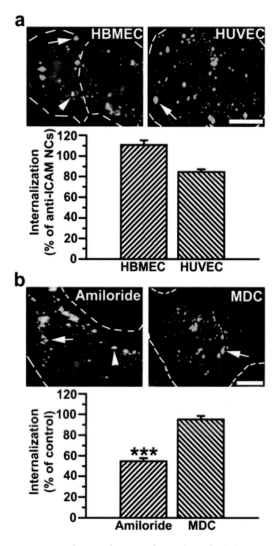

Figure 15.2. Efficient targeting and internalization of anti-ICAM/α-Gal NCs in micro- and macro-vascular endothelial cells. (a) Fluorescence microscopy images and quantification of tumor necrosis factor-α (TNF-α)-activated human brain microvascular endothelial cells (HBMECs) and human umbilical vein endothelial cells (HUVECs) incubated with fluorescein isothiocyanate (FITC)-labeled anti-ICAM/α-Gal NCs at 37°C for 30 minutes, washed and incubated in cell medium for 30 minutes. Cells were fixed and surface-bound NPs and nuclei were stained with Texas-Red-labeled anti-mouse immunoglobulin G (Ig G) and 4',6-diamidino-2-phenylindole (DAPI), respectively. (b) Uptake of anti-ICAM/α-Gal NPs was also tested in the presence of amiloride or monodansylcadaverine (MDC), which inhibit CAM- or clathrin-mediated endocytosis, respectively. In both (a) and (b), single-labeled green NPs are internalized (arrow) vs. double-labeled (green + red) yellow NPs which are located at the cell surface (arrow head). Dashed lines mark the cell border, determined by phase-contrast. Scale bar: 10 μm. Data are mean ± standard error of mean ($n \geq 55$, duplicated). *** is $p \leq 0.001$ by Student's t test. Reproduced with permission from Hsu et al. (2011). Copyright Elsevier B.V. (2011).

Conclusions

Biopharmaceuticals are continuously being researched against diseases. Particularly, in metabolic diseases there are some important advances that suggest the potential of these active agents. On the other hand, this field faces many challenges that need to be overcome in order to obtain formulations that are efficient, stable, non-toxic, and non-immunogenic. Moreover, metabolic diseases are chronic conditions that require health care during the entire life. In this context, it is crucial to develop formulations to improve patient compliance by non-injectable delivery of therapeutic proteins and peptides.

Acknowledgement

Financial support from Fundação para a Ciência e a Tecnologia (FCT, Portugal) (PTDC/SAU-FCF/70651/2006, SFRH/BPD/35996/2007 and PTDC/SAUFCF/104492/2008).

Abbreviations

ALG	:	alginate
ASM	:	acid sphingomyelinase
AUC	:	analytical ultracentrifugation
BP	:	bisphosphonate
CS	:	chitosan
CT	:	calcitonin
DAPI	:	4′,6-diamidino-2-phenylindole
DNA	:	deoxyribonucleic acid
FITC	:	fluorescein isothiocyanate
α-Gal	:	α-galactosidase
GI	:	gastrointestinal
GLP-1	:	glucagon-like peptide-1
HBMEC	:	human brain microvascular endothelial cell
hGH	:	human growth hormone
HTCC	:	N-(2-hydroxyl) propyl-3-trimethyl ammonium chitosan chloride
HUVEC	:	human umbilical vein endothelial cell
^{125}I	:	iodine-125
Ig G	:	immunoglobulin G
%ID/g	:	percent of injected dose per gram
IMD	:	inborn metabolic disorder
MDC	:	monodansylcadaverine
M_W	:	molecular weight
NC	:	nanocarrier
NP	:	nanoparticle

NPD	:	niemann-pick disease
PEG	:	poly(ethylene glycol)
Phe	:	phenylalanine
PLGA	:	poly(D,L-lactide-*co*-glycolide)
PTHrP1-34	:	parathyroid hormone-related protein 1-34
PKU	:	phenylketonuria
RNA*i*	:	ribonucleic acid interference
*sh*RNA	:	short hairpin ribonucleic acid
SEC	:	size exclusion chromatography
*si*RNA	:	small interfering ribonucleic acid
TNF-*α*	:	tumor necrosis factor-*α*

References

Al-Qadi, S. and A. Grenha, D. Carrión-Recio, B. Seijo and C. Remuñán-López. 2012. Microencapsulated chitosan nanoparticles for pulmonary protein delivery: *in vivo* evaluation of insulin-loaded formulations. J. Control. Release. 157: 383–390.

Balasundaram, G. and M. Sato and T.J. Webster. 2006. Using hydroxyapatite nanoparticles and decreased crystallinity to promote osteoblast adhesion similar to functionalizing with RGD. Biomaterials. 27: 2798–2805.

Bélanger-Quintana, A. and A. Burlina, C.O. Harding and A.C. Muntau. 2011. Up to date knowledge on different treatment strategies for phenylketonuria. Mol. Genet. Metab. 104: S19–S25.

Bhambure, R. and K. Kumar and A.S. Rathore. 2011. High-throughput process development for biopharmaceutical drug substances. Trends Biotechnol. 29: 127–135.

Bhandari, K.H. and M. Newa, J. Chapman and M.R. Doschak. 2012. Synthesis, characterization and evaluation of bone targeting salmon calcitonin analogs in normal and osteoporotic rats. J. Control. Release. 158: 44–52.

Bosquillon, C. and V. Préat and R. Vanbever. 2004. Pulmonary delivery of growth hormone using dry powders and visualization of its local fate in rats. J. Control. Release. 96: 233–244.

Butler, M. 2005. Animal cell cultures: recent achievements and perspectives in the production of biopharmaceuticals. Appl. Microbiol. Biotechnol. 68: 283–291.

Chaudhury, A. and S. Das. 2011. Recent advancement of chitosan-based nanoparticles for oral controlled delivery of insulin and other therapeutic agents. AAPS Pharm. Sci. Tech. 12: 10–20.

Cheng, Y.H. and A.M. Dyer, I. Jabbal-Gill, M. Hinchcliffe, R. Nankervis, A. Smith and P. Watts. 2005. Intranasal delivery of recombinant human growth hormone (somatropin) in sheep using chitosan-based powder formulations. Eur. J. Pharm. Sci. 26: 9–15.

Covic, A. and M. Kuhlmann. 2007. Biosimilars: recent developments. Int. Urol. Nephrol. 39: 261–266.

Erez, A. and O.A. Shchelochkov, S.E. Plon, F. Scaglia and B. Lee. 2011. Insights into the pathogenesis and treatment of cancer from inborn errors of metabolism. Am. J. Hum. Genet. 88: 402–421.

Florence, A.T. and D. Attwood. 2006. Physicochemical Principles of Pharmacy. 4th Ed. Pharmaceutical Press. London, UK.

Fröhlich, E. and E. Roblegg. 2012. Models for oral uptake of nanoparticles in consumer products. Toxicology. 291: 10–17.

Garnacho, C. and R. Dhami, E. Simone, T. Dziubla, J. Leferovich, E.H. Schuchman, V. Muzykantov and S. Muro. 2008. Delivery of acid sphingomyelinase in normal and niemann-pick disease mice using intercellular adhesion molecule-1-targeted polymer nanocarriers. J. Pharmacol. Exp. Ther. 325: 400–408.

Hsu, J. and D. Serrano, T. Bhowmick, K. Kumar, Y. Shen, Y.C. Kuo, C. Garnacho and S. Muro. 2011. Enhanced endothelial delivery and biochemical effects of α-galactosidase by ICAM-1-targeted nanocarriers for Fabry disease. J. Control. Release. 149: 323–331.

Illum, L. and F. Jordan and A.L. Lewis. 2012. CriticalSorb: a novel efficient nasal delivery system for human growth hormone based on Solutol HS15. J. Control. Release. 162: 194–200.

Jain, S. and S. Saraf. 2009. Influence of processing variables and *in vitro* characterization of glipizide loaded biodegradable nanoparticles. Diabetes Metab. Syndr. Clin. Res. Rev. 3: 113–117.

Jean, M. and M. Alameh, D. De Jesus, M. Thibault, M. Lavertu, V. Darras, M. Nelea, M.D. Buschmann and A. Merzouki. 2012. Chitosan-based therapeutic nanoparticles for combination gene therapy and gene silencing of *in vitro* cell lines relevant to type 2 diabetes. Eur. J. Pharm. Sci. 45: 138–149.

Katas, H. and H.O. Alpar. 2006. Development and characterisation of chitosan nanoparticles for siRNA delivery. J. Control. Release. 115: 216–225.

Krol, S. and R. Ellis-Behnke and P. Marchetti. 2012. Nanomedicine for treatment of diabetes in an aging population: state-of-the-art and future developments. Maturitas. 73: 61–67.

Mukhopadhyay, P. and R. Mishra and D. Rana. 2012. Strategies for effective oral insulin delivery with modified chitosan nanoparticles: a review. Prog. Polym. Sci. 37: 1457–1475.

Park, K. and I.C. Kwon and K. Park. 2011. Oral protein delivery: current status and future prospect. React. Funct. Polym. 71: 280–287.

Parkinson-Lawrence, E.J. and T. Shandala, M. Prodoehl, R. Plew, G.N. Borlace and D.A. Brooks. 2010. Lysosomal storage disease: revealing lysosomal function and physiology. Physiology (Bethesda). 25: 102–115.

Rekha, M.R. and C.P. Sharma. 2013. Oral delivery of therapeutic protein/peptide for diabetes—future perspectives. Int. J. Pharm. 440: 48–62.

Sarkissian, C.N. and T.S. Kang, A. Gámez, C.R. Scriver and R.C. Stevens. 2011. Evaluation of orally administered PEGylated phenylalanine ammonia lyase in mice for the treatment of Phenylketonuria. Mol. Genet. Metab. 104: 249–254.

Sarmento, B. and A. Ribeiro, F. Veiga and D. Ferreira. 2006. Development and characterization of new insulin containing polysaccharide nanoparticles. Colloids Surf. B Biointerfaces. 53: 193–202.

Sarmento, B. and S. Martins, D. Ferreira and E.B. Souto. 2007a. Oral insulin delivery by means of solid lipid nanoparticles. Int. J. Nanomedicine. 2: 743–749.

Sarmento, B. and A. Ribeiro, F. Veiga, P. Sampaio, R. Neufeld and D. Ferreira. 2007b. Alginate/chitosan nanoparticles are effective for oral insulin delivery. Pharm. Res. 24: 2198–2206.

Sarmento, B. 2010. Nanomedicines for delivery of therapeutic proteins and biopharmaceuticals. Ther. Deliv. 1: 231–235.

Soppimath, K.S. and T.M. Aminabhavi, A.R. Kulkarni and W.E. Rudzinski. 2001. Biodegradable polymeric nanoparticles as drug delivery devices. J. Control. Release. 70: 1–20.

Strohl, W.R. and D.M. Knight. 2009. Discovery and development of biopharmaceuticals: current issues. Curr. Opin. Biotechnol. 20: 668–672.

Tang, L. and A.M. Persky, G. Hochhaus and B. Meibohm. 2004. Pharmacokinetic aspects of biotechnology products. J. Pharm. Sci. 93: 2184–2204.

Vangala, S. and A. Tonelli. 2007. Biomarkers, metabonomics, and drug development: can inborn errors of metabolism help in understanding drug toxicity? AAPS J. 9: E284–E297.

Wagner, V. and A. Dullaart, A.K. Bock and A. Zweck. 2006. The emerging nanomedicine landscape. Nat. Biotechnol. 24: 1211–1217.

Walsh, G. 2005. Biopharmaceuticals: recent approvals and likely directions. Trends Biotechnol. 23: 553–558.

Wang, J. and Z. Lu, M.G. Wientjes and J.L. Au. 2010. Delivery of siRNA therapeutics: barriers and carriers. AAPS J. 12: 492–503.

Wang, Y. and D.W. Grainger. 2012. RNA therapeutics targeting osteoclast-mediated excessive bone resorption. Adv. Drug Deliv. Rev. 64: 1341–1357.

Wells, J.M. and A. Mercenier. 2008. Mucosal delivery of therapeutic and prophylactic molecules using lactic acid bacteria. Nat. Rev. Microbiol. 6: 349–362.

Wu, Z.M. and L. Zhou, X.D. Guo, W. Jiang, L. Ling, Y. Qian, K.Q. Luo and L.J. Zhang. 2012. HP55-coated capsule containing PLGA/RS nanoparticles for oral delivery of insulin. Int. J. Pharm. 425: 1–8.

Yuan, W. and Z. Hu, J. Su, F. Wu, Z. Liu and T. Jin. 2012. Preparation and characterization of recombinant human growth hormone–Zn2+-dextran nanoparticles using aqueous phase–aqueous phase emulsion. Nanomedicine. 8: 424–427.

Zhang, G. and B. Guo, H. Wu, T. Tang, B.T. Zhang, L. Zheng, Y. He, Z. Yang, X. Pan, H. Chow, K. To, Y. Li, D. Li, X. Wang, Y. Wang, K. Lee, Z. Hou, N. Dong, G. Li, K. Leung, L. Hung, F. He, L. Zhang and L. Qin. 2012. A delivery system targeting bone formation surfaces to facilitate RNAi-based anabolic therapy. Nat. Med. 18: 307–314.

Zhao, S.H. and X.T. Wu, W.C. Guo, Y.M. Du, L. Yu and J. Tang. 2010. N-(2-hydroxyl) propyl-3-trimethyl ammonium chitosan chloride nanoparticle as a novel delivery system for parathyroid hormone-related protein 1–34. Int. J. Pharm. 393: 269–273.

CHAPTER 16

Nanotechnology in Gene Knockdown and *mi*RNA Replacement *In Vivo*

Achim Aigner

ABSTRACT

Ribonucleic acid interference is a particularly efficient mechanism for the knockdown of virtually any given target gene, thus providing, in theory, abundant possibilities for therapeutic applications. It relies on the action of small interfering ribonucleic acids, and their delivery *in vivo* has become one of probably the most formidable obstacles in the exploration of ribonucleic acid interference. More recently, micro ribonucleic acids have been discovered as an important class of endogenous small ribonucleic acids. Since they specifically interfere in the expression of various genes, their aberrant down-regulation in many pathologies has led to the concept of micro ribonucleic acid replacement therapy, i.e., their re-introduction to restore physiological micro ribonucleic acid levels to inhibit the expression of disease relevant genes. Since the same pharmacokinetic issues apply, nanoparticles may offer a platform for small interfering ribonucleic acid as well as for micro ribonucleic acid delivery. Considerable progress in the development of novel non-viral strategies for nucleic acid delivery has been made, and preclinical *in vivo* studies have evaluated their therapeutic potential. This chapter provides an overview of various nanoparticle-based approaches for small interfering ribonucleic acid-mediated gene knockdown and micro ribonucleic acid replacement. After an introduction into small interfering ribonucleic acids and micro ribonucleic acids, their mechanisms of action and their therapeutic potential, various nanoparticulate systems are discussed, including liposomal and

Rudolf-Boehm-Institute for Pharmacology and Toxicology, Clinical Pharmacology, University of Leipzig, Haertelstrasse 16 – 18, D – 04107 Leipzig, Germany.
Email: achim.aigner@medizin.uni-leipzig.de

polymeric systems, and approaches for ligand-mediated targeted delivery. *In vivo* applications of the various nanoparticulate systems are exemplified by a comprehensive overview of preclinical studies.

Small Therapeutic Ribonucleic Acids

Small interfering ribonucleic acids for the induction of ribonucleic acid interference

Since the late 1970s, antisense oligonucleotides have been used for the specific inhibition of gene expression (Stephenson and Zamecnik 1978). Upon hybridizing to their target ribonucleic acid (RNA), they sterically inhibit messenger ribonucleic acid (*m*RNA) translation or the correct splicing of precursor RNAs, and/or mediate RNA degradation through the action of ribonuclease H. The idea of the specific knockdown of the expression of a given target gene was also explored after the discovery of ribozymes in the early 1980s: catalytically active RNAs that sequence-specifically bind to and cleave their target *m*RNA. Both approaches, including deoxyribonucleic acid (DNA)-based ribozymes, have been studied quite extensively with regard to the development of nucleic acid molecules with optimal chemical modifications, and strategies for their delivery *in vitro* and *in vivo*.

The initial observation of the silencing of an endogenous gene through a homologous double stranded ribonucleic acid (*ds*RNA) molecule, described first in petunia flowers more than 25 years ago (Jorgensen 1990, Napoli et al. 1990) and termed "post-transcriptional gene silencing" or "co-suppression", was mechanistically explained in 1998. Fire et al. (1998) demonstrated that the injection of *ds*RNAs into the nematode *Caenorhabditis elegans* led to a marked silencing of a gene. Importantly, subsequent studies showed that this process, that was termed ribonucleic acid interference (RNA*i*), also occurs in mammals (Hammond et al. 2000, Hannon 2002). In the last few years, it has become clear that RNA*i* represents a particularly efficient method of gene silencing. Meanwhile, it is an almost standard tool in biochemical and biomedical research *in vitro*, allowing the functional analysis of any selected gene *in vitro*. *In vivo* studies and in particular any therapeutic intervention, however, meet formidable obstacles that have already been issued in antisense and ribozyme targeting before, above all the delivery of the nucleic acids.

RNA*i* is mediated through short 21–23 nucleotide (nt) *ds*RNA molecules (small interfering ribonucleic acids, *si*RNAs). While these *si*RNAs can be generated intracellularly through the action of a ribonuclease type-III endonuclease enzyme complex called Dicer, that cleaves longer *ds*RNAs (Hammond et al. 2000, Parrish et al. 2000, Yang et al. 2000, Zamore et al. 2000, Elbashir et al. 2001a,b), it should be noted that the direct delivery of *si*RNAs as the RNA*i* effector molecules is sufficient for the induction of RNA*i* (Elbashir et al. 2001a). On their intracellular generation or delivery, *si*RNAs become part of a nuclease-containing multiprotein complex termed "ribonucleic acid-induced silencing complex" (RISC) (Hammond et al. 2000). Based on the sequence complementarity, the now single-stranded short RNA molecule, and with it the whole RISC complex, bind to the target *m*RNA. RISC also contains the endonuclease Argonaute2 that cleaves the target *m*RNA at the position directed by the guiding *si*RNA strand (Liu et al. 2004, Rand et al. 2004, Rivas et al. 2005). Due to the newly formed unprotected RNA ends, the cleaved *m*RNA is rapidly degraded by intracellular nucleases and is thus unavailable for translation. Since RISC on the other hand is recovered for further *m*RNA targeting, RNA*i* can be considered as a catalytical process which may well explain its comparably high efficacy.

Since the discovery of the pivotal roles of *si*RNA in mediating RNA*i*, several studies have defined criteria for optimal *si*RNA sequences against a given target (Reynolds et al. 2004, Ui-Tei et al. 2004). Beyond improved efficacy, this also includes the absence of unwanted non-specific effects. Off-target effects can occur when unwanted *m*RNAs are hit or when the passenger strand, rather than the guide strand, binds to a target *m*RNA molecule. This emphasizes the importance of efforts been made to increase *si*RNA specificities, including the so-called "strand bias", i.e., the use of *si*RNAs that ensure the preferential use of the correct strand as guide strand (Khvorova et al. 2003, Schwarz et al. 2003). Furthermore, effects unrelated to RNA*i* have been described like the activation of the innate immune system (e.g., Toll-like receptors), leading to stimulation of inflammatory cytokine release and inflammatory responses (Robbins et al. 2008, Jackson and Linsley 2010). These effects are based on certain sequence motives, which consequently should be avoided when defining optimal *si*RNAs (Judge et al. 2005, Robbins et al. 2009). Finally, chemical modifications have been explored, aiming at increased stability and/or improved binding to the target *m*RNA (Rettig and Behlke 2012). While all these studies have led to the development of highly efficient *si*RNAs, their delivery still poses a major challenge especially for their therapeutic application.

Micro (small non-coding) ribonucleic acids as regulators in physiological and pathophysiological processes

More recently, micro (small non-coding) ribonucleic acids (*mi*RNAs) have been discovered as an important class of small RNA molecules that regulate gene expression. Unlike *si*RNAs, *mi*RNAs are endogenous RNAs that are transcribed from the genome into large so-called primary *mi*RNAs of 1–3 kilobases in length (Lee et al. 2004, Rodriguez et al. 2004). The ribonuclease Drosha and DiGeorge critical region 8 (DGCR8) further process these primary transcripts in the nucleus to pre-*mi*RNAs, 70–100 nt hairpin intermediates that are then exported by exportin 5 in the cytoplasm (Bohnsack et al. 2004). Upon their Dicer-mediated processing into the mature 18–25 *mi*RNA (Hammond et al. 2000), the guide strand is incorporated into a complex called micro ribonucleic acid-induced silencing complex (*mi*RISC) and guides *mi*RISC to its target *m*RNA (Hutvágner and Zamore 2002, Bartel 2009). While this is reminiscent of *si*RNA-mediated RNA*i*, it should be noted that partial complementarity is sufficient for *mi*RNA action: translational repression or *m*RNA cleavage with subsequent degradation (Bartel 2004, Mathonnet et al. 2007, Pillai et al. 2007). Pivotal for *mi*RNA binding and activity are the nucleotides 2–8 of the *mi*RNA, the so-called "seed region", and while *in silico* analyses allow the prediction of target genes of a given *mi*RNA, this always needs experimental confirmation. Notably, since a partial complementarity is sufficient for *mi*RNA action, *mi*RNAs can well have several 100 target genes, with important implications for their therapeutic exploration.

Potential of small interfering ribonucleic acids or micro ribonucleic acids in therapy

In various diseases, gene products have been found to be overexpressed. Oncogenes in tumors are an example, leading to the hallmarks of cancer like uncontrolled proliferation, inhibition of apoptosis, or the capability to metastasize (Hanahan and Weinberg 2011). Here, the inhibition of the expression of the respective gene can revert cellular properties acquired during malignant transformation, thus leading, e.g., to growth arrest, induction of apoptosis, or increased sensitivity towards chemotherapy. One therapeutic approach may be the application of RNA*i* for the knockdown of gene expression. Additionally, in many pathologies mutated gene products have been identified and linked, e.g., to point mutations or chromosomal rearrangements, leading to an aberrant activity of the respective protein. Here, the inhibition on the protein level may be particularly difficult since it may be hard to find inhibitors that are specific only for the mutated protein, and some gene products are even considered "undruggable". Of note, the RNA*i*-mediated knockdown of the expression of the respective gene can provide a particularly high specificity since *si*RNAs act sequence-specifically and may be able to distinguish between wild-type and mutated genes.

Beyond their function as markers, numerous studies have identified certain *mi*RNAs as pathologically relevant, e.g., in cancer (Aigner 2011, Sayed and Abdellatif 2011, Lujambio and Lowe 2012). Here, *mi*RNAs inhibiting oncogenes can be down-regulated, and the replacement of these tumor suppressor *mi*RNAs may serve as a therapeutic approach. Similar results have been obtained in other pathologies, based on functional analysis and the identification of target genes of a given *mi*RNA *in vitro*, providing insight into the role of a given *mi*RNA in a certain pathology. The goal of the restoration of physiological *mi*RNA levels in the case of a pathological down-regulation can be achieved by delivering *mi*RNAs or *mi*RNA mimics. Compared to *si*RNAs, even a significant increase in *mi*RNA levels is expected to generate rather mild effects on their target genes. Unwanted "off-target effects" (non-specific effects), unwanted "on-target effects" (effects on unwanted target genes), the stimulation of the innate immune system or non-specific toxicities, however, still require detailed analysis.

Nanoparticles for Ribonucleic Acid Delivery

For the delivery of small RNA molecules (*si*RNA, *mi*RNA), various non-viral delivery strategies have been explored, thus avoiding the various issues associated with viral systems. In some cases, the injection of non-formulated RNAs can be considered, sometimes aided by physical methods like hydrodynamic injection (high speed injection of large volumes, leading to a transient increase in membrane permeability) (Merl et al. 2005), or electropulsation (Takahashi et al. 2005). Furthermore, the covalent conjugation of RNAs to antibodies, aptamers, cholesterol, lipids, peptides, and other moieties has been described.

Nanoparticles (NPs) are usually in the range of ≈ 20 to several 100 nanometers which allows their cellular endocytosis. They aim at the protection of the nucleic acid "payload" (*si*RNAs/*mi*RNAs are particularly prone to degradation and *si*RNA half-lives in serum have been found to be in the range of a few minutes) (Dowler et al. 2006), the delivery to the target organ, cellular entry and intracellular release, including the escape from endosomes/lysosomes and the release of the RNA from its formulation. Other issues that need to be taken into consideration are the absence of toxic and other non-specific effects of the NP and its components, and favorable pharmacokinetic properties. Routes of administration often rely on intravenous injections, however, various other local or systemic applications including intracardiac, intramuscular, intranasal, intraocular, intrapancreatic, intraperitoneal, intratesticular, intratracheal, intratumor, retroorbital/subretinal, subcutaneous, and transurethral injections, or injection/infusion into the brain (hypothalamus, ventricular system), the ear, joint, liver, optic nerve stump, renal artery, and the vagina have been explored as well.

NPs include liposomes and other lipid-based NPs, inorganic NPs like gold NPs, cationic polymers like polyamines or polyethylenimines (PEIs), atelocollagen, chitosan, or cyclodextrin (CD), and various derivatives and combinations of these. While some nanocarrier systems have initially been developed for DNA delivery and later adopted for small RNAs, other studies have aimed at NPs specialized for *si*RNAs. It should also be noted that DNA transfection efficacies do not necessarily correlate with *si*RNA knockdown performance, at least *in vitro* (Höbel et al. 2011). While this may be due to the different requirements with regard to the intracellular localization of the nucleic acids, it has also been shown that the different lengths of the nucleic acids (*si*RNAs are generally at least 200-fold shorter than plasmid DNA) translates into differences in physicochemical properties like the stability of polymeric nanoplexes (Malek et al. 2008). On the other hand, *in vitro* efficacies often poorly reflect the *in vivo* behavior of NPs, making it difficult to avoid their testing in animal experiments. A recent paper on the direct comparison of *in vitro* vs. *in vivo* effects revealed for *si*RNA-containing lipid NPs that it depends on the cell line if *in vitro* results correlate with the *in vivo* silencing potential, and that in fact only *si*RNA entrapment efficacy, but not NP size or zeta potential, are partially predictive of *in vivo* performance (Whitehead et al. 2012).

Liposomal/lipid-based nanoparticles

Liposomal NPs can be divided into neutral and cationic liposomes. Cationic lipids can be mixed with a co-lipid at different proportions, and different methods for liposome preparation can be employed, leading to different compositions and structures and thus different physicochemical and biological properties. When cationic NPs are formed on the basis of electrostatic interactions with nucleic acids, it needs to be kept in mind that *si*RNAs are smaller than DNA plasmids and may thus form less stable NPs with incomplete *si*RNA protection. As noted above, this leads to variations between liposomal formulations used for DNA vs. *si*RNA. The charge of cationic liposomes affects tissue distribution (Landen et al. 2005), and uptake by macrophages (Miller et al. 1998), and they may interact with biological materials *in vivo*, i.e., extracellular matrix components like glycosaminoglycans, lipoproteins, or serum proteins. Results can be NP aggregation or destabilization, binding to and uptake into non-target cells, or non-specific biological effects. To avoid these issues, the coating of cationic liposomes, e.g., with poly(ethylene glycol) (PEG) has been described to reduce interactions between NPs with biological structures, and to increase blood circulation and NP stability (Gomes-da-Silva et al. 2012).

Cationic lipids being used include 1,2-dioleoyl-3-trimethylammoniumpropane (DOTAP), *N*-(1-(2,3-dioleyloxy) propyl)-*N*,*N*,*N*-trimethyl-ammoniumchloride (DOTMA), or dioleoylphosphatidylethanolamine (DOPE). The toxicity of cationic lipids and their potential to induce interferon responses, however, can be limiting for their *in vivo* use, and chemical modifications have been introduced to address this issue (Tousignant et al. 2000, Dass 2002). Alternatively, neutral unilamellar nano-sized liposomes like 1,2-dioleoyl-*sn*-glycero-3-phosphatidylcholine (DOPC) have been employed, providing a hydrophobic surface and a hydrophilic core, thus mediating protection from outside endonucleases and internalization via membrane fusion or receptor-mediated endocytosis (Halder et al. 2006). These lipids can be envisaged as non-viral envelopes that encapsulate *si*RNAs. Again, this will protect *si*RNAs from nucleolytic degradation, increase serum half-lives, decrease renal excretion due to a size increase above the renal threshold, and mediate delivery and cellular uptake in target organs.

DOPE in combination with the cationic lipid RPR209120 has been used for the delivery of a *si*RNA that targets tumor necrosis factor. In an arthritis model in mice, knockdown of Tumor Necrosis Factor (TNF) levels increased after an intravenous injection resulting in the complete regression of the induced arthritis (Khoury et al. 2006, 2008). Staramine is a lipopolyamine functionalized with methoxy poly(ethylene glycol) (mPEG), and the intravenous injection of PEGylated Staramine NPs containing *si*RNAs demonstrated preferred uptake in the lung (Sparks et al. 2012). When using a monodisperse mPEG 515 Da, endothelial cells were identified as target cells (Polach et al. 2012).

*si*RNA cationic lipid (AtuFECT01) lipoplexes have been studied quite extensively. Notably, in tumor models they were shown to target the endothelium rather than the tumor cells (Santel et al. 2006a,b). When mice were intravenously injected with Atu027, an AtuFECT01-formulated modified *si*RNA targeting protein kinase N3, lung metastasis induced by tail vein injection of Lewis lung carcinoma or B16 melanoma cells was markedly decreased (Santel et al. 2010). Repeated bolus injections or infusions in mice, rats, and non-human primates resulted in the specific knockdown of protein kinase N3 expression, and in orthotopic mouse models for pancreatic or prostate cancer, a significant inhibition of tumor growth and lymph node metastasis formation was observed (Aleku et al. 2008).

Likewise, Stable Nucleic Acid Lipid Particles (SNALPs) have been used in several *in vivo* studies for *si*RNA delivery and are now also explored in clinical studies. SNALP-formulated *si*RNAs showed a longer half-life in the liver and plasma in an *in vivo* mouse model of Hepatitis B Virus (HBV) replication, and dose-dependently reduced serum HBV DNA after an intravenous injection into mice carrying replicating HBV (Morrissey et al. 2005). Protection from death was observed in guinea pigs when treated with a pool of SNALP-formulated *si*RNAs targeting the polymerase (L) gene of the Zaire species of Ebola virus shortly before the Ebola challenge. This was one study directly comparing SNALPs with polymeric NPs based on PEI (see below), with SNALPs here being more potent (Geisbert et al. 2006). SNALP-encapsulated *si*RNAs were also the first that were tested in non-human primates by intravenously injecting apolipoprotein B (Apo B)-specific SNALP/*si*RNAs into cynomolgus monkeys. A deep dose-dependent silencing of Apo B *m*RNA and protein levels was observed with concomitantly reduced low-density lipoprotein and serum cholesterol levels already 24 hours after treatment (Zimmermann et al. 2006). In a tumor study, chemically modified and SNALP-formulated *si*RNA targeting the essential cell-cycle proteins polo-like kinase 1 and kinesin spindle protein in mice exhibited potent antitumor efficacy in hepatic and subcutaneous tumor models (Judge et al. 2009).

Improvement of SNALPs was implemented using rational design strategies leading to specific alterations of lipid properties with regard to *si*RNA delivery. Based on the ionizable cationic lipid 1,2-dilinoleyloxy-3-dimethylaminopropane (DLinDMA), the key lipid component of SNALPs, DLinDMA-based lipids with superior delivery capacity were designed. The amino lipid 2,2-dilinoleyl-4-dimethylaminoethyl-[1,3]-dioxolane (DLin-KC2-DMA) as the best performing lipid displayed *in vivo* activity in SNALPs at low *si*RNA doses in rodents and non-human primates (Semple et al. 2010). Also, novel lipid-based formulations have been studied systematically by the screening of large combinatorial libraries and resulted in the identification of the so-called "lipoids" as promising new candidates. Chemical methods for the rapid synthesis of a large library of structurally diverse lipidoids allowed the screening of > 1,200 compounds, and the safety and efficacy of candidate lipidoids was evaluated in mice, rats, and non-human primates (Akinc et al. 2008, Love et al. 2010).

Polymers

Comparable to cationic liposomes, electrostatic interactions allow the formation of NPs comprising nucleic acids and cationic polymers. Candidate polymers include synthetic (e.g., PEI, CD-based polycations) or natural (e.g., atelocollagen, chitosan) polymers as well as cationic proteins/peptides like cationized human serum albumin, histones, poly(L-lysine), or poly(L-ornithine).

Atelocollagen

The first biomaterial introduced as a gene delivery system was atelocollagen, which is obtained by treatment of type I collagen of calf dermis with pepsin (Ochiya et al. 1999, 2001, Sano et al. 2003), in order to remove the immunogenic N- and C-terminal ends ("telopeptides"). Later studies showed that atelocollagen complexation leads to the protection of *si*RNAs, thus allowing their *in vivo* delivery (Aigner 2008). The complexes are based on electrostatic interactions and their size is dependent on the ratio between nucleic acids and atelocollagen.

Intratumor injection of atelocollagen/*si*RNA complexes was explored in subcutaneous prostate carcinoma xenograft models. The knockdown of the Vascular Endothelial Growth Factor (VEGF) receptor (Takei et al. 2004), or midkine (MK) (Takei et al. 2006) led to reduced tumor growth. In the latter study, antitumor effects could be augmented by combined treatment with paclitaxel, thus giving a good example for the possibility to incorporate knockdown strategies with established therapeutic regimens. MK as a target was also explored in intimal hyperplasia, which is a major obstacle to patency after vein grafting. The atelocollagen/*si*RNA-mediated knockdown of MK upon administration of the complexes to the external wall of grafted veins prevented this long-term progressive disease by leading to decreases of the intima-media ratio and the intima thickness, resulting in a significant reduction of inflammatory cell recruitment to the vessel walls and subsequent cell proliferation (Banno et al. 2006). An inhibition of orthotopic non-seminomatous germ cell tumor growth was achieved by site-specific injection of an atelocollagen/*si*RNA complex targeting the antisense oligonucleotide HST-1/FGF-4 (Minakuchi et al. 2004). Other examples include the suppression of Panc-1 pancreatic carcinoma xenograft growth through down-regulation of the proteinase-activated receptor-2 (Iwaki et al. 2008), antitumor effects upon HPV18 E6 and E7 gene knockdown in cervical xenografts (Fujii et al. 2006), increased apoptosis in a prostate cancer model upon the knockdown of glutathione S-transferase-pi (Hokaiwado et al. 2008), and the augmentation of cytostatic treatment through Epidermal Growth Factor Receptor (EGFR) knockdown in squamous cell carcinoma xenografts (Nozawa et al. 2006). The systemic administration of atelocollagen/*si*RNA complexes for tumor treatment was explored as well. The knockdown of candidate targets for inhibition of bone metastasis, the zeste homolog 2 and the phosphoinositide 3'-hydroxykinase p110-α-subunit, led to metastatic tumor growth inhibition in bone tissues (Takeshita et al. 2005). Increased muscle mass was determined on the intravenous or intramuscular injection of atelocollagen/*si*RNA complexes specific for myostatin (Kinouchi et al. 2008). Finally, as an example of antiviral treatment, inhibition of the John Cunningham virus agnoprotein expression was observed on local injection of atelocollagen/*si*RNA complexes in the mouse brain (Matoba et al. 2008), and the intravenous injection of atelocollagen-complexed *si*RNA targeting chemokine monocyte chemoattractant protein-1 (MCP-1) reduced recruitment of immune cells and symptoms of contact hypersensitivity in mice, as indicated by a significant decrease in ear swelling (Ishimoto et al. 2008).

Chitosan

Chitosan is a natural, biodegradable, positively charged polymer with low immunogenicity and low toxicity (Shu and Zhu 2002, Lee et al. 2005), that was initially used for *si*RNA delivery *in vitro* (Katas and Alpar 2006, Liu et al. 2007). It has also been found that the Molecular weight (M_w) and the degree of deacetylation of chitosan, the chitosan/*si*RNA ratio, the pH, as well as the method of ionic cross-linking (ionic gelation using sodium tripolyphosphate or simple complexation) determine the physicochemical properties and the targeting efficacies of the chitosan/*si*RNA NPs. Thus, optimal properties need to be determined when using chitosan for *si*RNA delivery (Katas and Alpar 2006, Liu et al. 2007, Xu et al. 2007).

Beyond *in vitro* studies, EGFR knockdown in bronchiole epithelial cells of transgenic mice was described after nasal administration of chitosan/*si*RNA NPs (Howard et al. 2006). As self-tracking delivery system for *si*RNAs, i.e., chitosan NPs with encapsulated fluorescent quantum dots and labeled with human epidermal growth factor receptor type-2 (HER-2) antibodies, were used to deliver HER-2/neu *si*RNA to HER-2-overexpressing SKBR3 breast cancer cells (Tan et al. 2007). Using chitosan derivatives, the intravenous administration of complexes comprising chitosan-coated poly(isohexylcyanoacrylate)/*si*RNAs targeting Rho A kinase resulted in tumor growth inhibition in breast cancer xenografts (Pille et al. 2006). Likewise, upon intratumor injection, the knockdown of ret/PTC1 oncogene led to thyroid carcinoma xenograft growth suppression (de Martimprey et al. 2008).

Cyclodextrin

CDs are highly biocompatible cyclic oligomers of glucose which, unlike atelocollagen or chitosan, do not carry a positive charge and, for nucleic acid delivery, can thus be combined with polymers (Heidel 2006). CD-containing polycations with transferrin as a ligand for preferential uptake into transferrin receptor-expressing tumor cells have been employed for *si*RNA delivery in a murine model of Ewing's sarcoma. The knockdown of the EWS-FLI1 gene product led to antitumor effects which, notably, were dependent on the targeting ligand transferrin (Hu-Lieskovan et al. 2005). In contrast, intravenously injected non-targeted NPs for the knockdown of the ribonucleotide reductase subunit M2 showed significantly lower effects in Neuro2A tumor xenografts (Bartlett and Davis 2008).

Polyethylenimine

PEIs are synthetic linear or branched polymers, showing partial protonation of the amino groups in every third position under physiological conditions. Thus, based on electrostatic interactions, the polymer molecules which are available at various M_ws are able to form complexes "polyplexes" with negatively charged nucleic acids (Boussif et al. 1995). This leads to the compaction of the nucleic acids (condensation), the shielding of their negative charges, and their complete protection from nuclease-mediated degradation. Complexes are internalized, dependent on the cell and the exact complex composition, via clathrin- or caveolae-dependent routes. Intracellularly, they are released from endosomes due to the so-called "proton sponge effect": PEI acts as proton acceptor and the osmotic imbalance leads to increased Cl$^-$ and subsequent water influx, osmotic swelling, and finally burst of the lysosomes with release of the complexes into the cytoplasm (Boussif et al. 1995, Behr 1997). Thus, PEI complexation combines the extracellular protection, cellular uptake, and intracellular release of nucleic acids including small RNAs. For still further improvement of complex release, membrane-destabilizing reagents have been introduced (Boeckle et al. 2006, Shir et al. 2006).

While all PEIs may be able to complex *si*RNAs, their suitability for *si*RNA delivery is determined by several parameters including toxicity and biological activity, complexation efficacy as well as stability, size and net charge of the complexes. Major determinants are thus the M_ws of the PEI and the nucleic acid, their molecular ratio (the so-called N/P ratio referring to the nitrogen atoms of PEI and the nucleic acid phosphates), the degree of branching of PEI, and the complexation buffer (Werth et al. 2006, Höbel et al. 2008). Regarding the M_w of *si*RNAs, the reversible concatemerization of *si*RNAs with short sticky overhangs was demonstrated to improve *in vivo* linear PEI/*si*RNA-mediated gene knockdown in the lung (Bolcato-Bellemin et al. 2007). This suggests that lacking cooperativity on complex formation and the rigidity of the *si*RNA may sometimes be problems in PEI/*si*RNA complexation formation.

PEIs that have been studied rather extensively with regard to the *in vivo* delivery of *si*RNAs include the linear, $\approx$ 22 kDa PEI and the branched $\approx$ 4–10 kDa PEI F25 low M_w. Studies using linear PEI demonstrated gene knockdown in brain and in the lung of luciferase-positive newborn mice (Hassani et al. 2005, Bolcato-Bellemin et al. 2007, Bonnet et al. 2008). Therapeutic studies showed the efficient delivery of intact *si*RNAs into subcutaneous SKOV-3 ovarian carcinoma mouse tumor xenografts and antitumor effects upon knockdown of HER-2 (Urban-Klein et al. 2005), or the inhibition of subcutaneous liver and lung xenografts upon knockdown of RecQL1 DNA helicase (Futami et al. 2008). Notably, biodistribution studies also showed that very different *si*RNA delivery profiles are obtained dependent on the route of administration, and with regard to the systemic application, intraperitoneal injection is the method of choice when targeting subcutaneous tumor xenografts. The same was true for the knockdown of the growth factor pleiotrophin in subcutaneous U87 glioblastoma xenografts, leading to reduced tumor growth and tumor angiogenesis (Grzelinski et al. 2006). In this study, the intrathecal injection of PEI/*si*RNA NPs was explored as well, with significant antitumorigenic effects compared to non-specific PEI/*si*RNA complexes or buffer control (Grzelinski et al. 2006). In the above mentioned paper on the post exposure protection of guinea pigs against a lethal Ebola virus challenge, the intraperitoneal injection of PEI/*si*RNA resulted in the knockdown of the polymerase (L) gene of the Zaire species of Ebola virus and to protective effects due to a significant reduction in plasma viremia, although SNALPs proved to be more efficient in this setting (Geisbert et al. 2006).

Beyond linear PEIs, certain branched PEIs have been employed as well for *si*RNA delivery *in vivo*. The low M_w PEI F25, derived from commercially available 25 kDa PEI through size exclusion chromatography (Werth et al. 2006), was used for the complexation of chemically modified or non-modified *si*RNAs targeting the tumor-relevant growth factor VEGF. In subcutaneous prostate and pancreatic carcinoma xenografts in mice, the intraperitoneal injection of the complexes resulted in tumor growth inhibition, based on the knockdown of VEGF expression (Höbel et al. 2010). Notably, the mode of injection was again critical for biological activity, and biodistribution studies of PEI-complexed 32P-labeled *si*RNAs supported the notion of marked differences between intraperitoneal and intravenous administration, with intraperitoneal injections being the method of choice in subcutaneous xenograft studies. Still, both approaches mediated systemic availability of the complexes, which was not the case upon intratracheal instillation. Here, complexes remained exclusively localized in the lung, thus offering the option of local therapy, and it should also be noted that PEI complexes can be nebulized. Intrathecal administration was explored by Hendruschk et al. (2011) targeting survivin. While the systemic treatment of subcutaneous glioblastoma xenograft bearing mice led to a marked reduction of tumor growth, the treatment of orthotopic glioblastomas with PEI/*si*RNA targeting survivin inhibitor apoptosis protein led to increased survival (Hendruschk et al. 2011). Systemic PEI/*si*RNA treatment was also explored for the targeting of the spindle checkpoint gene MAD2 in colon carcinoma xenografts, resulting in the inhibition of tumor xenograft growth (Kaestner et al. 2011). Despite the fact that PEI is not biodegradable, PEI accumulation or cumulative toxicity upon repeated injection of complexes or naked PEI was observed in none of these studies. Thus, in contrast to *in vitro* assays indicating that the free polymer can be somewhat more toxic (Malek et al. 2008), these results do not seem to apply for the *in vivo* situation.

Other PEIs have been employed for studies in the lung, relying on intravenous application. Examples include the treatment and prevention of lethal influenza infections in the mouse by injecting PEI/*si*RNA complexes for the knockdown of conserved regions of influenza virus genes. When the complexes were administered before or after initiation of the virus infection, reduced virus production in lungs of infected mice was observed (Ge et al. 2004). In agreement with the above mentioned biodistribution studies (Höbel et al. 2010), the lung was found to be one preferential organ of intravenously injected PEI/*si*RNA complexes (Ge et al. 2004).

Local administrations have been explored as well. Intratumor injections were employed for the knockdown of mutant K-ras gene in subcutaneous pancreatic carcinoma xenografts (Zhu et al. 2006). The local injection PEI/*si*RNA complexes for the knockdown of FCγ RIII receptors in arthritic temporomandibular joints led to decreased nociceptive and inflammatory responses (Yang et al. 2008). Other examples include the injection of PEI/*si*RNA complexes within the peritoneal cavity, aiming at the prevention of abdominopelvic adhesions upon generation of ischemic and serosal injury to the uterine horns in mice by knockdown of plasminogen activator inhibitor 1 and hypoxia inducible factor 1α (Segura et al. 2007), or the targeting of the N-methyl-D-aspartate receptor subunit protein NR2B in a rat model. In this study, intrathecal injection of PEI/*si*RNA complexes was employed with the primary goal of modulation of pain. Regarding receptor subtype specificity and hence the absence of non-selective binding, the advantages of the *si*RNA-mediated gene targeting over less selective N-methyl-D-aspartate antagonists become obvious in this study (Tan et al. 2005).

The biocompatibility of PEI complexes can be further increased by covalent coupling with non-ionic hydrophilic polymers like PEG (Bhadra et al. 2002) or other chemical modifications (Zintchenko et al. 2008). Surface modifications by using PEG-PEI copolymers for complex formation aim at shielding the positive surface charge of complexes with concomitant reduction of non-specific interactions of the complex with biological structures (Petersen et al. 2002). *In vivo*, some PEGylated PEI-based complexes show prolonged blood circulation times. This effect is dependent on the structure of PEG-PEI copolymer (Kunath et al. 2002), and physicochemical as well as biological properties of *si*RNA-copolymer complexes can be correlated with PEG-PEI structures and PEG grafting patterns (Mao et al. 2006, Malek et al. 2008, 2009, Merkel et al. 2009). Of note, the *in vivo* behavior of PEGylated PEI/*si*RNA complexes is also determined by physiological properties like, e.g., induction of hemorrhage in the lung or erythrocyte aggregation (Malek et al. 2009). In agreement with a recent study on liposomes (Whitehead et al. 2012), this demonstrates that it is hardly possible to conclude the *in vivo* behavior of a given NP only from physicochemical analyses or tissue culture data, without performing actual *in vivo* experiments. Another example of PEI modifications is the grafting of PEIs with maltose, maltotriose, or maltoheptaose, which has been shown to decrease cytotoxicities of those (oligo)maltose PEI-based complexes. While decreased zeta potentials led to poorer *si*RNA delivery *in vitro*, the systemic *in vivo* application of the complexes revealed differences in their biodistribution profiles, dependent on the pattern of (oligo)maltose grafting (Höbel et al. 2011). Another chemical modification is the full deacetylation of PEI. An increase in efficacy was shown by the knockdown of luciferase as a model gene or of the influenza viral nucleocapsid protein gene, leading to a 94% drop of virus titers in the lungs of influenza infected animals (Thomas et al. 2005).

Finally, chemical modifications may also apply to the *si*RNA. A polyelectrolyte complex micelle-based *si*RNA delivery system has been described, relying on the interaction between PEI and PEG-conjugated VEGF *si*RNAs. Intratumor or intravenous injection of the polyelectrolyte complex micelles decreased VEGF levels in the tumor tissue and tumor growth (Kim et al. 2008).

In addition to chemical modifications of PEI, the coupling of targeting ligands has been explored for a more target-specific uptake of PEI-based complexes into selected organs or tissues (see below).

Ligand-mediated targeted delivery

Since NPs usually do not provide target organ specificity, efforts have been made for their targeted delivery. Basically, one can distinguish between passive and active targeting. While passive targeting relies on the pathophysiology of the respective target organ or target cells, thus being based on NP size and shape as well as on the route of administration, active targeting is frequently achieved by chemical modification of NP surfaces. More specifically, it includes the covalent coupling of ligands or antibodies for specific recognition and binding to target structures on the surface of the target cells/target organ.

Liposomal nanoplexes decorated with anti-transferrin receptor single-chain antibody fragments (scFv) (immunoliposomes) were shown to preferentially bind to tumor cells with elevated transferrin receptor levels (Xu et al. 2001, 2002, Pirollo et al. 2006). Intravenously injected ≈ 100 nm-sized immunoliposomes delivered HER-2 specific *si*RNAs into subcutaneous breast carcinoma tumor xenografts in mice, leading to reduced HER-2 expression and induction of apoptosis (Hogrefe et al. 2006). Through inclusion of a pH-sensitive histidine-lysine peptide in the complex, the endosomal release of the payload was further increased (Yu et al. 2004). The immunoliposome/anti-HER-2 *si*RNA complex sensitized human tumor cells to chemotherapeutics, silenced HER-2, and affected HER-2 downstream pathway components *in vivo*, with a significant inhibition of tumor growth in a subcutaneous pancreatic carcinoma xenograft model (Pirollo et al. 2007).

In another study, PEG-PEI based self-assembling NPs were generated, with arginine-glycine-aspartic acid (RGD) peptides at the distal ends of the PEGs. This led to a preferential binding to the integrins on the tumor neovasculature. A selective uptake into subcutaneous tumor xenografts, target gene knockdown within the tumor as well as reduced tumor growth and angiogenesis was observed upon the intravenous injection of these NPs containing *si*RNAs against VEGF receptor type-2 (Schiffelers et al. 2004).

The tumor targeting ability of glycol chitosan-PEI/*si*RNA modified with hydrophobic 5-*β*-cholanic acid, was explored in tumor-bearing mice, and a significant inhibition of red fluorescent protein expression was observed (Huh et al. 2010). As a target-specific delivery system for the delivery of *si*RNAs into Hyaluronic Acid (HA) receptor-positive tumor cells, HA-modified PEI was explored. After intratumor injection, PEI-HA-based complexes delivered *si*RNAs for VEGF knockdown, leading to melanoma xenograft growth inhibition (Jiang et al. 2009).

Nanoparticles for *In Vivo* Micro Ribonucleic Acid Replacement

More recently, NPs have also been explored for the therapeutic delivery of *mi*RNAs under conditions of a pathologically low level of a given *mi*RNA (Table 16.1). Benefiting from the very similar structure of the RNAs, comparable or identical NP systems have been used.

An example is the *mi*RNA-143/145 family in colon carcinoma. Although no correlation between expression levels and clinical features was found (Wang et al. 2009, Akao et al. 2010), both *mi*RNAs are frequently down-regulated in cancer and adenoma specimens, and in mouse-based therapy studies the therapeutic effects of *mi*RNA replacement were demonstrated for both *mi*RNAs. More specifically, a synthetic, *mi*RNA-143 analog, chemically modified according to a previous study with *si*RNAs (Ueno et al. 2008) and mixed with cationic liposomes, led to the suppression of tumor xenograft growth when injected intravenously or intratumorally (Akao et al. 2010). Of note, the same group also showed the secreted microvesicles of monocytes/macrophages to deliver *mi*RNAs: when THP-1 human monocytic leukemia were *ex vivo* transfected with these *mi*RNA-143 and subsequently intravenously injected into mice, the secretion of the *mi*RNA-143 entrapped into microvesicles and *mi*RNA-143 delivery to the tumor xenografts was observed (Akao et al. 2011).

Chemically unmodified *mi*RNA-145 duplexes, formulated in polymeric NPs, were explored as well (Ibrahim et al. 2011). Upon complexation with low M_W PEI F25 (Werth et al. 2006), and intratumor injection, a significant reduction of tumor growth was observed in subcutaneous LS174T colon carcinoma xenografts in mice (Ibrahim et al. 2011). More importantly, PEI complexation

Table 16.1. *mi*RNA replacement therapy based on the NP-mediated delivery of *mi*RNAs.

Chemical composition/ formulation	Route of administration	*mi*RNA	*In vivo* model	Therapeutic effect	Reference
In vivo transfection reagent Entranster™	Intratumorally	let-7	Subcutaneous CRC DLD1 xenografts	Reduced tumor growth	Wang et al. 2012
Liposome-polycation-hyaluronic acid (LPHA) NPs with tumor targeting scFv	Intravenously	*mi*RNA-34a	Lung metastasis mouse model	Reduced metastatic tumor load	Chen et al. 2010
*mi*RNA mimics/Lipofectamine®	Intratumorally	*mi*RNA-29b	K562 xenografts	Suppression of tumor growth	Garzon et al. 2009
*mi*RNA-143BPx/cationic liposome	Intravenously	*mi*RNA-143	Subcutaneous colorectal cancer xenografts	Tumor suppression	Akao et al. 2010, Kitade and Akao 2010
*si*PORT™ amine transfection reagent	Intratumorally	let-7 *mi*RNA	Established non-small cell lung cancer in mice	Reduction of tumor burden	Trang et al. 2010
*mi*RNA-502 precursor/*si*PORT™ amine transfection reagent	Intratumorally	*mi*RNA-502	Established colorectal cancer in mice	Inhibition of tumor growth	Zhai et al. 2013
Atelocollagen	Intravenously	*mi*RNA-16	Bone metastasis model	Inhibition of prostate tumor growth in bone	Takeshita et al. 2010
PEI complexation	Intraperitoneally	*mi*RNA-33a, *mi*RNA-145	Subcutaneous colon carcinoma xenografts	Tumor growth inhibition	Ibrahim et al. 2011

also allowed the intraperitoneal application, leading to the delivery of intact *mi*RNA molecules into the xenograft tumors and profound antitumor effects. On the cellular and molecular level, decreased tumor proliferation and increased apoptosis was observed as well as inhibition of c-Myc gene and extracellular signal-regulated protein kinase 5 (ERK5) as a novel regulatory target of *mi*RNA-145 (Ibrahim et al. 2011). The same PEI NPs were employed for *mi*RNA-33a delivery. *mi*RNA-33a had been shown recently to directly regulate the constitutively active serine/threonine kinase Pim-1 (Thomas et al. 2012), which is a proto-oncogene overexpressed in various tumors and linked to poor prognosis. Indeed, antitumor effects were observed on the systemic injection of PEI-complexed *mi*RNA-33a. Notably, results were comparable with the direct RNA*i*-mediated knockdown of Pim-1 by PEI/*si*RNA complexes (Ibrahim et al. 2011).

Using atelocollagen *mi*RNA-16 replacement was explored by Takeshita et al. (2010). Three intravenous injections of atelocollagen/*mi*RNA-16 complexes into tumor-bearing mice every third day led to the inhibition of bone metastatic human prostate tumor growth in the mouse bone site.

Liposomal systems for *mi*RNA replacement were used in a xenograft leukemia model. The intratumor injection of *mi*RNA-29b mimics formulated with the transfection reagent lipofectamine led to antitumor effects, with two tumors going into complete remission (Garzon et al. 2009). Likewise, the intratumor injection of a *mi*RNA-502 precursor, formulated with the lipid-based transfection reagent *si*PORT™ Amine into established HCT-116 tumor xenografts decreased tumor growth (Zhai et al. 2013). In established subcutaneous H460 non-small cell lung cancer xenografts, the intratumor injection of the synthetic *mi*RNA let-7 complexed with *si*PORT™ Amine led to a robust decrease of tumor growth (Trang et al. 2010). *mi*RNA let-7 mixed with the transfection reagent Entranster™ and intratumorally injected in a study in subcutaneous colon tumor xenografts (Wang et al. 2012).

Conclusions

*si*RNAs allow the specific and efficient knockdown of any given target gene, with, in theory, abundant possibilities for therapeutic RNA*i* applications in various diseases. *mi*RNA-based therapies exhibit milder effects on a given target gene and rather lead to the reprogramming of whole molecular pathways. Consequently, both approaches are somewhat different with regard to biological and therapeutic results, and may be explored in parallel and in combination. In the last decade, the delivery of RNA molecules has become the probably most formidable obstacle in the exploration of RNA*i* and, more recently, of *mi*RNAs.

In both cases, NPs may offer a platform for *si*RNA/*mi*RNA protection and application. Approaches for their targeted, ligand-mediated delivery and uptake may have the potential to further improve pharmacokinetics and efficacies. However, issues that have been obstacles in antisense and ribozyme technologies need to be addressed here as well. While the design of NPs has to meet several criteria for *in vivo* applicability and efficacy, it should be noted that, from a viewpoint of clinical pharmacology and drug approval, complicated multi-component systems will be more likely to encounter obstacles in their transfer into the clinics. Also, after decades of working on targeted NPs, little success has been made with regard to their actual use in medicine. However, considerable progress regarding chemical modifications of RNA molecules, and the development of novel nanocarriers has been made. Once the problems related to the poor pharmacokinetics are solved, although probably more challenging than in the case of many low M_W drugs, novel strategies for individualized tailor-made therapies are feasible.

Acknowledgments

Original work from the Aigner laboratory on RNA*i* and *mi*RNA replacement was supported by grants from the Deutsche Forschungsgemeinschaft (German Research Foundation), the Deutsche Krebshilfe (German Cancer Aid), the Verein für Krebsforschung (VfK) and the Youssef Jameel Foundation. The author apologizes to colleagues whose excellent work has not been cited due to space restrictions.

Abbreviations

Apo B	:	apolipoprotein B
CD	:	cyclodextrin
DGCR8	:	DiGeorge critical region 8
DLinDMA	:	1,2-dilinoleyloxy-3-dimethylaminopropane
DLin-KC2-DMA	:	2,2-dilinoleyl-4-dimethylaminoethyl-[1,3]-dioxolane
DNA	:	deoxyribonucleic acid
DOPC	:	1,2-dioleoyl-*sn*-glycero-3-phosphatidylcholine
DOPE	:	dioleoylphosphatidylethanolamine
DOTAP	:	1,2-dioleoyl-3-trimethylammoniumpropane
DOTMA	:	*N*-(1-(2,3-dioleyloxy) propyl)-*N,N,N*-trimethyl-ammoniumchloride
*ds*RNA	:	double stranded ribonucleic acid
EGFR	:	epidermal growth factor receptor
ERK5	:	extracellular signal-regulated protein kinase 5
HA	:	hyaluronic acid
HBV	:	hepatitis B virus
LPHA	:	liposome-polycation-hyaluronic acid
MCP-1	:	chemokine monocyte chemoattractant protein-1
*mi*RISC	:	micro ribonucleic acid-induced silencing complex

miRNA	:	micro ribonucleic acid
MK	:	midkine
mRNA	:	messenger ribonucleic acid
mPEG	:	methoxy poly(ethylene glycol)
NP	:	nanoparticle
nt	:	nucleotide
PEG	:	poly(ethylene glycol)
PEI	:	polyethylenimine
RGD	:	arginine-glycine-aspartic acid
RISC	:	ribonucleic acid-induced silencing complex
RNA	:	ribonucleic acid
RNAi	:	ribonucleic acid interference
scFv	:	single-chain antibody fragments
siRNA	:	small interfering ribonucleic acid
SNALP	:	stable nucleic acid lipid particle
TNF	:	tumor necrosis factor
VEGF	:	vascular endothelial growth factor

References

Aigner, A. 2008. Cellular delivery *in vivo* of siRNA-based therapeutics. Curr. Pharm. Des. 14: 3603–3619.

Aigner, A. 2011. MicroRNAs (miRNAs) in cancer invasion and metastasis: therapeutic approaches based on metastasis-related miRNAs. J. Mol. Med. 89: 445–457.

Akao, Y. and Y. Nakagawa, I. Hirata, A. Iio, T. Itoh, K. Kojima, R. Nakashima, Y. Kitade and T. Naoe. 2010. Role of anti-oncomirs miR-143 and -145 in human colorectal tumors. Cancer Gene Ther. 17: 398–408.

Akao, Y. and A. Iio, T. Itoh, S. Noguchi, Y. Itoh, Y. Ohtsuki and T. Naoe. 2011. Microvesicle-mediated RNA molecule delivery system using monocytes/macrophages. Mol. Ther. 19: 395–399.

Akinc, A. and A. Zumbuehl, M. Goldberg, E.S. Leshchiner, V. Busini, N. Hossain, S.A. Bacallado, D.N. Nguyen, J. Fuller, R. Alvarez, A. Borodovsky, T. Borland, R. Constien, A. de Fougerolles, J.R. Dorkin, K. Narayanannair Jayaprakash, M. Jayaraman, M. John, V. Koteliansky, M. Manoharan, L. Nechev, J. Qin, T. Racie, D. Raitcheva, K.G. Rajeev, D.W. Sah, J. Soutschek, I. Toudjarska, H.P. Vornlocher, T.S. Zimmermann, R. Langer and D.G. Anderson. 2008. A combinatorial library of lipid-like materials for delivery of RNAi therapeutics. Nat. Biotechnol. 26: 561–569.

Aleku, M. and P. Schulz, O. Keil, A. Santel, U. Schaeper, B. Dieckhoff, O. Janke, J. Endruschat, B. Durieux, N. Roder, K. Loffler, C. Lange, M. Fechtner, K. Mopert, G. Fisch, S. Dames, W. Arnold, K. Jochims, K. Giese, B. Wiedenmann, A. Scholz and J. Kaufmann. 2008. Atu027, a liposomal small interfering RNA formulation targeting protein kinase N3, inhibits cancer progression. Cancer Res. 68: 9788–9798.

Banno, H. and Y. Takei, T. Muramatsu, K. Komori and K. Kadomatsu. 2006. Controlled release of small interfering RNA targeting midkine attenuates intimal hyperplasia in vein grafts. J. Vasc. Surg. 44: 633–641.

Bartel, D.P. 2004. MicroRNAs: genomics, biogenesis, mechanism, and function. Cell. 116: 281–297.

Bartel, D.P. 2009. MicroRNAs: target recognition and regulatory functions. Cell. 136: 215–233.

Bartlett, D.W. and M.E. Davis. 2008. Impact of tumor-specific targeting and dosing schedule on tumor growth inhibition after intravenous administration of siRNA-containing nanoparticles. Biotechnol. Bioeng. 99: 975–985.

Behr, J.P. 1997. The proton sponge: a trick to enter cells the viruses did not exploit. Chimia. 51: 34–36.

Bhadra, D. and S. Bhadra, P. Jain and N.K. Jain. 2002. Pegnology: a review of PEG-ylated systems. Pharmazie. 57: 5–29.

Boeckle, S. and J. Fahrmeir, W. Roedl, M. Ogris and E. Wagner. 2006. Melittin analogs with high lytic activity at endosomal pH enhance transfection with purified targeted PEI polyplexes. J. Control. Release. 112: 240–248.

Bohnsack, M.T. and K. Czaplinski and D. Gorlich. 2004. Exportin 5 is a RanGTP-dependent dsRNA-binding protein that mediates nuclear export of pre-miRNAs. RNA. 10: 185–191.

Bolcato-Bellemin, A.L. and M.E. Bonnet, G. CreU.S.A.t, P. Erbacher and J.P. Behr. 2007. Sticky overhangs enhance siRNA-mediated gene silencing. Proc. Natl. Acad. Sci. U.S.A. 104: 16050–16055.

Bonnet, M.E. and P. Erbacher and A.L. Bolcato-Bellemin. 2008. Systemic delivery of DNA or siRNA mediated by linear polyethylenimine (L-PEI) does not induce an inflammatory response. Pharm. Res. 25: 2972–2982.

Boussif, O. and F. Lezoualc'h, M.A. Zanta, M.D. Mergny, D. Scherman, B. Demeneix and J.P. Behr. 1995. A versatile vector for gene and oligonucleotide transfer into cells in culture and *in vivo*: polyethylenimine. Proc. Natl. Acad. Sci. U.S.A. 92: 7297–7301.

Chen, Y. and X. Zhu, X. Zhang, B. Liu and L. Huang. 2010. Nanoparticles modified with tumor-targeting scFv deliver siRNA and miRNA for cancer therapy. Mol. Ther. 18: 1650–1656.

Dass, C.R. 2002. Cytotoxicity issues pertinent to lipoplex-mediated gene therapy *in-vivo*. J. Pharm. Pharmacol. 54: 593–601.

de Martimprey, H. and J.R. Bertrand, A. Fusco, M. Santoro, P. Couvreur, C. Vauthier and C. Malvy. 2008. siRNA nanoformulation against the ret/PTC1 junction oncogene is efficient in an *in vivo* model of papillary thyroid carcinoma. Nucleic Acids Res. 36: e2.

Dowler, T. and D. Bergeron, A.L. Tedeschi, L. Paquet, N. Ferrari and M.J. Damha. 2006. Improvements in siRNA properties mediated by 2'-deoxy-2'-fluoro-beta-D-arabinonucleic acid (FANA). Nucleic Acids Res. 34: 1669–1675.

Elbashir, S.M. and J. Harborth, W. Lendeckel, A. Yalcin, K. Weber and T. Tuschl. 2001a. Duplexes of 21-nucleotide RNAs mediate RNA interference in cultured mammalian cells. Nature. 411: 494–498.

Elbashir, S.M. and W. Lendeckel and T. Tuschl. 2001b. RNA interference is mediated by 21- and 22-nucleotide RNAs. Genes Dev. 15: 188–200.

Fire, A. and S. Xu, M.K. Montgomery, S.A. Kostas, S.E. Driver and C.C. Mello. 1998. Potent and specific genetic interference by double-stranded RNA in Caenorhabditis elegans. Nature. 391: 806–811.

Fujii, T. and M. Saito, E. Iwasaki, T. Ochiya, Y. Takei, S. Hayashi, A. Ono, N. Hirao, M. Nakamura, K. Kubushiro, K. Tsukazaki and D. Aoki. 2006. Intratumor injection of small interfering RNA-targeting human papillomavirus 18 E6 and E7 successfully inhibits the growth of cervical cancer. Int. J. Oncol. 29: 541–548.

Futami, K. and E. Kumagai, H. Makino, A. Sato, M. Takagi, A. Shimamoto and Y. Furuichi. 2008. Anticancer activity of RecQL1 helicase siRNA in mouse xenograft models. Cancer Sci. 99: 1227–1236.

Garzon, R. and C.E. Heaphy, V. Havelange, M. Fabbri, S. Volinia, T. Tsao, N. Zanesi, S.M. Kornblau, G. Marcucci, G.A. Calin, M. Andreeff and C.M. Croce. 2009. MicroRNA 29b functions in acute myeloid leukemia. Blood. 114: 5331–5341.

Ge, Q. and L. Filip, A. Bai, T. Nguyen, H.N. Eisen and J. Chen. 2004. Inhibition of influenza virus production in virus-infected mice by RNA interference. Proc. Natl. Acad. Sci. U.S.A. 101: 8676–8681.

Geisbert, T.W. and L.E. Hensley, E. Kagan, E.Z. Yu, J.B. Geisbert, K. Daddario-DiCaprio, E.A. Fritz, P.B. Jahrling, K. McClintock, J.R. Phelps, A.C. Lee, A. Judge, L.B. Jeffs and I. MacLachlan. 2006. Postexposure protection of guinea pigs against a lethal ebola virus challenge is conferred by RNA interference. J. Infect. Dis. 193: 1650–1657.

Gomes-da-Silva, L.C. and N.A. Fonseca, V. Moura, M.C. Pedroso de Lima, S. Simoes and J.N. Moreira. 2012. Lipid-based nanoparticles for siRNA delivery in cancer therapy: paradigms and challenges. Acc. Chem. Res. 45: 1163–1171.

Grzelinski, M. and B. Urban-Klein, T. Martens, K. Lamszus, U. Bakowsky, S. Hobel, F. Czubayko and A. Aigner. 2006. RNA interference-mediated gene silencing of pleiotrophin through polyethylenimine-complexed small interfering RNAs *in vivo* exerts antitumoral effects in glioblastoma xenografts. Hum. Gene Ther. 17: 751–766.

Halder, J. and A.A. Kamat, C.N. Jr. Landen, L.Y. Han, S.K. Lutgendorf, Y.G. Lin, W.M. Merritt, N.B. Jennings, A. Chavez-Reyes, R.L. Coleman, D.M. Gershenson, R. Schmandt, S.W. Cole, G. Lopez-Berestein and A.K. Sood. 2006. Focal adhesion kinase targeting using *in vivo* short interfering RNA delivery in neutral liposomes for ovarian carcinoma therapy. Clin. Cancer Res. 12: 4916–4924.

Hammond, S.M. and E. Bernstein, D. Beach and G.J. Hannon. 2000. An RNA-directed nuclease mediates post-transcriptional gene silencing in Drosophila cells. Nature. 404: 293–296.

Hanahan, D. and R.A. Weinberg. 2011. Hallmarks of cancer: the next generation. Cell. 144: 646–674.

Hannon, G.J. 2002. RNA interference. Nature. 418: 244–251.

Hassani, Z. and G.F. Lemkine, P. Erbacher, K. Palmier, G. Alfama, C. Giovannangeli, J.P. Behr and B.A. Demeneix. 2005. Lipid-mediated siRNA delivery down-regulates exogenous gene expression in the mouse brain at picomolar levels. J. Gene Med. 7: 198–207.

Heidel, J.D. 2006. Linear cyclodextrin-containing polymers and their use as delivery agents. Expert Opin. Drug Deliv. 3: 641–646.

Hendruschk, S. and R. Wiedemuth, A. Aigner, K. Topfer, M. Cartellieri, D. Martin, M. Kirsch, C. Ikonomidou, G. Schackert and A. Temme. 2011. RNA interference targeting survivin exerts antitumoral effects *in vitro* and in established glioma xenografts *in vivo*. Neuro Oncol. 13: 1074–1089.

Höbel, S. and R. Prinz, A. Malek, B. Urban-Klein, J. Sitterberg, U. Bakowsky, F. Czubayko and A. Aigner. 2008. Polyethylenimine PEI F25-LMW allows the long-term storage of frozen complexes as fully active reagents in siRNA-mediated gene targeting and DNA delivery. Eur. J. Pharm. Biopharm. 70: 29–41.

Höbel, S. and I. Koburger, M. John, F. Czubayko, P. Hadwiger, H.P. Vornlocher and A. Aigner. 2010. Polyethylenimine/small interfering RNA-mediated knockdown of vascular endothelial growth factor *in vivo* exerts anti-tumor effects synergistically with Bevacizumab. J. Gene Med. 12: 287–300.

Höbel, S. and A. Loos, D. Appelhans, S. Schwarz, J. Seidel, B. Voit and A. Aigner. 2011. Maltose- and maltotriose-modified, hyperbranched poly(ethylene imine)s (OM-PEIs): physicochemical and biological properties of DNA and siRNA complexes. J. Control. Release. 149: 146–158.

Hogrefe, R.I. and A.V. Lebedev, G. Zon, K.F. Pirollo, A. Rait, Q. Zhou, W. Yu and E.H. Chang. 2006. Chemically modified short interfering hybrids (siHYBRIDS): nanoimmunoliposome delivery *in vitro* and *in vivo* for RNAi of HER-2. Nucleosides Nucleotides Nucleic Acids. 25: 889–907.

Hokaiwado, N. and F. Takeshita, A. Naiki-Ito, M. Asamoto, T. Ochiya and T. Shirai. 2008. Glutathione S-transferase Pi mediates proliferation of androgen independent prostate cancer cells. Carcinogenesis. 29: 1134–1138.

Howard, K.A. and U.L. Rahbek, X. Liu, C.K. Damgaard, S.Z. Glud, M.O. Andersen, M.B. Hovgaard, A. Schmitz, J.R. Nyengaard, F. Besenbacher and J. Kjems. 2006. RNA interference *in vitro* and *in vivo* using a novel chitosan/siRNA nanoparticle system. Mol. Ther. 14: 476–484.

Hu-Lieskovan, S. and J.D. Heidel, D.W. Bartlett, M.E. Davis and T.J. Triche. 2005. Sequence-specific knockdown of EWS-FLI1 by targeted, nonviral delivery of small interfering RNA inhibits tumor growth in a murine model of metastatic Ewing's sarcoma. Cancer Res. 65: 8984–8992.

Huh, M.S. and S.Y. Lee, S. Park, S. Lee, H. Chung, S. Lee, Y. Choi, Y.K. Oh, J.H. Park, S.Y. Jeong, K. Choi, K. Kim and I.C. Kwon. 2010. Tumor-homing glycol chitosan/polyethylenimine nanoparticles for the systemic delivery of siRNA in tumor-bearing mice. J. Control. Release. 144: 134–143.

Hutvágner, G. and P.D. Zamore. 2002. A microRNA in a multiple-turnover RNAi enzyme complex. Science. 297: 2056–2060.

Ibrahim, A.F. and U. Weirauch, M. Thomas, A. Grunweller, R.K. Hartmann and A. Aigner. 2011. MicroRNA replacement therapy for miR-145 and miR-33a is efficacious in a model of colon carcinoma. Cancer Res. 71: 5214–5224.

Ishimoto, T. and Y. Takei, Y. Yuzawa, K. Hanai, S. Nagahara, Y. Tarumi, S. Matsuo and K. Kadomatsu. 2008. Downregulation of monocyte chemoattractant protein-1 involving short interfering RNA attenuates hapten-induced contact hypersensitivity. Mol. Ther. 16: 387–395.

Iwaki, K. and K. Shibata, M. Ohta, Y. Endo, H. Uchida, M. Tominaga, R. Okunaga, S. Kai and S. Kitano. 2008. A small interfering RNA targeting proteinase-activated receptor-2 is effective in suppression of tumor growth in a Panc1 xenograft model. Int. J. Cancer. 122: 658–663.

Jackson, A.L. and P.S. Linsley. 2010. Recognizing and avoiding siRNA off-target effects for target identification and therapeutic application. Nat. Rev. Drug Discov. 9: 57–67.

Jiang, G. and K. Park, J. Kim, K.S. Kim and S.K. Hahn. 2009. Target specific intracellular delivery of siRNA/PEI-HA complex by receptor mediated endocytosis. Mol. Pharm. 6: 727–737.

Jorgensen, R. 1990. Altered gene expression in plants due to trans interactions between homologous genes. Trends Biotechnol. 8: 340–344.

Judge, A.D. and V. Sood, J.R. Shaw, D. Fang, K. McClintock and I. MacLachlan. 2005. Sequence-dependent stimulation of the mammalian innate immune response by synthetic siRNA. Nat. Biotechnol. 23: 457–462.

Judge, A.D. and M. Robbins, I. Tavakoli, J. Levi, L. Hu, A. Fronda, E. Ambegia, K. McClintock and I. MacLachlan. 2009. Confirming the RNAi-mediated mechanism of action of siRNA-based cancer therapeutics in mice. J. Clin. Invest. 119: 661–673.

Kaestner, P. and A. Aigner and H. Bastians. 2011. Therapeutic targeting of the mitotic spindle checkpoint through nanoparticle-mediated siRNA delivery inhibits tumor growth *in vivo*. Cancer Lett. 304: 128–136.

Katas, H. and H.O. Alpar. 2006. Development and characterisation of chitosan nanoparticles for siRNA delivery. J. Control. Release. 115: 216–225.

Khoury, M. and P. Louis-Plence, V. Escriou, D. Noel, C. Largeau, C. Cantos, D. Scherman, C. Jorgensen, and F. Apparailly. 2006. Efficient new cationic liposome formulation for systemic delivery of small interfering RNA silencing tumor necrosis factor alpha in experimental arthritis. Arthritis Rheum. 54: 1867–1877.

Khoury, M. and V. Escriou, G. Courties, A. Galy, R. Yao, C. Largeau, D. Scherman, C. Jorgensen and F. Apparailly. 2008. Efficient suppression of murine arthritis by combined anticytokine small interfering RNA lipoplexes. Arthritis Rheum. 58: 2356–2367.

Khvorova, A. and A. Reynolds and S.D. Jayasena. 2003. Functional siRNAs and miRNAs exhibit strand bias. Cell. 115: 209–216.

Kim, S.H. and J.H. Jeong, S.H. Lee, S.W. Kim and T.G. Park. 2008. Local and systemic delivery of VEGF siRNA using polyelectrolyte complex micelles for effective treatment of cancer. J. Control. Release. 129: 107–116.

Kinouchi, N. and Y. Ohsawa, N. Ishimaru, H. Ohuchi, Y. Sunada, Y. Hayashi, Y. Tanimoto, K. Moriyama and S. Noji. 2008. Atelocollagen-mediated local and systemic applications of myostatin-targeting siRNA increase skeletal muscle mass. Gene Ther. 15: 1126–1130.

Kitade, Y. and Y. Akao. 2010. MicroRNAs and their therapeutic potential for human diseases: microRNAs, miR-143 and -145. Function as anti-oncomirs and the application of chemically modified miR-143 as an anti-cancer Drug. J. Pharmcol. Sci. 114: 276–280.

Kunath, K. and A. von Harpe, H. Petersen, D. Fischer, K. Voigt, T. Kissel and U. Bickel. 2002. The structure of PEG-modified poly(ethylene imines) influences biodistribution and pharmacokinetics of their complexes with NF-kappaB decoy in mice. Pharm. Res. 19: 810–817.

Landen, C.N., Jr. and A. Chavez-Reyes, C. Bucana, R. Schmandt, M.T. Deavers, G. Lopez-Berestein and A.K. Sood. 2005. Therapeutic EphA2 gene targeting *in vivo* using neutral liposomal small interfering RNA delivery. Cancer Res. 65: 6910–6918.

Lee, Y. and M. Kim, J. Han, K.H. Yeom, S. Lee, S.H. Baek and V.N. Kim. 2004. MicroRNA genes are transcribed by RNA polymerase II. EMBO J. 23: 4051–4060.

Lee, M.K. and S.K. Chun, W.J. Choi, J.K. Kim, S.H. Choi, A. Kim, K. Oungbho, J.S. Park, W.S. Ahn and C.K. Kim. 2005. The use of chitosan as a condensing agent to enhance emulsion-mediated gene transfer. Biomaterials. 26: 2147–2156.

Liu, J. and M.A. Carmell, F.V. Rivas, C.G. Marsden, J.M. Thomson, J.J. Song, S.M. Hammond, L. Joshua-Tor and G.J. Hannon. 2004. Argonaute2 is the catalytic engine of mammalian RNAi. Science. 305: 1437–1441.

Liu, X. and K.A. Howard, M. Dong, M.O. Andersen, U.L. Rahbek, M.G. Johnsen, O.C. Hansen, F. Besenbacher and J. Kjems. 2007. The influence of polymeric properties on chitosan/siRNA nanoparticle formulation and gene silencing. Biomaterials. 28: 1280–1288.

Love, K.T. and K.P. Mahon, C.G. Levins, K.A. Whitehead, W. Querbes, J.R. Dorkin, J. Qin, W. Cantley, L.L. Qin, T. Racie, M. Frank-Kamenetsky, K.N. Yip, R. Alvarez, D.W. Sah, A. de Fougerolles, K. Fitzgerald, V. Koteliansky, A. Akinc, R. Langer and D.G. Anderson. 2010. Lipid-like materials for low-dose, *in vivo* gene silencing. Proc. Natl. Acad. Sci. U.S.A. 107: 1864–1869.

Lujambio, A. and S.W. Lowe. 2012. The microcosmos of cancer. Nature. 482: 347–355.

Malek, A. and F. Czubayko and A. Aigner. 2008. PEG grafting of polyethylenimine (PEI) exerts different effects on DNA transfection and siRNA-induced gene targeting efficacy. J. Drug Target. 16: 124–139.

Malek, A. and O. Merkel, L. Fink, F. Czubayko, T. Kissel and A. Aigner. 2009. *In vivo* pharmacokinetics, tissue distribution and underlying mechanisms of various PEI(-PEG)/siRNA complexes. Toxicol. Appl. Pharmacol. 236: 97–108.

Mao, S. and M. Neu, O. Germershaus, O. Merkel, J. Sitterberg, U. Bakowsky and T. Kissel. 2006. Influence of polyethylene glycol chain length on the physicochemical and biological properties of poly(ethylene imine)-graft-poly(ethylene glycol) block copolymer/siRNA polyplexes. Bioconjug. Chem. 17: 1209–1218.

Mathonnet, G. and M.R. Fabian, Y.V. Svitkin, A. Parsyan, L. Huck, T. Murata, S. Biffo, W.C. Merrick, E. Darzynkiewicz, R.S. Pillai, W. Filipowicz, T.F. Duchaine and N. Sonenberg. 2007. MicroRNA inhibition of translation initiation *in vitro* by targeting the cap-binding complex eIF4F. Science. 317: 1764–1767.

Matoba, T. and Y. Orba, T. Suzuki, Y. Makino, H. Shichinohe, S. Kuroda, T. Ochiya, H. Itoh, S. Tanaka, K. Nagashima and H. Sawa. 2008. An siRNA against JC virus (JCV) agnoprotein inhibits JCV infection in JCV-producing cells inoculated in nude mice. Neuropathology. 28: 286–294.

Merkel, O.M. and A. Beyerle, D. Librizzi, A. Pfestroff, T.M. Behr, B. Sproat, P.J. Barth and T. Kissel. 2009. Nonviral siRNA delivery to the lung: investigation of PEG-PEI polyplexes and their *in vivo* performance. Mol. Pharm. 6: 1246–1260.

Merl, S. and C. Michaelis, B. Jaschke, M. Vorpahl, S. Seidl and R. Wessely. 2005. Targeting 2A protease by RNA interference attenuates coxsackieviral cytopathogenicity and promotes survival in highly susceptible mice. Circulation. 111: 1583–1592.

Miller, C.R. and B. Bondurant, S.D. McLean, K.A. McGovern and D.F. O'Brien. 1998. Liposome-cell interactions *in vitro*: effect of liposome surface charge on the binding and endocytosis of conventional and sterically stabilized liposomes. Biochemistry. 37: 12875–12883.

Minakuchi, Y. and F. Takeshita, N. Kosaka, H. Sasaki, Y. Yamamoto, M. Kouno, K. Honma, S. Nagahara, K. Hanai, A. Sano, T. Kato, M. Terada and T. Ochiya. 2004. Atelocollagen-mediated synthetic small interfering RNA delivery for effective gene silencing *in vitro* and *in vivo*. Nucleic Acids Res. 32: e109.

Morrissey, D.V. and J.A. Lockridge, L. Shaw, K. Blanchard, K. Jensen, W. Breen, K. Hartsough, L. Machemer, S. Radka, V. Jadhav, N. Vaish, S. Zinnen, C. Vargeese, K. Bowman, C.S. Shaffer, L.B. Jeffs, A. Judge, I. MacLachlan and B. Polisky. 2005. Potent and persistent *in vivo* anti-HBV activity of chemically modified siRNAs. Nat. Biotechnol. 23: 1002–1007.

Napoli, C. and C. Lemieux and R. Jorgensen. 1990. Introduction of a chimeric chalcone synthase gene into petunia results in reversible co-suppression of homologous genes in trans. Plant. Cell. 2: 279–289.

Nozawa, H. and T. Tadakuma, T. Ono, M. Sato, S. Hiroi, K. Masumoto and Y. Sato. 2006. Small interfering RNA targeting epidermal growth factor receptor enhances chemosensitivity to cisplatin, 5-fluorouracil and docetaxel in head and neck squamous cell carcinoma. Cancer Sci. 97: 1115–1124.

Ochiya, T. and Y. Takahama, S. Nagahara, Y. Sumita, A. Hisada, H. Itoh, Y. Nagai and M. Terada. 1999. New delivery system for plasmid DNA *in vivo* using atelocollagen as a carrier material: the Minipellet. Nat. Med. 5: 707–710.

Ochiya, T. and S. Nagahara, A. Sano, H. Itoh and M. Terada. 2001. Biomaterials for gene delivery: atelocollagen-mediated controlled release of molecular medicines. Curr. Gene Ther. 1: 31–52.

Parrish, S. and J. Fleenor, S. Xu, C. Mello and A. Fire. 2000. Functional anatomy of a dsRNA trigger: differential requirement for the two trigger strands in RNA interference. Mol. Cell. 6: 1077–1087.

Petersen, H. and P.M. Fechner, A.L. Martin, K. Kunath, S. Stolnik, C.J. Roberts, D. Fischer, M.C. Davies and T. Kissel. 2002. Polyethylenimine-graft-poly(ethylene glycol) copolymers: influence of copolymer block structure on DNA complexation and biological activities as gene delivery system. Bioconjug. Chem. 13: 845–854.

Pillai, R.S. and S.N. Bhattacharyya and W. Filipowicz. 2007. Repression of protein synthesis by miRNAs: how many mechanisms? Trends Cell Biol. 17: 118–126.

Pille, J.Y. and H. Li, E. Blot, J.R. Bertrand, L.L. Pritchard, P. Opolon, A. Maksimenko, H. Lu, J.P. Vannier, J. Soria, C. Malvy and C. Soria. 2006. Intravenous delivery of anti-RhoA small interfering RNA loaded in nanoparticles of chitosan in mice: safety and efficacy in xenografted aggressive breast cancer. Hum. Gene Ther. 17: 1019–1026.

Pirollo, K.F. and G. Zon, A. Rait, Q. Zhou, W. Yu, R. Hogrefe and E.H. Chang. 2006. Tumor-targeting nanoimmunoliposome complex for short interfering RNA delivery. Hum. Gene Ther. 17: 117–124.

Pirollo, K.F. and A. Rait, Q. Zhou, S.H. Hwang, J.A. Dagata, G. Zon, R.I. Hogrefe, G. Palchik and E.H. Chang. 2007. Materializing the potential of small interfering RNA via a tumor-targeting nanodelivery system. Cancer Res. 67: 2938–2943.

Polach, K.J. and M. Matar, J. Rice, G. Slobodkin, J. Sparks, R. Congo, A. Rea-Ramsey, D. McClure, E. Brunhoeber, M. Krampert, A. Schuster, K. Jahn-Hofmann, M. John, H.P. Vornlocher, J.G. Fewell, K. Anwer and A. Geick. 2012. Delivery of siRNA to the mouse lung via a functionalized lipopolyamine. Mol. Ther. 20: 91–100.

Rand, T.A. and K. Ginalski, N.V. Grishin and X. Wang. 2004. Biochemical identification of Argonaute 2 as the sole protein required for RNA-induced silencing complex activity. Proc. Natl. Acad. Sci. U.S.A. 101: 14385–14389.

Rettig, G.R. and M.A. Behlke. 2012. Progress toward *in vivo* use of siRNAs-II. Mol. Ther. 20: 483–512.

Reynolds, A. and D. Leake, Q. Boese, S. Scaringe, W.S. Marshall and A. Khvorova. 2004. Rational siRNA design for RNA interference. Nat. Biotechnol. 22: 326–330.

Rivas, F.V. and N.H. Tolia, J.J. Song, J.P. Aragon, J. Liu, G.J. Hannon and L. Joshua-Tor. 2005. Purified Argonaute2 and an siRNA form recombinant human RISC. Nat. Struct. Mol. Biol. 12: 340–349.

Robbins, M. and A. Judge, E. Ambegia, C. Choi, E. Yaworski, L. Palmer, K. McClintock and I. Maclachlan. 2008. Misinterpreting the therapeutic effects of siRNA caused by immune stimulation. Hum. Gene Ther. 19: 991–999.

Robbins, M. and A. Judge and I. MacLachlan. 2009. siRNA and innate immunity. Oligonucleotides. 19: 89–102.

Rodriguez, A. and S. Griffiths-Jones, J.L. Ashurst and A. Bradley. 2004. Identification of mammalian microRNA host genes and transcription units. Genome Res. 14: 1902–1910.

Sano, A. and M. Maeda, S. Nagahara, T. Ochiya, K. Honma, H. Itoh, T. Miyata and K. Fujioka. 2003. Atelocollagen for protein and gene delivery. Adv. Drug Deliv. Rev. 55: 1651–1677.

Santel, A. and M. Aleku, O. Keil, J. Endruschat, V. Esche, G. Fisch, S. Dames, K. Loffler, M. Fechtner, W. Arnold, K. Giese, A. Klippel and J. Kaufmann. 2006a. A novel siRNA-lipoplex technology for RNA interference in the mouse vascular endothelium. Gene Ther. 13: 1222–1234.

Santel, A. and M. Aleku, O. Keil, J. Endruschat, V. Esche, B. Durieux, K. Loffler, M. Fechtner, T. Rohl, G. Fisch, S. Dames, W. Arnold, K. Giese, A. Klippel and J. Kaufmann. 2006b. RNA interference in the mouse vascular endothelium by systemic administration of siRNA-lipoplexes for cancer therapy. Gene Ther. 13: 1360–1370.

Santel, A. and M. Aleku, N. Roder, K. Mopert, B. Durieux, O. Janke, O. Keil, J. Endruschat, S. Dames, C. Lange, M. Eisermann, K. Loffler, M. Fechtner, G. Fisch, C. Vank, U. Schaeper, K. Giese and J. Kaufmann. 2010. Atu027 prevents pulmonary metastasis in experimental and spontaneous mouse metastasis models. Clin. Cancer Res. 16: 5469–5480.

Sayed, D. and M. Abdellatif. 2011. MicroRNAs in development and disease. Physiol. Rev. 91: 827–887.

Schiffelers, R.M. and A. Ansari, J. Xu, Q. Zhou, Q. Tang, G. Storm, G. Molema, P.Y. Lu, P.V. Scaria and M.C. Woodle. 2004. Cancer siRNA therapy by tumor selective delivery with ligand-targeted sterically stabilized nanoparticle. Nucleic Acids Res. 32: e149.

Schwarz, D.S. and G. Hutvagner, T. Du, Z. Xu, N. Aronin and P.D. Zamore. 2003. Asymmetry in the assembly of the RNAi enzyme complex. Cell. 115: 199–208.

Segura, T. and H. Schmokel and J.A. Hubbell. 2007. RNA interference targeting hypoxia inducible factor 1alpha reduces post-operative adhesions in rats. J. Surg. Res. 141: 162–170.

Semple, S.C. and A. Akinc, J. Chen, A.P. Sandhu, B.L. Mui, C.K. Cho, D.W. Sah, D. Stebbing, E.J. Crosley, E. Yaworski, I.M. Hafez, J.R. Dorkin, J. Qin, K. Lam, K.G. Rajeev, K.F. Wong, L.B. Jeffs, L. Nechev, M.L. Eisenhardt, M. Jayaraman, M. Kazem, M.A. Maier, M. Srinivasulu, M.J. Weinstein, Q. Chen, R. Alvarez, S.A. Barros, S. De, S.K. Klimuk, T. Borland, V. Kosovrasti, W.L. Cantley, Y.K. Tam, M. Manoharan, M.A. Ciufolini, M.A. Tracy, A. de Fougerolles, I. MacLachlan, P.R. Cullis, T.D. Madden and M.J. Hope. 2010. Rational design of cationic lipids for siRNA delivery. Nat. Biotechnol. 28: 172–176.

Shir, A. and M. Ogris, E. Wagner and A. Levitzki. 2006. EGF receptor-targeted synthetic double-stranded RNA eliminates glioblastoma, breast cancer, and adenocarcinoma tumors in mice. PLoS Med. 3: e6.

Shu, X.Z. and K.J. Zhu. 2002. The influence of multivalent phosphate structure on the properties of ionically cross-linked chitosan films for controlled drug release. Eur. J. Pharm. Biopharm. 54: 235–243.

Sparks, J. and G. Slobodkin, M. Matar, R. Congo, D. Ulkoski, A. Rea-Ramsey, C. Pence, J. Rice, D. McClure, K.J. Polach, E. Brunhoeber, L. Wilkinson, K. Wallace, K. Anwer and J.G. Fewell. 2012. Versatile cationic lipids for siRNA delivery. J. Control. Release. 158: 269–276.

Stephenson, M.L. and P.C. Zamecnik. 1978. Inhibition of Rous sarcoma viral RNA translation by a specific oligodeoxyribonucleotide. Proc. Natl. Acad. Sci. U.S.A. 75: 285–288.

Takahashi, Y. and M. Nishikawa, N. Kobayashi and Y. Takakura. 2005. Gene silencing in primary and metastatic tumors by small interfering RNA delivery in mice: quantitative analysis using melanoma cells expressing firefly and sea pansy luciferases. J. Control. Release. 105: 332–343.

Takei, Y. and K. Kadomatsu, Y. Yuzawa, S. Matsuo and T. Muramatsu. 2004. A small interfering RNA targeting vascular endothelial growth factor as cancer therapeutics. Cancer Res. 64: 3365–3370.

Takei, Y. and K. Kadomatsu, T. Goto and T. Muramatsu. 2006. Combinational antitumor effect of siRNA against midkine and paclitaxel on growth of human prostate cancer xenografts. Cancer. 107: 864–873.

Takeshita, F. and Y. Minakuchi, S. Nagahara, K. Honma, H. Sasaki, K. Hirai, T. Teratani, N. Namatame, Y. Yamamoto, K. Hanai, T. Kato, A. Sano and T. Ochiya. 2005. Efficient delivery of small interfering RNA to bone-metastatic tumors by using atelocollagen *in vivo*. Proc. Natl. Acad. Sci. U.S.A. 102: 12177–12182.

Takeshita, F. and L. Patrawala, M. Osaki, R.U. Takahashi, Y. Yamamoto, N. Kosaka, M. Kawamata, K. Kelnar, A.G. Bader, D. Brown and T. Ochiya. 2010. Systemic delivery of synthetic microRNA-16 inhibits the growth of metastatic prostate tumors via downregulation of multiple cell-cycle genes. Mol. Ther. 18: 181–187.

Tan, P.H. and L.C. Yang, H.C. Shih, K.C. Lan and J.T. Cheng. 2005. Gene knockdown with intrathecal siRNA of NMDA receptor NR2B subunit reduces formalin-induced nociception in the rat. Gene Ther. 12: 59–66.

Tan, W.B. and S. Jiang and Y. Zhang. 2007. Quantum-dot based nanoparticles for targeted silencing of HER2/neu gene via RNA interference. Biomaterials. 28: 1565–1571.

Thomas, M. and J.J. Lu, Q. Ge, C. Zhang, J. Chen and A.M. Klibanov. 2005. Full deacylation of polyethylenimine dramatically boosts its gene delivery efficiency and specificity to mouse lung. Proc. Natl. Acad. Sci. U.S.A. 102: 5679–5684.

Thomas, M. and K. Lange-Grunweller, U. Weirauch, D. Gutsch, A. Aigner, A. Grunweller and R.K. Hartmann. 2012. The proto-oncogene Pim-1 is a target of miR-33a. Oncogene. 31: 918–928.

Tousignant, J.D. and A.L. Gates, L.A. Ingram, C.L. Johnson, J.B. Nietupski, S.H. Cheng, S.J. Eastman and R.K. Scheule. 2000. Comprehensive analysis of the acute toxicities induced by systemic administration of cationic lipid: plasmid DNA complexes in mice. Hum. Gene Ther. 11: 2493–2513.

Trang, P. and P.P. Medina, J.F. Wiggins, L. Ruffino, K. Kelnar, M. Omotola, R. Homer, D. Brown, A.G. Bader, J.B. Weidhaas and F.J. Slack. 2010. Regression of murine lung tumors by the let-7 microRNA. Oncogene. 29: 1580–1587.

Ueno, Y. and T. Inoue, M. Yoshida, K. Yoshikawa, A. Shibata, Y. Kitamura and Y. Kitade. 2008. Synthesis of nuclease-resistant siRNAs possessing benzene-phosphate backbones in their 3'-overhang regions. Bioorg. Med. Chem. Lett. 18: 5194–5196.

Ui-Tei, K. and Y. Naito, F. Takahashi, T. Haraguchi, H. Ohki-Hamazaki, A. Juni, R. Ueda and K. Saigo. 2004. Guidelines for the selection of highly effective siRNA sequences for mammalian and chick RNA interference. Nucleic Acids Res. 32: 936–948.

Urban-Klein, B. and S. Werth, S. Abuharbeid, F. Czubayko and A. Aigner. 2005. RNAi-mediated gene-targeting through systemic application of polyethylenimine (PEI)-complexed siRNA *in vivo*. Gene Ther. 12: 461–466.

Wang, C.J. and Z.G. Zhou, L. Wang, L. Yang, B. Zhou, J. Gu, H.Y. Chen and X.F. Sun. 2009. Clinicopathological significance of microRNA-31, -143 and -145 expression in colorectal cancer. Dis. Markers. 26: 27–34.

Wang, F. and P. Zhang, Y. Ma, J. Yang, M.P. Moyer, C. Shi, J. Peng and H. Qin. 2012. NIRF is frequently upregulated in colorectal cancer and its oncogenicity can be suppressed by let-7a microRNA. Cancer Lett. 314: 223–231.

Werth, S. and B. Urban-Klein, L. Dai, S. Hobel, M. Grzelinski, U. Bakowsky, F. Czubayko and A. Aigner. 2006. A low molecular weight fraction of polyethylenimine (PEI) displays increased transfection efficiency of DNA and siRNA in fresh or lyophilized complexes. J. Control. Release. 112: 257–270.

Whitehead, K.A. and J. Matthews, P.H. Chang, F. Niroui, J.R. Dorkin, M. Severgnini and D.G. Anderson. 2012. *In vitro-in vivo* translation of lipid nanoparticles for hepatocellular siRNA delivery. ACS Nano. 6: 6922–6929.

Xu, L. and W.H. Tang, C.C. Huang, W. Alexander, L.M. Xiang, K.F. Pirollo, A. Rait and E.H. Chang. 2001. Systemic p53 gene therapy of cancer with immunolipoplexes targeted by anti-transferrin receptor scFv. Mol. Med. 7: 723–734.

Xu, L. and C.C. Huang, W. Huang, W.H. Tang, A. Rait, Y.Z. Yin, I. Cruz, L.M. Xiang, K.F. Pirollo and E.H. Chang. 2002. Systemic tumor-targeted gene delivery by anti-transferrin receptor scFv-immunoliposomes. Mol. Cancer Ther. 1: 337–346.

Xu, S. and M. Dong, X. Liu, K.A. Howard, J. Kjems and F. Besenbacher. 2007. Direct force measurements between siRNA and chitosan molecules using force spectroscopy. Biophys. J. 93: 952–959.

Yang, D. and H. Lu and J.W. Erickson. 2000. Evidence that processed small dsRNAs may mediate sequence-specific mRNA degradation during RNAi in Drosophila embryos. Curr. Biol. 10: 1191–1200.

Yang, Y.D. and H. Cho, J.Y. Koo, M.H. Tak, Y. Cho, W.S. Shim, S.P. Park, J. Lee, B. Lee, B.M. Kim, R. Raouf, Y.K. Shin and U. Oh. 2008. TMEM16A confers receptor-activated calcium-dependent chloride conductance. Nature. 455: 1210–1215.

Yu, W. and K.F. Pirollo, B. Yu, A. Rait, L. Xiang, W. Huang, Q. Zhou, G. Ertem and E.H. Chang. 2004. Enhanced transfection efficiency of a systemically delivered tumor-targeting immunoplex by inclusion of a pH-sensitive histidylated oligolysine peptide. Nucleic Acids Res. 32: e48.

Zamore, P.D. and T. Tuschl, P.A. Sharp and D.P. Bartel. 2000. RNAi: double-stranded RNA directs the ATP-dependent cleavage of mRNA at 21 to 23 nucleotide intervals. Cell. 101: 25–33.

Zhai, H. and B. Song, X. Xu, W. Zhu and J. Ju. 2013. Inhibition of autophagy and tumor growth in colon cancer by miR-502. Oncogene. 32: 1570–1579.

Zhu, H. and Z.Y. Liang, X.Y. Ren and T.H. Liu. 2006. Small interfering RNAs targeting mutant K-ras inhibit human pancreatic carcinoma cells growth *in vitro* and *in vivo*. Cancer Biol. Ther. 5: 1693–1698.

Zimmermann, T.S. and A.C. Lee, A. Akinc, B. Bramlage, D. Bumcrot, M.N. Fedoruk, J. Harborth, J.A. Heyes, L.B. Jeffs, M. John, A.D. Judge, K. Lam, K. McClintock, L.V. Nechev, L.R. Palmer, T. Racie, I. Rohl, S. Seiffert, S. Shanmugam, V. Sood, J. Soutschek, I. Toudjarska, A.J. Wheat, E. Yaworski, W. Zedalis, V. Koteliansky, M. Manoharan, H.P. Vornlocher and I. MacLachlan. 2006. RNAi-mediated gene silencing in non-human primates. Nature. 441: 111–114.

Zintchenko, A. and A. Philipp, A. Dehshahri and E. Wagner. 2008. Simple modifications of branched PEI lead to highly efficient siRNA carriers with low toxicity. Bioconjug. Chem. 19: 1448–1455.

CHAPTER 17
Nanotheranostics

Benjamin Theek,[1,a] *Sijumon Kunjachan,*[2]
Fabian Kiessling[1,b] *and Twan Lammers*[1,3,4,*]

ABSTRACT

Theranostics refers to the combination of disease diagnosis and therapy. Nanomedicines, i.e., submicrometer-sized carrier materials designed to improve the biodistribution and target site accumulation of low molecular weight (chemo)therapeutics, are excellent tools for combining disease diagnosis and therapy, since they can be easily functionalized both with drugs and with imaging agents. Many different nanomedicine formulations have been designed and evaluated over the years, including, e.g., liposomes, polymers, and micelles, which accumulate in tumors and at sites of inflammation via the so-called enhanced permeability and retention effect. In recent years, imaging has started to play an ever more important role in nanomedicine, e.g., to enable the non-invasive visualization of drug delivery, drug release, and drug efficacy. In this chapter, some of the most relevant constructs and concepts will be introduced. In addition, the advantages of nanomedicines and nanotheranostics over conventional pharmacotherapeutic interventions will be discussed, as will be their ability to individualize and personalize chemotherapeutic treatments.

---

[1] Department of Experimental Molecular Imaging, Helmholtz Institute for Biomedical Engineering, RWTH – Aachen University, Aachen, Germany.
[a] Email: btheek@ukaachen.de
[b] Email: fkiessling@ukaachen.de
[2] Department of Radiation Oncology, Brigham and Women's Hospital, Dana-Farber Cancer Institute and Harvard Medical School, Boston, Massachusetts 02115, USA.
 Email: sijumon@gmail.com
[3] Department of Targeted Therapeutics, MIRA Institute for Biomedical Technology and Technical Medicine, University of Twente, Enschede, The Netherlands.
[4] Department of Pharmaceutics, Utrecht Institute for Pharmaceutical Sciences, Utrecht University, Sorbonnelaan 16, 3584 CA Utrecht, The Netherlands.
[*] Corresponding author: tlammers@ukaachen.de; t.lammers@uu.nl

Introduction

Nanometer-sized objects have attracted enormous attention in recent years. Especially in the field of (bio)medical sciences, advances in nanotechnology have been promising, in terms of the potential benefits they might provide to improve disease diagnosis and therapy. Strictly speaking, nanotechnology relates to the study of objects smaller than 1 μm. However, most nanomaterials used for biomedical purposes have sizes less than 100 nm in diameter. Nanomaterials used for diagnostic or therapeutic applications are generally termed nanomedicines, and nanomaterials in which diagnostic and therapeutic applications are combined are routinely referred to as nanotheranostics.

In recent years, ever more nanotheranostics have been designed and evaluated, e.g., to enable the non-invasive visualization of drug delivery, drug release, and drug efficacy. Longitudinal and non-invasive imaging of such processes allows optimization of drug delivery systems and drug targeting strategies, as well as a better analysis of potential therapeutic responses. In this chapter, after briefly introducing the need for and the rationale of drug targeting (to tumors), we summarize some of the recent progress made with regard to nanotheranostics and image-guided drug delivery. In this regard, we describe several proof-of-principle studies showing how theranostic systems and strategies can be used to facilitate, foster, and further improve nanomedicine-mediated drug targeting.

Drug Therapy and Drug Delivery Systems

Most routinely used (chemo)therapeutic agents are small and hydrophobic, and have a large volume of distribution. These suboptimal physicochemical and pharmacokinetic properties often result in improper *in vivo* behavior, including, e.g., rapid clearance from systemic circulation, low target site accumulation, and/or high drug levels in healthy organs and tissues, generally leading to low efficacy and high toxicity. Such effects are most obvious for standard low Molecular weight (M_w) anticancer agents. Two exemplary classes of chemotherapeutics routinely used in the clinic are alkylating agents (such as cisplatin) and anthracycline antibiotics (such as doxorubicin, DOX). In order to be effective, these compounds have to accumulate in the nuclei of cancer cells to exert their action, i.e., deoxyribonucleic acid (DNA) alkylation and intercalation, respectively. Alkylation and intercalation damage the DNA of proliferating cells, and cause them to undergo apoptosis. Because cancer cells proliferate more rapidly than most healthy cells, the damage done is somewhat specific. Due to their small size and/or their high hydrophobic character, however, chemotherapeutics agents often accumulate much stronger in healthy tissues than in tumors. This, together with the fact that their mechanism of action is not absolutely specific to malignant cells, generally leads to severe side effects, in particular in organs exposed to high peak concentrations of the drug (such as the heart), as well as in tissues characterized by a high degree of proliferation (such as hair cells, the gastrointestinal lining, and the bone marrow).

To reduce the toxicity and improve the efficacy of chemotherapeutic agents, a large number of drug delivery systems have been designed and evaluated over the years (Peer et al. 2007, Lammers et al. 2010a, Al-Jamal and Kostarelos 2011, Ambrogio et al. 2011). These formulations are nowadays routinely referred to as nanomedicines. Among the first nanometer-sized carrier materials designed for drug delivery purposes were liposomes, invented more than 40 years ago by Bangham et al. (1965). In the decade that followed, liposomes became established as delivery vehicles for low M_W drugs (Gregoriadis et al. 1974), and additional carrier materials started to be developed, in particular natural and synthetic macromolecules. Advances in polymer chemistry, which had actually already started several years earlier with the development of local depot devices for the sustained release of proteins, provided a solid basis for macromolecular drug delivery, and also stimulated the design of a number of other carrier materials, including, e.g., dendrimers, micelles, and nanoparticles (NPs) (Fig. 17.1A, 1B, 1C, 1D, and 1E). Depending on their size, shape, chemical properties and the method of drug conjugation/incorporation, important parameters, such as blood half-life, target site accumulation, and drug release kinetics, can be adjusted. Whereas the size and shape of drug delivery systems generally has a major impact on the pharmacokinetic properties of the drug (such as blood half-life, distribution, extravasation, renal clearance, liver metabolism, etc.), also the nature of drug encapsulation or conjugation (in)to nanomedicine formulation plays an important role, determining, e.g., its release kinetics, its bioavailability, its efficacy, and its toxicity.

Drug targeting strategies

As opposed to low M_W chemotherapeutic drugs, intravenously administered nanomedicine formulations circulate for prolonged periods of time. The former generally have blood half-life times in the order of minutes, whereas the latter circulate for hours to days. Their much larger size not only attenuates the extravasation of nanomedicines into healthy tissues, but it also enables them to accumulate relatively efficiently and specifically by means of the so-called Enhanced Permeability and Retention (EPR) effect (Maeda et al. 2009, Maeda 2012). The EPR effect is based on the high leakiness and the loose or absent pericyte coverage of tumor blood vessels (Hobbs et al. 1998, Fukumura et al. 2010, Raza et al. 2010), both of which result from rapid tumor growth and permanent exposure to pro-angiogenic signals. In addition, the absence of a proper lymphatic system enables the retention of the drug within tumors (Maeda et al. 2009, Fukumura et al. 2010, Maeda 2012). These pathophysiological properties allow long-circulating nanomedicines with sizes of from ≈ 1 nm to ≈ 200 nm to passively accumulate in tumors over

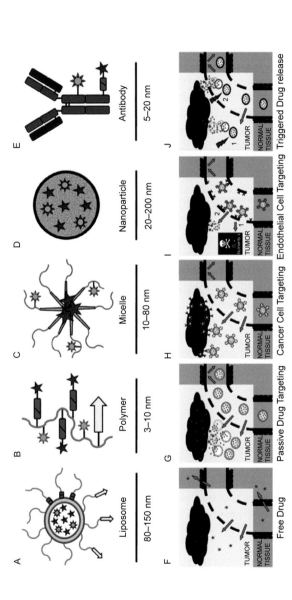

Figure 17.1. Drug delivery systems and drug targeting strategies. (A-E) clinically relevant drug delivery systems, co-loaded with drugs (red) and imaging agents (orange). Targeting ligands are shown in yellow, and cleavable linkers in blue. (F-J) drug targeting strategies. (F) upon the intravenous injection of a low M_W chemotherapeutic agent, which is generally rapidly cleared from the blood, only low levels of the drug accumulate in tumors and in tumor cells, while its localization in healthy organs and tissues tends to be high. (G) upon using a passively targeted drug delivery system, by means of the EPR effect, the accumulation of drugs in tumors can be increased, while its localization to healthy tissues can be attenuated. (H) active targeting to receptors (over)expressed by cancer cells generally intends to improve the cellular uptake of nanomedicine formulations, and is particularly useful for the delivery of otherwise poorly internalized agents, such as DNA and small interfering ribonucleic acid (siRNA). (I) active targeting to receptors (over)expressed by angiogenic endothelial cells either aims to eradicate tumor blood vessels (1, thereby depriving tumors from oxygen and nutrients), or to increase overall drug delivery to tumors (2). (J) stimuli-responsive nanomedicines can be triggered to release their contents upon exposure to external stimuli, such as hyperthermia, ultrasound, or light. Drug release can be triggered either upon EPR-mediated passive accumulation in tumors (1), or during circulation in tumor blood vessels (2). Adapted with permission from Lammers et al. (2008a, 2010a). Copyright Nature Publishing Group (2008), and ACS Publications (2010), respectively.

time (Fig. 17.1G). In this regard, it is important to take into account that the degree of EPR significantly varies between different tumor types, and also between animal models and patients (Jain and Stylianopoulos 2010, Bae and Park 2011, Lammers et al. 2012a). Some degree of EPR has been observed in the majority of malignancies, but there is always a very high inter- and intra-individual variability. Current efforts aiming to improve our understanding of the pathophysiological properties contributing to EPR, to image (the functionality of) tumor blood vessels and to visualize EPR-mediated drug targeting in individual patients (see below), might assist in overcoming such shortcomings related to low and/or highly variable passive drug targeting.

Active targeting is based on the incorporation of recognition motifs, such as antibodies or peptides, into nanomedicine formulations, which are directed against receptor structures (over)expressed at the pathological site. Active targeting strategies can either be directed to cancer cells, or to endothelial cells (e.g., to induce anti-angiogenic effects, see Fig. 17.1H and 17.1I). One should be aware that in case of active targeting to cancer cells, the tumor accumulation primarily relies on the EPR effect; after this, antibody or peptide moieties might influence cellular uptake, intratumor distribution, and/or therapeutic efficacy, but they generally do not increase overall tumor concentrations (Lammers et al. 2012a). An interesting example is this regard was published by Choi et al. (2010), who showed there is no difference in overall tumor concentration of transferrin (Tf)-targeted vs. untargeted gold NPs. The uptake of Tf-targeted NPs by tumor cells in Neuro2A xenografts, however, was considerably higher, and their intratumor distribution was more homogenous than that of Tf-free NPs. Targeting to receptors overexpressed by angiogenic endothelial cells, such as integrins, might improve early accumulation within tumors, as well as uptake by endothelial cells, but whether this results in significantly higher concentrations accumulating in tumors over time remains elusive. In this regard, it is important to take into account that the incorporation of targeting ligands into nanomedicine formulations generally strongly influences their pharmacokinetics and biodistribution. Because of enhanced recognition by the Mononuclear Phagocytic System (MPS), which is responsible for clearing long-circulating nanomedicines from the blood, half-life times often are reduced for actively targeted formulations, resulting in less efficient EPR-mediated passive drug targeting, and somewhat lower overall tumor concentrations. In addition, in particular for polymer-drug conjugates, the incorporation of antibodies or peptides changes their flexibility and their conformation properties, resulting, e.g., in shorter circulation times and in much stronger accumulation in the kidney (Lammers et al. 2005, 2010a).

Clinical translation

A large number of nanomedicine formulations have been evaluated in patients over the years, and several of them have been approved for routine clinical use (Allen and Cullis 2004, Wang et al. 2012). Examples of the latter are Myocet® and Doxil®, i.e., liposomes and liposomes surface functionalized with poly(ethylene glycol) (PEG) chains (PEGylated) containing DOX, which are used in the treatment of metastatic breast cancer (both), multiple myeloma, ovarian carcinoma, and Kaposi sarcoma (only Doxil®). Additional examples are Abraxane®, i.e., albumin NPs containing paclitaxel (PTX), which has been approved for metastatic breast cancer, and Genexol® PM, i.e., polymeric micelles containing PTX, which has been approved for breast, lung, and ovarian cancer in Korea. Regarding polymer-drug conjugates, several constructs have been approved for treating hematological malignancies (e.g., Oncaspar®), and a number of others are in clinical trials (e.g., Opaxio® and ProLindac™). Virtually all of these formulations have been shown to beneficially affect the pharmacokinetics and the biodistribution of the conjugated or entrapped chemotherapeutic drug. Furthermore, virtually all of them have been shown to significantly reduce the side effects associated with systemic chemotherapy (e.g., cardiotoxicity induced by DOX). Importantly, however, thus far, significant improvements in therapeutic outcome, such as response rates, and progression-free and overall survival times, have been rare. This shortcoming may be overcome in the near future using more optimal formulations (e.g., pH-responsive vs. cathepsin-dependent drug release), by establishing more efficient targeting strategies [e.g., MRI and High-Intensity Focused Ultrasound (MRI-HIFU)-triggered drug release from temperature-sensitive liposomes], by integrating nanomedicine formulation in combination therapies, or by rationally combining drug targeting with imaging (Lammers et al. 2012a). The latter possibility will be addressed in more detail below.

Image-Guided Drug Delivery

Besides with drugs, NPs can also be easily functionalized with imaging agents. This enables image-guided drug delivery, in which theranostic nanomedicines can, e.g., be used to non-invasively assess biodistribution, target site accumulation, drug release kinetics, and treatment efficacy. Depending on the process to be visualized, on the imaging agent incorporated, and on the physicochemical composition of the carrier material, various different imaging modalities can be used. Each imaging modality has its specific pros and cons, related, e.g., to sensitivity, spatial resolution, and the type of information that can be obtained.

Among the imaging modalities routinely used in nanomedicine and theranostics research are Positron Emission Tomography (PET), Single Photon Emission Computed Tomography (SPECT), Magnetic Resonance Imaging (MRI), Computed Tomography (CT) and ultrasound (US). In recent years, also Optical Imaging (OI), which comprises various different sub-techniques such as Fluorescence Reflectance Imaging (FRI), Fluorescence Molecular Tomography (FMT) and intravital microscopy, has been used more often.

Because of its relatively simple and straightforward principles and procedures, currently OI is the most extensively used imaging modality in the drug delivery field (in spite of limitations with regard to quantification) (Hodenius et al. 2012, Hoffmann et al. 2012).

As mentioned before, each imaging modality has several drawbacks, and tradeoffs need to be made with regard to the qualitative and quantitative nature of the information that can be obtained. Hybrid imaging techniques can help to overcome some of these limitations. The missing anatomical information of PET/SPECT devices can, e.g., be overcome using setups combining anatomical, functional and/or molecular information, such PET-CT and PET-MRI. Similarly, CT-based co-registration and reconstruction can be employed to improve the information (and the quantification) obtained using OI (Fu et al. 2011, Ale et al. 2012).

All in all, imaging modalities, either standard or hybrid, hold significant potential for better understanding and optimizing nanomedicine research. Below, several examples will be given exemplifying how such theranostic approaches can be used to monitor biodistribution, target site accumulation, drug release, and drug efficacy. Given the progress made in both the nanomedicine and the imaging field, such strategies are expected to substantially expand in the next couple of years, not only at the preclinical level, but also in patients, eventually ideally resulting in more individualized treatment regimens, with improved efficacy and reduced toxicity (Lammers et al. 2012b).

Imaging pharmacokinetics, biodistribution, and target site accumulation

As standard low M_W drugs neither have intrinsic (non-invasive) imaging properties, nor can be readily modified with an imaging agent (without completely changing their physicochemical, their pharmacokinetic, and their pharmacological properties), the combination of imaging and therapy can be optimally exploited using nanomedicines. This is because nanomedicines can be easily functionalized both with drugs and with imaging agents, in many cases without substantially altering their properties (Fig. 17.1A, 1B, 1C, 1D, and 1E).

As noted above, nanomedicines are primarily developed to increase the therapeutic index, i.e., the balance between the efficacy and the toxicity of systemic chemotherapeutic interventions. To understand, visualize, and validate higher target site accumulation and/or lower levels in potentially endangered healthy tissues, co-incorporating drugs and imaging agents within a single nanomedicine formulation is highly advantageous. The same drug delivery systems modified either with an imaging agent or with a drug, however, can result in different pharmacokinetic behavior. This would mean that the analyzed biodistribution and target site accumulation changes when the therapeutic agent is replaced by an imaging agent. Besides changes in conformation, induced by attaching different agents to polymer-drug conjugates (Lammers et al. 2010b), also the presence vs. absence of a pharmacologically active moiety (i.e., the drug itself) can have an impact on the pharmacokinetics, the biodistribution, and the target site accumulation of the formulation in question. Contrast agent-containing but drug-free nanomedicines, when used in biodistribution analyses, do not affect macrophages and clearance by the MPS. In case of the presence of a drug, in particular a chemotherapeutic drug, macrophage function and/or survival, and thereby also clearance from systemic circulation, is often changed quite substantially. For radiolabeled PEGylated liposomes lacking a drug, for instance, significantly more rapid blood clearance is observed at low lipid doses and upon repeated injection (via accelerated blood clearance); upon entrapping DOX into the same radiolabeled PEGylated liposomes, however, no accelerated blood clearance is observed (Dams et al. 2000, Laverman et al. 2001). Therefore, it is very important to take such physiological phenomena and co-formulation issues into account when evaluating the *in vivo* potential of nanotheranostics.

Because of their high sensitivity and the quantitative nature of the information they provide, in particular nuclear medicine techniques, such as PET and SPECT, are suitable for non-invasive biodistribution monitoring. Because of this, many different drug delivery systems, including, e.g., liposomes, polymers, and micelles, have been labeled with radionuclides, and their biodistribution and target site accumulation has been visualized and quantified. The circulation half-life of unmodified (i.e., non-PEGylated) liposomes is known to depend on size and surface charge, but is generally relatively short, due to significant protein opsonization, resulting in rapid macrophage recognition and high uptake in the liver and spleen. A successful approach to increase the circulation time of liposomes is the incorporation of PEG into their shell, to attenuate (the kinetics of) protein opsonization. The biodistribution of PEGylated liposomes has been imaged by Harrington et al. (2001), who visualized drug delivery to tumors in patients, suffering from different types of solid malignancies. They used indium-111-diethylenetriaminepentaacetic acid (^{111}In-DTPA)-labeled PEGylated liposomes, and reported different accumulation patterns for breast, lung, and head and neck cancers (Fig. 17.2A, 2B, 2C, 2D, 2E, 2F, and 2G). Whereas a relatively high accumulation was observed in head and neck cancer (Fig. 17.2A, 2B, 2C, and 2D), the tumor localization in breast cancer was much less (Fig. 17.2E, 2F, and 2G). This tumor type-specific accumulation pattern and imaging strategy might help to categorize tumors and to pre-select patients, subdividing them into those likely to respond (i.e., with high EPR-mediated tumor accumulation) and those unlikely to respond (i.e., those with no/low tumor accumulation), thereby potentially paving the way for personalized nanomedicine (Lammers et al. 2012b).

Another interesting study in this regard has been published by Awasthi et al. (2004): instead of preparing PEGylated liposomes via the "classical" way, i.e., of producing PEGylated lipids before mixing them with other lipids during

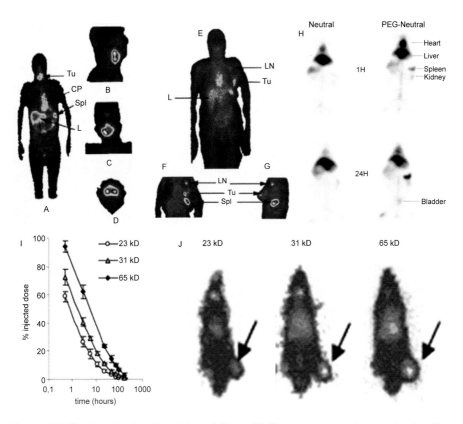

Figure 17.2. Non-invasive imaging of drug delivery. (A-G) gamma camera images showing the biodistribution of ^{111}In-labeled PEGylated liposomes at 72 hours after intravenous injection into a grade 3 squamous cell carcinoma (A-D) and a grade 4 ductal breast carcinoma (E-G) patient. (A-D) in the squamous cell carcinoma patient, it can be seen that, even after three days, a substantial amount of the liposomes is still present in systemic circulation (i.e., in the cardiac blood pool, *CP*), while a significant amount has also already accumulated at the target site (i.e., in a tumor localized at the tongue base, *Tu*). Significant accumulation was also observed in organs of the MPS, like the liver (*L*) and spleen (*Spl*), which are known to be involved in the clearance of long-circulating nanomedicines. (E-G) in the ductal breast carcinoma patient, besides localization to blood, tumor (*Tu*), liver (*L*), and spleen (*Spl*), also accumulation in left axillary lymph node (*LN*) could be clearly observed, indicative of metastasis and of effective drug targeting to this pathological site. (H) scintigraphic images of rabbits injected with post-loaded PEGylated liposomes. PEGylated liposomes show a longer blood half-life compared to non-PEGylated liposomes, indicated by the stronger signal coming from the heart. (I-J) influence of increasing M_w of ^{131}I-labeled HPMA copolymers on their pharmacokinetics and biodistribution. (I) percentage of the injected dose present in blood after intravenous injection at several different time points during follow up. (J) target site accumulation of the three differently sized HPMA copolymers in rats bearing subcutaneously transplanted Dunning AT1 tumors. Scintigraphic images were obtained 168 hours after intravenous injection. Adapted with permission from Harrington et al. (2001), Awasthi et al. (2004), and Lammers et al. (2005). Copyright American Association for Cancer Research (2001), American Society for Pharmacology and Experimental Therapeutics (2004), and Elsevier B.V. (2005), respectively.

liposome formation, they established a post-insertion technique, in which PEGylated lipids are introduced into the bilayer after initial liposome self-assembly. Thereby they could improve PEG-loading efficiency as well as drug loading capacity, e.g., hemoglobin for liposome-encapsulated hemoglobin, used as an oxygen carrier. Both are important parameters to optimize liposomes as theranostic agents. To show that their post-insertion strategy was efficient, they imaged the biodistribution of technetium-99m (^{99m}Tc)-labeled PEGylated liposomes and control liposomes, and obtained γ-scintigraphy images for mice injected with PEGylated and non-PEGylated liposomes (Fig. 17.2H). After one hour and also after 24 hours, they observed a substantially higher signal in the heart region for the PEGylated liposomes, representative for the fraction still circulating in the blood. By this means, they non-invasively demonstrated that PEGylated liposomes possessed advantageous long-circulating properties, providing the basis for EPR-mediated passive drug targeting to tumors.

Many comparable studies have been performed using radiolabeled and image-guided polymers. To improve the understanding of tumor-targeted drug delivery using polymeric drug carriers, we therefore radiolabeled with iodine-131 (^{131}I) 13 physicochemically different N-(2-hydroxypropyl) methacrylamide (HPMA) copolymers, varying in M_w and chemical modification, and monitored their circulation kinetics, tissue distribution, and tumor accumulation (Lammers et al. 2005). As exemplified by Fig. 17.2I and 2J, it was found that physicochemical modification substantially impacted the biodistribution of the polymeric carrier materials. Increasing their M_w from 23.4 to 64.5 kDa, for instance, resulted in a ≈ four-fold increase in circulation half-life time and tumor accumulation. Chemical modifications, on the other hand, such as the introduction of charged groups, drugs, and peptides, significantly decreased blood half-life, and resulted in lower overall levels accumulating in tumors. Interestingly, however, it was also noticed that the functionalization of HPMA copolymers does not affect the overall biodistribution of the polymers (apart from levels in kidney), with in the majority of cases, the highest levels observed in tumors and spleen, and significantly lower levels in all other organs. These image-guided insights indicate that the intrinsic tumor targeting potential of HPMA copolymers is retained even upon functionalization and/ or physicochemical modification. They thereby not only exemplify the high potential of HPMA copolymers for use as tumor-targeted drug delivery systems, but also the need for nanotheranostic approaches and non-invasive imaging techniques to better understand drug targeting to tumors in general.

Besides cancer, nanotheranostics can also be used to visualize and quantify drug targeting to inflammatory disorders, such as Rheumatoid Arthritis (RA). A drug delivery system based on Human Serum Albumin (HSA), covalently coupled to methotrexate (MTX, an antiproliferative drug used to treat both cancer and RA), has undergone phase I/II clinical trials in patients (Vis et al. 2002, Bolling et al. 2006), and it has also been used for RA therapy in mice (Wunder et al. 2003). Regarding the latter, to assess HSA-MTX accumulation in inflamed joints, a radionuclide and a fluorescent dye were co-incorporated, thereby enabling the visualization of the carrier system by γ-scintigraphy and optical methods, respectively. Figure 17.3A shows a representative scintigraphic image obtained using this construct, clearly indicating stronger accumulation in RA-affected paws than in control paws. Also the fluorescence image in Fig. 17.3C clearly shows the accumulation of double-labeled HSA in the inflamed paw.

In a similar setup, Wang et al. (2004) convincingly demonstrated that gadolinium (Gd)-labeled HPMA copolymers efficiently accumulate in

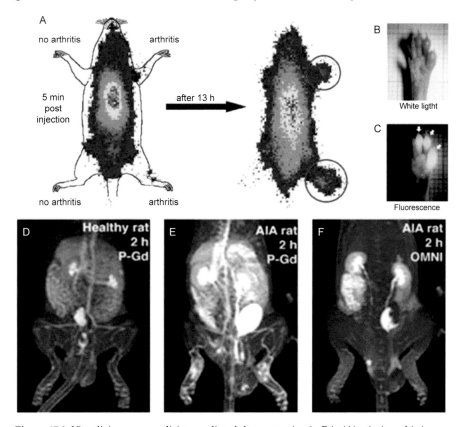

Figure 17.3. Visualizing nanomedicine-mediated drug targeting in RA. (A) scintigraphic image of a mouse injected with ^{111}In-DTPA-HSA, directly after intravenous injection and 13 hours later. After 13 hours, a high accumulation of the formulation is observed in inflamed paws (red circles). (B-C) supporting data were obtained by aminofluorescein-labeled HSA, three hours after aminofluorescein-labeled HSA injection, a strong fluorescent signal was seen in three arthritic toes. (D-E) a Gd-labeled HPMA copolymer (*P-Gd*) was injected into healthy and adjuvant induced arthritis (*AIA*) rats. Two hours after an injection, a positive signal was observed in arthritic joints (E), indicating an accumulation of the *P-Gd*. The positive signal in the arthritic joints could be detected for more than 24 hours. (F) an image taken from an *AIA* rat, two hours after the injection of the low M_W control contrast agent gadodiamide (*OMNI*), showing no specific accumulation in arthritic joints. Adapted with permission from Wunder et al. (2003), and Wang et al. (2004). Copyright The American Association of Immunologists, Inc. (2003), and Springer Science+Business Media, Inc. (2004), respectively.

inflamed joints in mice with RA (Fig. 17.3E), but failed to do so in healthy mice (Fig. 17.3D). They have in the meantime taken these efforts several steps further, showing very high efficacy in RA and several additional inflammatory disorders (Liu et al. 2010). These proof-of-principle preclinical experiments demonstrate that also in case of non-cancerous disorders, nanomedicines can be used to target drugs to pathological sites, and they exemplify that nanotheranostics and non-invasive imaging techniques can be used to visualize, quantify, better understand, and improve drug targeting to pathological sites.

Imaging drug release

When drug delivery systems present with a proper target site accumulation and overall biodistribution profile (i.e., low levels localizing in potentially endangered healthy organs), further important parameters, such as drug release kinetics, can be visualized and quantified, to evaluate their eventual suitability for clinical translation. It is important to realize in this regard that without a proper drug release kinetic, even the best nanocarrier would be of no use. Therefore, different nanotheranostics have been developed over the years, which allow for the visualization and quantification of drug release. Whereas *in vitro* drug release can be assessed with relative ease, e.g., by means of High Performance Liquid Chromatography (HPLC), determining *in vivo* drug release is much more difficult, in particular in case of liposomes (since they are also disrupted when degrading the tumor matrix and/or lyzing tumor cells). The possibility to image and quantify drug release is very important to assess the potential of triggerable drug delivery systems, and to analyze bioavailable drug concentration at the target site.

In this respect, an interesting and elegant approach is based on Low Temperature-Sensitive Liposomes (LTSLs), first described more than 30 years ago (Yatvin et al. 1978). The rationale for using such lysolipid-containing liposomes is that during mild hyperthermia ($\approx$ 40–42°C), LTSLs undergo a phase transition and encapsulated substances are released, whereas minimal leakage occurs at temperatures < 37°C. Intending to visualize and quantify drug release from LTSLs, de Smet et al. (2011) co-encapsulated DOX and the MRI contrast agent gadoteridol into them, and used a combination of MRI-HIFU to analyze the efficiency of this approach. During HIFU therapy, tumors were mildly heated to 40–42°C, and LTSLs entering the tumor microcirculation locally released both DOX and gadoteridol, resulting in a quantifiable decrease in the T_1 signal (Fig. 17.4A), which was shown to correlate very well with DOX release.

Similar LTSLs were used by Langereis et al. (2009); however, they established a protocol exploiting Chemical Exchange Saturation Transfer (CEST) and ^{19}F to generate contrast in MRI upon HIFU-mediated content release from LTSLs. To this end, they co-encapsulated ^{1}H CEST and ^{19}F MRI contrast agents in LTSLs, enabling MRI of intact LTSLs, even before hyperthermia. In this case, the physical properties of intact liposomes and their

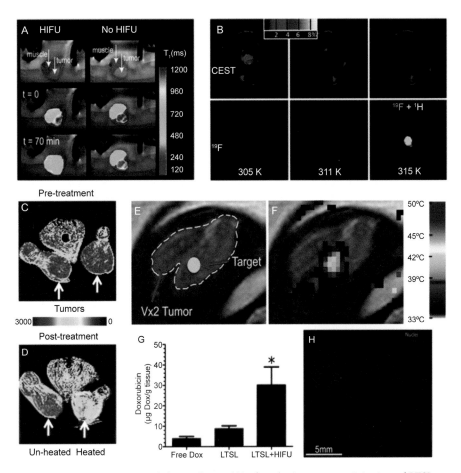

Figure 17.4. Imaging triggered drug release. (A) after the intravenous injection of LTSLs, a shortening of the T_1 relaxation can be observed in a HIFU-treated tumor. In contrast, no changes were observed in a tumor not treated with HIFU. (B) LTSLs co-loaded with ^{1}H CEST and ^{19}F contrast agents. At low temperatures, the LTSLs are intact and generate a ^{1}H CEST signal. Upon heating, the liposomes disintegrate, the CEST signal vanishes, and the ^{19}F signal can be visualized and quantified, correlating to liposomal content release. (C-D) visualization of contrast agent release from cytotoxic LTSLs upon HIFU-mediated hyperthermia. (E-F) MRI-guided HIFU treatment of Vx2 tumors, showing the benefit of using MR temperature mapping for optimizing HIFU-mediated hyperthermia. (G) DOX accumulation in tumors upon intravenous administration of free DOX, DOX-loaded LTSLs, and DOX-loaded LTSLs plus HIFU-mediated hyperthermia. (H) fluorescence image, detailing DOX distribution within a tumor upon DOX-loaded LTSLs plus HIFU-mediated hyperthermia. Reproduced with permission from Langereis et al. (2009), de Smet et al. (2011), Tagami et al. (2011b), and Ranjan et al. (2012). Copyright ACS Publications (2009), Elsevier Ltd. (2011), Elsevier Ltd. (2011b), and Elsevier Ltd. (2012), respectively.

selective saturation allows the generation of a ^{1}H CEST signal, which can, e.g., be used to visualize and quantify the target site accumulation of liposomes. During and after hyperthermia, i.e., upon content release, the CEST signal vanishes and the ^{19}F MRI signal starts appearing, enabling the quantification of drug release (Fig. 17.4B).

Comparable LTSLs were developed by Tagami et al. (2011a,b). They used a different lipid composition for their hyperthermia-activated cytotoxic liposomes, to make them somewhat more stable at physiological temperatures, while maintaining phase transition properties at 40–42°C. As exemplified by Fig. 17.4C and 4D, this formulation conveys rapid release properties, and retains the ability to correlate Gd-DTPA release with DOX release. In line with these findings, Ranjan et al. (2012) recently confirmed that the application of DOX-loaded LTSLs plus MRI-HIFU substantially increases DOX concentrations in mildly heated vs. control Vx2 tumors (Fig. 17.4E and 4F). Note that HIFU was performed under MRI-guidance to tailor the intensity and the location of hyperthermia. Even though only certain parts of the tumor were heated, the overall concentration of DOX could be significantly increased (Fig. 17.4G). Furthermore, not only drug concentrations increased, but also the penetration and the spatial distribution of the drug within tumors could be enhanced (Fig. 17.4H). Together, these insights convincingly demonstrate that non-invasive imaging information can be used to visualize and quantify drug release, and that it might be very useful for optimizing the properties of stimuli-responsive nanomedicine formulations.

Imaging nanomedicine activity

Besides for imaging drug delivery and drug release, nanotheranostics can also be used to visualize drug efficacy. They might thereby help to decide whether the formulation in question is suitable for a specific application or not, and whether or not drug doses should be adapted. Imaging anti-angiogenic treatment efficacy can for instance be performed using MRI angiography and Gd-labeled HPMA copolymers (Kiessling et al. 2006, Lammers et al. 2008b). This formulation enables the non-invasive assessment of tumor perfusion and tumor blood vessels (Fig. 17.5A and 5B), and when envisioning that an anti-angiogenic agent, such as TNP-470, is coupled to that copolymer, direct feedback on treatment efficacy can be obtained during the course of therapy.

Based on a similar rationale, nanotheranostics can be used to assess the efficacy of anti-angiogenic therapy via non-invasive imaging information on receptor expression by tumor blood vessels. The peptide sequence arginine-glycine-aspartic acid (RGD), for instance, targets angiogenesis-specific $\alpha_v\beta_3$ integrins, which are highly expressed on activated endothelium. Consequently, the coupling of such peptide motifs to drug- and imaging agent-containing nanomedicines allows for the determination of areas of active angiogenesis within tumors, and for the monitoring of anti-angiogenic therapy responses. As an example of this, magneto-optical near-infrared dye-containing iron oxide NPs were functionalized with RGD-based targeting ligands, and were shown to be able to sensitively detect integrin expression *in vivo* (by intravital microscopy, MRI and FMT; Fig. 17.5C and 5D; Montet et al. 2006).

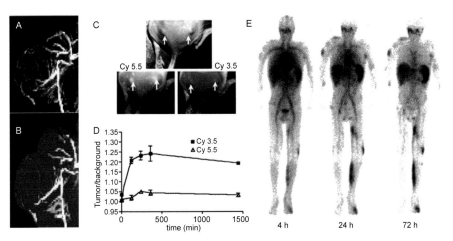

Figure 17.5. Theranostic strategies to visualize and personalize nanomedicine treatment. (A-B) Gd-labeled HPMA copolymers can be used to visualize tumor blood vessels and the efficacy of anti-angiogenic therapy. (C-D) fluorescence reflectance images (C) showing the tumor accumulation of iron oxide NPs labeled with the cyanine dyes Cy5.5 (RGD) and Cy3.5 (control, scrambled RGD). Non-invasive imaging enables feedback on the time dependence of tumor accumulation and on angiogenic marker expression in tumor blood vessels (D). (E) accumulation of ^{111}In-DTPA-labeled PEGylated liposomes in primary (lower left leg) and metastatic (facial region) Kaposi sarcoma lesions. Such imaging information can be used to pre-select patients and monitor therapeutic responses. Adapted with permission from Harrington et al. (2001), Montet et al. (2006), and Lammers et al. (2008b). Copyright American Association for Cancer Research (2001), Elsevier Inc. (2006), and Nature Publishing Group (2008), respectively.

Upon co-loading therapeutic/anti-angiogenic agents into such formulations (note that this was not done in this particular study), they could be used to provide important information on the level of tumor angiogenesis before, during, and after therapy. Therfore, they may be very useful for adapting drug doses and dosing regimens, and for pre-selecting patients (i.e., those with particularly high levels of integrin expression), together leading to optimized and individualized (chemo)therapeutic interventions. The concept of non-invasive target screening and follow up assessment during therapy can be easily transferred to other disease- and angiogenesis-associated markers, and might therefore be very valuable for establishing personalized nanomedicine treatments.

Analogously, also other nanotheranostic systems and strategies can be used for simultaneously inducing and imaging therapeutic effects, as well as for pre-selecting patients and individualizing interventions. Taking, e.g., the above mentioned studies by Harrington et al. (2001) with ^{111}In-DTPA-labeled PEGylated liposomes into account (Figs. 17.2A, 2B, 2C, 2D, 2E, 2F, 2G, and 17.5E), and the intra- and interindividual differences in tumor accumulation in patients suffering from different types of malignancies, it can be reasoned that on the basis of such non-invasive imaging insights, patients can be pre-selected. In such setups, patients with high levels of (passive) tumor accumulation can be identified early on during the course of therapy, and to optimize therapeutic outcome, nanomedicine treatments would only be continued in these patients. By doing this, patients showing significant EPR-mediated drug targeting to tumors can likely be efficiently treated, whereas those that do not can be spared from potential side effects, and can be forwarded to treatment with other established or experimental therapeutic interventions (Lammers et al. 2012b). In addition, non-invasive imaging information on EPR, tumor size, and metastatic burden can be employed to adjust drug doses and/ or discontinue therapy, if necessary. Such theranostic systems and strategies are considered to be very useful for personalizing and optimizing tumor-targeted nanomedicine treatment.

Conclusions

Non-invasive imaging has many potential benefits, not only for basic biomedical research and preclinical experiments, but also for routine clinical practice and clinical translation. Similarly, non-invasive imaging also substantially facilitates basic and (pre)clinical nanomedicine research. In recent years, significant progress has been made in the area of nanotheranostics and image-guided drug delivery. These efforts have thus far primarily focused on the visualization and quantification of drug delivery and drug release, to better understand and improve drug targeting to pathological sites. Imaging drug efficacy and pre-selecting patients on the basis of non-invasive imaging information are areas which are expected to start attracting ever more attention in the years to come. Rationally and more extensively combining drug targeting and imaging is considered to be very useful for the future development of the nanomedicine field, not only because it might aid in the establishment of more effective and more selective drug delivery systems, but also because it might pave the way for personalized and individually optimized nanomedicine treatments.

Abbreviations

CEST	:	chemical exchange saturation transfer
CT	:	computed tomography
DNA	:	deoxyribonucleic acid
DOX	:	doxorubicin
DTPA	:	diethylenetriaminepentaacetic acid
EPR	:	enhanced permeability and retention
FMT	:	fluorescence molecular tomography
FRI	:	fluorescence reflectance imaging
Gd	:	gadolinium
HIFU	:	high intensity focused ultrasound
HPLC	:	high performance liquid chromatography

HPMA	:	N-(2-hydroxypropyl)methacrylamide
HSA	:	human serum albumin
^{131}I	:	iodine-131
^{111}In	:	indium-111
LTSL	:	low temperature-sensitive liposome
MPS	:	mononuclear phagocytic system
MRI	:	magnetic resonance imaging
MTX	:	methotrexate
M_W	:	molecular weight
NP	:	nanoparticle
OI	:	optical imaging
PEG	:	poly(ethylene glycol)
PET	:	positron emission tomography
PTX	:	paclitaxel
RA	:	rheumatoid arthritis
RGD	:	arginine-glycine-aspartic acid
siRNA	:	small interfering ribonucleic acid
SPECT	:	single photon emission computed tomography
^{99m}Tc	:	technetium-99m
Tf	:	transferrin
US	:	ultrasound

References

Al-Jamal, W.T. and K. Kostarelos. 2011. Liposomes: from a clinically established drug delivery system to a nanoparticle platform for theranostic nanomedicine. Acc. Chem. Res. 10: 1094–1104.

Ale, A. and V. Ermolayev, E. Herzog, C. Cohrs, M.H. de Angelis and V. Ntziachristos. 2012. FMT-XCT: in vivo animal studies with hybrid fluorescence molecular tomography-X-ray computed tomography. Nat. Methods. 9: 615–620.

Allen, T.M. and P.R. Cullis. 2004. Drug delivery systems: entering the mainstream. Science. 5665: 1818–1822.

Ambrogio, M.W. and C.R. Thomas, Y.L. Zhao, J.I. Zink and J.F. Stoddart. 2011. Mechanized silica nanoparticles: a new frontier in theranostic nanomedicine. Acc. Chem. Res. 10: 903–913.

Awasthi, V.D. and D. Garcia, R. Klipper, B.A. Goins and W.T. Phillips. 2004. Neutral and anionic liposome-encapsulated hemoglobin: effect of postinserted poly(ethylene glycol)-distearo ylphosphatidylethanolamine on distribution and circulation kinetics. J. Pharmacol. Exp. Ther. 1: 241–248.

Bae, Y.H. and K. Park. 2011. Targeted drug delivery to tumors: myths, reality and possibility. J. Control. Release. 3: 198–205.

Bangham, A.D. and M.M. Standish and J.C. Watkins. 1965. Diffusion of univalent ions across the lamellae of swollen phospholipids. J. Mol. Biol. 1: 238–252.

Bolling, C. and T. Graefe, C. Lubbing, F. Jankevicius, S. Uktveris, A. Cesas, W.H. Meyer-Moldenhauer, H. Starkmann, M. Weigel, K. Burk and A.R. Hanauske. 2006. Phase II study of MTX-HSA in combination with cisplatin as first line treatment in patients with advanced or metastatic transitional cell carcinoma. Invest. New Drugs. 6: 521–527.

Choi, C.H. and C.A. Alabi, P. Webster and M.E. Davis. 2010. Mechanism of active targeting in solid tumors with transferrin-containing gold nanoparticles. Proc. Natl. Acad. Sci. U.S.A. 3: 1235–1240.

Dams, E.T. and P. Laverman, W.J. Oyen, G. Storm, G.L. Scherphof, J.W. van der Meer, F.H. Corstens and O.C. Boerman. 2000. Accelerated blood clearance and altered biodistribution of repeated injections of sterically stabilized liposomes. J. Pharmacol. Exp. Ther. 3: 1071–1079.

de Smet, M. and E. Heijman, S. Langereis, N.M. Hijnen and H. Grull. 2011. Magnetic resonance imaging of high intensity focused ultrasound mediated drug delivery from temperature-sensitive liposomes: an *in vivo* proof-of-concept study. J. Control. Release. 1: 102–110.

Fu, J. and X. Yang, K. Wang, Q. Luo and H. Gong. 2011. A generic, geometric cocalibration method for a combined system of fluorescence molecular tomography and microcomputed tomography with arbitrarily shaped objects. Med. Phys. 12: 6561–6570.

Fukumura, D. and D.G. Duda, L.L. Munn and R.K. Jain. 2010. Tumor microvasculature and microenvironment: novel insights through intravital imaging in pre-clinical models. Microcirculation. 3: 206–225.

Gregoriadis, G. and E.J. Wills, C.P. Swain and A.S. Tavill. 1974. Drug-carrier potential of liposomes in cancer chemotherapy. Lancet. 7870: 1313–1316.

Harrington, K.J. and S. Mohammadtaghi, P.S. Uster, D. Glass, A.M. Peters, R.G. Vile and J.S. Stewart. 2001. Effective targeting of solid tumors in patients with locally advanced cancers by radiolabeled pegylated liposomes. Clin. Cancer Res. 2: 243–254.

Hobbs, S.K. and W.L. Monsky, F. Yuan, W.G. Roberts, L. Griffith, V.P. Torchilin and R.K. Jain. 1998. Regulation of transport pathways in tumor vessels: role of tumor type and microenvironment. Proc. Natl. Acad. Sci. U.S.A. 8: 4607–4612.

Hodenius, M. and C. Wurth, J. Jayapaul, J.E. Wong, T. Lammers, J. Gatjens, S. Arns, N. Mertens, I. Slabu, G. Ivanova, J. Bornemann, M.D. Cuyper, U. Resch-Genger and F. Kiessling. 2012. Fluorescent magnetoliposomes as a platform technology for functional and molecular MR and optical imaging. Contrast. Media Mol. Imaging. 1: 59–67.

Hoffmann, S. and L. Vystrcilova, K. Ulbrich, T. Etrych, H. Caysa, T. Mueller and K. Mader. 2012. Dual fluorescent HPMA copolymers for passive tumor targeting with pH-sensitive drug release: synthesis and characterization of distribution and tumor accumulation in mice by noninvasive multispectral optical imaging. Biomacromolecules. 3: 652–663.

Jain, R.K. and T. Stylianopoulos. 2010. Delivering nanomedicine to solid tumors. Nat. Rev. Clin. Oncol. 11: 653–664.

Kiessling, F. and M. Heilmann, T. Lammers, K. Ulbrich, V. Subr, P. Peschke, B. Wängler, W. Mier, H. Schrenk, M. Bock, L. Schad and W. Semmler. 2006. Synthesis and characterization of HE-24.8: a polymeric contrast agent for MR Angiography. Bioconjug. Chem. 17: 42–51.

Lammers, T. and R. Kuhnlein, M. Kissel, V. Subr, T. Etrych, R. Pola, M. Pechar, K. Ulbrich, G. Storm, P. Huber and P. Peschke. 2005. Effect of physicochemical modification on the biodistribution and tumor accumulation of HPMA copolymers. J. Control. Release. 1: 103–118.

Lammers, T. and W.E. Hennink and G. Storm. 2008a. Tumour-targeted nanomedicines: principles and practice. Br. J. Cancer. 3: 392–397.

Lammers, T. and V. Subr, P. Peschke, R. Kuhnlein, W.E. Hennink, K. Ulbrich, F. Kiessling, M. Heilmann, J. Debus, P.E. Huber and G. Storm. 2008b. Image-guided and passively tumour-targeted polymeric nanomedicines for radiochemotherapy. Br. J. Cancer. 6: 900–910.

Lammers, T. and F. Kiessling, W.E. Hennink and G. Storm. 2010a. Nanotheranostics and image-guided drug delivery: current concepts and future directions. Mol. Pharm. 6: 1899–1912.

Lammers, T. and V. Subr, K. Ulbrich, P. Peschke, P.E. Huber, W.E. Hennink, G. Storm and F. Kiessling. 2010b. HPMA-based polymer therapeutics improve the efficacy of surgery, of radiotherapy and of chemotherapy combinations. Nanomedicine (Lond.). 10: 1501–1523.

Lammers, T. and F. Kiessling, W.E. Hennink and G. Storm. 2012a. Drug targeting to tumors: principles, pitfalls and (pre-) clinical progress. J. Control. Release. 2: 175–187.

Lammers, T. and L. Yokota-Rizzo, G. Storm and F. Kiessling. 2012b. Personalized nanomedicine. Clin. Cancer Res. 18: 4889–4894.

Langereis, S. and J. Keupp, J.L. van Velthoven, I.H. Roos, D. Burdinski, J.A. Pikkemaat and H. Grüll. 2009. A temperature-sensitive liposomal 1H CEST and 19F contrast agent for MR image-guided drug delivery. J. Am. Chem. Soc. 4: 1380–1381.

Laverman, P. and M.G. Carstens, O.C. Boerman, E.T. Dams, W.J. Oyen, N. van Rooijen, F.H. Corstens and G. Storm. 2001. Factors affecting the accelerated blood clearance of polyethylene glycol-liposomes upon repeated injection. J. Pharmacol. Exp. Ther. 2: 607–612.

Liu, X.M. and S.C. Miller and D. Wang. 2010. Beyond oncology—application of HPMA copolymers in non-cancerous diseases. Adv. Drug Deliv. Rev. 62: 258–271.

Maeda, H. and G.Y. Bharate and J. Daruwalla. 2009. Polymeric drugs for efficient tumor-targeted drug delivery based on EPR-effect. Eur. J. Pharm. Biopharm. 3: 409–419.

Maeda, H. 2012. Macromolecular therapeutics in cancer treatment: the EPR effect and beyond. J. Control. Release. 164: 138–144.

Montet, X. and K. Montet-Abou, F. Reynolds, R. Weissleder and L. Josephson. 2006. Nanoparticle imaging of integrins on tumor cells. Neoplasia. 3: 214–222.

Peer, D. and J.M. Karp, S. Hong, O.C. Farokhzad, R. Margalit and R. Langer. 2007. Nanocarriers as an emerging platform for cancer therapy. Nat. Nanotechnol. 12: 751–760.

Ranjan, A. and G.C. Jacobs, D.L. Woods, A.H. Negussie, A. Partanen, P.S. Yarmolenko, C.E. Gacchina, K.V. Sharma, V. Frenkel, B.J. Wood and M.R. Dreher. 2012. Image-guided drug delivery with magnetic resonance guided high intensity focused ultrasound and temperature sensitive liposomes in a rabbit Vx2 tumor model. J. Control. Release. 3: 487–494.

Raza, A. and M.J. Franklin and A.Z. Dudek. 2010. Pericytes and vessel maturation during tumor angiogenesis and metastasis. Am. J. Hematol. 8: 593–598.

Tagami, T. and M.J. Ernsting and S.D. Li. 2011a. Efficient tumor regression by a single and low dose treatment with a novel and enhanced formulation of thermosensitive liposomal doxorubicin. J. Control. Release. 2: 303–309.

Tagami, T. and W.D. Foltz, M.J. Ernsting, C.M. Lee, I.F. Tannock, J.P. May and S.D. Li. 2011b. MRI monitoring of intratumoral drug delivery and prediction of the therapeutic effect with a multifunctional thermosensitive liposome. Biomaterials. 27: 6570–6578.

Vis, A.N. and A. van der Gaast, B.W. van Rhijn, T.K. Catsburg, C. Schmidt and G.H. Mickisch. 2002. A phase II trial of methotrexate-human serum albumin (MTX-HSA) in patients with metastatic renal cell carcinoma who progressed under immunotherapy. Cancer Chemother. Pharmacol. 4: 342–345.

Wang, D. and S.C. Miller, M. Sima, D. Parker, H. Buswell, K.C. Goodrich, P. Kopeckova and J. Kopecek. 2004. The arthrotropism of macromolecules in adjuvant-induced arthritis rat model: a preliminary study. Pharm. Res. 21: 1741–1749.

Wang, A.Z. and R. Langer and O.C. Farokhzad. 2012. Nanoparticle delivery of cancer drugs. Annu. Rev. Med. 63: 185–198.

Wunder, A. and U. Muller-Ladner, E.H. Stelzer, J. Funk, E. Neumann, G. Stehle, T. Pap, H. Sinn, S. Gay and C. Fiehn. 2003. Albumin-based drug delivery as novel therapeutic approach for rheumatoid arthritis. J. Immunol. 9: 4793–4801.

Yatvin, M.B. and J.N. Weinstein, W.H. Dennis and R. Blumenthal. 1978. Design of liposomes for enhanced local release of drugs by hyperthermia. Science. 4374: 1290–1293.

Index